PSYCHIATRIC INTERVIEWING

PSYCHIATRIC INTERVIEWING
The Art of Understanding

A Practical Guide
for Psychiatrists, Psychologists, Counselors, Social Workers,
Nurses, and Other Mental Health Professionals

2nd Edition

SHAWN CHRISTOPHER SHEA, M.D.

Adjunct Assistant Professor
Dartmouth Medical School
Department of Psychiatry
Lebanon, New Hampshire
Private Practice
Keene, New Hampshire

with illustrations by Meg Maloney

SAUNDERS
An Imprint of Elsevier

SAUNDERS
An Imprint of Elsevier
The Curtis Center
Independence Square West
Philadelphia, PA 19106

Library of Congress Cataloging-in-Publication Data

Shea, Shawn C.

Psychiatric interviewing: the art of understanding / Shawn Christopher Shea; with
illustrations by Meg Maloney.—2nd ed.

p.   cm.

Includes bibliographical references and index.

ISBN-13: 978-0-7216-7011-9   ISBN-10: 0-7216-7011-3

1. Interviewing in psychiatry.   I. Title.   [DNLM: 1. Interview, Psychological—
   methods.   2. Physician-Patient Relations.   WM 141 S539p 1998]

RC480.7.S54   1998   616.89—dc21

DNLM/DLC   97–36788

ISBN-13: 978-0-7216-7011-9
ISBN-10: 0-7216-7011-3

PSYCHIATRIC INTERVIEWING: The Art of Understanding

Printed in the United States of America.

Last digit is the print number: 19 18 17 16 15

*T*o my father who showed me the door of creativity,

In fondest memory of my mother who urged me
to open it,

And to Susan, Brenden, and Ryan who were waiting
on the other side.

This beautiful and immensely useful book is a great gift. It should stand as the best starting clinical text for all mental health professionals, because the ultimate success of our clinical interventions is determined directly by the information we must sensitively garner from the interview. Einstein remarked that in early sciences, examples serve better than concepts; indeed, they form the earliest concepts. Shea introduces the beginning clinician to the work by means of concrete situations and particular examples of actual clinical dialogue. There could be no sounder starting point. Later, I predict, beginning clinicians, and many experienced ones, too, will return to this book the way people return to the books that they find deepest and most evocative, reading a few pages at a time, to be savored and enjoyed, so its wisdom enters their bones.

The book starts where all interviewers start, in the dark, knowing that they must gently feel their way. This is a necessity not only because valid psychological data are extremely difficult to secure but also because our first job is to establish an effective relationship to carry on the work. In other words, Shea takes the interview with deep seriousness, which is the same as taking the relationship seriously and the importance of uncovering valid findings.

On the other hand, in a particularly refreshing light, Shea does not take himself too seriously. He draws our attention to his own mistakes, reflecting on them with a gentle humor, demonstrating directly what can be learned from them. No better model for learning could be demonstrated for the beginning, and often frightened student, allowing the student immediately to feel more at home both with himself or herself and with the author. Moreover, Shea knows that an interview and a relationship can be at cross purposes, so he doesn't want patients to feel that they are "being interviewed," but rather that they are "talking with someone." He states his goal early, "to gather the necessary clinical information efficiently while powerfully engaging the patient."

The focus is on assessment, not ongoing psychotherapy, but there is much here for all psychotherapists. For instance, throughout the book Shea emphasizes the point that a well-crafted initial interview, although it is not psychotherapy, is always therapeutic. He proceeds to demonstrate with practical illustrations, including an entire transcript of one of his own interviews, exactly how to accomplish this complex task.

With "facilics," his innovative set of principles for studying and understanding the methods by which clinicians structure interviews and manage their time, he provides a wonderfully practical method for gracefully navigating the tight time constraints of modern clinical practice. He manages to artfully wed the process of data gathering with compassionate listening. He furthers this integrative task by highlighting the many practical interviewing techniques that other authors have developed from a myriad of disciplines, including analytic, interpersonal, self-psychological, cognitive-behavioral, and existential schools of thought. In short, this is a sophisticated, deeply informed work, the hands-on emphasis of which does not belie a profound understanding.

Too often clinical discussions have a pretentious, high theoretical cast, whether of putative brain processes or unconscious ones. In our mission to help others, unlike theoretical physicists, it is not our main goal to penetrate the secrets of nature and society. Rather, in clinical care, we are more like engineers whose task is to construct the practical bridges and strong foundations that foster the healing process. We need to get from A to B, from meeting to connecting, from guessing to surmising, from sensing to feeling deeply. Shea breaks down the steps, makes the distinctions, and lets us build our own working methods from the various examples he provides. We are to practice techniques and create new ones, until a wide range of possible actions becomes second nature to us all.

This is where clinical work must begin. We could not be in better hands.

Leston Havens, M.D.

PREFACE

The purpose of life is to serve and to show compassion and the will to help others. Only then have we ourselves become true human beings.

Albert Schweitzer, M.D.

It is with true pleasure that I sit down to write the Preface for the second edition. Much has changed in our field of mental health since the book first appeared 10 years ago—some of it good and some of it not so good. My pleasure arises from the fact that the cornerstone principles of the first edition—sensitivity and compassion—still resonate in our field today; in fact, in the age of managed care and tight time constraints, they may play an even more important role as guideposts than before.

One of my biggest pleasures over the past 10 years has been the warm reception given to the system of "facilics," introduced in the first edition. Facilics has been adopted as a core component of graduate training programs across disciplines—from masters' programs in counseling and social work to psychiatric residencies. For those not familiar with it, facilics is an approach for understanding how we, as front-line clinicians, can most sensitively structure our interviews and effectively manage time constraints during the initial assessment. An innovative aspect of the facilic system is an easily learned system of schematics for supervisors to utilize while tracking the structuring and engagement strategies of the clinician. These schematics function as a supervisory shorthand and provide a direct visual platform for individual supervision and class discussion. Although developed long before the pressures of managed care, facilics has proved to be a popular method for allowing clinicians and supervisors to discover new ways of sensitively handling those very same pressures. For these reasons once again, in the second edition, facilics has been highlighted.

I have tried to keep intact whatever elements of the book that reader feedback has suggested were most effective. Indeed, other than updates to the DSM-IV, most of the chapters have relatively minor changes. On the other hand, Chapter 8 on suicide and violence assessment has been greatly expanded and introduces a new system for eliciting suicidal ideation, which I hope you will find practical and immediately useful. Furthermore, a good deal more time has been spent on practical tips and strategies for assessing violent ideation, an area of relative weakness in the first edition.

The biggest changes in the book are to be found in the appendices, in which more than 100 pages of new information appear. In speaking with readers at my workshops throughout the United States, perhaps the most common suggestion for improvement has been for the addition of an annotated transcript of an actual 60-minute intake. The second most common request has been for the inclusion of practical information on how to write up an assessment that is both clinically useful and forensically sound. Both requests have been fulfilled in the appendices of the second edition.

In addition, there is an appendix that gives specific quality assurance guidelines and "dictation prompts" for the written document. For those who like to record the initial database on a standardized clinical form, a prototypic clinical assessment form is provided. There is also a copy of the actual written document derived from the database of the annotated interview itself, thus allowing the reader to see the interview unfold, in actual practice, from the first greeting of the interview to the last period in the written document.

Over the years, I have often been approached by young psychiatrists who ask whether or not the book would help them to prepare for the oral boards. Although the first edition was not designed specifically for that purpose, in my heart I have always thought it would help, because I strongly believe that good clinical principles are at the core of the oral boards. In the second edition, however, I can now confidently answer "yes" to this question, because I have included an entire appendix that is devoted to practical tips and strategies for passing the oral boards.

I hope that the reader enjoys reading this book as much as I enjoyed revising it. In the final analysis, interviewing should be fun. I think it is important to emphasize that this book does not pretend to show the "correct" way of interviewing, because there is no correct way. Instead, I offer suggestions that will hopefully provide the reader with the principles to develop his or her own creative style of interviewing, always flexibly matching the interview to the needs of the patient, not the dictates of a school of thought.

In closing, this is a book about knowledge—knowledge applied to the art of healing. In the last analysis, as students of this art, it will always remain our great privilege to ensure that the knowledge of our minds is guided by the compassion of our hearts.

Shawn Christopher Shea, M.D.

PREFACE

to the 1st Edition

*A*fter all, there is nothing in the world as interesting as people, and one can never study them enough.

Vincent Van Gogh

The initial psychiatric interview is a creative act. It is a study of movement and change. It is unique. The circumstances, the environment, and the people involved can never be duplicated. Even if the interviewer and interviewee wanted to replicate their own interaction, they could not; for with each sentence their relationship has subtly changed. With each sentence they define a new phenomenon. This creativity is harnessed by two pivotal principles: (1) the patient must be powerfully engaged, and (2) a thorough and valid database must be gathered in a limited amount of time. These two principles form the basis of the initial therapeutic encounter. They represent a complementary pair. When performed with sensitivity, thorough data gathering mirrors effective engagement.

Rapid advancements in the field of mental health have necessitated an evolution in the craft of assessment interviewing. In the past 40 years an impressive array of new therapeutic interventions has emerged. These revolutionary advances include modalities such as tricyclic antidepressants, antipsychotic medications, behavior modification, family therapy, group therapy, and more sophisticated forms of dynamic and hypnotic psychotherapies, to name only a few.

The development of so many new tools has presented a startling challenge to the initial interviewer, especially when the interviewer is functioning as a triage agent or consultant who may never see the patient again. More specifically, in order to determine an effective treatment plan and disposition, the interviewer must gather an amount of information in 50 minutes, which might have staggered an interviewer of 40 years ago. At that time, one did not need to elicit the neurovegetative symptoms of depression, because tricyclic antidepressants did not exist. One did not have to carefully delineate the diagnosis of agoraphobia, because behavioral tools such as flooding were unavailable. It did not matter whether the interviewee had symptoms suggestive of mania, because lithium was a dream waiting to crystallize in John Cade's mind. In short, the therapeutic explosion has created an impressive need for more effective and thorough data gathering in the initial encounter.

The challenge of the interview currently revolves around the manner in which the initial interviewer collects critical data, while constantly attending to rapport. With each unique pairing of interviewer and interviewee, this tension must be creatively resolved. A skilled interviewer is remarkably flexible. As has always been the case, the validity of the data depends directly on the strength of the therapeutic engagement. In fact, if anything, the importance of the therapeutic alliance has increased over the years. In the long run, reliable diagnosis, effective treatment planning, treatment compliance, and family support of therapeutic intervention are all limited by a common factor: the therapist's ability to engage the patient. Consequently, the initial interview remains the foundation of all mental health interventions. This book focuses the attention on this craft that it rightfully deserves.

The text developed from my work as the medical director and instructor of interviewing at the Diagnostic and Evaluation Center (DEC) of the Western Psychiatric Institute and Clinic of the University of Pittsburgh. Our 3-month interviewing program emphasizes didactic teaching, live interviewing, role playing, and direct feedback by fellow students, as well as videotaped and direct supervision. I felt that a practical textbook, emphasizing the integration of engagement, diagnosis, and treatment planning, would be very helpful. To my surprise, I could not find such a book. Indeed, excellent books exist, but each tends to be primarily based on a specific style of interviewing, such as the psychodynamic approach or the behavioral approach. *Psychiatric Interviewing: The Art of Understanding* attempts to fill this void, providing a synthesis of many perspectives, including various schools of psychiatry, psychology, and counseling.

More to the point, students seemed eager to read a book that integrated many different concerns, such as body language, engagement techniques, differential diagnosis by DSM-III-R criteria, treatment planning, and the internal structure of the interview. Students also repeatedly emphasized the usefulness of hearing the specific phrases and questions that different interviewers employed to explore distinct areas of information.

In the interviewing class (consisting of psychiatric residents, psychiatric nurses, psychology interns, social work interns, family practice residents, emergency room residents, and medical students), this practical exposure was accomplished by the experiential methods mentioned earlier. In this book, the same goal is approached by the generous use of sample questions, case vignettes, direct transcripts of actual interviews, and numerous mock interviews created to demonstrate specific teaching points. This textbook is a clinician's book, focusing directly on the practical issues of sensitive interviewing.

As a field guide, this text reflects the concern of any professional asked to perform the initial interview. Therefore, it is primarily written with psychiatric residents, counselors, clinical psychologists, social workers, psychiatric nurses, and psychiatrists in mind. The format allows flexible use as a guide for individual study, a classroom textbook, or a seminar springboard. With regard to flexibility, the book may be read as a whole or in parts. Each chapter tends to function as a unit unto itself, thus allowing readers to pick and choose relevant material for their particular needs.

The book was also written to be a core textbook for medical and nursing students as they studied psychiatry. All physicians and nurses, no matter which field they choose as a specialty, must be able to effectively engage patients and determine whether major types of psychopathology are present and require treatment. All physicians and nurses should be adept at detecting critical processes such as suicidal ideation or the presence of psychosis. This text provides the groundwork for these critical skills. Moreover, many textbooks of psychiatry provide the facts but not the methods. Consequently, medical students and nurses know what a major depression is but do not have any idea how to explore for it in an actual clinical setting. This book provides the practical bridge that can lead students from the classroom into practice. With regard to medical and nursing students, the critical chapters for study are Chapters 1, 4, 5, 6, 7, and 8. The section on the mental status in Chapter 9 is also very useful for the students moving on to the clinical wards.

The text can also be used as a unique supplementary reading source in abnormal psychology, because it functions as a clinical reference point. It illustrates the human aspect of psychopathology, as evidenced by the interviewing experience. The interviewee appears as an individual, not a textbook label. In this regard, Chapters 4, 5, 6, and 7 are most relevant.

Concerning structure, the book is organized into three sections: (I) Fundamentals of Interviewing, (II) The Interview and Psychopathology, and (III) Advanced Techniques of Interviewing.

In Part I, Fundamentals of Interviewing, the first two chapters center around core issues challenging the assessment interviewer, such as the structure and tasks of the interview, the validity and reliability of the data gathered, and basic types of resistance such as overly talkative patients or adamantly shut-down patients. In essence, these issues determine the nature of the interview itself. The understanding of how one should interview grows from an understanding of why one is interviewing.

The third chapter explores the fascinating world of body language, emphasizing the nonverbal dialogue that occurs throughout the interview process. It pays particular attention to the powerful impact of the clinician's own body language and paralanguage on the interview process, influencing a diversity of factors such as patient engagement, validity of data, and the pacing of the interview itself.

The fourth chapter focuses on treatment planning and the organization of clinical data. It also introduces the reader to a simplifying and practical approach to utilizing the DSM-III and DSM-III-R, describing in detail the five diagnostic axes. Equally important approaches, such as the perspective of family systems and the patient's framework for meaning, are also explored in depth.

In Part II, The Interview and Psychopathology, the principles discussed earlier are viewed in the context of their application to three major areas of psychopathology: (1) affective disorders, (2) schizophrenia and psychotic process, and (3) personality disorders. A chapter is devoted to each of these areas. By intensively studying interviewing principles in these three circumscribed areas it is hoped that a variety of core principles will be delineated, which are generalizable to many other areas of psychopathology such as anxiety disorders and substance abuse. Thus, Chapters 5, 6, and 7 magnify the subtle nuances of the interviewing process, providing a more sophisticated understanding from which to develop one's own interviewing style.

To facilitate this exploration, Chapters 5 and 6 are split into two complementary sections. In the first section, interviewing techniques useful in the process of differential diagnosis by DSM-III and DSM-III-R criteria are examined in detail. These principles are explored through discussions of interviews based on actual case histories or hypothetical case histories created to enhance learning. In the second section, an attempt is made to understand the phenomenology of each pathologic state, emphasizing the ramifications of these states on various systems pertinent to treatment planning in the initial interview itself.

Chapter 7 is devoted to personality disorders and emphasizes the need to understand not only diagnostic criteria but also the world view of the patients suffering from character psychopathology. A concerted effort is made to help the reader feel what it is like to be in the world as these patients experience their worlds. To this end, topics such as sensitively eliciting "difficult histories," including the sexual history and the drug and alcohol history, are examined in detail. Many other troublesome areas are discussed, such as performing a formal mental status and dealing with a tearful or angry patient.

In Part III, Advanced Techniques of Interviewing, the emphasis shifts to more sophisticated methods of analysis and interviewing. An entire chapter is devoted to the critical issue of evaluating suicidal and homicidal ideation. Besides examining the many pertinent risk factors through case histories, this chapter carefully explores many of the specific interviewing techniques useful in uncovering suicidal and homicidal ideation. The ninth chapter deals with shifting perspectives during the interview itself, as exemplified by looking at one's own emotional responses, fantasies, and countertransference. In the final chapter, the thorny issue of patient resistance is addressed directly, including both general principles and specific methods of handling awkward situations, which use actual patient questions as jumping-off points for discussion.

As this introduction draws to a close, I am reminded that if someone asked me to define the major goal of this book, I would be flooded with many possibilities. To begin with, it is not an attempt at an exhaustive study, which unfortunately can often transform into a study in exhaustion for the reader. Instead, I have attempted to produce a quick reading field guide that examines carefully many of the core practical and clinical issues surrounding the first clinical encounter. From this exploration I hope to achieve my major goal, the stimulation of intellectual excitement. Hopefully this excitement will entice readers to proceed upon their own ongoing exploration of this craft long after they have put this book down.

I would like to add that the style of interviewing described here represents only one of many effective styles. I do not present this style as "correct interviewing." Instead, I offer this material as an invitation to readers to develop their own styles, by borrowing some methods, discarding others, and creating new ones.

In closing, I want to say that interviewing has provided me with many fascinating moments. I believe we are studying a very special human interaction, one in which we are privileged to be participants. In the last analysis, interviewing is an ultimate art, a shared work of creativity, undertaken in the service of a person in need.

Please note that the names of all patients have been changed, and at times distinguishing characteristics or facts have been altered to further protect their identity.

Shawn Christopher Shea, M.D.

ACKNOWLEDGMENTS

I would like to begin by expressing my deep gratitude, once again, to all those who helped with the first edition.

With regards to the second edition, I would like to begin by expressing my appreciation to the Department of Psychiatry at the Dartmouth Medical School. Many thanks for the administrative support provided for my interviewing training ideas from the Chairman of the Psychiatry Department, Peter Silberfarb, M.D., and to Leighton Huey, M.D., and David Budlong, Ph.D., both of whom have offered gracious support to the interviewing training program.

My greatest thanks, in this regard, goes to Ron Green, M.D., the Director of Residency Training at Dartmouth, who for the past 10 years has given me unqualified support in building an interviewing training program that expresses the ideals of this book. Toward the fulfillment of these educational ideals at the Dartmouth Program, all third-year psychiatry residents are assigned an "interviewing mentor" who watches them perform initial intakes, in a 2-hour block, every other week for a year. This intensive mentorship includes videotaping, direct supervision, modeling, role-playing, and an individualized learning program for each resident.

Naturally, I would also like to thank all the Dartmouth faculty who have served as interviewing mentors over the years—the so-called "Phantom Gate Club." I offer a very special thanks to those mentors who, like Ron Green, have been providing mentorship since the very first year of the Dartmouth program. This select group includes Bruce Baker, Ph.D., Christine Barney, M.D., and Stephen Cole, Ph.D. They have provided the feedback, challenges, and innovations that are reflected in the pages of this edition. Furthermore, they have been great colleagues and friends, whom I genuinely admire.

Since the writing of the first edition, most of my time has been spent working in community mental health. In a direct sense, the special clinicians with whom I worked, both within the Community Support Programs and the Adult Services, have helped me to grow as a clinician and as a person, which, I hope, is reflected in the second edition. I thank all of you. In particular, I would like to express a deep-felt gratitude to two groups—first, the wonderful clinicians of the Continuous Treatment Team (CTT) and second, to the CTT patients and their family members. Each group, respectively, showed me the true meaning of the words "compassion" and "courage." I will forever remain in debt to both sets of people.

One of the most significant improvements in the second edition is the work on the interviewing strategy known as the Chronological Assessment of Suicide Events (CASE) Approach. I would like to convey gratitude to David Jobes, Ph.D., for reviewing the chapter describing the CASE Approach and to Thomas Ellis, Ph.D., for his enthusiastic support of the CASE Approach over the years.

A debt of gratitude goes to the W.B. Saunders team, including Judith Fletcher, Paul Fry, and Bob Keller, which has helped to shape my ideas into a polished product. I give special thanks to Marjory Fraser, whose gifted editing has clearly improved the text.

Naturally, I would like to thank Leston Havens, M.D., for his enthusiastic support of my work and for taking the time out of a very busy schedule to write his gracious Foreword to the second edition.

Finally, I cannot thank enough my wife Susan for her love, understanding, and support. As she was with the first edition, Susan has been a wonderful sounding board and a source of editorial support, but, more important, she has been the strongest believer in the mission and ideals of this book.

Thanks again, to all.

Shawn Christopher Shea, M.D.

ACKNOWLEDGMENTS
to the 1st Edition

I would like to begin by expressing my deep gratitude to Thomas Detre, M.D., Director of Western Psychiatric Institute and Clinic, and David Kupfer, M.D., Chairman of the Department of Psychiatry at Western Psychiatric Institute and Clinic, for their enthusiastic support of the book. Both Dr. Detre and Dr. Kupfer have also given their strong support to my attempts to develop a training program dedicated to interviewing and to the development of an interviewing laboratory in which the interviewing process can be given the empirical study that it deserves. I would also like to thank the remaining administration of Western Psychiatric Institute and Clinic for their key support of our interviewing program, many of whom also provided invaluable feedback on the book, including Carol Anderson, Ph.D., George Board, Dr. PH, Richard Cohen, M.D., George Huber, J.D., Joan Kyes, M.S.N., Joaquim Puig-Antich, M.D., Jeffrey Romoff, M.Phil., Loren Roth, M.D., Duane Spiker, M.D., and Jack Wolford, M.D.

I would like to thank the following clinicians, each of whom reviewed various chapters from the book and whose comments were greatly appreciated, including Cleon Cornes, M.D., Peter Fabrega, M.D., Rohan Ganguli, M.D., Tom Horn, M.D., Stan Imber, Ph.D., Paul Pilkonis, Ph.D., and Grady Roberts, Ph.D. A warm thanks to Val Brown, Ph.D., and Mimi Brown, M.S.N., for both their constructive feedback and their delightful friendship. Thanks should also be given to Jeff Wilson, M.D., who allowed me to utilize various quotations he had discovered related to the phenomenology of psychotic process. The quotations greatly enhance Chapter Six.

I would like to give a special thanks to Richard Simons, M.D., a man I tracked down as he was racing to leave for the airport, after giving his keynote address at the Annual Meeting of the Association for Academic Psychiatry, who quickly agreed to review several chapters and proceeded to provide enthusiastic support. His willingness to help a young academician, whom he had never met before, represents a model of the academic spirit at its best.

I would like to also give a very special thanks to Juan

Mezzich, M.D., Ph.D., who has served as my mentor over the years and without whom the book would never have developed. A special thanks is given in memory to the late Peter Henderson, M.D., whose dedication to training will always remain as a source of inspiration and whose support of my career and this book will never be forgotten.

As the author of a book dedicated to teaching, perhaps my strongest debt is to those who taught me. Many of them have already been mentioned, but I would also like to thank the following clinicians, whose compassion and excellence created a stimulating learning experience during my residency at Western Psychiatric Institute and Clinic: Anselm George, M.D., Carol Heape, R.N., M.S.N., Diane Holder, M.S.W., George Hsu, M.D., Tony Mannarino, Ph.D., Bob Marin, M.D., Swami Nathan, M.D., Elaine Portner, Ph.D., Al Rossi, M.D., Mike Shostack, M.D., Paul Soloff, M.D., Susan Stewart, M.S.W., Rick Tomb, M.D., Paul Weiss, M.D., Gerhard Werner, M.D., and Bob Wittig, M.D.

I would also like to thank my editor, Bill Lamsback, for his belief in the text and his efforts to achieve a book that would not only be enjoyable to read but a pleasure to the eyes. I would also like to thank Jack Farrell of the Marketing Department whose enthusiastic support for the book and whose creative ideas will hopefully ensure its success. I would also like to thank my secretary, Maria Antonich, for her patient help in preparing the text and correspondence associated with the book.

Before closing, a few more particularly important thanks are warranted. Working with Meg Maloney was a true treat. Her creativity and imagination, as well as her ability to bring our ideas to visual fruition, were a continuing source of excitement. I believe her illustrations bring a true feeling of awe and sensitivity to the written word.

I would like to thank all my students, from whom I am always learning and whose provocative questions provide a constant source of growth. A particular thanks to two former students, Barb McCann, Ph.D., and Scott Bohon, M.D., who have become my colleagues, working together with me towards a better understanding of the art of interviewing.

Ultimately a clinician and educator is only as good as the people with whom he works; people who provide a constant source of creative ideas and emotional support. In this respect I would like to thank Karen Evanczuk, R.N., Anita Zeiders, M.S., and Patty McHugh, M.S.W., the clinical/administrative arm of the Diagnostic and Evaluation Center, for their continued support. And a special thanks to the staff nurses and telephone counselors of the Diagnostic and Evaluation Center; a more dedicated and talented staff cannot be found. They are a pleasure to work with, and it is with a great sense of gratitude that I have found a home in our work together.

A warm thanks also goes to my sister, Sandy, who showed me the beauty of teaching and to my brother, Chuck, who has always been a model in the art of compassion.

Finally, all my thanks goes to my wife, Susan, for her love, understanding, and support. She has believed in the book from the beginning, and her insight and editorial comments were invaluable in improving the text. Her help with word processing was also greatly appreciated.

Thanks again, to all.

NOTICE

Mental Health Care is an ever-changing field. Standard safety precautions must be followed, but as new research and clinical experience broaden our knowledge, changes in treatment and drug therapy become necessary or appropriate. Readers are advised to check the product information currently provided by the manufacturer of each drug to be administered to verify the recommended dose, the method and duration of administration, and contraindications. It is the responsibility of the treating physician, relying on experience and knowledge of the patient, to determine dosages and the best treatment for the patient. Neither the publisher nor the editor assumes any responsibility for any injury and/or damage to persons or property.

THE PUBLISHER

CONTENTS

PART 1

Fundamentals of Interviewing

CHAPTER 1

Interviewing: The Principles Behind the Art

*W*hen a doctor tells me that he adheres strictly to this or that method, I have my doubts about his therapeutic effect. . . . I treat every patient as individually as possible, because the solution of the problem is always an individual one . . .

Carl G. Jung
Memories, Dreams, Reflections

*I*n the following pages, we will begin a study of the interviewing process. We will be examining the craft in which one human attempts the formidable task of understanding another human. By way of analogy, this task is not unlike exploring a darkened room in an old Victorian house, holding only a candle as a source of illumination. Occasionally, as one explores the shadows, a brisk wind may snuff the candle out and the room will grow less defined. But with patience, the explorer begins to see more clearly. The outlines of the family portraits and oil lamps become more distinct. In a similar fashion, the subtle characteristics of a patient begin gradually to emerge. This quiet uncovering is a process with which some clinicians appear to familiarize themselves more adeptly than others. It is as if these more perceptive clinicians had somehow known the layout of the room before entering it—and indeed, in some respects, they had.

Their a priori knowledge is the topic of this chapter. We will attempt to discern some of the underlying principles that determine whether an initial interview fails or succeeds. As Jung suggests in the epigraph to this chapter, these principles do not harden into rigid rules. Instead they represent flexible guidelines, providing structure to what at first appears structureless.

Perhaps a second analogy may be clarifying at this point. A recent book on 19th century art by Rosenblum and Janson provides some useful insight.[1] In it, the authors attempt to describe the numerous processes that lead to the creation of a work of art, including environmental influences, political concerns, and the goals and limitations of the artist. With each painting these historians appeared to question themselves vigorously concerning concepts such as color, composition, originality, perspective, and theme. In short, Rosenblum and Janson utilized a specific language of art consisting of concisely defined terms. This language provided them with the tools to conceptualize and communicate their understanding. Since the language was one understood by most artists, the concepts of Rosenblum and Janson could be widely discussed and debated.

The work of the art historian is not at all unlike our own; as clinicians, however, we are concerned with a living art. We can study the characteristics of this living art once we possess a language with which to conceptualize our interviewing styles. With this language, the principles that seem to provide an experienced clinician with a "map of the Victorian room" naturally evolve.

In this chapter we will begin to develop a language with which to describe the interviewing process. Towards this goal the chapter itself is divided into two parts: (1) an operational definition of interviewing, and (2) a concrete conceptualization of the major goals of the interview. This foray into the language of interviewing will shed new light on familiar faces, providing a chance for the development of a more flexible and penetrating style of interviewing.

IN SEARCH OF A DEFINITION

There probably exists no better method for uncovering a definition of interviewing than by analyzing a brief piece of clinical dialogue. Even in a short excerpt, clarifying principles may begin to emerge.

The following dialogue was taken from a videotaped diagnostic interview. Of particular note is the fact that the supervisee was disturbed by a not uncommon problem faced by an interviewer, "the wandering patient." Specifically, the supervisee commented, "I couldn't really even get a picture of her major problem, because she took off on every subject that came to her mind." In this excerpt, the interviewer was attempting to discover whether the patient was suffering from the symptoms of a major depression. The patient, a middle-aged woman, had been describing some problems with her son, who was suffering from an attention deficit disorder.

Pt.:   . . . He's a behavior problem; maybe a phase he's going through. (Interviewer writes note.) He's exhibiting crying spells, which don't necessarily have a reason. The teacher is trying to interview him to see what exactly is wrong with the child because he's tense and crying, which isn't like him; he's been a happy-go-lucky kid.

Clin.:   Is he still kind of hyperactive?

Pt.:   Oh yeah . . . now that we've lowered the medication he's a little bit better, but I was just mad at the doctor; you know, one of them should have explained it to me.

Clin.:   I would think that must be very frustrating to you.

Pt.:   It was.

Clin.:   And how has this affected your mood?

Pt.:   Ah . . . I have a husband who works shifts (interviewer takes note), and he wants to be in charge of everything. I had a job until last February, when I got laid off. I was working more than full time. My husband does not pitch in at all. I was working about 60 hours a week. He wouldn't lift a dish, which really gets to you.

Clin.:   Uh huh; I'm sure.

Pt.:   Especially when you're working Saturdays and Sundays and you start at 6:30 in the morning and don't get home 'til 8:00 at night.

Clin.:   What kind of work?

Pt.:   I was working in electronic assembly. I was an x-ray technician for 10 years and then we decided to settle down and have a family. I was working at the hospital up in Terryhill. And, uh, he said, and I can see his point . . .

At first glance, one can quickly empathize with the interviewer's frustration, for indeed this patient is in no hurry to describe her mood or her depressive symptoms. Instead, when asked directly about her mood, she immediately darts down a side alley into a belittlement of her husband. She appears to wander from topic to topic. But with a second glance, an interesting observation is apparent concerning the communication pattern between these two co-participants. It is unclear who is wandering more, the patient or the interviewer. It is as if the two had decided to take an evening stroll together, hand in hand.

Specifically, the interviewer had intended to explore for information concerning depression. But when the interviewer asked about mood, the patient chose to move tangentially. At this crucial point, where the patient left the desired topic, the interviewer left with her. Unintentionally the clinician may have immediately rewarded the patient for leaving the desired topic by taking notes. Her scribbling may have inadvertently told the patient to continue by suggesting that what the patient was saying was important enough for the clinician to jot down. The interviewer further rewarded the tangentiality of the patient by proffering an empathic statement, "Uh, huh; I'm sure." As if this were not enough, the clinician follows the patient down the alley by asking a question about the new topic.

Thus, both the patient and the clinician had an impact upon each other, their interface defining a dyadic system unconsciously committed to the perpetuation of a tangential interview.

This example illustrates the point that interviews define interactional processes, some of which facilitate communication and others which inhibit communication. These processes are so distinctive that one can name them. For instance, the above process could be named "feeding the wanderer." If one is trying to uncover specific information within a set topic, then the process of feeding the wanderer represents a maladaptive technique. Curiously, if one were attempting to foster an atmosphere conducive to free association, the same technique might be beneficial. In either case, the interviewer can and should be consciously aware of this technique, implementing it when desirable and avoiding it when it would not be efficacious.

For example, in the next chapter we will discover that the interviewer may have been able, in the above dialogue, to lead this patient effectively into a less digressive mode of speech through the use of focusing statements. However, our most immediate concern involves the hint provided by this excerpt with regard to the nature of the interviewing process itself, a definition of which is beginning to crystalize. This definition would be equally true for an assessment interview by a social worker or a television interview by a talk show host. The clinical definition reads as follows:

An interview represents a verbal and nonverbal dialogue between two participants, whose behaviors affect each other's style of communication, resulting in specific patterns of interaction. In the interview one participant, who labels himself or herself as the "interviewer," attempts to achieve specific goals, while the other participant generally assumes the role of "answering the questions."

This definition emphasizes the interactional process of the interview. It also allows one to refine the definition depending on the desired goals and the context of the interview. To make this definition more specific to the clinical assessment, one has only to look for the goals particular to the clinical situation.

In a broad sense, these assessment goals are as follows:

1. To establish a sound engagement of the patient in a therapeutic alliance
2. To collect a valid database
3. To develop an evolving and compassionate understanding of the patient
4. To develop an assessment from which a tentative diagnosis can be made
5. To develop an appropriate disposition and treatment plan
6. To effect some decrease of anxiety in the patient
7. To instill hope and ensure that the client will return for the next appointment

Furthermore, the goals of the initial interview will vary depending on the demands of the assessment situation, including issues such as time constraints and the interviewer's determination of what type of data seems clinically necessary in order to make an appropriate disposition. For instance, a crisis worker called into an extremely busy emergency room to interview a rape victim will clearly sculpt a different interview than an analyst asked to spend an hour or two with a well-educated patient requesting psychotherapy for chronic depression. In short, the needs of the clinical situation should determine the style of the interview but can do so only if the clinician remains willing to flexibly alter his or her approach.

In any case, the above consideration emphasizes one of the frequent challenges facing the initial interviewer, namely to gain a thorough and valid database in a limited amount of time while sensitively engaging the patient. The shorter the time period provided, the more complex the task appears. To return to our Victorian room, it is as if a clinician were being asked to make an inventory of a darkened room in a restricted amount of time while being careful not to disturb the decor too much. No easy task, even for a master of parlor games. Perhaps this challenge reaches its most formidable peak when an interviewer or consultant is placed in the unenviable role of performing an intake assessment. From his or her assessment, frequently limited to about 60 minutes by the numerous time pressures present in a busy clinic, the interviewer must determine the treatment disposition of the patient.

I have chosen to focus on this particularly challenging type of interview in this book, for the principles needed to perform it gracefully can be generalized to most other types of interviews, where more time may be available, resulting in a more leisurely pace. In short, the difficulties presented by the assessment interview provide tremendous opportunities for learning skills critical to understanding the core issue of most interviews, the delicate interplay between engagement and data gathering. Many of these same skills will ultimately also be of use in psychotherapy itself.

The discussion so far has provided an operational definition of an assessment interview. From this definition, a map of sorts can be formulated as shown in Figure 1.

This map, delineating the various goals of the assessment interview, begins with the engagement process, which, in many respects, determines whether the other goals will be successfully achieved. As engagement proceeds, the data gathering process unfolds, leading to a progressive understanding of the patient. This understanding of the patient as a unique person depends on the clinician's ability to see the patient's view of the world and recognize the patient's fears, pains, and hopes. As the interview progresses, the clinician begins to formulate a clinical assessment, including a tentative differential diagnosis. From both the assessment of the patient's situation and

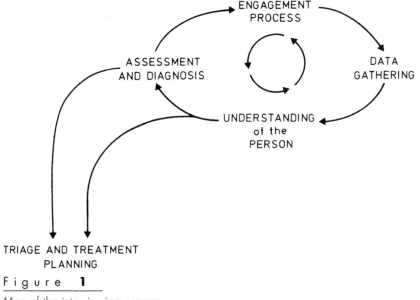

Figure 1

Map of the interviewing process.

an understanding of the patient as a person the clinician can formulate a treatment plan suited to the individual needs of the interviewee, while acknowledging the constraints placed on treatment by the limitations of the mental health system itself.

These processes of engagement, data gathering, understanding, and assessment are in actuality parallel processes. The reverse arrows in the center of the map emphasize this fact, highlighting the clinician's need to attend to engagement activities throughout the first 60 minutes.

CREATION OF AN INTERVIEW: GOALS AND VARIATIONS

Engagement Process

BLENDING AND EMPATHY

From the first moment they see, hear, smell, and touch each other, the clinician and the patient begin the engagement process. In this complex interplay they reflect their sensory information onto the slippery screen of their memories. From these comparisons, both the clinician and the patient attempt to determine where each will fit into the other's life. Even as simple a gesture as a handshake can lead to lasting impressions. The experienced clinician may note whether he or she encounters the iron fingers of a Hercules bent upon establishing control or the dampened palm of a Charlie Brown expecting imminent rejection.

Ironically, at this same moment, the patient will have begun his or her own mental status on the clinician. This process can be seen clearly in the patient who greets the clinician's outstretched hand not with a handshake but with a look of disdain. As the clinician responds to the patient's rejection of a simple social amenity, who can doubt that the patient will be gaining some hints about the psychological workings of the clinician. For example, one interviewer, perhaps with an obsessive need to "do things my way," may further extend his or her hand, testily adding, "Don't you want to shake?" Another clinician, perhaps jaded from overwork, may dryly comment, "Not in the mood for shaking today, are we?"

In either case, the patient has struck a rich vein from which to mine answers to questions such as the following: (1) Will this interviewer get angry with me?, (2) Will this interviewer make me do things I don't want to do?, and (3) Am I safe here? This example hints at the complex and mutual activities affecting the engagement process, during which territorial issues are initially addressed.

Before proceeding it is important to define two terms, *engage-*

ment and *blending*. Engagement refers to the ongoing development of a sense of safety and respect from which patients feel increasingly free to share their problems, while gaining an increased confidence in the clinician's potential to understand them. Blending represents the behavioral and emotional clues from the interview that suggest that this engagement process is proceeding effectively. Stated differently, engagement defines a set of goals, and the concept of blending provides a method of monitoring the effectiveness of the strategies utilized to achieve those goals.

Not all writers emphasize the distinction between engagement and blending, but I feel it is an important one. Its significance lies in the fact that it does one little good to study engagement techniques if one does not develop a reliable method of measuring the effectiveness of these techniques in the interview itself. The concept of blending provides an avenue for active self-monitoring by the clinician. Problems in blending can alert the interviewer to the need to change interview strategies before serious damage to the clinician-patient alliance has developed.

One can assess blending by utilizing three complementary approaches: a subjective method, an objective method, and a patient's self-report. With regard to the subjective technique, an interviewer can learn what sensations he or she experiences when engagement is optimal—in essence, what a good interview feels like. Educators have suggested that once this internal and idiosyncratic feeling stage has been identified, the clinician can use it as a type of thermometer, to determine the intensity of blending at any given moment.[2]

Naturally, this subjective feeling will vary from one interviewer to another. Consequently it may help to examine some of the descriptions clinicians have related concerning this feeling state.

a. "To me good blending feels more like a conversation and a lot less like an interview or interrogation."
b. "I know blending has occurred when suddenly I realize during the interview that I'm actually talking with a person with real pain, not a case with imagined defenses."
c. "When the blending is good, I notice that I feel more relaxed, sometimes even giving off a sigh. Curiously I also feel more interested."

These descriptions suggest the personal uniqueness of the blending process. It is this personal uniqueness that allows the concept of blending to function as such a reliable and sensitive tool for monitoring the degree of engagement. If clinicians can train themselves to intermittently check the progress of blending, they will have discovered a window from which to study the unfolding engagement process. To this extent, the interview becomes less nebulous and more tangible. It evolves into something that can be modified.

This increased tangibility can be furthered by utilizing the second major avenue for monitoring the blending process, an objective look at the behavioral characteristics of the interview itself. The behavioral clues suggested by body language will be discussed in Chapter 3. In this chapter an examination of the timing and structural characteristics of the verbal exchange will be highlighted.

The issue facing the interviewer involves finding concrete behavioral cues from the verbal exchange that indicate the presence of good blending. Wiens[3] and colleagues have provided some simple but fascinating methods of analyzing the temporal characteristics of speech by studying three major speech variables: duration of utterance (DOU), reaction time latency (RTL), and the percentage of interruptions. The DOU can be roughly equated with the length of time taken up by the interviewee's response following a question. The RTL represents the length of time it takes an interviewee to respond to a question. The percentage of interruptions represents the tendency for the interviewee to cut the clinician off before a question has been finished. One can look at all of these variables in relation to the clinician's speech patterns as well.

With regard to blending, these variables offer a potentially more objective measure of effectiveness, because certain patterns of exchange may suggest weak blending. For instance, a guarded or suspicious patient often produces curt responses to questions (a short DOU), long pauses before answering (long RTL), and occasional cut-offs as the patient corrects the interviewer for inaccuracies in his or her statements. If an interviewer spots such a pattern emerging, it may be a clue to ineffective engagement.

Another example at the opposite end of a continuum concerns the hypomanic, histrionic, or anxious patient who tends to wander. These wandering patients frequently present with a long DOU and a very brief RTL and may actually cut the interviewer off frequently. Interestingly, the interviewer may find himself or herself reciprocating with cut-offs in a vain effort to get a word in edgewise.

Moreover, with histrionic, hypomanic, or manic patients, the blending is frequently marked by a peculiar superficial quality. With regard to spontaneity of speech these patients open up inappropriately quickly, as opposed to the gradual increase in blending seen with most patients. Consequently, the observed blending possesses a one-sided and shallow quality, aptly called by one student "unipolar blending."

In the above two examples, we have seen that variations in basic patterns of verbal output, such as a DOU and RTL, can provide objective indications of the adequacy of the blending process. One might ask whether this objective technique offers any advantage over the subjective approach described previously. I believe that it does. But one method does not appear more valuable than another; rather each method complements the other. For instance, not infrequently clinicians are duped into missing the psychopathology of histrionic or hypomanic patients.

One of the reasons this problem occurs is that the clinician feels at a subjective level that the blending is unusually good. Indeed, the clinician is fascinated by the patient's story. In actuality, the blending is artificially good, representing the unipolar blending just described. In fact, unipolar blending, if recognized by the clinician, could provide the clue that "something is wrong here." The patient's engaging style and subtle dramatics are misleading the clinician. If in this instance the clinician could step back to look at the DOU and RTL, the clinician might recognize the hallmarks of a unipolar blending and consequently evaluate the possible psychopathologic causes of it. In this case the objective technique sidesteps the confusion created by judging the blending process solely by the subjective method.

The other advantage of paying attention to more concrete parameters such as DOU and RTL is the ability to use these criteria to judge the effectiveness of a specific technique employed by the clinician. If, for example, the clinician attempts to actively engage a patient who seems hesitant to talk, one of the earliest and most easily recognized markers of success will be an increase in DOU. Correspondingly, changes in the subjective feeling of increased blending may appear only later and may be less easily recognized.

A third method of determining the degree of blending consists of the patient's self-report. Occasionally, a patient will spontaneously tell an interviewer to what degree the interaction is enjoyable. More commonly, the interviewer may inquire, as the interview winds down, "What was it like talking with me today?" Often, because of a hesitancy to appear unappreciative or rude, patients will reply that everything was fine, even if it was not. On the other hand, patients may pointedly discuss specific concerns, which sometimes provides appropriate and constructive criticism.

In other instances, the patient's self-report may provide unexpected insights, especially when the self-report contradicts the subjective and objective methods of evaluating blending. For instance, I am reminded of a young man who appeared somewhat disinterested as we spoke. He talked softly and with little animation. As we proceeded, I felt awkward, as if this were going to be a bad mix of personalities. Although both the objective and subjective signs of blending suggested poor engagement, to my surprise, at the end of the interview he reported feeling very at home with me.

He stated that he had enjoyed the interview, and he appeared sincere.

His diagnosis was paranoid schizophrenia in remission. It was a residual blunting of affect that was creating both an outward and an inward suggestion of poor blending; the engagement was not, in truth, weak. This disparity highlighted the type of miscommunication that this patient could easily convey to other people, an aloofness that was both disarming and misleading. Attention to blending by self-report greatly enhanced my understanding of the manner in which this patient embraces the world. It also suggested the possible utility of social skills training.

Thus, the clinician can benefit from learning to judge blending by the subjective, objective, and self-report approaches. With these three techniques in mind, the interview becomes at once less mystifying and more gratifying. The gratification arises from the realization that the interviewer can learn to creatively alter the interview process itself.

Once blending has been analyzed, the clinician possesses a concrete idea of the strength of the engagement process with any particular patient at any given moment. Weak engagement may imply that invalid data is more likely and compliance more problematic. Moreover, a weak engagement process suggests one of the following three conditions:

1. The interviewer's actions are actively disengaging the patient.
2. The interviewee's psychopathologic processes or defenses are interfering with engagement.
3. A combination of the above.

If the clinician feels that the damaged blending can be attributed to the first condition, then the clinician can attempt to consciously alter his or her style of interaction. For instance, a paranoid patient may be put off by an extroverted style of interviewing. In such an instance, the clinician may decide to tone down the interview in an effort to ease the patient's fears.

If the weak blending can be ascribed to the second condition, then the clinician may be alerted to the types of psychopathology that could be blocking the blending, such as with the histrionic process described earlier. Naturally, if the third condition is the issue, increased attention to both style of interaction and psychopathology can be brought into play.

At this point we have reviewed three methods of directly assessing blending that indirectly assess engagement itself. It is valuable to reflect on the map of the interviewing process delineated earlier. On this map, the interviewer begins with the engagement process for a good reason. The engagement process affects all subsequent goals of the interview.

More specifically, poor engagement raises significant doubts about the validity of the database, because patients generally do not freely share with people they do not like. Moreover, without effective engagement, one will seldom gain knowledge of the private corners of the patient's room alluded to in our comparison of an interview with an exploration of a dark Victorian room. Hence, the clinician leaves with only a superficial understanding of the patient's pain. Furthermore, without valid data falling into place, the clinician's assessment and diagnosis are frequently in significant jeopardy. Finally, if the engagement process proceeds poorly, the patient may never return for a second appointment, casting the shadow of irrelevance over the work of the first interview.

Thus one is left with the realization that this somewhat nebulous concept of engagement appears to be the pivotal process on which much of clinical practice turns. Fortunately, this process is not as mercurial as it first appears. Upon a more searching exploration specific principles for engagement emerge, including: (1) the assessment of blending, (2) the effective conveyance of empathy, (3) the ability to foster a safe environment in which the patient can share, (4) the ability to appear genuine and natural to the patient, and (5) the ability to appear reassuringly competent. In the following pages we will attempt to get beyond the obvious meanings of these terms in an effort to recognize their practical applications. We shall begin with the term *empathy*.

CONVEYING EMPATHY: STRATEGIES AND PITFALLS

Many clinicians assume that empathy is a simple concept. It is not. The large number of research papers devoted to its capture testifies to its elusiveness. Fortunately, over the years insights have been achieved that help to demystify empathy, a quality that all people feel they naturally possess but that in reality may be less ubiquitous than imagined. It seems only appropriate to begin our story with Carl Rogers, who developed the field of client-centered counseling. He conceptualized empathy as the clinician's ability "to perceive the internal frame of reference of another with accuracy, and with the emotional components and meanings which pertain thereto, as if one were the other person, but without ever losing the 'as if' condition."[4] Stated more simply, empathy is the ability to accurately recognize the immediate emotional perspective of another person while maintaining one's own perspective.

As Rogers pointed out, there is an important distinction between empathy and identification, although they can overlap. In the latter process the clinician not only recognizes the emotional state of the other but also proceeds to feel it. The importance of this distinction lies in the fact that identification often marks the pathway toward such unrecognized therapeutic gremlins as burn out and unidentified countertransference. The persistent appearance of strong feelings of identification may alert clinicians to the need to begin or return to their own therapy, because such identification can quickly destroy the therapeutic process.

One feels compelled to say a silent prayer for the poor patient with borderline features who meets a clinician who boldly proclaims, "I can feel your pain." Borderline patients have enough problems with identity diffusion without finding "silly putty" coating the edges of their clinician. Thus a simple but important lesson to be learned from the study of empathy is that most patients are not searching for a person who feels as they do; they are searching for someone who is trying to understand what they feel.

G. T. Barrett-Lennard sheds further light on the concept of empathy by recognizing the fact that empathy is effective only if it involves both the interviewee and the interviewer.[5] He calls this shared response the "empathy cycle," a concept providing an excellent framework with which to study the practical application of empathy. Consequently we will look at each phase of this cycle in detail.

The empathy cycle consists of the following phases: (1) the patient expresses a feeling, (2) the clinician recognizes this feeling, (3) the clinician conveys recognition of the feeling to the patient, (4) the patient receives this conveyance of recognition, and (5) the patient provides feedback to the clinician that the recognition has been received.[5] With this cycle in mind, the empathic process begins to make significantly more sense. In fact, one can see that a breakdown in empathy can arise at each of these five stages.

First Phase of the Empathy Cycle. In the first phase of the empathy cycle, in which the patient expresses a specific feeling, a variety of processes can disrupt empathy. For instance, both conscious and unconscious defenses may block the patient from expressing his or her actual emotions. A poignant example of this process is illustrated by the following dialogue, in which a mother of a mildly retarded 7-year-old discusses her son:

Clin.: Tell me a little about John's behavior with other children.

Pt.: Oh there is really little wrong there, he's really quite normal, just like the other kids. He doesn't like to play games very much or sports, but then he has a mind of his own, maybe someday he'll be a star golfer or skier.

Clin.:   You had mentioned something about his speech earlier.

Pt.:   Oh, hmm, you must be thinking of his lisp. Well I think we all went through that phase as children. In a few years it'll all work out. You know, I have trouble understanding most little kids when they talk, it's part of being a little person.

One feels the pathos of this situation, in which the mother's defenses of denial and rationalization prevent the expression of core feelings of pain. If the interviewer should attempt to make an empathic statement such as, "It sounds like you're really going through a lot with John," I doubt the response would be positive. In this case the patient's own unconscious defenses have prevented the empathy cycle from spontaneously unfolding.

Second Phase of the Empathy Cycle. But phase 1 does not have a monopoly on the common breakdowns that prevent the establishment of an empathic contact. In phase 2, the recognition of the patient's feeling, problems may arise if the clinician's perceptual or intuitive skills fall short, perhaps related to his or her own defenses or psychopathologic undertow. In particular, interviewers need to be aware of the impact of their immediate emotional status on their ability to empathize accurately. For example, a clinician who has recently experienced an unsettling session in supervision may have significant trouble attending to a patient's subtle clues of inner pain. At the other extreme, a recently divorced clinician could easily project his own feelings of betrayal onto a patient undergoing a trial separation, when, in fact, the patient is not experiencing such feelings at all. In both situations, the clinician's emotional state prevents an accurate perception of the interviewee's feelings.

In this light, it can be stated that interviewers have only themselves to serve as measuring instruments. The clinician has no microscope or computed tomography (CT) scan to provide insight. However, like the sophisticated machine, interviewers can unintentionally bias their data. Before beginning an interview, it is often useful to check the bias of the instrument by pausing for a moment of reflection, asking what feelings are present before proceeding to meet the patient. Such a simple process may alert the clinician to potentially distorting factors such as feeling rushed, angry, sad, or simply weary. Once alerted to their biases, interviewers may hope to stand one step further away from invalid data.

The second phase of the empathy cycle also raises several interesting questions concerning the actual nature of intuition. Margulies and Havens[6, 7] have emphasized two frames of mind that appear to be integral aspects of the empathic process. In the first place, the clinician must possess the ability to listen with an attitude of disciplined naiveté, literally attempting to feel the world of the patient without seeking cause and effect, classification, or moral judgment. This receptive listening perspective was masterfully developed by the psychological school of phenomenology, which we shall discuss at greater length later in this chapter. But the bottom line can be simply stated: The clinician must learn to suspend analytic thought when such thought may be destructive to the engagement process.

The second frame of mind that Margulies discusses concerns the ability of the clinician to imagine the inner experiences of the patient by creatively projecting himself or herself into the patient's world. He likens this ability to the poetic imagination of artists, emphasizing the ability to move actively into the patient's world, or "inscape," as this phenomenon has been called.[8] When the clinician does this well, he or she not only paints a picture of the patient's world, but also enters it.

The ability to listen while suspending analysis and the ability to sensitively project what another person may be experiencing can be viewed as two skills from which intuition is born. They remain pivotal to effective clinical practice, typically reaching powerful proportions when clinicians achieve a high degree of blending.

Here we stumble upon a fascinating irony, because one of the characteristics of a gifted interviewer is the ability to know not only when to use these intuitive skills but also when not to use them. Phrased slightly differently, a skilled clinician draws from both intuition and analysis. In a matter of a few minutes the skilled interviewer may juxtapose periods of intuitive listening with moments of analytic thought. Indeed, the two processes, in the hands of a seasoned clinician, tend to guide each other. For example, a clinician may intuitively sense a patient's extreme fear of a disintegration of the self. Besides immediately helping the clinician to blend with the patient, this intuitive feeling might prompt the clinician to later explore, in a diagnostic sense, whether the patient may represent a borderline personality or a narcissistic personality.

Similarly, an analytic process can lead a clinician to a higher level of empathy. For instance, a clinician may observe that as the interview proceeds, the patient avoids eye contact and becomes increasingly anxious. This analytic observation may prompt the clinician to be more empathically aware of the patient's feeling of being ill at ease. At such moments the clinician may gently ask, "I'm wondering what it has been like for you coming to see a psychiatrist?" Subsequently an empathic mode of listening may significantly help the patient to relieve his or her sense of guilt or embarrassment. The important point remains that intuition and analysis are complements, not antagonists. Both skills are utilized frequently during the first encounter.

Third Phase of the Empathy Cycle. In the third phase of the cycle, the clinician's actual phrasing of the empathic statement, the complexities of human interaction further manifest themselves. Here is a phase in which some surprises may appear. One such unexpected twist arises from the fact that not all empathic statements work equally effectively with all patients. In order to understand why, close inspection of this phase is warranted.

One of the more puzzling aspects of empathic statements remains their uncanny ability to promptly disengage a small subset of patients, in short, to achieve the exact opposite of their intended use. One is reminded of the varying fashions in which people accept compliments in everyday situations. Some people take compliments well, whereas others take them poorly. Members of the latter group often become decidedly ill at ease following a sincere compliment, shrugging it off with "Thank you, but it's really nothing."

One manner of interpreting this peculiar phenomenon consists of viewing the compliment as pushing the recipient towards one of two uncomfortable states: (1) accepting a view of himself or herself that seems inaccurate, or (2) feeling an emotional state (e.g., a pleasant sense of self-worth) that he or she does not want to experience, as may be seen in a person burdened by a chronically punitive superego. So it is with empathic statements, which backfire when they push people into interpersonal niches they do not wish to occupy.

The question is whether or not this situation can be avoided. To a large extent I think it can be. Preventing such undesirable repercussions represents one of those areas in which analytic thinking can be of considerable help. More specifically, one can categorize patients, with some degree of caution, into two types, those who are trusting and those who feel guarded. It is with the latter patient, the so-called guarded patient, that empathic statements most frequently display the nasty habit of disrupting the engagement process. The guarded quality of these patients may arise from a variety of sources, including a fear of the clinician, a long-standing character trait of suspiciousness, or frankly prepsychotic or psychotic paranoia.

Empathic statements made to guarded patients from whatever etiology frequently decrease the interpersonal distance between these patients and the clinician. This interpersonal intimacy is exactly what guarded or paranoid patients do not want. Stripped of their "buffer zones" by the well-intentioned clinician, these patients have only one option: to escape through retreat or attack. In short, guarded patients need "distance," a fact too frequently overlooked by interviewers.

So far we have delineated the concept that patients may respond to empathic overtures in different manners secondary to their degree of guardedness, ranging from a trusting bias to frank paranoia. Our understanding can be developed even more fully if we look at three of the characteristic qualities of empathic statements in general, for a change in these characteristics can affect the responses of guarded patients.

In this regard, empathic statements appear to vary along the following three axes: (1) the degree of implied certainty of the interviewee's feelings by the interviewer, (2) the degree of implied intimacy between the interviewer and the interviewee, and (3) the degree of intuited attribution made by the interviewer from statements offered by the interviewee. As one would expect, these axes overlap considerably. However, for purposes of acquiring a more sophisticated understanding, it will be worthwhile to look at them separately, their unique qualities offering the structural foundation from which to understand the impact of empathic statements in general. Along each of these axes one can move from *basic* to *complex empathic statements.*

To begin our inquiry let us speculate on the first axis, the degree of certainty implied by an empathic statement. Put simply, one considers to what degree the clinician implies that he or she knows exactly what the patient is experiencing. In basic statements, the interviewer expresses considerable uncertainty. In contrast, in complex empathic statements the interviewer conveys a high degree of certainty, as illustrated in the following dialogue, in which the patient, a poetic young man, has just suffered the cruelities of an unwanted divorce. This same man had lost his mother to leukemia when he was 13 years old. Following the patient's statement, an example of both a basic and a complex response along the axis of implied certainty will be given.

> **Pt.:**   After my wife left, it was like a star exploded inward, everything seemed so empty . . . she seemed like a memory and my life began to fall apart. Very shortly afterwards I began feeling very depressed and very tearful.

> **Clin.:**   [Basic Empathic Statement] (said gently) It *sounds like* everything seemed to be collapsing around you.

> **Clin.:**   [Complex Empathic Statement] (said gently) *You were* feeling like everything was collapsing around you.

As a general rule, basic empathic statements, which tend to possess a "sounds-like" quality, can be used effectively to enhance blending with *both* a trusting and a guarded patient. In the case of a trusting patient, the complex empathic statement may represent an even more effective device, because it may indicate to the patient a higher degree of seeing things through their eyes, in a phenomenological sense. On the other hand, complex empathic statements may disengage a guarded patient, as shown in the following:

> **Pt.:** I can't believe how cruel people can be. My ex-boss won't even talk with me, won't even give me a minute of his damn time. It hurts, yes it does. But at this point I've got a million problems and nobody to help me.
>
> **Clin.:** *You are feeling very hurt.*
>
> **Pt.:** How would you know what it feels like, have you ever been fired?
>
> **Clin.:** No, I can't say I have, but it surely must be a devastating process.
>
> **Pt.:** To some people perhaps (slight glare from patient).

In this passage, the clinician's attempt at a complex empathic statement with regard to certainty seems to have unsettled the paranoid patient, a verbal boomerang of sorts. Perhaps this backfire has its origins in the patient's desire for a private and hence safe world. More explicitly, this patient appears to dislike the process of being told what he is feeling or should be doing, for that world is his world, and trespassers are not encouraged.

This trespass has led to a rather awkward moment, in which the patient challenges the clinician's ability to understand him, which is not exactly the response desired by the interviewer, who suddenly finds himself dodging the cutting edge of a paranoid accusation.

One can speculate that if the clinician had used a basic empathic phrase such as, "It *sounds like* you have been feeling pretty hurt" instead of the complex phrase, "*You are* feeling hurt," perhaps the interaction may have been less antagonistic.

The second axis of empathy concerns the degree to which the clinician's response implies emotional intimacy to the patient. It specifically evaluates the degree to which the clinician suggests that "I am or probably would be experiencing at this very moment the same emotion you are." In this sense, it implies a feeling of "our world" as opposed to "your world" and "my world," as seen below, using the patient discussed earlier as a model.

> **Pt.:** After my wife left, it was like a star exploded inward, everything seemed so empty . . . she seemed like a

memory and my life began to fall apart. Very shortly afterwards I began feeling very depressed and very tearful.

Clin.:   [Basic Empathic Response] *To me it seems as if you may be* feeling a whole set of intensely painful emotions.

or

Clin.:   [Complex Empathic Response] It hurts to lose someone like her.

Once again the basic empathic response will frequently foster the blending process with both trusting and guarded patients. Furthermore, with the guarded patient, the basic empathic response seems to provide ample distance or breathing room, a quality much in demand by guarded patients.

For a moment, let us focus on the ramifications and potential advantages and disadvantages of complex empathic responses with regard to the axis of intimacy. With trusting patients, another example of a complex empathic statement begins with phrases such as "It is" or "There is." These phrases can sometimes be unusually effective for engagement purposes.[9] Such third-person singular impersonal phrases tend to suggest a shared experience to the patient, in the sense that the clinician acknowledges the validity of the patient's experience while simultaneously suggesting one would (or even has) experienced similar emotions. When well-timed, these phrases can shore up a faltering alliance. Of course the difficulty surfaces when complex statements are poorly timed, as with some paranoid patients. In such cases complex phrases can precipitate unwanted misunderstandings, as suggested by the following:

Pt.:   My husband is a strange man. You might call him evil. It's the "divorce game," him trying to drive me nuts so that he can divorce me.

Clin.:   How do you mean?

Pt.:   For about 3 months he's had them on me. I know they're watching, every night at 6 o'clock. I feel their presence. I think they use telescopes and maybe mind probes to see me, a terrible terrible position to be in.

Clin.:   *It is* frightening to be constantly watched by others.

Pt.:   Just what do you mean by that? How would you know what I'm feeling? (said testily)

Clin.:   Well, in the situation you're describing I think it would be frightening.

Pt.:   Frightening enough to make one lose one's mind?

Clin.:   Well . . . that's difficult to say, it's not . . .

Pt.:   It's *what* Dr. Jones? Frightening enough to make one crazy, well I'm not crazy Dr. Jones, no matter what you think, and trust me I'm not defenseless.

In this example, the clinician's complex empathic statement has suggested a shared intimacy that has been rudely rejected by the patient. In fact, for the patient, fleeing from a world studded with "mind probes," the clinician's unsolicited entry into her world seems most poorly timed. Indeed, the unintended invasiveness resulting from the phrasing has formed a paranoid rage of no small proportion, perhaps placing this patient near the edge of violence. Once again, with this type of paranoid process, it may have been wiser for the clinician to employ a basic empathic statement or perhaps no empathic statement at all. Along the third axis of empathy, we will once again see that the impact of empathic statements can vary depending on the mental state of the patient.

The third axis, concerning the degree of implication of specific qualities to the patient, warrants considerable attention. Along this axis how much the clinician reads into the patient is compared with how much the clinician repeats back exactly what he or she has heard. The opposing ends of this spectrum appear in the following:

Pt.:   After my wife left, it was like a star exploded inward, everything seemed so empty . . . she seemed like a memory and my life began to fall apart. Very shortly afterwards I began feeling very depressed and very tearful.

Clin.:   [Basic Empathic Response] (said softly) It sounds as if your whole life began falling apart.

or

Clin.:   [Complex Empathic Response] (said softly) It is very frightening to lose her so suddenly, so similar to the pain you felt when your mother died.

In the basic empathic response, the clinician, essentially employing the same wording as the patient, has truly mirrored back the patient's thoughts. No intuition is displayed here. Consequently there exists little chance that the statement will be perceived as inaccurate or too invasive by either a trusting or a guarded patient. Moreover, if said in a caring tone, this basic response can convey concern while demonstrating an attentive listening style. It may represent a rudimentary level of empathy, but it does convey caring when done well. This statement has significant limitations, because it does not particularly demonstrate great sensitivity or understanding by the clinician.

To the contrary, the complex response to a *trusting* patient may suggest to the patient that he or she is dealing with a keenly perceptive individual. For instance, in our example this sensitivity was suggested by the clinician's use of the term "frightening," a feeling never mentioned by the patient but nevertheless felt to be present by the clinician. When accurate, such empathic connections can be powerful indeed. Moreover, the second part of the clinician's response, suggesting a relationship of the current grief to an earlier mourning for the patient's mother, also represents an attribute made by the clinician to the patient that may suggest to the patient that he has found an understanding and insightful listener. The presence of such comments often characterizes the dialogue of an experienced clinician.

Once again, however, one must ask whether or not this complex empathic statement can get a clinician into trouble. Not surprisingly, the answer is "yes," especially with guarded patients. By way of example, paranoid process is often associated with an inordinate attention to details, demonstrated by an unexpected value on accuracy. This need for *accurate* understanding at all costs is bolstered by the paranoid fear that "no one understands what I'm really feeling." With these two processes in mind, one can easily imagine potential traps awaiting the clinician who unwittingly uses a complex empathic response with a paranoid patient, as displayed in what follows:

> **Pt.:** After my wife left, it was like a star exploded inward, everything seemed so empty . . . she seemed like a memory and my life began to fall apart. Very shortly afterwards I began feeling very depressed and very tearful.

> **Clin.:** It sounds terribly frightening to lose her so suddenly, so similar to the pain you felt when your mother died.

> **Pt.:** No . . . no, that's not right at all. My mother did not purposely abandon me. That's simply not true.

> **Clin.:** I did not mean that your mother purposely abandoned you, but rather that both people were unexpected losses.

> **Pt.:** I suppose . . . but they were very different. I never was afraid of my mother . . . they're really *very* different.

Needless to say, this attempt at empathic connection leaves something to be desired. The patient's attention to detail and fear of misunderstanding have obliterated the intended empathic message, leaving the clinician with a frustrating need to mollify a patient who has successfully twisted an empathic statement into an insult of sorts. At this point some relatively simple patterns are emerging, which can act as practical guidelines to effective phrasing of empathic statements.

1. In general, empathic statements represent extremely valuable methods for strengthening engagement. Consequently, the clinician will usually employ such statements intermittently throughout an interview.
2. The statements themselves vary in degree of implied certainty, intimacy, and attribution of qualities, which represent three axes of empathy.
3. Along these three axes, one can characterize empathic statements as either basic or complex.
4. Basic statements are generally useful with *both* trusting and guarded patients. Their weakness lies in the fact that they do not convey a particularly sensitive understanding to the patient, although they do demonstrate concern. Their strength lies in the fact that they seldom backfire.
5. With guarded patients it is frequently best to utilize basic empathic statements. At other times it is best to avoid empathic statements. If one attempts to use a more complex statement and discovers some evidence of resulting disengagement, then further complex statements should probably be avoided.
6. On the other hand, with trusting patients, interviewers frequently begin with basic statements and progress to more complex empathic statements, for such complex statements may prove more effective in producing a deepening sense of trust.

In our survey of the empathic axes, we have uncovered an important principle of interviewing: empathic statements may disengage guarded or paranoid patients, a breakdown in communications that is called "the paranoid spiral," in which meaningful interaction spirals downward towards a cool silence. This acute decrease in blending may show itself by a disavowal or correction of the empathic statement or by various nonverbal communications. Being aware of this principle can allow the clinician to consciously avoid the inappropriate use of empathy. However, this principle provides another service to the clinician if looked at from the diagnostic perspective. If a clinician is in the midst of an interview and finds that the patient disengages when offered empathic statements, then the clinician should be aware that a hostile or paranoid process may be present, a process that may have been masked until that moment in the interview. Of course, not all patients who disavow empathic statements are guarded or paranoid. At times, patients who feel a need to appear strong will also refuse empathy. With such patients, it is often wise to emphasize their strengths as opposed to utilizing empathic statements.

At this juncture in our discussion of the third phase of the empathy cycle, the actual conveyance of empathy, three further variables determining the effectiveness of empathic statements warrant attention: frequency, timing, and length. With regard to frequency, no magic number exists. I do not think anyone can authoritatively state the number of optimal empathic comments per interview, because this number must surely vary for each paired interviewer and interviewee. On the other hand I would estimate that well-received clinicians frequently seem to scatter empathic statements throughout their interview, perhaps averaging one statement every 5 to 20 minutes. Moreover, it seems likely that one could either potentially overuse or underuse empathic statements. In the former case the clinician runs the risk of sounding superficially caring or paternalistic. In the latter case, the interviewer may be perceived to be as inscrutable as a sphinx, hardly an effective tool for ensuring a follow-up appointment.

This discussion of frequency naturally leads into the issue of timing. One underlying principle, perhaps the most important, remains that of using at least one or two empathic statements during the first 5 to 10 minutes. Generally speaking, I would suspect that many patients often determine whether they like or dislike the clinician during these initial minutes, and their decision frequently rests upon whether the clinician seems accepting or not. Specifically, patients may fear that the clinician will not understand them or will think they are silly or weak. No better tool exists in the clinician's repertoire for decisively allaying such fears than an empathic statement. Although an easy maneuver, this technique can set the tone for an entire interview.

Of course, even with the best of intentions, empathic statements can miss their mark, as illustrated below:

Pt.: Well I don't really think it's right for the university to be so upset with me for not paying back the loan. I mean it was 7 years ago and I simply don't have the money. It really hurts me too.

Clin.: It sure sounds like a difficult spot to be in, what with all those pressures and financial responsibilities. I bet it seems like you have no place to go, you know, sort of

> stranded, probably makes you feel like everyone is against you.
>
> **Pt.:**   Uh-huh (painful pause).
>
> **Clin.:**   What are you thinking of doing?

In this example the empathic statement has all the power of a two-page descriptive paragraph in an adventure story. It is far too long. In general, empathic comments display their engagement best when they are concise and unambiguous.

This example also points out one method of determining the effectiveness of any given empathic comment. Put succinctly, effective statements usually result in an increased verbal production by the patient. Shut-downs, as shown earlier, often follow an ineffective comment. Leston Havens describes this process elegantly:

A more exacting test of successful empathy is the extent to which our responses stimulate and deepen the other's narrative flow. Does the speaker stop or change subjects? Are the expressions of feeling increased or decreased? One of the moments of greatest clinician drama occurs when a strong empathic flow encounters a memory heretofore forbidden to consciousness or denied.[10]

There remains one last comment to make before leaving the discussion of the third phase of the cycle. Empathy is probably not primarily conveyed through empathic statements. Large amounts of empathy appear to be communicated through facial expressions, body language, tone of voice, and other "empathic noises," as Havens calls them.[10] These nonverbal elements will be given the attention they deserve in Chapter 3.

Fourth Phase of the Empathy Cycle. In the fourth phase of the empathy cycle, in which the patient receives the conveyed empathic statement, problems can also arise. Specifically, the patient's psychopathology may limit his or her ability to perceive empathy or even to understand language itself. Such a situation can occur with delirious patients or severely psychotic patients. In extreme cases, empathic statements can be malignantly transformed into an auditory illusion, perhaps becoming a derogatory statement or threatening insult.

Another case in point concerns manic patients who quite simply are sometimes too busy talking to even register an empathic statement. Indeed, at times it is not clear whether they care if the clinician is being empathic or not. With these patients, attempts to empathize may actually be counterproductive, being in some respects contrary to what they most want at that moment, an audience.

Fifth Phase of the Empathy Cycle. In the fifth phase of the empathic cycle, in which the patient provides feedback to the clinician that the empathic statement was received, difficulties may once again surface. As before, the patient's psychopathology may prevent acknowledgment of the clinician's empathic communications. This is perhaps most poignantly demonstrated by the patient ravaged by a severe, regressive depression or a catatonic stupor. Such patients sometimes seem almost hollow, as if our words pass through them unheard and unanswered. But I think it is important not to be misled by this sensation, because these patients may very well be hearing and even responding to empathic statements despite their inability to convey their reception. Clinician statements such as, "I have no real way of knowing what you are feeling, but if you are feeling lonely or sad or want to talk, I will be available, just let me know," can be very important, perhaps even pivotal in providing a new bridge for communication, the first resonation in the empathy cycle.

Through this review of the empathy cycle, we have, it is hoped, moved from a cliché-like understanding of empathy towards a more sophisticated understanding of one of the most practical tools available to the initial interviewer. Furthermore, our discussion has indirectly led us to our next topic, the establishment in the interview of a feeling of safety.

INDUCEMENT OF A SAFE RELATIONSHIP

The patient's waiting room period before meeting his or her clinician may pass with an urgent slowness. It is frequently teeming with fears of rejection and with self-recrimination. It is often accompanied by ruminations such as, "Well, it's finally come to this, I'm so weak I need a shrink." As professionals we would like to think patients do not feel this way about us, but we should not deceive ourselves. For most people (including most mental health professionals), it is genuinely upsetting to admit the need for help with a psychological problem. The sensitive handling of this anxiety represents one of the main tasks of the initial interviewer. In fact, if it is not handled well, there may not be a second interview.

In his insightful book *The Psychiatric Interview* Harry Stack Sullivan describes a novel idea he calls "the self-system." This self-system consists of "a vast system of processes, states of alertness, symbols, and signs of warnings," which protects us from a lowering of self-esteem as we meet new people.[11] This self-system, consisting of both conscious and unconscious coping mechanisms, becomes activated in an effort to decrease the anxiety generated by fears of rejection. It is this self-system that rises to a high pitch as a patient absent-mindedly turns the pages of a magazine in the waiting room.

Three ideas immediately come to mind. First, one of the primary goals of the clinician in the initial interview consists of attempting to decrease the patient's anxiety and hence the need for an extremely active self-system. Second, the activation of the self-system offers the clinician an excellent preview of the patient's defenses against interpersonal anxiety. Thus, the opening 10 minutes of the interview provide an unexpected window into the workings of the patient's mental guard dogs, both healthy and rabid. And third, in most cases, the clinician's own self-system is also aroused when the clinician meets a new patient. The interplay of these three processes lies at the very heart of the engagement process.

As we have seen, to some extent the conveyance of empathy can significantly decrease the patient's need for an active self-system, but other specific processes can also reassure the interviewee. In the 1950s and 1960s, Carl Rogers developed the concept of "unconditional positive regard," which he defines as follows: "The therapist communicates to his client a deep and genuine caring for him as a person with potentialities, a caring uncontaminated by evaluations of his thoughts, feelings, or behaviors."[12] It is a powerful statement. It is not unlike the suspension of analytic thought seen in the process of intuition.

Placed into the context of the initial interview, as opposed to ongoing therapy, unconditional positive regard translates as a suspension of moral opinion by the interviewer in respect to the interviewee. In short, the patient comes away with the feeling that the clinician is not going to pass judgment on him. In many cases, this safe feeling contrasts starkly with the patient's recent experience (and at times lifelong experience) of encountering a long string of raised eyebrows on the faces of friends, family members, and employers. It is up to the interviewer not to follow this parade of frowns.

In this regard, it becomes important for the clinician to work out the potentially disturbing feelings raised by emotionally charged issues such as divorce, religion, sexual preference, violence, rape, and abortion. No matter what the clinician's view of these activities, in the initial interview, the goal remains to show no judgment to the patient. Instead, the interviewer attempts to convey interest in finding out the significance of these ideas to the patient, recognizing the truth in the very wise statement of Armond Nicholi, Jr., that "whether the patient is young or old, neatly groomed or disheveled, outgoing or withdrawn, articulate, highly integrated or totally disintegrated, of high or low socioeconomic status, the skilled clinician realizes that the patient, as a fellow human being, is considerably more like himself than he is different . . ."[13]

Practically, one effective method of spotting potentially disruptive topics for oneself consists of monitoring interviews for topics that one consistently avoids. For instance, one interviewer may discover that he or she seldom knows anything about the religious beliefs of the patient, whereas another interviewer never asks about sexuality. Such gaps in data gathering may point to precisely those topics about which the interviewer has strong opinions. It is in these areas that conveying unconditional positive regard may be problematic.

It is not only controversial issues that can disrupt the conveyance of unconditional positive regard. In fact, as clinicians we may unwittingly sound like parents at the most unlikely times. In the following dialogue with a young man suffering from paranoid schizophrenia, this disconcerting process rears its head in a subtle form:

Clin.: Tell me more about what you've been doing since your last hospitalization.

Pt.: Things are going well. I'm getting along much better at home, and I haven't needed all those drugs the doctor told me to take.

Clin.: (pause, clinician looks up from clipboard) So you haven't been taking your medications like you're supposed to.

Pt.: No, I just think they fog up my mind.

Clin.: We'll need to talk about that a little later.

This clinician's choice of words has created an atmosphere potentially suggestive of a parent's reprimand. Indeed the interviewer's last statement sounds suspiciously like a threat to go to the principal's office.

As a contrast, in the following dialogue, a different approach yields a different interaction with significantly less activation of the patient's self-system:

Clin.: Tell me more about what you've been doing since your last hospitalization.

Pt.: Things are going well. I'm getting along much better at home, and I haven't needed all those drugs the doctor told me to take.

Clin.: What were some of the medications you were using?

Pt.: I think it was called Haldol and a little pill . . . Cogentin or something like that.

Clin.: Tell me a little bit about what you felt like while you were on these medications.

Pt.: It was strange. I don't know which one was doing it, but I always felt doped up, like I was in a fog.

Clin.: That sounds like an unpleasant side effect.

Pt.: Yes, it was.

This interviewer has successfully conveyed concern without a price tag of obedience. Ironically, later in the interview, I would suspect the latter clinician would be in a more favorable position to persuade the patient to try a neuroleptic again.

This discussion suggests another characteristic, nondefensiveness, that contributes to a feeling of safety for the patient. Patients are very quick to perceive defensiveness in an interviewer. Defensive posturing by the clinician may create in the interviewee the feeling that "I've got to watch what I say here." The following example illustrates a defensive position by the clinician, as a woman describes her anguish concerning her son's problems with schizophrenia:

Moth.: I just don't know what to do with him. Nothing the doctors do ever helps. It's always the same. I don't think they know what they are doing. They haven't tried megavitamin therapy, and I hear that sometimes works miracles. I want you to try that treatment.

Clin.: Well, let's get something straight, these kinds of therapies are simply unproven and maybe unsafe. So we don't use those here.

Moth.: But some people claim they've been helped.

Clin.: Don't believe everything you read Mrs. Jones.

Here we see the paternalistic tone that can so readily destroy a patient's trust. The clinician's self-system has been activated, resulting in a defensive, "educational" posture, which only serves to reciprocally activate the patient's own self-system. This interaction might have been avoided with the following approach:

Moth.: . . . They haven't tried megavitamin therapy and I hear that sometimes works. I want you to try that treatment.

Clin.: It sounds like you've really gone through a lot of frustration, Mrs. Jones. In a little while we'll talk about the pros and cons of different treatments, including megavitamin therapy, but first I want to hear more about your son so that I have a better understanding of exactly what we are dealing with here.

Moth.: Sure. It's long and complicated. But it all started about 3 years ago . . .

Our discussion of the principles behind the development of a safe alliance began with the words of Harry Stack Sullivan. Sullivan also provided an important note upon which to close our discussion. One of the contributing factors to the development of an overactive self-system is the not so maladaptive fear that strangers may harbor ulterior motives. In short, a patient may fear that he or she is going to be used, or even abused.

It is hoped that conscious abuse of a patient is a rarity in our field, but less sinister abuse may enter the picture unconsciously. Clinicians may have ulterior motives of which they have little if any awareness. For example, a clinician may depend on a patient for the gratification of the clinician's need to feel liked or important. If the patient feels that the clinician needs something from them, such as respect, caring, or fondness, the relationship is no longer a safe one. Once again the patient is faced with watching what he or she says, from the fear that professional help will be withdrawn if certain needs are not satisfied.

Sullivan stated this principle elegantly.

*H*e [the clinician] is an expert having expert knowledge of interpersonal relations, personality problems, and so on; he has no traffic in the satisfactions which may come from interpersonal relations, and he does not pursue prestige or standing in the eyes of his clients, or at the expense of his clients. In accordance with this definition, the psychiatrist is quite obviously uninterested in what the patient might have to offer, temporarily or permanently, as a companion, and quite resistant to any support by the patient for his prestige, importance, and so on. It is only if the psychiatrist is very clearly aware of this taboo, as it were, on trafficking in the ordinary commodities of interpersonal relations, that many suspicious people discover that they can deal with him and can actually communicate to him their problems with other people.[14]

Besides offering a safe relationship, the initial interviewer also actively engages the patient in a positive fashion, utilizing those gestures and words that suggest to the patient that future interaction will be enjoyable and rewarding, as seen in our next topic.

CLINICIAN GENUINENESS

The term "genuineness" has been described by a variety of researchers.[15, 16] As was the case with empathy, genuineness appears to be a nebulous term at first glance. Once again, an operative definition provides clarification. One can state that "being genuine" occurs when the following is present:

The behavioral characteristics of the clinician suggest to the patient that the clinician is feeling at ease both with himself and with the patient. It is frequently marked by three characteristics in the clinician: (1) responsiveness, (2) spontaneity, and (3) consistency.

Perhaps there exists no better arena for examining these characteristics of clinician genuineness than looking at the reactions of a clinician to patient humor.

When faced with humor some clinicians display a curious sense of awkwardness, as if humor should not be allowed during an interview. In essence these clinicians "run-over" the moment of humor. Rather than responding with a smile or a chuckle, they maintain a somber expression.

This rather extreme form of nonresponsiveness can produce an immediate increase in patient anxiety, not unlike the discomfort many of us have had the misfortune of experiencing in a social setting, when one of our jokes is followed by an absence of laughter. Ironically, such clinicians may argue that their nonresponsiveness reprsents professionalism, but it seems odd that professional behavior should result in increased patient anxiety during the early stages of an interview. Moreover, this same lack of clinician responsiveness may be uniformly provided in response to a variety of patient affects, including tearfulness, anger, and fear, all in the name of professionalism.

Many patients balk at such pseudoprofessionalism, preferring a clinician who interacts with a gentle responsiveness. In the final analysis, the mark of a true professional seems to be his or her lack of a need to feign professionalism. Such clinicians quickly and easily appear at ease with both their body language and their reactivity. They are attentively relaxed. Moreover, they bring to the interview a sense of appropriate spontaneity, the second characteristic of genuine interaction as described in our definition.

This spontaneity does not exist as a license for sharing whatever comes to mind. To the contrary, a skilled clinician consistently assesses the potential impact of all statements but also possesses the ability to share some spontaneous feelings if they are deemed appropriate for the patient. This spontaneous quality often demonstrates itself in characteristics such as a well-timed sense of humor, a flexible method of structuring the interview, and a nondefensive attitude towards questions voiced by the patient.

As just mentioned, one must be careful about the degree of responsiveness and spontaneity one displays. Both too much and too little can present problems. For instance, a bouyant interviewer can intimidate certain patients, whereas a wooden interviewer may frighten them. In the latter regard, if the frightened patient feels too uncomfortable with the clinician to share suicidal ideation, then the unresponsive interviewer may truly regret having presented a wooden attitude. The clinician needs to nurture a flexible style. The degree of spontaneity and responsiveness will probably vary from one patient to another and with the clinical setting.

In this regard, the myth of "professional blandness" may have evolved from a misinterpretation of the psychoanalytic concept of presenting a neutral screen, upon which the patient could project his or her transference. This neutral screen concept does not represent a dictum for unresponsiveness. In the first place, an expressionless presentation hardly represents a neutral stance, as Ryle[17] has commented, for such a bland reaction typically suggests that the nonresponder dislikes the other participant. This supposed "neutral stance" is, in actuality, potentially very disengaging. Moreover, rather than providing a blank screen, it seems to bias the patient towards negative transference.

Even if one adhered to this neutral stance theory for therapeutic application, and few talented analysts I have met do so in a strict sense, it does not necessarily follow that the neutral stance is effective for assessment interviewing. Indeed, as we have seen, one of the major goals of the initial interview remains the development of a powerful blending, which will, it is hoped, lead to both powerful compliance and a second appointment. A wooden interview hardly lends itself to the facilitation of engagement.

It seems timely to examine consistency, the third element commonly characterizing a genuine interaction. Gerard Egan has emphasized the importance of consistency as demonstrated by the clinician's willingness to explore the patient's world in a shared manner, while respecting the patient's present limitations and defenses. More specifically, the clinician avoids discordant actions, such as appearing warmly responsive in part of the interview and cooly distant later; nor does the clinician suddenly become confrontative, as demonstrated by Counselor A in the following example provided by Egan.[18]

Client: I want to know what you really think of me.

Counselor A.: I think you're lazy and that you would like things to get better if that could happen by magic.

Counselor B.: Frankly, I don't find a great deal of value in such direct evaluation, but I think it's good to talk about this directly. Maybe we can take a look at what's happening between you and me.

The response of Counselor B demonstrates a willingness to share exploration, including a foray into the developing interviewer-interviewee relationship.

Together, the traits of appropriate responsiveness, spontaneity, and consistency coalesce to create an appealing milieu for the sharing of problems. When adroitly blended, these three traits of genuineness convey a sense of emotional balance in the clinician, a balance that suggests a possible source of help to the person in need.

In the following dialogue, these traits as well as a sense of nondefensiveness are elegantly displayed in a situation in which a therapist could easily have swallowed his or her foot. In this interaction, the clinician, a physician, had determined from the preceding conversation that the patient was pleasant and well integrated but very anxious. Consequently, the interviewer felt that humor could be safely employed.

> **Clin.:** What has it been like coming down to the emergency room today?
>
> **Pt.:** Unsettling, to say the least. I feel very awkward here, sort of like I'm vulnerable. To be honest, I've had some horrible experiences with doctors, I don't like them.
>
> **Clin.:** I see, well, they scare the hell out of me too (smiles, indicating the humor in his comment).
>
> **Pt.:** (chuckle) I thought you were a doctor.
>
> **Clin.:** I am (pause, smiles), that's what's so scary.
>
> **Pt.:** (smiles and laughs)
>
> **Clin.:** Tell me a little more about some of your unpleasant experiences with doctors, because I want to make sure I'm not doing anything that is upsetting you or frightening you. I don't want that to happen.
>
> **Pt.:** Well, that's very nice to hear. My last doctor didn't give a hoot about what I said and he only spoke in huge words.

In this example, the clinician has skillfully transformed a potentially "loaded moment" into a shared resolution through humor. If patients realize that avenues for discussing their needs and complaints are open, they frequently feel less frightened. The presence of pathways for "filing complaints" paradoxically often decreases the need for their use.

This excerpt also illustrates the common finding that experienced interviewers frequently appear to enjoy the process of interviewing itself. Experienced clinicians feel at home in the interviewing process, their own self-systems purring quietly. It is this sense of natural balance in the clinician that remains one of the most powerful of engagement tools. This balance is complemented by the next trait to be discussed, yet another important tool in the engagement process.

CLINICIAN EXPERTISE

In order to explain the concept of clinician expertise most effectively, it may be best temporarily to view the interviewing process solely from the patient's perspective. To the patient, certain questions are of paramount importance. The answer to one of these questions in particular holds unusually powerful significance, perhaps even determining the degree of final compliance. It is a logical question. It is a natural question. And it can be paraphrased simply as follows: "Can this person help me?"

To ignore the reality that the patient is attempting to answer this question can lead to serious problems in engagement. To begin with, the act of hanging out our shingles as mental health professionals suggests that we have something to offer to patients for which they are exchanging money, time, and trust. On a basic level, they are generally expecting to find a good listener, albeit a "paid ear" of sorts. But at a deeper level, they are also expecting something else, something more. They are expecting to find an expert, a term I find mildly threatening, because it comes preseasoned with more than a pinch of pride. One feels hesitant to declare oneself an expert in so vast a field as human behavior, feelings, and psychophysiology.

But the term becomes more palatable, and indeed appropriate, if one keeps in mind two of the principles behind it. First, being an expert does not mean that one has all the answers or, for that matter, can necessarily provide relief. And second, being an expert does suggest that we have been rigorously schooled in an effort to consolidate a body of knowledge found useful in our field. It is the presence of this body of knowledge that may most successfully answer the patient's pressing question, "Can this person help me?"

In this regard, it is also useful to remember that in an anthropological sense, the initial clinician is fulfilling the role of a healer, and whether one is a shaman or a social worker, as a healer one is expected to possess knowledge not commonly available to the patient. From the above discussions, it should be apparent that at both a personal and a societal level, the clinician's expertise as perceived by the patient is critical to the engagement process.

The next logical question is, "How does one convey expertise effectively during an initial interview?" The answer lies primarily not in what we tell the patient but in what we ask the patient. It is the quality of our questions, not the quantity of our words, that generally convinces a patient that the clinician knows something that might help.

Questions, like empathic statements, can be categorized along a number of continua, including: (1) open-ended versus closed-ended, (2) probing versus nonprobing, (3) fact-finding versus opinion-finding, and (4) structured versus unstructured. Questions along the full range of these continua can be clinically useful, and all can be surprisingly ineffective as well. Their effectiveness or ineffectiveness seems to depend upon their timing as well as the appropriateness of the type of question for the task of the interviewer at any specific moment.

In the next chapter a great deal of time will be spent discussing the flexible use of questions at different phases of the interview. But at this point, I want to focus on an especially useful question, a type of question that can unobtrusively yet effectively convey expertise to the patient: the fact-oriented question.

By a fact-oriented question, I am referring to questions concerned with the concrete realities of the patient's situation, symptoms, and problems. Questions such as, "Are you having any problem falling asleep?" or "Has your appetite changed?" represent typical examples of fact-oriented questions. Frequently, fact-oriented questions concern diagnostic issues, and they are generally closed-ended in nature.

Some initial interviewers shy away from fact-oriented questions, because they believe that such questions are generally disengaging. In this regard I agree that they can be disengaging when used at the wrong moments, too frequently, or in checklist fashion. And an interviewer should learn to avoid these pitfalls. But when asked sensitively, fact-oriented questions are powerful engagement tools, which also yield large amounts of valuable information for triage decisions.

To illustrate the point, let us look at the mid-phase of an initial interview with a woman in her late 20s. Rather than just going with the patient, the interviewer begins a more structured effort to tease out the symptoms upsetting this patient in an effort to arrive at a useful diagnosis.

>**Pt.:** I am terribly frightened about going back for my masters, I mean, is it worth it? . . . When I think about it, I get all uptight.
>
>**Clin.:** How do you mean?
>
>**Pt.:** I start to fret and worry. I feel extremely tense and wound up like a crazy alarm clock, ready to explode.
>
>**Clin.:** Over the course of any given day, say over the last month, how much of your day do you spend worrying like that?
>
>**Pt.:** Oh, I'd say at least 70%, sometimes almost the whole day.

Clin.:   (said gently) Sounds miserable.

Pt.:   It really is, and the bad part is, I can't stop it.

Clin.:   Sounds like you find it difficult to relax.

Pt.:   Oh my god, yes! Even when I come home I feel like I've got to do something, something needs to be done and if I don't do it I'm a bad person. It's strange.

Clin.:   People develop a lot of tensions during the day, especially in a job like yours. I'm wondering if you find yourself having muscle aches, trembling sensations, or eye twitches related to your tension.

Pt.:   Funny you should ask. You may have noticed, but my left eye twitches when I'm tense, drives me nuts.

Clin.:   How long has that been going on?

Pt.:   I've had it . . . let's see . . . maybe 5 or 6 years, but ever since deciding on grad school it's been really much worse.

Clin.:   How do you mean?

Pt.:   I look like a "mad winker" (patient and clinician chuckle). It really can be embarrassing.

Clin.:   I'm sure it can be (warmly chuckles again). Tell me, have you noticed any other evidence of tension in your body, other than the twitching?

Pt.:   I've had a lot of diarrhea lately, I don't know if that's related or not and I also have been feeling flashes of feeling real hot, makes me think of my mother and menopause, but I've had those kinds of flashes off and on for years.

Clin.:   With these hot flashes do you notice any change in your pulse rate or breathing rate?

Pt.:   No, I can't say I have.

Clin.:   Have you ever found yourself suddenly having an abrupt episode of being extremely anxious, all at once?

Pt.:   No . . . let me think, . . . not really.

Clin.:   When you say "not really," what have you experienced?

Pt.:   About a week ago I really got upset about Bob, but I wasn't really anxious, I was mad.

Clin.: What about periods when you suddenly became very frightened, perhaps of dying, without any apparent reason?

Pt.: No, that I can clearly say I've never had.

Clin.: Any periods when you suddenly found yourself panicking and perhaps short of breath or noticing tingling sensations in your fingers or around your mouth?

Pt.: No, I don't get that either.

Clin.: What about your concentration?

Pt.: Now that's shot. I can't concentrate at all. I've particularly noticed that when doing the books at work. Math comes simple to me and usually I fly through that stuff, but over the past 2 months I feel really frazzled. It takes forever.

Clin.: Earlier you mentioned the relationship of these feelings to your fears about grad school. What are some of the connections you see?

Pt.: Well, in the first place, I don't think I can do it. I mean I'm smart, at least I think I'm reasonably intelligent, but I don't know about the discipline I'd need. I think that worries me most.

Clin.: What else worries you?

Pt.: What would happen to Bob and me, I mean, when would I see him? I don't know, maybe never . . .

I have used a rather lengthy example because I want to emphasize the usefulness of sensitively utilized fact-oriented questions. In this excerpt, their gentle structuring, while clearly providing answers to diagnostic questions concerning anxiety disorders, may have also helped to convey a variety of important metacommunications to the patient, such as the following:

1. This interviewer is obviously interested in finding out exactly what symptoms and experiences I have been feeling.
2. This interviewer must have worked with similar problems before because the questions asked hit upon a lot of the feelings I have had.
3. This interviewer seems to be thorough and is actively exploring many different issues.

In short, all of these metacommunications serve to increase the patient's confidence in the clinician's expertise and ultimately in the clinician's potential to provide help. Good friends can provide sensitive listening, but only good clinicians can provide both sensitive listening and knowledgeable questioning.

It is also informative to see the frequent peppering of this fact-oriented dialogue with unstructured questions and basic empathic comments. In fact, it looks as if the interviewer was about to leave structured questioning in order to pursue a region of open-ended inquiries into psychodynamic issues. Once again the art lies in a flexible attitude, a suiting of the most effective form of questioning to the task at hand.

It is interesting to note that an interviewer who gets stuck on the idea of open-ended questioning throughout the entire initial interview potentially robs himself or herself of the chance to be perceived not only as a good listener but also as a skilled caregiver. In addition, it goes without saying that the clinician limited to an open-ended approach may also come away with an inadequate database for triage purposes. The use of fact-oriented questions in the previous example has provided a sound exploration of the symptoms of a generalized anxiety disorder and a panic disorder by DSM-IV criteria. The treatment may vary for these two disorders, especially if the questioning around panic episodes had uncovered entities such as agoraphobia or a simple phobia, in which case specific treatment modalities are available.

In a last note concerning clinician expertise, we can see the complementary functions of all the factors discussed so far under the rubric of engagement. Indeed, the ability to blend effectively with a patient is mirrored by the clinician's ability to blend a variety of techniques, such as: (1) the skilled use of empathic statements; (2) the creation of a safe environment; (3) the ability to convey genuineness through spontaneity, responsiveness, and consistency; and (4) the conveyance of a reassuring knowledge base. These four attributes lay the groundwork for quickly establishing an effective therapeutic alliance.

At this point we have completed our exploration of the engagement process, the first goal in our map of the interview. The reader will recall that the next way station concerns the process of effective data gathering.

Subtleties of Collecting a Database

In many respects the major goal of the initial interview remains the elicitation of information. At first glance, this process sounds simple enough, perhaps too simple. Earlier we had likened the initial interview to a person exploring an old Victorian room with only a candle in hand, the limited light source representing an exterior hindrance to the endeavor at hand. However, a weak light source does not represent the only barrier to a familiarization with the antique furniture scattered about, because the method of exploration can provide internal barriers to the effectiveness of gathering an accurate picture of the room. For instance, one explorer may walk about with his hands held only at shoulder level, hence missing all the curios lying upon a well-varnished table. A second explorer may underuse her sense of hearing, thus ignoring the presence of a clock tucked away in a quiet niche beside Sarah Bernhardt's portrait. A third explorer may be afraid of dark corners, thus never spotting the elaborately carved chess set hidden away in the shadows. Thus, it is not only a matter of gathering data, it is also a question of realizing that one alters the database by the very act of gathering the data. For these reasons it is beneficial to explore the issues of validity and reliability, because both of these factors can be altered by the idiosyncratic traits of each clinician's style.

VALIDITY

Statisticians discuss a variety of forms of validity, including content validity, empirical validity, and construct validity. To discuss all three of these concepts remains beyond the scope of our study, however. Instead, we will look at an admittedly simplified concept of validity, which nevertheless sheds considerable light on its clinical application. In a clinical sense, validity can be formulated as a question, "Are we actually eliciting the information we are trying to elicit?" From a slightly different perspective, the issue of validity can be conceptualized as the question, "Is the database accurate?"

Clearly, because of psychological defenses, predispositions for deceit, fading memories, and actual cognitive deficits (as seen in dementia), patients may not provide accurate histories. For instance, a patient suffering from schizophrenia, who wants to return to work quickly, may not readily tell the interviewer about the persistence of auditory hallucinations. On the other hand, a different patient, not suffering from schizophrenia but actively seeking disability, may tell the clinician about a plethora of tormenting yet nonexistent voices.

Along these lines, it is important for the interviewer to be alert for signs that the patient harbors a hidden agenda, such as needing a mental health professional to appear in court or to provide addictive drugs. For instance, in an emergency room setting, it is not uncommon for people with imminent court appearances to seem unusually interested in hospital admission, because hospitalization may represent a clever and logical excuse for missing the court date. In such cases, the tip-off is often the spontaneous request for admission from a patient who is typically noncompliant and indeed antagonistic towards health care. This example stands as one of many instances in which the patient may be actively distorting information.

However, it is frequently not the patient's resistances or deceits that alter validity. It may be the clinician who stands in the way of accurate information.

To focus on this issue, we will look at a validity technique known as "the behavioral incident," which was developed by Pascal and Jenkins and presented in an imminently useful fashion by Pascal in his book *The Practical Art of Diagnostic Interviewing*.[19] The basic concept can be delineated as follows.

When a clinician is particularly concerned about gaining accurate information, it is often best to ask the patient to describe specific historical details as opposed to asking the patient his or her opinions about these details. Once a patient is asked to make an opinion, the validity of the data becomes more suspect, because the clinician does not know how accurate the patient's perceptions may be.

All kinds of resistances may predispose a patient to distort information. For instance, if the clinician wants to determine whether a patient dates frequently, a patient may respond to a question such as "Do you date fairly regularly?" with a simple "yes," because the patient may be embarrassed to relate a sparse dating pattern. To sidestep this problem, the clinician could specifically ask about the frequency of dates over the past several years and ultimately the past several months. If the clinician finds only several dates spanning 5 or 6 months, then the clinician will have discovered a lack of dating activity without necessarily embarrassing the patient. As Pascal states, in general it is best for clinicians to make their own judgment based on the details of the story itself, for it seems unwise to assume that patients can objectively describe matters that have strong subjective implications.

Pascal calls the discrete historical behaviors elicited "behavioral incidents." There are two styles of questioning for behavioral incidents. In the first style, the clinician simply asks for the client to "chronologically" unfold the story with questions such as, "What happened next?" or "What did he do then?" In the second style, the clinician asks for a specific and concrete bit of information such as "Did you load the gun?" or "What thoughts were going through your mind at that moment?" Pascal believes that interviewers frequently collect invalid data by not asking for such concrete information, an extremely useful principle worthy of clarification.

Let us assume that an interviewer is interested in accurately determining the amount of open affection shared between a woman and her husband. We will look at two hypothetical dialogues with the same woman but with different interviewers. In the first excerpt, the interviewer asks primarily for the patient's opinions, a process that yields invalid data. In the second excerpt, the sensitive search for behavioral incidents provides a different story.

Interview 1

Pt.: Basically I've been very busy, what with the kids and my mother getting sick.

Clin.: Do you feel happy with your husband's support?

Pt.: Yes . . . yes he's been fairly good about it all.

Clin.: Is he very affectionate?

Pt.: (pause) Uh huh, affectionate enough.

Clin.: Have there been any financial strains?

Pt.: No, not really. Although the past several months have been a little tight, what with decreased benefits and a new school year starting.

Interview 2

Pt.: Basically I've been very busy, what with the kids and my mother getting sick.

Clin.: What kinds of things does your husband do to support you?

Pt.: Well, he's been a little less demanding, he doesn't get upset if the dirty dishes stack up a little longer or a shirt is a little wrinkled.

Clin.: When he comes home from work, what is his typical routine?

Pt.: That's pretty simple. He'll walk in the door, I usually don't see him come in and he goes straight back to his room to change clothes.

Clin.: And then?

Pt.: Well, let's see, I usually knock on the door and let him know dinner will be ready.

Clin.: Do you go in and talk with him then?

Pt.: No, I go straight back. Oh I usually peek in and say hello, but I have to get back to the stove.

Clin.: During the course of the night, is he the type of man who likes to hug, or does he prefer to keep a little more to himself?

Pt.: Well, let me see, he really doesn't hug a lot. No I can't say he does.

Clin.:   Do you remember the last time he hugged you?

Pt.:   I honestly can't remember (patient's affect is becoming more sad).

Clin.:   You look a little sad. Has it been some time since the two of you felt close?

Pt.:   (patient looks at interviewer and pauses with a little sigh) I think the last time he hugged me was about 6 months ago near Christmas. I remember because I was so pleased by it. It's rare for him to touch me like that any more. (pause) It didn't used to be this way . . . (breaks into tears).

Clearly, the second interviewer seems to have uncovered a different and more valid story than the first one. Through the gentle use of behavioral incidents, the second clinician has gathered evidence that problems exist in the marriage, a situation the first interviewer missed.

The apparent loss of validity caused by the first interviewer's reliance on patient opinion, as opposed to behavioral incidents, can be seen in many areas, ranging from simple questions such as "Do you have problems falling asleep?" to more critical questions such as "Do you ever want to kill yourself?" Consequently, the usefulness of listening for behavioral incidents when seeking valid data speaks for itself. There remain a few points worth mentioning, however. First, this form of questioning can be time consuming, and in initial triage interviews the clinician will probably utilize it judiciously in areas in which the clinician deems validity to be of particular importance. Second, the idea of a behavioral incident does not mean that patient opinions are not to be sought. Quite to the contrary, the patient's perspective often yields revealing insights into various dynamic issues. The point is not that one should avoid patient opinions, but rather that one should not rely solely on them. In short, different styles of questioning tend to yield differing degrees of validity.

Over the years, in addition to the "behavioral incident," a variety of powerful validity enhancing techniques, such as shame attenuation, gentle assumption, and denial of the specific have been developed. Because these validity techniques are of such immense importance to uncovering personality dysfunction, they are described in Chapter 7. The interested reader can turn to page 392 for a preview of both these techniques and their strategic use.

RELIABILITY

With the advent of the concept of reliability, a new factor awaits the self-attentive interviewer. In a statistical sense, reliability can be defined as follows:

Reliability is an indication of the extent to which a measure contains variable errors; that is, *errors* that differed from individual to individual using any one measuring instrument and that varied from time to time for a given individual measured twice by the same instrument. For example, if one measures the length of a given object in two points of time with the same instrument—say, a ruler—and gets slightly different results, the instrument contains variable errors.[20]

One can translate the above concept into practical interviewing terms by remembering that our own interviewing style functions as our measuring instrument. The question then becomes: Does our way of asking questions change from one individual to another and, if so, do we bias patients towards certain answers?

This issue of interviewer reliability can be framed within two problem areas, although many other areas also exist: (1) The interviewer changes his or her style of asking a question and is not aware of the impact of this change, and (2) the interviewer has good reliability but unfortunately reliably evokes invalid information. We will briefly examine each of these potential pitfalls.

Specific clinical settings predispose to the problem of inadvertently changing styles. This issue appears to frequently shadow the presence of countertransference or emotional strains in the clinician. For example, if an interviewer feels pushed for time or begins to dislike an interviewee, subtle changes in interviewing style frequently emerge. For instance, the interviewer may cut off the patient's responses or actually cast a disarming scowl. In other cases in which a clinician may have gently requested a pleasant patient to explain a vague response further, the same clinician might ask for no further clarification from a sarcastic patient, resulting in a shortened interview.

In any case, such changes in style can significantly decrease the reliability of the interviewing instrument, with subsequent deficits in the validity of the data. All clinicians will experience such negative emotions. There is nothing innately wrong with these feelings as long as their potential impact is considered. Indeed, at times an awareness of such emotions may provide us with clues to the inner workings of both the clinician and the patient.

The second area of concern focuses on the knotty issue that I shall loosely label as being "reliably invalid." In brief, one wonders whether interviewers can develop habits that consistently increase the risk of obtaining invalid data. Actually we have already seen an example of this process, because an interviewer who never uses behavioral incidents is probably reliably invalid. Furthermore, as normal humans, most of us have developed other rather clever ways of not hearing what we do not want to hear. Such ingenious devices may get us through some touch-and-go dinners with in-laws, but if unchecked, these habits may cause problems during a clinical interview. In a more precise fashion, I am describing processes such as cajoling desirable answers from patients through choices of words and tone of voice.

Interviewers may not want to hear positive responses to questions concerning sensitive topics such as suicidal ideation, homicidal ideation, child abuse, or even the emergence of certain target symptoms such as depression. The hesitancy to uncover positive replies to such questions probably results from the fact that such responses may demand increased time from the clinician or legal action or even generate fear or a sense of failure in the clinician. Consequently, clinicians may unconsciously develop methods of decreasing the risk of a positive reply by beginning their questions with a negative (e.g., not), as follows:

a. You don't really feel more depressed, do you?
b. You're not feeling any chest pain today, are you?
c. You're not having thoughts of hurting yourself, are you?
d. (Said to your mother or father-in-law) You're not really thinking of spending the whole week here, are you?

An unusually sophisticated clinician will reinforce the negative bias by adding a subtle shake of the head from side to side. In essence, this negative approach to asking for a yes or no answer strongly biases the patient to say no. The reason for this negative bias most likely relates to the fact that the patient feels a need to please the clinician with a negative response. This biasing remains one of the most common errors I see during supervision. It represents a particular nemesis when employed around issues of high sensitivity such as sexuality or lethality, areas in which patients are hesitant to share positive answers to begin with, and answers which clinicians are occasionally afraid to hear.

Another reliably invalid type of questioning consists of habitually asking multiple questions disguised as a single query, so-called "cannon questions" because they are rapidly "fired off," as demonstrated below:

> **Pt.:** I just don't feel the same, there's no question about that. Even my weekends seem bland.
>
> **Clin.:** When did you begin to feel depressed, to feel hopeless like life was not worth living?
>
> **Pt.:** Probably back around May. Everything seemed to be collapsing back then, near our anniversary.

In this excerpt the clinician has unwittingly set up a confusing situation. He or she does not know if the patient's depression *or* the patient's hopelessness began back in May. It is possible, even probable, that the patient's depression began much earlier than the deep sense of hopelessness. Only further questioning could clarify this issue that resulted from the cannon question. In addition, cannon questions are frequently employed during a review of physical systems, such as:

Clin.:   Are you having any problem with your eyes, ears, heart, or stomach?

Pt.:   No.

Clin.:   Have you noticed any coughing, constipation, diarrhea, headache, backache, or change in bowel habits?

Pt.:   No, I don't think so.

Although time constraints may necessitate such cannon questions, it remains important to realize that such questions may be confusing to patients. Only one of the words may stick out in their minds, and such confusion can cause considerable problems with validity.

For supervision purposes, errors in validity and reliability can be conveniently labeled as type A or type B errors. Type A errors consist of all errors associated with the verbal content of the clinician's speech, including omission of behavioral incidents, lack of persistent probing when a patient seems to falter, negative questions, and cannon questions. Type B errors relate to nonverbal biasing elements, such as the shaking of the head from side to side while asking a question and many others, which are discussed in Chapter 3.

Towards an Understanding of the Patient

As the clinician integrates the processes of engagement and data gathering, a curious phenomenon emerges. Gradually, the clinician begins to gain an understanding of the world through another person's eyes. This process does not happen suddenly or dramatically. Instead, like the imperceptible clearing of a mist, the clinician's conceptualization of the patient's perspective crystallizes. To return to our analogy of the Victorian room, the nooks and crannies of the environment gradually become more familiar. As interviewers we are no longer strangers. In the concluding section of this chapter, we will look at three areas that may enrich our ability to understand the patient, and perhaps ultimately our ability to offer compassion. These three areas are: (1) interpersonal dynamics, (2) parataxic distortion, and (3) phenomenological perspective.

INTERPERSONAL PERSPECTIVE

It seems naive to assume a simple causative agent for most examples of human anxiety. For instance, future research will probably unmask many physiologic as well as psychosocial precipitants to anxiety. In this section we focus on some of the interpersonal forces at work in the creation of anxiety as it unfolds in an initial interview. Much of the following discussion is borrowed directly from the work of John Whitehorn[21] and Harry Stack Sullivan,[11] both pivotal explorers of interpersonal psychology.

To begin our discussion, the following question is worth considering as the interview proceeds: "How does this patient feel that he or she is viewed by others?" In many instances, the answers to this question will provide clues to the patient's immediate presence in our office. Guilt, shame, inadequacy, and fear of failure—these concerns are the stuff of neurosis. Many of the paralyzing defenses developed by people are erected to deflect such painful feelings. Whitehorn cogently expressed this idea, "Even in deadly warfare one's greatest apprehension is not of death but of being maimed or of failing in one's duty, and that, in large part, because one dreads the reactions of other persons. This is not to downplay the fear of death but rather to emphasize the fear of life."[22]

In another sense, developmentally speaking, the child appears to incorporate its sense of self-worth through a synthesis of perceived parental and family attitudes towards it. Indeed, persons demonstrating poorly developed personality states, such as the borderline personality and the narcissistic personality, have frequently evolved from chaotic childhoods. These developmental issues highlight the importance of interpersonal issues in the birth and feeding of unpleasant affects such as anxiety and depression. An actress has told me, "I can play any role once I understand what the character feels guilty about."

With regard to the art of understanding in the initial interview, these concerns suggest the utility of a sensitive search for answers to the questions discussed earlier. In particular, certain questions concerning the adolescent years may help to open the interpersonal door a bit, such as:

a. What were some of your teachers like?
b. Tell me a little bit about the kids in your neighborhood where you grew up.
c. What was it like for you to walk home from school or go on the bus?
d. Which of your brothers or sisters are you most like?
e. Who do you think is the happiest in your family?
f. Who do you admire most in your family?
g. What do you think are some of your parents' concerns for you?
h. What was gym class like for you?
i. What was report card day like for you?

Most likely this list could be endless, but these questions represent samples of pathways into interpersonal affect related to past and perhaps current symptomatology. Of course, besides these reflections on the past, the interviewer will also pay heed to the patient's immediate concerns about spouse, family members, friends, bosses, and fellow employees.

Of even more immediate concern to the interviewer is the generalization of the patient's interpersonal fears to the interview itself. As mentioned earlier, the patient's self-system may be activated by the perceived threat of rejection or disapproval from the interviewer. Whitehorn once again crystallizes the idea, "The patient's attitudes are not likely to appear at first, in answer to prepared questions, but later, in reaction to what he feels is the interviewer's response to his statements."[22] In this regard the clinician may be aptly rewarded by reflecting upon the following two queries: (1) How is this particular patient trying to come across to me? and (2) Why does he or she feel a need to present himself or herself in this fashion?

Some patients may feel that either the clinician or their friends think that they must be weak or "nuts" to be "seeing a shrink." This anxiety can seriously hamper engagement and may be partially alleviated by allowing some ventilation later in the interview with questions such as, "What has it been like for you to come to see a mental health professional?" Such a question may provide reassuring feelings of interpersonal safety for the patient, because he or she realizes that the clinician is aware of the all too human anxieties associated with admitting a need for help.

Another possible method of gaining insight into interpersonal issues arises from asking patients to describe their attitudes toward others. As Whitehorn states, "A fruitful field of study lies in a consideration of his sentiments or prejudices, that is, his attitudes toward father, mother, siblings and other significant others, toward church and state, toward his home town and toward secret societies, antisemitism, Socialism, Fascism, and other 'isms.' In the discussion of such matters, the patient reveals more clearly than in response to direct questions the character of his ideals and the way in which he has come to dramatize his role in life."[22]

During an interview with an adolescent boy of about 14 years of age, the wisdom of this approach became apparent to me. The boy was suffering from a severe depression and seemed reluctant to talk about himself, but to my surprise he was not reluctant to talk about others. The request, "Tell me about some of the things you would change at school," led to a long and revealing discussion of complex social issues such as his school's policy towards racial integration and his own contempt for prejudice. Clearly this was not a boy interested only in the next football game or party. His detailed analysis suggested that he was a person preoccupied with powerful moral concerns, which, when on overtime, could transform into harsh superego admonishings. His world was tense and dotted with rights and wrongs, creating an intrapsychic field of land mines.

This boy's interview also raises another pertinent issue, "Can an interviewer probe too much or too quickly?" Generally speaking, when questioning is done sensitively, it infrequently goes too far. But the trick lies in being attuned to the degree of interpersonal guilt generated by the patient's responses. If the questions generate too much guilt, the initial interviewer may find that an impressively thorough database has been developed but that there is no patient present with whom to discuss this database at the second appointment.

To avoid this problem, the clinician watches vigilantly for signs of embarrassment or shame in the patient, perhaps indicated by an averted gaze or a hesitant first step into speech. This awareness is combined with a common sense attitude towards which subject areas typically produce anxiety. When present, these signs may suggest the presence of potentially disengaging guilt, at which point the clinician may opt to reduce the tension by gently asking questions such as, "What has it been like for you to share such complicated material today?"

Asked calmly and sincerely, such questions demonstrate Rogers' unconditional positive regard while allowing patients to ventilate fears of clinician rejection, discovering to their surprise that such rejection is not imminent. The clinician can further decrease tension by positively reinforcing the patient's courage for sharing delicate material with phrases such as, "You've done an excellent job of sharing difficult material. It's really helping me to understand what you've been experiencing."

A combination of these techniques was useful in allaying the intense interpersonal anxieties generated in a man about 30 years of age who had presented for an initial assessment. Ostensibly requesting self-assertiveness training, he eventually related a striking list of paraphilias, including voyeurism, exhibitionism, and frotteurism (rubbing one's genitals against people in crowded public places). As he spoke, eye contact vanished, while his hands picked at one another. Near the end of the session, the dialogue evolved roughly as follows:

Clin.: John, I've been wondering what it has been like for you to share this material? You look like you're feeling a little upset.

Pt.: It's been very unsettling. I have never shared this stuff with anybody, it's so weird, . . . uh . . . uh . . . I, I feel

ashamed every time I meet someone new, afraid of
. . . what they might think.

Clin.: What have you been afraid I might be thinking?

Pt.: Oh that I'm really sick or disgusting.

Clin.: Has there been anything I've done or said that has
conveyed that to you?

Pt.: (pause) No, no, I can't say there has been.

Clin.: Good, because I have a feeling there is only one
person in this room who feels you are sick or
disgusting, and that person isn't me.

Pt.: (patient nods head and smiles gently) That could be
(patient visibly relaxes).

Clin.: Why don't we try to find out more about why these
unwanted behaviors developed so that we can look at
potential ways of changing them. It's important we
can talk about them openly and you've done an
excellent job so far.

Pt.: Oh, that sounds real good to me.

Clin.: Tell me what you were feeling the last time you
exposed yourself.

Pt.: I had had a bad day, I was really angry at a sales
clerk . . .

John went on to be successfully treated using cognitive/behavioral
techniques. The above interaction had helped him to dismantle a
powerful projection, a projection that threatened to disrupt the therapy before it even began.

Thus as clinicians we need to consider carefully the impact of
our probings, recognizing that certain patients may not be ready to
discuss certain issues, whereas others might actually benefit from
our exploration. At these moments, during the initial assessment, we
must rely upon our ever-growing experience to guide us, keeping in
mind a most relevant statement made by a wizened monk in the
novel *The Name of the Rose* by Umberto Eco: "Because learning does
not consist only of knowing what we must or we can do, but also
of knowing what we could do and perhaps should not do."[23]

PARATAXIC DISTORTION

So far we have been examining the generation of interpersonal
perceptions primarily via conscious or preconscious processes. If it
could be so simple! Unfortunately, the patient's developing image

of the clinician and, for that matter, the clinician's developing image of the patient are influenced by unconscious processes. Unknown to the clinician, he or she may resemble a family member of the patient or an ex-spouse or fill a stereotype of a concrete prejudice. As Sullivan put it, "The *real* characteristics of the other fellow at that time may be of negligible importance to the interpersonal situation. This we call parataxic distortion."[24]

This distorting process can affect the patient or the clinician and sometimes both parties. In actuality, parataxic distortion may evolve from the early seeding of both transference and countertransference; as such, its formation and resolution may play a pivotal role in subsequent therapy. But, in the initial interview such undetected early distortions may beleaguer an already fragile alliance.

Fortunately, such intense parataxic distortion is atypical. But when it does occur, it generally displays itself either through unusually poor blending or by atypically high levels of anxiety in the patient, perhaps even frank antagonism. This weakening of the blending process represents one more area in which monitoring of the blending process can provide important clues to the engagement process. Once such weak blending is recognized, the clinician can begin repair work. The first step in the repair process consists of questioning whether one's own actions are somehow disengaging the patient. At times these self-defeating behaviors may be related to countertransference issues with the patient (parataxic distortion on the part of the clinician).

If free of such processes, the clinician can then legitimately wonder whether parataxic distortion is at work in the patient's mind. If such distortion is suggested, an open exploration may decrease the growing resistance. For instance, the clinician can ask, "I'm wondering what you're feeling as we are talking," or "I sense you are feeling a little displeased with the interview so far, and I'm wondering what's going on?"

This type of nondefensive statement may seem to defuse the situation, because it brings hostile feelings into the open where they can at least be approached. Moreover, the clinician should not be afraid to uncover specific feelings of ill will, such as, "I find you very controlling," because these feelings can be tapped for clues of dynamic significance with questions such as, "When are some times you've felt similar feelings in the past?" Once again the emphasis rests upon allowing the patient to openly express his or her view of the world, in this case, of the interview itself. This emphasis upon understanding the patient's view of the world provides the focus for our last topic in this chapter.

PHENOMENOLOGICAL INQUIRY

We now have a moment to re-examine the process of blending. At times, blending can be improved by utilizing a style of questioning that can lead directly to a clearer understanding of the patient. This style has its roots in the fields of existentialism and phenomenological psychology to which the book, *Existence*, by Rollo May,[25] remains an excellent introduction. While employing a more phenomenological style, the clinician attempts to see the world as the person experiences it, to literally see the world through the patient's eyes, to understand the phenomenon of being that person.

The emphasis rests upon what Medard Boss called "Daseinsanalysis," a German word translatable as "analysis of being-in-the-world."[26] In short, the clinician attempts to know what it *would* be like and what it *is* like to be the person sitting across from himself or herself. To this end, it is often useful to emphasize the world of the senses by asking specifically about what the patient is seeing, hearing, feeling, smelling, or tasting. From this sensate inquiry, doors may open into the patient's feelings, attitudes, and thoughts. To borrow a phrase from Aldous Huxley and William Blake, it is "through the doors of perception" that one may enter a patient's unique way of being, the patient's inner home. Indeed, this home may be turbulent, beautiful, or terrifying, but once experienced, the clinician's understanding cannot help but be clearer.

Moreover, such sensitive questioning can convey to the patient that the clinician remains interested in the patient as a person, not merely as a new case. In this regard, in the first interview the clinician may decide to include brief (sometimes not so brief) forays into the phenomenology of the patient. These dialogues may be similar to the following one involving an overweight woman, reflecting a string of suicidal gestures in her eyes:

> **Pt.:** I guess I was just sick of everything . . . everything . . . so I wanted to get away, to be by myself away from everybody who can hurt me. So I went into my room and shut off the light. I lit a few candles and I sat there.
>
> **Clin.:** What were you looking at as you sat there?
>
> **Pt.:** Nothing really . . . occasionally I watched the candle light flickering, it made the shadows of the vase dance around on the wall.
>
> **Clin.:** Do you remember anything else that caught your eye?
>
> **Pt.:** Uh huh, I remember looking at my high school prom picture.
>
> **Clin.:** And?
>
> **Pt.:** I thought how cruel it was the way relations have to break up. The person in that picture meant nothing to

me now, and I don't think I really meant anything to him ever (patient sighs).

Clin.: What else are you feeling in the room?

Pt.: Lonely and empty. I just wanted to crawl up into a tiny ball like a cocoon.

Clin.: What does the world feel like to you in your cocoon?

Pt.: It feels distant, dark, and numb. I feel, feel sort of blank, but I also am angry. I'm angry at my mother for never really caring, for putting me in the cocoon in the first place. I don't ever remember her hugging me (begins crying gently). I remember going away for the summer once to stay with my grandparents. And at the train station I felt very frightened and sad. I kept wondering what my mother would do when she said good bye—would she hug me or kiss me, and for how long? And you know what she did? She did nothing. She said good-bye.

Clin.: That must have hurt.

Pt.: It really did, it really hurt . . . (perks up) But that's the way it's always been.

Clin.: Do you expect people to hurt you?

Pt.: . . . Yes, yes I do, maybe I'm growing accustomed to it, maybe I even like it.

Clin.: Going back to that night in the room with the candle flickering, did you have any thoughts of wanting to hurt yourself?

Pt.: Yes, I did. As I sat there it all seemed sort of silly, so I began thinking about taking some pills. I'd stored up some Valium.

Clin.: What thoughts went through your mind?

From this dialogue the clinician can begin to feel the resounding hollowness of this patient's world, the intensity of her pain. One gains a sense of her neediness and her latent expectation of rejection, an expectation that may very well create the very bitterness that seeds actual antagonistic behavior from others put off by the patient's hostility. In any case the patient seems somehow more "real." Moreover, this phenomenological excursion has provided many hints for the clinician of potentially productive regions of future exploration, another example of intuition guiding further analysis. Indeed one wonders if this hollow world represents one petal in the abated flower we call a borderline personality.

This excerpt began with an active investigation of the room with the patient, moving into associations generated by this phenomenological exploration. Sometimes the patient will share associations experienced at the time being discussed, while at other times new associations stirred by recounting the experience may surface. In either case, rich material may become accessible to the clinician. Phenomenological inquiries are not necessarily based on questions dealing with the five senses. Frequently the patient's experience of the world is entered by questions exploring attitudes, opinions, recollections, and by an immediate sharing of feelings as they arise within the clinician-patient dyad.

Before leaving this excerpt a quick perusal reveals an interesting twist. The clinician has switched tenses from past tense to present tense with the phrase, "What else are you feeling in the room?" Such a switch sometimes facilitates a regression in the patient to a point at which images become more real and less memory-derived. This type of maneuver can unlock repressed memories and emotions, as witnessed here by the unexpected emergence of anger directed towards a parent figure perceived as cool and distant. Naturally, if one feels the patient cannot tolerate such a regression, as in an unstable patient or a psychotic patient, one would not utilize such a technique. In conclusion, phenomenological inquiry provides one more powerful method by which understanding may be increased.

CONCLUDING STATEMENTS

In this chapter we have attempted to develop a practical language through which we can study the interviewing process. We began with an operative definition and proceeded to study various aspects of that definition, including the engagement process, the ramifications of data collection such as validity and reliability, and, finally, the subtleties of understanding another person's pains.

It is hoped this new language offers us a chance to explore effectively our own styles of interviewing, while greatly increasing the opportunity to learn from observing others. This language of the interview has revealed the fact that interviewing is an art, and like the art historian mentioned in the introduction, one can discuss this craft precisely and concretely. Indeed the language we have uncovered, utilizing words such as engagement, blending, behavioral incidents, and parataxic distortion, provides us with the map of the interviewing process discussed earlier. The interior of our Victorian room now appears considerably less foreboding.

At this point, we have developed a language with which to begin our study of the interviewing process. But this language is incomplete, for an exploration of the interplay between clinician and patient represents a pressing matter not yet fully examined. It is this interaction that creates the structure of the interview. This structure provides the passageway to clinical effectiveness.

References

1. Rosenblum, R., and Janson, H. W.: *19th Century Art*. New York, Harry N. Abrams, 1984.
2. Ward, N. G., and Stein, G.: Reducing emotional distance: A new method to teaching interviewing skills. *Journal of Medical Education* 50:605–614, 1975.
3. Wiens, A. N.: The assessment interview. In *Clinical Methods in Psychology*, edited by Irving Weiner. New York, John Wiley, 1976.
4. Barrett-Lennard, G. T.: The empathy cycle: Refinement of a nuclear concept. *Journal of Counseling Psychology* 28:2, 91–100, 1981.
5. Barrett-Lennard, G. T., 1981, p. 94.
6. Margulies, A.: Toward empathy: The uses of wonder. *American Journal of Psychiatry* 141(9):1025–1033, 1984.
7. Margulies, A., and Havens, L.: The initial encounter: What to do first. *American Journal of Psychiatry* 138(4):421–428, 1981.
8. Margulies, A., 1984, p. 1031.
9. Havens, L.: Exploration in the uses of language in psychotherapy: Simple empathic statements. *Psychiatry* 41:430, 1978.
10. Havens, L., 1978, p. 338.
11. Sullivan, H. S.: *The Psychiatric Interview*. New York, W. W. Norton, 1970.
12. Egan, G.: *The Skilled Helper: A Model for Systematic Helping and Interpersonal Relating*. Monterey, Brooks/Cole Publishing Company, 1975, p. 97.
13. Nicholi, A. M., Jr.: The Therapist-Patient Relationship. In *The Harvard Guide to Modern Psychiatry*, edited by A. M. Nicholi, Jr. Cambridge, CA, Belknap Press of Harvard University Press, 1978.
14. Sullivan, H. S., 1970, p. 12.
15. Rogers, C. R., and Traux, C. B.: The therapeutic conditions antecedent to change: A theoretical view. In *The Therapeutic Relationship and Its Impact*, edited by Carl Rogers. Madison, University of Wisconsin Press, 1967, pp. 97–108.
16. Egan, G., 1975, p. 90.
17. Ryle, A.: *Psychotherapy: A Cognitive Integration of Theory and Practice*. New York, Grune & Stratton, 1982, p. 103.
18. Egan, G., 1975, p. 93.
19. Pascal, G. R.: *The Practical Art of Diagnostic Interviewing*. Homewood, IL, Dow Jones-Irwin, 1983.
20. Nachmias, D., and Nachmias, C.: *Research Methods in the Social Sciences*. New York, St. Martin's Press, 1976.
21. Whitehorn, J. C.: Guide to interviewing and clinical personality study. *Archives of Neurology and Psychiatry* 52:197–216, 1944.
22. Whitehorn, J. C., 1944, pp. 197–216.
23. Eco, U.: *The Name of the Rose*. San Diego, Harcourt Brace Jovanovich, 1983.
24. Sullivan, H. S., 1970, p. 25.
25. May, R. (ed.): *Existence*. New York, Simon & Schuster, 1958.
26. Hall, C. S., and Lindzey, G.: *Theories of Personality*, 3rd ed. New York, John Wiley, 1978, p. 320.

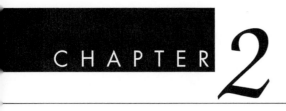

CHAPTER 2

Dynamic Structure of the Interview

*I*nsecurity and uncertainty are everywhere. If you don't let it become part of your flow, you will always be resisting and fighting . . . If the ground here suddenly shakes and trembles, can you give with it and still maintain your center? If you can become fluid and open even when you are standing still, then this fluidness and openness makes you able to respond to changes.[1]

Al Chung-liang Huang
Embrace Tiger, Return to Mountain

*T*he clinical interview manifests as a relationship. As with all relationships, it undergoes a continuous process of change, evolving like a delicate landscape by a Chinese artist or the movements of a T'ai Chi Master like Al Chung-liang Huang. It will change as the needs and the fears of the two participants evolve. This metamorphosis occurs whether either participant wants it to occur or not. The clinician must choose whether to move with these changes gracefully or to struggle against them.

In this chapter we will examine one method of conceptualizing the structure of the interview. This conceptualization focuses on the naturally occurring phases of the interview. By uncovering the structure of the interview, clinicians can develop methods of utilizing the natural flow of the interview to their benefit.

The five phases of the interview are as follows: (1) the introduction, (2) the opening, (3) the body, (4) the closing, and (5) the termination. Categorizing the stages of the interview in this fashion is somewhat artificial, but this separation temporarily provides an avenue for a more sophisticated study. In reality, like the movement of a Chinese martial arts practitioner, these stages merge with one another, a process at least partially determined by the pathways chosen by the clinician. Appreciating that the clinician has a choice creates both a more efficient interview and a more exciting one. The ability to consciously guide the interview is one of the differences between a good clinician and an outstanding one. It lies at the core of what has been called the art of interviewing.

INTRODUCTION: PHASE 1

The introduction begins when the clinician and the patient first see one another. It ends when the clinician feels comfortable enough to begin an inquiry into the reasons why the patient has sought help. When done well, it lasts a minute or two. When done poorly, it hardly occurs at all, or worse yet, the clinician regrets having been a part of it. The introduction represents one of the most important phases of the interview, because patients will frequently have formed their initial impression of the clinician by its end. This initial impression, whether justified or not, may help to determine the remaining course of the interview and perhaps even of therapy itself.

The goal of the interviewer during the introduction remains relatively simple: engage the patient by decreasing the patient's anxiety. Employing one of Sullivan's terms mentioned earlier, we can state the goal as follows: the clinician attempts to decrease the patient's need for an overactive self-system. In a similar vein, the goal of the patient is also relatively easy: "to find out what is going on here," because many patients are encountering a mental health professional for the first time.

The patient's need to understand the process tends to be rather intense, because it is rooted in some of the following basic fears:

1. Who is this clinician?
2. Is he or she competent?
3. Is this person understanding?
4. What does he or she already know about me?
5. Whose side is this clinician on?
6. How long will this assessment take?
7. Am I going to be hurt?
8. Do I have any control in this matter? (Am I going to be "mind-raped"? as one patient described her initial fear.)

Not all patients are dealing with all these fears, but most patients are probably coping with a good number of them either consciously or unconsciously. The goal of the clinician and the goal of the patient are really the same at this moment in the interview: in short, to help the patient to feel more at ease. To achieve this more comfortable state of affairs, the clinician may want to answer some of these questions either directly or indirectly. If done sensitively, the patient's initial anxiety should begin to decrease and the interview should begin to move.

There exists no correct method for handling these fears. Consequently, each clinician needs to determine a comfortable style of addressing these issues in his or her own fashion. I shall give two examples. The first example is the work of an inexperienced clinician. The second dialogue demonstrates one method that addresses the issues more smoothly.

[The clinician enters brusquely, shaking the patient's hand very firmly. The clinician does not smile.]

Clin.: Well John, my name is Dr. James, I'll be conducting the interview. I understand you have some problems. Tell me about them.

Pt.: Let me see, I'm not really sure where to begin.

Clin.: Why don't you start at the beginning. I understand you've been acting a little odd.

Pt.: Who told you that?

Clin.: Your wife, but that's neither here nor there, I need to know when it all began.

It is hard not to chuckle at this exchange, for the interviewer has successfully aroused almost all of the anxieties mentioned earlier. Even such word choices as "I'll be conducting the interview" suggest that the patient should expect no control here, although the clinician's overpowering handshake may have already served as a premonition of this fact.

The following dialogue represents a more satisfying solution to the demands of the situation.

[The patient knocks. The clinician says "Come in." The patient enters the room. The clinician smiles warmly and spontaneously. He walks over to the patient at a normal pace and shakes the patient's hand with a gentle firmness.]

Clin.: Hello, my name is Dr. James. I'm one of the senior psychiatrists at the clinic here. Why don't we sit over here. By the way, if you like, I can hang your coat up (gestures toward wall).

Pt.: Thank you (patient passes coat and sits down).

Clin.: Did you have any trouble finding a parking space?

Pt.: No, not really. It's not that bad at this time of the day.

Clin.: Good. Sometimes people have some problems with it . . . Why don't we begin by my giving you some idea of what to expect today.

Pt.: That sounds good to me.

Clin.: First of all, do you like to be called Mr. Fenner or William or Bill?

Pt.: I don't like the name William. "Bill" would be just fine.

Clin.: Good. Your wife had called earlier . . . were you aware she had called ahead?

Pt.: Well, sort of. She said she would, and I told her to go ahead. I didn't know if she had or not.

Clin.: Let me summarize my impression from her call. She certainly seems concerned and a little confused about what you've been thinking and feeling recently. She seems to feel that you may be somewhat depressed. What I'd like to do is begin by hearing from you and getting your perspectives on what, if anything, has been going on. Perhaps we could start with your telling me a little about how you see things at this point.

Pt.: It takes a second to get in gear here . . . well . . . let's see . . . In the first place, I must admit I've been feeling sort of down, not depressed mind you, but down.

Clin.: Uh-huh.

Pt.: Things have been going poorly at work. My boss left and he was replaced by a, let me just say, someone more difficult to get along with. The end result has been that I'm not enjoying my work like I used to.

Clin.: And where is it you work?

Pt.:   Down at the lumber company.

Clin.:   Go on (said gently).

Pt.:   Well, about 3 weeks ago I did something I've never done in all my 20 years of work (pause) (clinician waits)—I called in sick without actually being sick.

Clin.:   Uh-huh.

Pt.:   It's really unusual for me to do that.

Clin.:   O.K.

In this introduction, which has imperceptibly moved into the opening phase, the clinician has smoothly addressed many of the potential resistances mentioned earlier. In particular, a large element of respect has been conveyed to the patient by the simple gesture of offering to hang up the patient's coat and by asking the patient whether he had been aware of the call from his wife. The clinician also clearly appears to be on no one's side, emphasizing the desire to hear the patient's opinions and even stating that the issue of a problem with the patient has not been determined yet by the comment "and getting your perspectives on what, if anything, has been going on."

Anthony Storr points out that the situation may be slightly different if the patient has been referred by a fellow professional. In these cases, Storr adds a nice touch, as follows:

Clin.:   I've read your notes and I have some idea of your background and your present trouble, but I would be grateful if you would go over some of it again. I know that you have told it all before to various people and that it must be very tedious for you to repeat it, but I find it difficult to remember details from notes made by other people. I understand that your present trouble is depression. . . . Could we start there? What is your kind of depression really like?[1]

In this example Storr conveys respect and concern, essentially acknowledging that he, too, might find repeating the story again somewhat difficult. The last statement also indicates the clinician's desire to understand the patient as a unique individual, not just a case. Some clinicians also prefer to end the introduction by asking, "Before we go on, do you have any questions?" Such a question once again conveys a sense of respect, while checking for possible resistances.

Going back to our own example of an effective introduction, we find that the clinician has also managed to give a sense of control to the patient with phrases such as, "Perhaps we could start with your telling me a little about how you see things at this point."

The clinician also asked the patient how he would like to be addressed. One can find many vehemently written pages both for and against using a patient's first name. I shall not add many pages to this debate, because I think the intensity of the debate has led to overstated arguments on both sides.

I, personally, feel that one should not assume a first name basis without asking first. Some patients may find a first name threatening or a "put down," especially if the patient is a young adult or much older than the clinician. Consequently, when first greeting a patient I always use his or her last name.

On the other hand, the ability to use the patient's first name can be a powerful asset in engagement. When used sparingly and with good timing, it can effectively help patients to share difficult material. In a cultural sense, first names are generally used by people who care about us and are privy to our private thoughts.

Consequently, I have found it both satisfying and rewarding to simply ask the patient how he or she would like to be addressed. This question accomplishes several tasks:

1. It conveys respect.
2. It gives the patient direct control over an important ego issue. (Some patients do not like to be called by last names and others do not like to be called by first names.)
3. One may learn a significant amount concerning the dynamics of the patient as revealed by the patient's preference.

For instance, very strong opinions voiced by the patient may represent the presence of character pathology or defensive posturing, thus offering the clinician immediate grist for the mill. A patient developing grandiose thinking as part of a manic episode may adamantly insist on being called "Dr. Jones." At the other extreme, patients with regressive tendencies may sheepishly smile while stating, "Please just call me Jim." With experience one can begin to discern the sense of self-identity implied by the patient's response to this simple question. Indeed, one wonders what dynamic issues may lie beneath ambivalent responses such as, "It doesn't really matter, you can call me Jim, Jack, or Jimmy."

There are some exceptions to the above guidelines. If the clinician knows beforehand that the patient has a history of paranoia, it may be advisable to use the last name throughout the interview, because such "distance" may be more comfortable for the paranoid patient. Patients who are much older than the clinician may prefer to be addressed by the last name. In the opposite direction, children and early adolescents generally should be addressed on a first name basis from the start. In these cases, though, it is often useful to ask the child which first name to use. For instance, the family may call the child "Johnny," yet the child would prefer being called "John." Such a simple show of respect can go a long way towards ensuring a powerful engagement.

I should add that with regard to addressing the patient, I have yet to find any problem arising in either the initial interview or subsequent psychotherapy using the above approach. In the end, the reader must decide, from his or her own experience, what feels most comfortable.

In familiarizing the patient with the ensuing interview process, some clinicians go one step further than illustrated above. They specifically describe for the patient what to expect, depending on the goals of the interview. After the clinician and patient have introduced themselves, the dialogue may proceed as follows:

Clin.: Perhaps it would be of value to describe what we'll be doing today.

Pt.: I would really appreciate that.

Clin.: Of course, first, I'd like to get an idea of what some of your concerns are and what types of stresses you're coping with. I'll try to get a clear idea of your symptoms with an idea of seeing how we may be able to help you. Later in the interview, I'll try to get a better idea of what has been happening by asking some background questions about your family, your health, your schooling, and any previous symptoms you've had. I find that getting an understanding of your background can really help me understand your current problem better. Do you have any questions?

Pt.: Not really, no . . . not really.

Clin.: Then let's begin by looking at what brought you here today.

Pt.: (sigh) I'll tell you, it's a long story.

Clin.: I have big ears (smiles).

Pt.: (chuckles) Well, it has to do with some problems with my wife and me. It began about 2 months after our first child, Jenny . . .

The purpose of a more extended description of the process is two-fold. First, it is hoped that the patient's fear of the unknown will be decreased. Second, the description of the process serves as an educational ploy, subtly alerting the patient to the fact that large amounts of data will be covered. This may allow the clinician to structure the ensuing interview more effectively and with less resistance. It also provides one method for smoothly switching gears later with transitions such as, "As I mentioned earlier, I'd like to learn a little more about your family. How many children do you have besides Jenny?" At the end of this interaction, the clinician also demonstrated the use of well-timed humor to break the anxiety of the first meeting.

Before moving on, one final point may be of value. As with all the other aspects of interviewing we have discussed so far, the format of the introduction varies from one patient to another. In some instances in which the patient is extremely psychotic, the patient may quickly cut short the introduction. In such cases, it is wise to follow the patient's lead, because clearly such patients have a need to tell their story quickly. It would be inappropriate to adhere rigidly to the typical format of the introduction with such patients. The format is a guide, not a rule.

In any case, the previous statements serve as a foundation for an exploration of the introduction. When performed well, this phase can provide the beginnings of a powerful blending, because patients truly appreciate the sense of acceptance created by a sensitive clinician. In the next phase the patient does most of the talking while the clinician listens attentively.

OPENING: PHASE 2

With the clinician's first inquiry into the patient's immediate state of affairs, the opening phase begins. It ends when the clinician begins to focus his or her questions on specific topics deemed important by the clinician, after listening to the patient nondirectively. Whether a 30-minute emergency room interview or a 60-minute diagnostic assessment, the opening phase lasts about 5 to 7 minutes, because it is the cornerstone of engagement.

Combined with the introductory phase, the opening phase probably represents the most critical area for establishing rapport with the patient. If the end of the introduction marked the formation of the patient's initial impression of the clinician, the end of the opening phase represents the solidification or rejection of that impression. For the most part, patients have determined by the end of the opening whether they basically like or dislike the interviewer.

These patient opinions are not irrevocably etched in stone, but it would take a rather large chisel to change them. In many instances when patients abandon therapy after two or three sessions, their disapproval may have been planted in the opening 10 minutes of the first interview.

The patient has two primary goals during the opening phase: (1) to determine whether it is "okay" to share personal matters with this particular clinician, and (2) to determine which personal matters to share. A third major goal of the patient also surfaces, namely "to tell my story right, so that the clinician understands me." Despite a well-handled introduction, the patient's self-system will usually be activated during this phase, because it is here that self-exposure begins.

With these ideas in mind, one of the complementary goals of the interviewer becomes apparent: The engagement process begun in the introduction must be secured during the opening. The durability and elasticity of this engagement bonding, to a large degree, determine the depth of probing and the degree of structuring that the patient will tolerate in the subsequent phases of the interview. It is at this time that many of the engagement skills discussed in Chapter 1 meet their greatest challenge and yield their highest reward.

The approach to the opening phase generally proceeds along the following lines. Once the clinician has ended his or her introduction, an open-ended technique is used to turn the interview over to the patient on a verbal level. Frequently used openings include the following:

a. Tell me a little about what brought you here today.
b. Perhaps you can begin by letting me know what some of your concerns have been recently.
c. To start with, tell me a little about what has been happening in the past couple of weeks.
d. What are some of the stresses you have been coping with recently?

Such open-ended questions or statements provide the patient with a chance to begin talking at a comfortable point. Broadly speaking, the goals are to decrease the patient's anxiety while beginning to uncover the patient's viewpoint. Both of these goals are generally met by giving the patient plenty of room to wander during the opening phase.

During this facilitating opening phase, one hopes to begin to see outward signs of good blending, such as the patient's assumption of a more relaxed body posture and a reasonably long duration of utterance (DOU) by the patient following the clinician's questions.

This facilitation can be nurtured by the use of phrases such as "Go on," "And then what happened," and frequent short convey-ances of the clinician's interest such as "Uh-huh." Generally it ap-pears useful to employ at least one or two basic empathic statements during the opening phase, because such phrases frequently circum-vent the patient's fear of imminent rejection.

The opening phase bears a characteristic that distinguishes it from other phases of the interview. In sharp contrast to the introduc-tion, in the opening phase the clinician speaks very little. To the contrary, there exists a strong emphasis on open-ended questions or open-ended statements in an effort to get the patient talking. In an uncomplicated opening phase, approximately 30 to 90% of the clinician's questions or statements will be open-ended. During an assessment interview, the opening phase will probably represent the least verbally active phase for the clinician, because in the subse-quent body of the interview, clinicians tend to increase the frequency of their questions as they attempt to clarify diagnostic and triage questions.

With regard to this open-ended emphasis, two frequent prob-lems are encountered: (1) premature structuring of the interview before the patient has begun to relax, and (2) the too frequent use of closed-ended questions. Both of these tendencies remove control of the interview from the patient, a policy that serves only to heighten the patient's interpersonal anxiety. Perhaps equally im-portant, these activities represent an increased amount of clinician speech, and at this early stage of the interview a direct correlation can be drawn between clinician confusion and the amount of time that the clinician spends with his or her mouth open. In short, the opening phase is a time for reflection, not action, unless a specific resistance needs to be transformed.

Before proceeding, it is worth noting that some clinicians like to employ a bridge between the introduction and the opening. This bridge consists of a brief series of demographic questions that function to provide a cursory background while not intimidating the patient. The clinician may state, "As we get started I'd like to ask a few background questions that can help give me some perspec-tive. For instance, how old are you, Mr. Jones?" Further questions may concern the place of residence, occupation, or a description of the patient's family. Following these questions, the clinician may proceed with the opening as described above. Once again, the em-phasis is on effective and rapid engagement.

However, active engagement techniques are not the only activi-ties of the clinician during the opening phase. Much of the activity cannot be seen, because it is mental in nature. More specifically, the opening phase represents an intensely productive assessment period for the clinician. During these initial minutes, the clinician scours the interpersonal countryside in search of clues that may lead to the most effective engagement techniques for this particular patient. Simultaneously, the clinician determines the best manner in which to structure the body of the interview itself. In short, the clinician develops a tentative game plan, in the sense that a strategy for the interview will be developed, hand-tailored to the needs of the patient.

This early assessment process, which may be significantly revised as the interview proceeds, represents a mental "scouting period." This scouting period actually encompasses both the introduction phase, already discussed, and the opening phase. But since the main work of the scouting period occurs during the opening phase, it seems most appropriate to explore its intricacies at this time.

In the scouting period, usually encompassing the first 6 to 9 minutes of the interview, the clinician receives a rare opportunity to assess four vital areas: (1) the patient's conscious view of his or her problems, as well as the patient's conscious agenda for the interview itself (e.g., What does the patient want from the interview?); (2) the patient's mental status, which can influence the type of interview the clinician feels would be most clinically effective for this particular patient; (3) the clinician's conceptualization of the patient's problems as well as the clinician's view of the patient's *unconscious* agenda for the interview (e.g., What, in reality, does this patient desire from this interview?); and (4) an evaluation of the interview process itself.

Through an understanding of these four variables, the clinician can begin the delicate matter of matching the patient's agenda with his or her own agenda. If these agenda cannot be resolved, the resultant interview may prove to be relatively unproductive. It is interesting to note, just as Lazare[2] states that outpatient psychotherapy has a contractual nature, that in a sense each interview shares this contractual element. The contract can be either implicit or explicit—but it always occurs. Indeed, interviews break down when the participants cannot agree to shared goals. Many of these communication breakdowns result when the clinician does not recognize the goals of the patient, or worse yet, knows the goals but does not acknowledge them.

The four analytic tasks of the scouting period are creatively coupled with the intuitive skills of the clinician. Armed with this interplay between analysis and intuition, the clinician quickly begins a "knowing" of the patient. In an attempt to sharpen the analytic skills of the scouting phase, the following acronym, PACE, is useful in reminding the clinician of the goals of this phase:

Patient's perspectives and conscious agenda
Assessment of the patient's mental status
Clinician's perspective of the patient's problems and the
    patient's unconscious agenda
Evaluation of the interview itself

An ability to make these assessments quickly and accurately often signifies the presence of a skilled clinician. To develop this ability, one must first understand its utility.

Patient's Perspective and Conscious Agenda

Each patient brings a unique set of perceptions and opinions to the initial interview. Two patient perspectives appear to be particularly crucial in determining whether contractual agreement will occur: (1) the patient's concept of what is wrong, and (2) the patient's expectations of the interview or the interviewer. Many resistances to the interview process arise when these parameters are not understood by the clinician. On the other hand, if the interviewer is aware of these concerns, some resistances may be diminished, worked through, or perhaps even nipped in the bud.

To illustrate this aspect of the scouting period it may be useful to look at a short piece of dialogue. We will picture a man in his mid-30s, who has scheduled an appointment at the strong urges of his wife. He nervously looks about the office, as if anticipating the appearance of a Grand Inquisitor. He has a small mustache and a nervous nose. Early in the scouting period the following interaction develops:

Clin.:   Tell me a little bit about some of the reasons you came here today.

Pt.:   It is very difficult to say. I don't know what Jane thinks is happening, but I'm not nuts. It's all got something to do with my chemistry, of that I'm sure. Somehow or other I'm a little speeded up.

Clin.:   In what sense do you feel you're speeded up?

Pt.:   I'm feeling excitable, ready to roll, very creative, but maybe a little too juiced up. That's why I think it's biologic, not mental. I've been doing some reading about physical fitness and its impact on emotions, and

I think I've got some understanding of what the hell is going on here.

The art inherent in the scouting period consists of listening not only to what the patient says but also to what the patient implies. A careful delineation of this patient's opening dialogue may yield some pertinent information.

His opening gambit, "It is very difficult to say," suggests a fear of being misunderstood by the interviewer. This phrase is followed by the statement, "I don't know what Jane thinks is happening, but I'm not nuts." Paradoxically, the patient relates that he does not know what his wife thinks yet he implies that she has labeled him as "nuts." The connection with his fear of being misunderstood seems clearer. More specifically, he may be worried that the clinician will immediately view him as irrational. He probably also fears that the clinician will not value his opinions. These opinions he openly shares with the phrase, "It's all got something to do with my chemistry, of that I'm sure."

With this last statement, he offers an explanation for his problem on one level but also provides two more important pieces of information: (1) At some plane of awareness, he recognizes a problem, and (2) he has a need not to view the problem as psychological. With the subsequent phrase, "Somehow or other, I'm a little speeded up," he further describes his perception of the problem. In the next question, the clinician demonstrates a desire to understand the patient's world by requesting a more phenomenological description of his stated symptom. The patient's reply once again confirms his immediate need to conceptualize the problem in physical terms, betraying his fear that the "clinician-inquisitor" will not share this perspective. Of course, the patient's insistence on a physical cause may represent an example of a person who "doth protest too much." Even the patient may subconsciously fear a psychological problem.

Although short in length, this excerpt provides a variety of pertinent clues for engagement. At one level, some unconscious agenda and needs have been delineated, but such unconscious needs will be discussed later. At this point, we are interested in the patient's conscious views of his problem. These can be summarized as follows:

1. The problem is physiologic, not psychological
2. A conscious desire to discuss his own view during the hour
3. A conscious desire to convince the clinician of his view

The next question arises: What can be done with this information? First, one can easily imagine what not to do, as would be exemplified by the clinician's proceeding with questions such as, "Perhaps you can start by telling me about some of your stresses with your son, since your wife seems to feel these stresses are at the root of your problem," or "Physiology may play a part here, but first let's look at the real problem." Such blundering inquiries must represent the clinician's hidden masochistic needs, because the clinician is adamantly refusing to explore the patient's world through the patient's eyes. A reciprocal desire by the patient not to accommodate the clinician's agenda should not be unexpected. In contrast, let us look at a possible line of questioning that attempts to move with these needs while ultimately joining both agenda:

> **Pt.:** I'm feeling excitable, ready to roll, very creative, but maybe a little too juiced up. That's why I think it's biologic, not mental. I've been doing some reading about physical fitness and its impact on emotions, and I think I've got some understanding of what is going on here.
>
> **Clin.:** Oh, what kinds of things have you come up with?
>
> **Pt.:** Well, some people have found that running and jogging can release substances in the brain called endorphins that help people feel good. I'm thinking that maybe that is why I'm speeded up.
>
> **Clin.:** Hmm, that's interesting. How frequently do you run?
>
> **Pt.:** About 3 miles every day, sometimes up to 5 miles.
>
> **Clin.:** It sounds like you must be in pretty good shape. How did you get interested in physical fitness to begin with?
>
> **Pt.:** I guess you could say it runs in the family, no pun intended (patient and clinician smile). My father was a jock, and my two brothers both went to college on football scholarships.
>
> **Clin.:** Tell me a little bit about them.
>
> **Pt.:** Oh, they are both high-powered people, both very successful, (pause) more successful than me, but I do okay. John is a corporate lawyer in Dallas, and Jack is a physician.

As opposed to a denial of the patient's overt needs, this interviewer has implicitly acknowledged them. For example, the clinician picks up on the patient's hint, ". . . and I think I've got some understanding of what is going on here," by asking what the patient has discovered, thus allowing the patient to discuss his view openly. One of the most useful techniques with which to increase blending consists of asking patients for their opinions. Here is an example in which an opinion-oriented question, as opposed to a behavioral incident, is the technique of choice. This emphasizes the point that interview techniques are neither good nor bad. They are either "more useful" or "less useful" depending on the interview task at hand. In the scouting period, opinion-oriented questions frequently open up patients, because most people have a need to be heard.

This particular choice of topics by the interviewer has also reinforced the issue of physiology, which symbolizes an area in which this patient feels safe. By moving with this patient's needs, the conversation transforms itself gracefully into an exploration of family relations.

This example stands merely as an illustration. Patient needs and perspectives change with each individual. But certain conscious patient agenda items are fairly common, and the interviewer may want to listen attentively for their presence. The following list includes some of the more common needs:

1. Somebody to listen to their story (e.g., "I've got to get this off my chest.")
2. Somebody to give them medications
3. Somebody to "discover secrets" such as suicidal intent or a history of incest, which the patient has been afraid to share previously
4. Somebody to confirm that they are sane
5. Somebody to confirm that they are not sane
6. Somebody to "tell me what's happening to me"

Naturally, some of these agenda items may or may not be compatible with the goals of the clinician. In particular, problems arise when the patient's agenda may not originate from a sincere motivation for help, as with the following more manipulative needs:

1. A desire for addictive drugs
2. A desire to be hospitalized secondary to a need for shelter
3. A desire to have the clinician help him or her in a legal hassle by proving the patient is "seeing a therapist"
4. A desire to appear mentally ill for legal purposes
5. A desire to have the clinician confirm that the patient's regular therapist is "all wrong"
6. A desire simply to get a relative "off their back" by "seeing a specialist"

7. A desire for the clinician to tell relatives and friends that there is "nothing wrong"

All of these conscious agenda items can realistically lead to significant areas of resistance during the initial interview. Surprisingly, when one of these items is suspected by the interviewer, it may surface with the simple question, "At this point in our talk, it might help both of us to clarify what we want to accomplish today. I'm wondering what you were hoping might be done today." Some clinicians find this type of question to be routinely useful during the opening phase. In a literal sense, one can agree to a contract of shared goals for the first hour.

In any case, an attentive assessment of the patient's perspectives and conscious agenda provides valuable information during the scouting period. The usefulness of this information can be increased when it is added to a keen observation of the patient's behavior and appearance. A talented clinician develops the type of sensitivity to details that a good Agatha Christie detective like Miss Marple would admire. This quick-witted ability to observe leads to the second letter in the acronym PACE.

Assessment of the Patient's Mental Status

Much can be learned from a single glance if the glance has years of experience behind it. Although the formal mental status examination will generally occur in the body of the interview, during the scouting period a quick and informal assessment of mental status can provide invaluable information. (Note that a detailed discussion of the mental status and its written record is presented in Chapter 9, starting on page 521.) In the scouting period, the clinician searches for mental status clues that suggest a need for changing the strategy of the interview itself.

These clues are of three major types: (1) clues suggesting possible diagnoses and, hence, suggesting future areas for more extensive exploration; (2) clues suggesting significant resistances in the patient that need to be addressed; and (3) clues indicating that rather radical changes in the interview format may be needed. In a later chapter, we will look at the mental status in more detail, but for now we will briefly survey these three topics as they pertain to the scouting period.

With regard to diagnostic clues, one of the more interesting findings revolves about the issue of psychosis. If a patient presents with a smoldering psychotic process, it is not unusual for subtle signs to be present during the scouting period. Such subtle signs may include processes such as an infrequent loosening of associations, a slightly inappropriate affect, or an over-riding intensity to the patient's feelings and affects. The presence of such clues may suggest that questions dealing with psychosis may yield a rich harvest later in the interview.

Concerning the second area, evidence of resistance, the scouting period remains of vital importance. If strong resistance is present, it generally becomes necessary to work through this resistance, if possible, before proceeding into the main body of data gathering. Unresolved resistance may leave the clinician with an unresolved database, because invalid data often lie in its wake.

To this end, the clinician keeps a wary eye out for behavioral evidence suggesting unspoken resistance. As discussed earlier, interpersonal anxiety is to be expected, but unusually high anxiety states may indicate intense fears of rejection, embarrassment, or ridicule. If the clinician suspects the presence of these fears, the following, said gently, may bring the resistance to the surface, where it can be dealt with more effectively: "It's somewhat anxiety provoking to be interviewed. I'm wondering what types of things you may be concerned or worried about as we are talking here today."

James Morrison, in his informative book, *The First Interview: A Guide for Clinicians*, takes this one step further in a technique that he refers to as "naming emotions." If a patient appears to be stalled, secondary to resistance, Morrison suggests addressing this process by naming several emotions that could be behind the resistance. His gentle yet direct approach is as follows:

I can see that you are having a real problem with that question. Sometimes people have trouble with questions when they feel ashamed. Or sometimes it's anxiety or fear. Are you having any of those feelings now?[3]

This technique can open the gate to transform a potentially damaging communication impasse. It should also be kept in mind that resistance may be quite direct, as evidenced by purposefully vague answers, an irritated or hostile affect, or no answer at all.

With regard to the third area, the discovery of a need to significantly change the structure of the interview, the issue of disruptive psychopathology rears its head. The question becomes whether a given patient can tolerate a standard initial interview. This question, frequently relevant to the emergency room setting, focuses directly upon the patient's immediate impulse control. A good clinician becomes facile at recognizing the situation in which the best interview may be a short one.

For instance, the clinician may happen upon a patient whose thinking has become laced with delusional ideation. The patient may be furiously pacing about the waiting room, shaking a fist at voices heard only in the private world of a psychotic nightmare. When questioning begins, this type of patient may rapidly escalate towards violence.

As such a rapid escalation begins to unfold, the clinician may decide to alter the strategy of the interview drastically, including its length. This type of agitated behavior may also suggest the wisdom of interrupting the interview briefly in order to alert the charge nurse of the possibility of impending violence. In any case, during the scouting period, mental status observations provide valuable clues as to which directions to take in the interview. These mental status observations may also provide clues related to the third letter of the acronym PACE.

Clinician's Perspective of the Patient's Problems and the Patient's Unconscious Agenda

A significant chasm may separate the patient's perspective from the clinician's perspective. For example, a patient may feel that the central problem consists of a vicious harassment devised by the FBI. The clinician may view this patient's problem as the development of a paranoid delusion. In other instances, the clinician and the patient may share similar views concerning the nature of the problem but differ upon its etiology. Fortunately, at times, both the clinician and the patient may share similar conceptualizations.

The clinician needs to begin a clinical and diagnostic formulation early in the interview, because this tentative formulation may help determine the basic strategy of the interview itself. By way of illustration, the clinician may be interviewing an elderly man brought by his family because "he can't take care of himself any more." During the scouting period, the clinician may notice thought disorganization, thought blocking, and an apparent memory deficit. Normally, the cognitive mental status examination is brief and generally appears late in the body of the interview. But in this instance, the clinician may decide that a determination should be made of the severity of this patient's cognitive deficit early in the interviewing process. Moreover, with this type of patient the cognitive examination may be lengthened in an effort to explore the degree of cognitive deficit.

If severe memory deficits are recognized, then little can be gained by a lengthy and tiring inquiry with the patient about the course of his illness. Instead, this time may be more profitably spent with members of the patient's family, because they may provide a more reliable history. Once again, the clinician moves flexibly, adjusting to the needs of the clinical situation. However, such a creative change in strategy can follow only in the footsteps of a conscious awareness of the patient's condition by the clinician.

Of equal importance is the determination made by the clinician of the patient's unconscious agenda. It is worth emphasizing repeatedly that much of the art of interviewing consists not of analyzing what the patient said but of speculating on what was not said and why it was not said. In a similar vein, patients often "half mention" issues, and the clinician needs to uncover what has been left partially clad. In particular, the issue of unconscious agenda remains one of the major tasks of the scouting period.

The unconscious agenda includes those drives of which the patient may be partially or totally unaware. These needs, frequently arising from core psychological pains, may represent the most telling reasons why the patient has come for help or may also cause significant resistance to the task of the initial assessment. An example will help to clarify this concept.

In this illustration the patient is a young man about 30 years of age. His speech has a pressured quality, as if his words need to escape his mouth. He has been brought by his father, who threatened to commit him, after the patient squirted his father with tear gas during a family squabble.

Clin.: Tell me some more about what brought you here today.

Pt.: (Patient looks away disdainfully.) I'll tell you what brought me here today . . . No! Before I tell you that, let me reassure you that I'm not crazy! My father's crazy, yeah, crazy, a real nut. . . . I'm an important person with important business, I don't have time to waste and I don't belong here, my father belongs here, you should see him, let's wrap this thing up here quickly.

Clin.: Perhaps we could (patient interrupts).

Pt.: I need an ashtray, you got a light?

Clin.: Yes, I do (clinician offers matches and places an ashtray near the patient).

Pt.: Look, I need to be out of here by 4 o'clock . . . the bottom line, the goal line is that there is nothing wrong with me that a little peace and quiet won't help, too many people do all the talking and no one listens. I'm a man whose time is worth big bucks, here, look at this (patient shows clinician business card).

Clin.: Let me take a closer look at that (inspects card). I see you are a vice president, no wonder your time is valuable. Perhaps we should start to get to the point.

Pt.: No kidding, that's a good idea. I think you and I could work this thing out logically. We are both professionals, so professional to professional is the way to work this out. There is a big misunderstanding here. He's got it all wrong, I didn't want to squirt him in the face but he attacked me, he needed a lesson, a whopper, something to put him in his place, always talking, always telling me what to do. That's the way he's always been and I'm sick of it.

Clin.: Tell me more about the misunderstanding, the way you see it, and take as much time as you need.

Pt.: The way I see it, no one appreciates me. I just started a mail order business with my fiancée, she is wonderful, she understands. It's a dog eat dog world out there and the old man doesn't give a damn, he lives in the age of horse-hoofs, the Stone Age.

Clin.: What are some of the specific stresses you are handling right now?

Pt.: Financial strain, paying the rent, getting ready for the wedding, this, that, and the other.

Clin.: Sounds like a lot of bills to pay.

Pt.: You're darn right. The trouble is my landlord is a jerk. All he thinks about is money and payments. I've been a good tenant, and he has no right to throw me out.

Clin.: When is he threatening to throw you out?

Pt.: Two weeks from now, the man's got a lot of nerve. To think I used to say nice things about him.

Clin.: How have all these pressures affected your sleep?

Pt.: I don't need much sleep, I get along with very little sleep because I'm energized.

Clin.: What time do you go to sleep roughly?

Pt.: Well, that varies. Usually around 12 or 1 o'clock, but recently I've been staying up later to do my work.

Clin.: And what kinds of things do you do when you stay up?

In this vignette, one can see the subtle maneuverings of the opening phase. The art lies in the interviewer's ability to recognize the unstated needs of the patient, while subsequently attending to some of these same needs. The passage warrants a closer look.

On a conscious level, the patient's agenda includes items such as convincing the clinician that nothing is wrong, convincing the clinician that the patient's father is wrong, and making a quick exit subsequent to an equally quick interview. But it is the unconscious agenda that yields the most fertile engagement secrets.

Two of these unstated needs could be described as follows:

1. The need to appear important, possibly related to an underlying fear of inferiority
2. The need to be in control, perhaps generated by the impending threat of an involuntary commitment, which would represent a total loss of control

The first need, the need for praise, manifests itself early in the dialogue. For instance, the patient immediately raises himself by putting down his father, "the nut," and the interviewer with a disdainful look. These defiant steps, indicative of a frightened ego, are quickly followed by a blunt request for praise, "I'm an important person who has important business." Later we hear, "I'm a man whose time is worth big bucks," at which point he proceeds to display his business card.

It is at this point that the clinician plays a gentle gambit. Specifically, he goes out of his way to provide the much needed praise. The clinician does not merely glance at the offered business card, he calmly admires it. Indeed, it is this quiet admiration that represents the real and immediate business of this interview, for with its presence the engagement process can begin to unfold. This quiet praise is furthered by a simple but elegantly effective acknowledgment of the patient's importance, "I see you are a vice president, no wonder your time is valuable." At last, the patient's self-system receives a chance to relax. Someone has seen his worth. Defenses, such as pressured speech and accusation, may become less necessary.

Further acknowledgment of the patient's importance resides in the clinician's recognition of the patient's stated time needs, "Perhaps we should start to get to the point." With this apparently appeasing statement, the clinician, in reality, is beginning to structure the interview. In a relatively short time this patient will be providing diagnostic information related to mania instead of demanding a shorter interaction.

The second hidden need, the need for control, begins with a

subtle redirecting of the clinician's attention by the patient, ". . . my father belongs here, you should see him . . ." and ends with a not so subtle directive, ". . . let's wrap this thing up here quickly."

The patient continues to control the interview by interrupting the clinician's question by stating a demand, "I need an ashtray . . ." It is not so hard to imagine that someone close to involuntary commitment would feel threatened, because he is in reality threatened with an imprisonment of sorts. Fortunately, the interviewer recognizes this need and focuses attention on helping this patient regain some semblance of self-determination. This release of control in the service of gaining control is accomplished by the phrase, "Tell me more about the misunderstanding, the way you see it, and take as much time as you need." This conveyance of control is gently bolstered by suggesting that the patient has been appropriately managing at least some aspects of his life as implied by the wording, "What are some of the specific stresses you are handling right now?" How different this phrase must sound compared with a similar content message, "What problems are unsettling you right now?" a phrase that would have ignored the patient's need to feel confident.

This dialogue represents only one of numberless interactions. It is not the specific words that are important here. It is the underlying principle of listening for the hidden needs that warrants emphasis. It is this third assessment of the scouting period, the search for the pains that drive the patient, that opens the door to engagement. Understanding this aspect of the scouting period is akin to understanding resistance itself, but that topic awaits future discussion. Presently, the fourth assessment, the fourth letter in the acronym PACE, deserves attention.

Evaluation of the Interview Itself

Interviews, like the people creating them, tend to develop personalities of a sort. The personality of the interview appears to be determined by the quality and quantity of the communication evolving between the participants. Ideally, a clinician would like to become a co-participant in an interview characterized by a patient who produces relatively large amounts of pertinent and valid information, while easily focusing on issues raised by the clinician. This ideal patient would become increasingly at ease as the interview proceeded, becoming the proverbial open book. Within minutes, an adequate level of blending would be achieved, the patient and clinician working together towards unified goals. Someday, I would like to be a participant in such an interview.

In reality, ideal interviews are hard to find. Fortunately, good interviews are not. One of the keys to developing consistently productive interviews remains the ability to spot bad interviews before they become painful lessons in frustration. By consciously evaluating the interview process, the clinician opens the door to control and flexibility. Phrased more accurately, once the clinician has determined the personality of the interview, the clinician may gain control by adaptively altering technique. To this end, during the scouting period, the clinician needs to attempt a conscious assessment of the progress of the interview. If pleased with its nascent development, then the clinician may continue with similar strategies. If displeased, the clinician may consider new options.

The interviewer should be on the lookout for a variety of less productive patterns in communication, three of which are the shut-down interview, the wandering interview, and the rehearsed interview. All three of these interview types can lead to serious problems with engagement and data gathering. All three, once spotted, warrant a change in strategy (Table 1).

SHUT-DOWN INTERVIEW

In the shut-down interview, the patient displays a short duration of utterance, a long response time latency, and usually a variety of body language clues indicating that things are not going well. In particular, eye contact is often poor. I am reminded of a patient who I observed during supervision who sat morosely, her legs propped up on a stool, her own crossed arms representing the main objects of interest to her eyes. As if to place appropriate exclamation points in her nonverbal communication, she yawned with impeccable timing. She represented the ideal persona of a shut-down in communication.

However, shut-down interviews are not the creation of the patient alone. As emphasized earlier, all interviews represent interaction. In this respect, the action of the patient just described suggests the possibility that the interview will become a shut-down interview. But for this process to unfold fully, the interviewer must feed it.

This feeding occurs when the interviewer fosters the shut-down pattern by utilizing a low ratio of open-ended to closed-ended questions. These closed-ended questions tend to decrease patient spontaneity and, hence, hinder the blending process. This tendency becomes further entrenched when the interviewer uses a high proportion of focusing statements and other structuring techniques. It may be even further entrenched if the clinician tends to utilize facilitating maneuvers poorly, such as head nodding, empathic statements, and an encouraging tone of voice.

During shut-down interviews, it is not uncommon for clinicians to feel frustration, which often manifests itself in a sharpness to the

▤ TABLE 1 ❙ INTERVIEW TYPOLOGIES

Interview Type	Characteristics of Patient			Characteristics of Interviewer		
	Duration of Utterance (DOU)	Response Time Latency (RTL)	Natural Body Language such as Eye Contact	Ratio of Open-Ended Questions to Closed-Ended Questions	Focusing Statements	Facilitating Maneuvers, Empathic Statements
Shut-down interview	↓	↑	↓	↓	↑	↓
Wandering interview	↑	↓	↑	↑	↓	↑
Rehearsed interview	↑	↓	↕	↕	↓	↑

KEY: ↑ = increased; ↓ = decreased; ↕ = either increased or decreased.

tone of voice and a distinct lack of empathic communication. Ironically, such action merely fosters the further development of the shut-down process itself. Thus, the dyadic nature of the interview surfaces once again.

If the interviewer spots the characteristics in the patient that may lead to a shut-down in communications, certain steps may be taken to reverse the process. This issue of practical interview management brings us directly to the topic of open-ended questioning.

The concept of an open-ended question appears at first glance as so self-explanatory that it warrants little discussion. But one could not be more mistaken. In actual practice, the open-ended question is frequently not utilized effectively. Moreover, numerous references to the technique in both research literature and interviewing texts tend to disagree with each other about the definition of open-endedness and about which questions are open versus closed.[4-19] The following approach clarifies these discrepancies and provides a practical approach to the application of open-ended techniques in shut-down interviews.

Open-Ended Verbalizations. Both questions and statements can be classified as open-ended or closed. For example, the statement, "Tell me something about your old high-school girlfriend" is significantly more open-ended than the question, "Did you have a high-school girlfriend?" Any question or statement can be classified along the continuum of openness. Three variables seem to influence where a verbalization sits on this continuum: (1) the degree to which the verbalization tends to produce spontaneous and lengthy responses, (2) the degree to which the verbalization does not limit the patient's answer set, and (3) the degree to which the verbalization opens up a moderately shut-down interviewee.

At this juncture let us examine the continuum of openness more closely. In general, verbalizations can, by referring to the above variables, be classified into one of three broad categories: open-ended verbalizations, closed-ended verbalizations, and variable verbalizations, which lie somewhere between the two poles. In the following discussion these three categories will be defined and examples of each type given.

By definition, open-ended verbalizations are difficult to answer with one word or a short phrase even if the interviewee is moderately guarded or resistant. It is extremely difficult to respond to open-ended verbalizations with a simple "yes" or "no." Moreover, questions that provide or imply possible answers, or ask for specific items, places, dates, numbers, or names are closed-ended, for they limit the patient's freedom of choice. Broadly speaking, with patients in whom the blending is high, open-ended verbalizations tend to produce relatively large quantities of speech.

Open-ended verbalizations appear in one of two forms—open-ended questions or gentle commands. A classic example of an open-ended question would look as follows, "What would you do if your wife decided to leave you?" (See Table 2 for further examples.) This question does not guide the patient towards any specific answer nor can it easily be answered tersely. It invites the patient to share personal experience.

TABLE 2	DEGREE OF OPENNESS CONTINUUM
Verbalization	Example
Open-Ended	
1. Open-ended questions	1. What are your plans for the future?
	2. How will you approach your father?
	3. What are some of your thoughts about the marriage?
2. Gentle commands	1. Tell me something about your brother.
	2. Describe your initial reaction to me.
	3. Share with me some of your hopes about the marriage.
Variable	
1. Swing questions	1. Can you describe your feelings?
	2. Can you tell me a little about your boss?
	3. Can you say anything about the marriage?
2. Qualitative questions	1. How's your appetite?
	2. How's your job going?
	3. How's your mood been?
3. Statements of inquiry	1. You have never smoked marijuana?
	2. You say you were fifth in your class?
	3. So you left the marriage after 3 years?
4. Empathic statements	1. It sounds like a troubling time for you.
	2. It's difficult to end a marriage after 10 years.
	3. It looks like you're feeling very sad.
5. Facilitatory statements	1. Uh-huh.
	2. Go on.
	3. I see.
Closed-Ended	
1. Closed-ended questions	1. Do you think your son will pass?
	2. Are you feeling happy, sad, or angry?
	3. What medication is he taking?
2. Closed-ended statements	1. Please sit over there.
	2. I read the letter Dr. Smith wrote.
	3. Anxiety can be helped with behavioral therapies.

We have already seen one example of a gentle command. They consist of statements such as, "Tell me something about your old high-school girlfriend," which direct the patient to speak but do not limit the potential answer. Gentle commands begin with words such as "Tell me . . ." or "Describe for me . . . ." They are stated with a gentle tone of voice while expressing a genuine interest. A series of such gentle commands or a mixture of these statements with open-ended questions frequently increases the blending and spontaneity of even the most shut-down interaction. Generally speaking, gentle commands represent one of the most powerful tools available to the clinician for opening up resistant patients.

Closed-Ended Verbalizations. At the other end of the openness continuum one encounters closed-ended verbalizations. With closed-ended techniques it is extremely easy for a moderately shut-down patient to answer with one word, a short phrase, or a simple "yes" or "no." Even in instances in which the blending is high, these techniques may tend to decrease interviewee response length. Indeed, as we shall see shortly, closed-ended inquiries are frequently useful in focusing wandering patients.

Closed-ended verbalizations come in two types, closed-ended questions and closed-ended statements (see Table 2). Closed-ended questions frequently are of a yes/no format such as, "Did you seek therapy at the time of the accident?" or ask for specific details such as, "Which hospital were you at in 1982?" Although frequently hunting for facts, they may also seek out opinions and emotions as seen with, "Do you think your husband is hard working?"

Closed-ended statements do not suggest that any response is expected from the patient and frequently are of an explanatory or educational slant as with, "We will begin by looking at some of your symptoms."

Variable Verbalizations. Thus far we have examined both open and closed techniques, but what should we make of a question such as, "Can you tell me something about your first date?" This question seems to lie somewhere in between, for it is open-ended in the sense of suggesting no specific answer set but also appears closed-ended, for it can be easily brushed aside with a short phrase such as, "not much to say." This type of question, "the swing question" represents one of five variable verbalizations. Variable verbalizations represent a middle ground with regard to openness, because they tend to vary in the responses they create depending upon the degree of blending. When blending is high, these types of questions often result in the production of large amounts of spontaneous speech. But when blending is low and the patient is resistant, the very same questions can be easily answered tersely. And therein lies their danger for the clinician, for these questions are tickets towards monologue when used in a shut-down interview. Consequently, we will examine the five variable verbalizations: swing questions, qualitative questions, statements of inquiry, empathic statements, and facilitatory statements, more closely.

Swing questions are characterized by the quality of asking the patient whether he or she wants to answer. They often begin with phrases such as, "Would you tell me . . ." or "Can you describe . . ." (see Table 2). The impact of such questions literally swings from open to closed depending on the degree of blending present. When blending is high, a patient may merrily chatter away following such a question. But when a patient feels resistant, these questions can be curtly answered with statements such as, "not really," "don't feel like it," or simply "no." Consequently, as mentioned above, they generally should not be used in a shut-down interview.

A second type of variable verbalization is the qualitative question, with which the clinician inquires about the quality of the state of the patient, his symptoms, or his relations and activities. They frequently begin with the words, "How is your . . .?" Qualitative questions such as, "How's your relationship with your son?" have the potential to produce a significant elaboration if the blending is high. But, as was the case with swing questions, a resistant patient could easily answer tersely with a phrase such as, "Just fine." Operationally speaking, if a question begins with the word "how," has a form of the verb "to be" within it, and can be answered by the single word "fine," then it is by definition a qualitative question.

The third type of variable verbalization, the statement of inquiry, is represented by a complete sentence followed by a question mark. Unlike closed-ended statements, they are intended to stimulate a response from the patient as seen with, "You were working at the factory right after college?" or "You're viewed as the black sheep in the family?" The tone of voice of the clinician has a lot to do with the transformation of these statements into questions. The clinician's tone of voice can also move these statements from a gentle probing to a blunt confrontation. Statements of inquiry tend to perform one of several functions: clarification, summarization, confrontation, or interpretation by reflecting the patient's words back to him or her so that the patient can hear the implication of what was just said. As with the two previous variable verbalizations, statements of inquiry can be easily shut-down by resistant patients, whereas in situations of high blending these statements may function as springboards for further patient elaboration.

It should also be noted that leading questions frequently take the form of statements of inquiry. If a clinician uses statements of inquiry too frequently or at the wrong moment, then errors in validity may result. Statements of inquiry that are leading in nature often begin with the word "so," as seen with "So, you began drinking even in junior high?"

The final two types of variable verbalizations, empathic statements and facilitatory statements, can be usefully discussed together, because they generally tend to open patients up, although with guarded or hostile patients they may backfire, as discussed in Chapter 1. By definition, empathic statements are attempts to convey to clients that one is gaining an understanding of their feelings and perceptions of the world (see Table 2). Facilitatory statements include the wide range of single utterances or short phrases used to signal that the clinician is carefully listening such as, "Uh-huh" and, "Go on." Although these facilitatory phrases tend to urge the patient towards more speech, looked at on an individual basis they are not as powerfully open as a gentle command or an open-ended question. With hostile patients they may even backfire. I recall one instance in the emergency room, when an intoxicated alcoholic began angrily aping both my facilitatory statements and my head nodding, saying, "Yeah, you're a shrink all right, yeah, you're a shrink." Several minutes later he attacked a safety officer.

Unlocking Shut-Down Interviews. Now that we have surveyed the types of questions along the continuum of openness, it is valuable to look at a frequent problem encountered with shut-down patients. Specifically, variable verbalizations such as swing questions and statements of inquiry tend to become a habit. And as an interview becomes more shut-down, maladaptive habits have a tendency to return, just when they are least useful. As the patient grunts out short answers and begins to appear aggravated, the natural tendency is to ask questions even faster. These questions are frequently of a swing nature, asked almost apologetically. Closed-ended questions also seem to appear more frequently, probably because they are easier to formulate than open-ended questions. The unpleasant result may be as follows:

Clin.: How long were you in prison? (closed question)

Pt.: (looking somewhat disgusted) Two years.

Clin.: Was it a bad experience? (closed question)

pt.: What do you think? (said sarcastically)

Clin.: Were the guards tough? (closed question)

Pt.: Yeah.

Clin.: Did they get on your nerves? (closed question)

Pt.: Yeah.

Clin.: Did you get time for exercise? (closed question)

Pt.: Sometimes.

Clin.: Pretty bad food, I bet. (empathic statement)

Pt.: Yeah.

Clin.: Did you get very lonely there? (closed question)

Pt.: Yep.

Clin.: Could you tell me a little about what that felt like? (swing question)

Pt.: Not much to tell you.

Clin.: Well, I, uh, was it tough being away from your wife? (closed question)

Pt.: Sort of.

Clin.: Would you be able to tell me how she felt about it? (swing question)

Pt.: Don't really know.

Clin.: Can you tell me if she still loves you? (swing question)

Pt.: Don't really know that either.

Clin.: What do you think? (open-ended question)

Pt.: I think she might.

Clin.: How's the communication between you two? (qualitative question)

Pt.: Just dandy.

Clin.: How do you mean? (open-ended question)

Pt.: I mean she still writes and visits.

Clin.: Ah, how often does she visit? (closed question)

Pt.: About twice a year.

Clin.: When is that? (closed question)

Pt.: Take a guess . . . around Christmas and on my birthday.

The only person probably less comfortable than the patient is the clinician. Indeed, here is a classic shut-down interview moving into a spiral of silence. It illustrates several errors that are frequently made by clinicians. In the latter half, one sees the use of swing questions, under the mistaken thought that they are open-ended. The result proves otherwise. Then one sees the use of two true open-ended questions, "What do you think?" and "How do you mean?" But two open-ended questions are too few. For the open-ended effect to really take hold, the clinician generally needs to ask a series of open-ended questions or use a series of gentle commands, not just a couple. In fact, following the first couple of open-ended questions, the patient's responses will probably still be brief. But after five or six open-ended questions in a row, many patients will start to yield to the awkwardness of not responding appropriately. The above exchange also illustrates how easily other variable verbalizations, such as qualitative questions, can be shut down by resistant patients.

In the following example, we will see the course the previous dialogue might have taken if handled differently:

Clin.: How long were you in prison? (closed question)

Pt.: (looking somewhat disgusted) Two years.

Clin.: Huh . . . Most people hate being in prison but some find it less upsetting. What did you do to keep yourself busy? (open-ended question)

Pt.: Sports and cards, sports and cards, but it grows old real fast.

Clin.: I really don't know much about what a prison is like; tell me something about it (gentle command).

Pt.: Let me put it this way. You wouldn't last a day (patient smiles). Yeah, they'd get you fast.

Clin.: Tell me what it's really like in there (gentle command).

Pt.: Well, it's boring, day after day of the same shit. And time goes much slower. Everything, everything changes for you, man. Eating dinner is something to do, a movie is a scene, man. And you become a "con" man, not a jerk-off.

Clin.: How do you mean, a "con"? (open-ended question)

Pt.: A "con" is no one's fool. We don't come on to the guards or anyone. You can't survive unless you watch out for yourself.

This clinician is cleverly engaging the patient by utilizing open-ended questions and gentle commands. In particular, the clinician has avoided the pitfall of utilizing swing questions and other variable verbalizations, which could function in a closed role, as evidenced in the earlier example. This clinician also wisely went into an area in which the patient felt comfortable and, indeed, could "instruct" the clinician.

The following list reviews the techniques we have discussed for working through a shut-down interview and suggests as well a few more tips:

1. Employ large numbers of combinations of open-ended questions and gentle commands in a series. Too frequently interviewers ask one or two open-ended questions followed by a close-ended question or a variable verbalization, which can immediately defeat the gains made by the open-ended approach.
2. Follow up any topic that the patient gives the slightest hint that he or she wants to discuss (i.e., any topic on which the patient shows an increasing DOU, even for a brief period of time).
3. Avoid, in general, difficult or sensitive topics such as lethality, drugs and alcohol abuse, and sexual history.
4. Pick topics that gather general background information such as, "Tell me a little bit about the neighborhood you live in?" or "What are the people like where you work?" Or choose topics about which the patient has strong opinions as with, "What are some of the things your boss does that seem unfair?"
5. Avoid initiating questions with phrases such as, "Can you tell me . . ." or "Would you tell me. . . ." Such swing questions are easily answered with silence or frowns. Instead, it is frequently best to use gentle commands to instruct the patient to answer.
6. Increase attempts at eye contact, while increasing the reinforcement of verbal output with head nodding, empathic sounds, and phrases such as, "Go on," except with hostile patients, with whom a less frequent use of such techniques may be advisable.
7. Avoid long pauses before asking the next question. Long pauses are effective techniques for eliciting information from reasonably well-engaged patients who stop their flow because of their desire to avoid a topic. On the other hand, long pauses in shut-down patients frequently create further resistance and resentment. Effective use of long pauses depends on effective timing and good common sense.

It should also be kept in mind that the above techniques are generally applicable not only in shut-down interviews but also during the opening phase of any interview. In contrast, in interviews with good blending, patients may spontaneously talk about a variety of painful or sensitive areas fairly early. In even sharper contrast, the first principle outlined above is specific to shut-down interviews. In naturally evolving interviews, open-ended techniques are interwoven with statements of empathy and closed-ended questions, both of which serve to clarify issues and demonstrate the clinician's interest. Thus it is uncommon in interviews with good initial blending to employ overly long strings of open-ended techniques, remembering that about 30 to 90% of verbalizations in the opening phase are open.

This list offers some of the guiding principles with which to approach stalled interviews. Most important, a concentrated effort should be made to increase patient output before proceeding with information gathering. If these techniques do not work, then a more deep-rooted resistance may have formed. Approaches to resolving such deep-rooted resistances will be discussed in Chapter 10. Another method of approaching shut-down interviews is to address the underlying resistance almost immediately. This technique is also discussed in Chapter 10. The most telling point remains that the presence of a shut-down interview indicates a need for an active change in interviewing style. These changes frequently and rapidly result in a more fruitful dialogue.

As with any interview, one must work flexibly and creatively with the individual patient. In some instances of a shut-down interview, the above techniques may actually hinder progress. In particular, some patients, whose thinking is grossly disorganized, secondary to either psychotic process or interpersonal anxiety, may respond poorly to open-ended questions or gentle commands. These techniques force these patients to conceptualize at a level at which they may not be capable, further increasing anxiety.

In these instances, very structured and concrete questions may help the patient with organization. In this effort, the clinician may employ a higher number of closed-ended questions and statements of inquiry. With experience one quickly learns which technique works best with which type of patient.

In a similar vein, some adolescents and adults need to "warm up" with a higher ratio of closed-ended questions, because these tend to be less probing and can be more quickly answered. Two other types of questions merit attention. At first glance they seem like classic open-ended techniques and they are open-ended, but they tend to perplex patients and should be avoided in shut-down interviews.

The first problematic question begins with the word "why" such as, "Why did you stop going to your classes?" As Alfred Benjamin has cogently discussed, questions beginning with "why" frequently sound judgmental and break the feeling of unconditional positive regard, especially if the tone of voice is even mildly harsh.[20] They also seem to suggest that there exists one answer to the question, and it may be difficult for the patient to sort through all the confounding factors to produce the single right answer. Instead of beginning with "why" one can rephrase the question in one of several ways, such as, "What were some of the things going through your mind when you decided that it would be best to leave school?" or "What were the pros and cons of leaving school when you made your decision?"

The second troublesome question that tends to hinder dialogue in a shut-down interview may represent the all-time stereotypical "shrink question," and it reads something like this, "What are you feeling as we talk?" In actuality, it is both uncommon and difficult for most people to be aware of their inner feelings. Thus in shut-down interviews this type of question is particularly good at producing looks of consternation on patients' faces. Avoid it. It may be of use later in therapy or with patients with whom the blending is high, but not in shut-down interviews. By the way, children and adolescents, in particular, find this question puzzling.

FOCUSING THE WANDERING INTERVIEW

At this point we have spent a large amount of time discussing methods of working through a shut-down interview, because this type of interaction is both common and frustrating. At the other end of the continuum, one may be unfortunate enough to become a participant in a wandering interview, one of the most feared gremlins in a managed care setting or a busy clinic. We met this entity at the very beginning of the book. As we saw then, in the wandering interview, the patient displays a tendency toward mildly tangential and circumstantial thought, and his or her serpentine meanderings swallow the interviewer's train of questioning in a cloud of spicy irrelevancies. The patient's loquaciousness is often characterized by a mild pressure to speech, resulting in a long DOU, almost tempting the interviewer not to ask questions, because each question creates a new verbal leak. The response time latency (RTL) is short, and eye contact is often good.

A variant of the wandering interview, "the loquacious interview," occurs when the patient demonstrates pressured speech but does not stray off the topic. In fact, at times the patient becomes lost in a mass of related details. The characteristics described above represent the attributes of a patient that predispose the patient towards the development of a wandering interview. But once again, a true wandering interview remains the joint creation of both the patient and the clinician. Clinicians foster the wandering by asking open-ended questions and by not utilizing focusing statements. In short, as the patient extends his or her hand, the clinician accepts it. And the rambling walk begins.

Frequently clinicians unwittingly further their own demise by employing many facilitatory gestures and sounds, which only serve to reward the patient's abundant flow of speech. Note-taking can also serve to reward this process, functioning as a metacommunication such as "What you just said is important, keep going." Interviewers can learn to quiet all of these facilitatory activities in the service of closing off a runaway interview, if the clinician is aware of them in the first place.

The patient's contribution to the wandering interview has many etiologies. Such an interpersonal style may accompany histrionic personality structure or indicate the earliest stages of a mania; or this style may represent something much less serious, as seen with a patient who is simply anxious. In any case, several principles may be of value in transforming such an interview into a more productive exchange. While moving out of the scouting phase, begin to help the patient structure his or her answers as follows:

a. Gently increase the ratio of closed-ended questions to open-ended ones.
b. Avoid reinforcing the wandering pattern by excessive head nodding or paralanguage cues to "go on." This process was referred to earlier as "feeding the wanderer."
c. Begin with a gentle structuring by immediately returning to the topic of the question that led to the tangential thought.
d. If the wandering continues, become progressively more structured with statements such as, "For a moment, let's focus on what your mood was like back then."
e. With further wandering, one can further increase the focusing with statements such as, "This is such an important area I would like to focus on it alone for a few minutes."
f. If the above techniques fail, one can simply tell the patient what is needed: "We have a limited amount of time. Consequently, I'm going to focus on some of the very important areas you mentioned in an effort to understand more clearly. It's important for us to focus on one topic at a time."
g. Another approach consists of addressing the resistance itself, "I have noticed that when I ask questions we quickly seem to wander off the subject. What do you think may be going on"?
h. Finally, one can become very structured: "Because of time, we need to focus directly on the last 2 weeks of your mood. It will be important not to wander on to other topics because learning specifically about your mood is so important for our understanding. In fact, if we wander off, you'll notice that I'll bring us back

to the last 2 weeks. Is that all right with you? . . . Let's start with your sleep. Over the past 2 weeks how long has it been taking you to fall asleep?"

Generally speaking, unless the patient has some serious underlying psychopathology, such as a manic process, the first several techniques will decrease the wandering process.

At times it may also be necessary to literally cut a patient off in mid-sentence. This technique is fairly forceful and consequently should only be utilized after less aggressive focusing techniques have failed, although clinicians frequently don't use it enough. Frequently cut-offs are less disengaging if piggybacked onto empathic statements as shown below:

Clin.:   Exactly how depressed have you been feeling?

Pt.:   Well, let's see, in the past several months a lot has been happening to me, you know, what with the move and everything. I was very upset by my mother's nagging and the bills are really mounting, much as they did when I was living with Aunt Louise. Fortunately, I'm not quite as bad off as with Aunt Louise because . . .

Clin.:   (clinician cuts off patient) It really sounds like you've been through a lot. Have you been feeling depressed over the past 2 weeks?

Pt.:   Oh, I've been feeling very depressed.

Clin.:   Have you cried or felt like crying?

In this example the cut-off included an empathic statement, which provided a softening touch without decreasing the effectiveness of the cut-off. Another method of effectively using a cut-off is to include a comment acknowledging the importance of what the patient is saying such as, "So much of what you are saying is important that we need to focus a bit to ensure we get the most important points. Has your mood been depressed over the past 2 weeks?" Once again the patient was cut off in mid-stream, but the opening line acknowledges the importance of what the patient is saying while focusing the conversation.

I would like to emphasize that the recognition of a wandering interview occurs during the scouting period, but the attempt to transform this process actually occurs somewhere in the body of the interview. This point warrants emphasis because one of the major deterrents to focusing a patient effectively is the attempt to focus too early. Ironically, such premature focusing can leave the patient and the clinician in a duel for control. In such a duel, both partici-pants may go home wounded, because the patient responds by talking even more profusely. The main point remains: Facilitate first, structure second.

A second major factor in successfully focusing a patient lies in the effective use of paralanguage and body language during the structuring process. The art is not so much in the choice of words but in the method of presentation. For instance, if said with a concerned tone of voice, a phrase such as, "Let's look again at what your mood was like over the past 2 weeks," will seldom be inter-preted as a structuring ploy. On the other hand, the same phrase said harshly or in frustration may quickly disengage a timid patient.

At present, it may be valuable to examine an interviewer suc-cessfully working with a persistent wanderer. The interviewer recog-nized the wandering pattern during the scouting period and, conse-quently, began to structure as the scouting period ended and the body of the interview began.

> **Clin.:** Tell me what your sleep has been like (gentle command).
>
> **Pt.:** My sleep, now that's a good question. Nobody in my family has ever been a sound sleeper. I remember my father always talking about his restless nights. Same way with Uncle Harry, although, personally, I think Uncle Harry was a drunk. They say drunks, I shouldn't call him that (patient giggles), have really bad sleep.
>
> **Clin.:** How has your sleep been over the past 2 weeks? (qualitative question)
>
> **Pt.:** Pretty bad, more wound up, what with all the worries on my mind. I'm really upset about my decrease in pay. I don't think my boss should have cut my salary.
>
> **Clin.:** It sounds like you've had a lot of worries. How many hours do you think it takes you to fall asleep? (closed question)
>
> **Pt.:** Oh, maybe 2 or 3.
>
> **Clin.:** Once you're asleep, do you stay asleep the whole night or do you tend to wake up occasionally? (closed question)
>
> **Pt.:** No, no, once I'm out, I'm really out, just like the night after my chem final. I was so tired I literally slept like a log, but fortunately I was alert enough to pack up

> for home, although I don't know why I should want to go home, why . . .

Clin.: Before talking about home, let us get an even clearer picture of how your sleep has been affected. For instance, over the past 2 weeks have you been awakening earlier than usual for yourself? (closed question)

Pt.: No, I can't say that I have.

Clin.: Do you sleep at all during the day? (closed question)

Pt.: No, once I'm up, I'm really up.

Clin.: How has your energy been recently? (qualitative question)

Pt.: Up and down, mostly down. I guess I'm not as interested in things as I used to be.

Clin.: How do you mean? (open-ended question)

Pt.: Well, I used to be into jazz dance and ballet. On Wednesday nights I did aerobics. My sister, Jane, had gotten me into aerobics, she was always a super athlete.

Clin.: What about your own interest in things like dance now—has it increased or decreased? (closed question)

Pt.: Definitely decreased. I'm finding it harder and harder to enjoy all my hobbies. I'm even having a hard time reading . . .

In this illustration, the clinician has begun structuring this interview without disengaging the patient. This toning down of a wound-up wanderer was accomplished using a variety of techniques, including focusing statements, closed-ended questions, and even interrupting the patient with a cut-off statement at one point. Note that variable verbalizations, such as qualitative questions, though more effective than open-ended questions at focusing the patient, are not as effective as closed-ended questions in this regard. Consequently, when focusing, it is best to stick with closed-ended questions most of the time. The art lies in focusing while sensitively monitoring the blending.

Even when using a patient cut-off, the clinician maintained blending by conveying the importance of gaining a clear picture of exactly what the patient had been experiencing. Moreover, the clinician also emphasized the importance of what the patient was discussing by implying that the topic would be examined later in the interview. Both of these goals were accomplished with a single phrase, "Before talking about home, let us get a clearer picture of how your sleep has been affected." Even the use of the pronoun "us" helps to convey to the patient a shared goal and task.

Not surprisingly, working with a wandering patient is one of the most frequent problems for which clinicians request supervision, probably because we are often hesitant to structure, anticipating a rebuff from the patient. This hesitancy prevents us from learning how to structure effectively. In a sense, a wandering interview reminds one of an unchecked nuclear reaction; its ultimate result is a chaotic and sparse understanding of the patient. On the other hand, the ability to structure the flow of the interview offers the clinician a method of controlling the reaction, much as nuclear fission is controlled in a reactor.

Later, in the body of the interview, the clinician may find good reasons to unleash the reaction again while exploring the patient's dynamics or feelings. The important point remains that the clinician can modify the interview process in either direction, depending on what the goals of the interview are at the moment.

To end this discussion of the wandering interview, it is of value to list some of the most common errors that clinicians commit while handling a wandering patient:

1. Continuing to "feed the wanderer" instead of beginning to structure gently as one enters the main body of the interview
2. Being afraid to focus or interrupt the patient. When done effectively focusing statements are generally well tolerated by patients.
3. Structuring too early. During the scouting period one generally lets the patient go wherever the patient wants to go. The interview, at this stage, is highly unstructured. This facilitation period allows one to increase blending, while letting the clinician assess the various areas of PACE, as mentioned earlier.
4. Focusing too bluntly before trying more subtle approaches. It is best to begin with subtle focusing techniques, increasing the firmness as needed.

BREAKING THROUGH THE REHEARSED INTERVIEW

At this point, it seems pertinent to examine briefly another problematic style of interview, keeping in mind that many other styles exist and that many interviews represent mixtures of these three styles. This third type can be labeled as "the rehearsed interview." It commonly appears when working with a chronic mental health patient who "knows the system." In this process, the patient tells a story that may even bore the patient himself or herself, because it has been told so often. The history seems pat and simple, and therein lies the problem.

Both the patient and the clinician can be lulled into a joint acceptance of half truths. No person's life history or history of their present illness is simple. To get at the appropriate facts, both the patient and the clinician need motivation and involvement. Without these features, the validity and thoroughness of the database may be seriously jeopardized.

To do something about the rehearsed interview one must first recognize it. It frequently announces itself with early diagnostic statements by the patient and a quick and unsolicited review of the history of the present illness. Sometimes a patient will reel off a list of symptoms pertinent to the disorder with which the patient wants to present. These monologues frequently result in a long DOU and a short RTL. Eye contact varies depending on the situation. It is generally good, but if the patient is feeling guilt or covering something up, eye contact may be poor.

On the interpersonal level, the patient may be quick to tell his or her side, while dismantling opposing views before the clinician can even think of them. This last phenomenon also illustrates that the rehearsed interview does not always arise from indifference. Quite the opposite, rehearsed interviews may grow from the patient's need to control the interview. The clinician colludes with a rehearsed interview by focusing poorly or by providing an abundance of facilitation activities, as seen in the wandering interview. A rehearsed interview can be unfortunately fed by the use of open-ended, variable, or closed-ended verbalizations, for any question that tracks with the patient can reinforce the direction of the interview.

The following brief vignette conveys a feeling for such an interview:

Clin.: Tell me what brings you here today?

Pt.: Well, I got out of St. Joseph's hospital 2 months ago. After I got out, I moved to a new catchment area, so I need new doctors. I've been feeling a little edgy and need to be on lithium. You see I'm manic depressive.

Clin.: I see.

Pt.: Now, I'm not having racing thoughts or problems sleeping and my energy is just fine. You'll probably be hearing from my sister and don't listen to a word she says. She over-reacts and she doesn't understand this disease. Other than my ediginess everything is fine.

The problem here is the validity of these data. All angles are being covered so quickly that one can feel hedged in by the patient's story, almost as if one should not ask any more questions. To break this mechanical storytelling a variety of methods can be used.

One of the methods consists of disrupting the flow of patient opinion by asking for behavioral incidents, as discussed in Chapter 1. This type of behavioral questioning serves the dual purpose of forcing the patient to reflect, while also helping the clinician to gain a more effective database.

A second method consists of interrupting the twice-told tale by getting the patient to discuss areas that require new conceptualization or bringing the patient face to face with affectively charged topics.

For instance, later in the above interview, perhaps as the clinician was leaving the scouting phase, the patient could be led into more immediate material as follows:

Clin.: You mentioned your sister several times, tell me a little bit about her.

Pt.: She's sort of a jerk and I'll tell you one thing, I want her to keep her nose out of my affairs.

Clin.: What has she been doing recently that has been so upsetting?

Pt.: She's been mouthing off, getting me in trouble.

Clin.: What sort of ways?

Pt.: She got me into the hospital, when I didn't want to go. I didn't need to be in there, but she called the cops and the next thing I know, I'm committed. She claims I'm a danger to her children. I would say the greatest danger to her children is their mother.

In this instance, the patient has been led away from his rehearsed story, through the gate of affect. With this side trip, important information that may not have been intended for psychiatric ears has surfaced, namely that the patient was recently committed involuntarily. Perhaps things are not as cut and dried as the patient wanted the clinician to believe.

At this juncture, we have concluded our survey of the various assessments that occur during the scouting period as summarized by the acronym PACE. This rapid assessment occurs during the first two phases of the interview, the introduction and the opening.

It is hoped that the above information explains why a large amount of time has been devoted to the scouting period. Its importance would be hard to exaggerate, because in it the first hints of understanding are born in the clinician. The interviewer may have intuited some of the core pains and needs of the patient. Aware of these issues, the clinician is now prepared to enter the patient's world more fully. If the scouting period is done effectively, the clinician will generally be asked to enter the patient's world as an invited guest, and there will be no need for a "break in." The question now becomes an issue of finding the most effective method to gather the necessary clinical information efficiently while powerfully engaging the patient.

BODY OF THE INTERVIEW: PHASE 3

The chapter began with a quotation concerning the ability to move flexibly, as seen with a martial artist, and it can be as directly applied to the clinician's movements in the body of the interview. It seems only appropriate to look at another Eastern quotation, from Chang Chung-Yuan, which concerns the ability to make flexible transitions gracefully, because a sense of timing and naturalness represents the essence of our approach in the body of the interview:

> It was said that Wang Hsia's [a Chinese painter] brush sometimes waves and sometimes sweeps. The color of his ink is sometimes light and sometimes dark. Following the splotches of the ink he shapes them into mountains, rocks, clouds, and water. His action is so swift as if it were from Heaven. Spontaneously, his hand responds and his mind follows. All at once clouds and mists are completed; wind and rain are painted. Yet, when one looks carefully, one cannot find any marks of demarcation in the ink.[21]

Like those of the Chinese artist, the goals of the clinician vary during the body of the interview depending on the various clinical landscapes with which the clinician is presented.

If the interviewer intends to see the patient numerous times, then the data needed from the first interview may represent a relatively small body of knowledge, because several sessions are available before a treatment plan will be evolved. Consequently, the clinician's pace can be correspondingly leisurely, the emphasis being on a less structured approach that is similar in many respects to the processes seen during a dynamic-oriented psychotherapy.

On the other end of the continuum, the clinician may frequently face a true intake interview, in which both triage decisions and initial treatment plans are expected, at times demanded, by the end of 60 minutes. In this situation, perhaps the most demanding of all interviews, the database requirements are considerably more extensive and require a corresponding shift in the interviewer's style.

In this section, the focus will be on these full intake assessments. To begin the inquiry, we must first acknowledge that one of the major dilemmas confronting the intake clinician concerns the realization that large volumes of data often need to be gathered in short periods of time. Stated differently, good clinicians do not merely empathically listen, they actively explore. Patients do not necessarily know which information is relevant for their treatment planning. It is the clinician who must provide the gentle structuring and guidance that will establish a valid foundation for action.

The apparent "magic" with which a skilled interviewer accomplishes this task is not really magic. It is a skill. It is a skill based on the knowledge of which questions to ask and when to ask them during the body of the interview. This craft emerges directly from a study of the dynamic interactions creating the informational flow of the interview. These principles determine why one interviewer moves smoothly and efficiently, while another proceeds more awkwardly.

In Chapter 1 we discussed the observation that an interview in which the blending is high seems to take on some of the characteristics of a conversation. A natural flow emerges. The two participants appear to move with one another. Common hallmarks of a flowing conversation appear, such as humor and natural body posturing, as the two become "engaged" in conversation.

The engagement process, spontaneously developed during natural conversation, holds within itself some pertinent clues as to methods of enhancing the flow of a clinical interview. Consequently it is valuable to look briefly at the processes involved in an everyday conversation because they may pertain to the clinical interview itself.

To begin with, if one observes two close friends chatting over some coffee and cheesecake, one will quickly notice, depending on whether one possesses a habit of eavesdropping, that their conversation is not simply a potpourri of unrelated statements. Quite to the contrary, such conversation usually possesses a gentle structure, determined, albeit unconsciously, by its participants. In general, one friend brings up a topic, which both friends animatedly expand. Often the second member of the conversation will ask questions in an effort to more thoroughly understand the first while also showing an appropriate increase in interest.

Once the topic has been discussed, one of the friends will move the conversation to a new topic. This transition is often prompted by something that has already been discussed. Frequently the new topic is triggered directly by a preceding statement. And so the conversation between the friends moves, swelling and ebbing, as more or less interesting topics arise. The basic structure of the conversation consists of succeeding topics connected by transitions.

A smoothly flowing interview possesses many of these same structural elements. One of the keys to generating a natural flow of speech during the body of the interview consists of learning to move gracefully from one topic to another while taking cues from the interviewee's statements. The interviewer is aware of which topics are most pertinent for a triage interview and can gently guide the conversation to these topics. Once within a desired topic, the interviewer takes advantage of the natural conversational mode in order to fully expand that topic. When done well, the interviewer has structured the interview imperceptibly. The clinician establishes a powerful engagement with the interviewee while efficiently gathering a strategic database for decision-making.

This ability to structure patients naturally is one of the most, if not the most, difficult set of skills for most clinicians to acquire. The problem is that many trainees have no method to their madness, in the sense that no principles or techniques for structuring are utilized. Without a concrete language with which to understand the process of structuring, the trainee is faced with vague admonitions, such as "Work faster," hardly a useful criticism.

The trick for successful structuring lies in developing and understanding a language of structuring that spells out practical applications. This conceptual framework can be gained from a study of the everyday conversation described above.

Specifically, we will focus on a series of concepts, including topics on which information is needed during a clinical interview (called "regions"), the method of exploring these topics once they are entered (a process referred to as "expansion"), and the methods of transition used between topics (a structure called a "gate"). This language, which allows us to study the intricate movements and transitions used to structure the interview process, while also noting how a clinician manages his or her time during the interview, is called "facilics." The term "facilics" is derived from the Latin root *facilis* indicating grace in movement. An understanding of facilic principles provides the sound framework that allows interviewers to structure effectively.

Region of Dialogue

One of the first problems facing the novice interviewer remains the issue of what information is important in a full intake assessment. In this regard the first facilic concept to investigate is the region.

A region is defined as any section of an interview, lasting at least several sentences, in which there exists a unified topic of discussion or a unified process of interaction. In this general sense, a region may be described as either a content region or a process region.

CONTENT REGIONS

As discussed earlier, as with a conversation, an interview tends to revolve around discrete topics. Ten general content regions of frequent practical use in an assessment interview are as follows: (1) the history of the present illness, (2) the diagnostic explorations, (3) the psychological perspectives of the interviewee, (4) the formal mental status examination, (5) the social history, (6) the family history, (7) the determination of suicidal/homicidal potential, (8) the past psychiatric history, (9) the developmental and psychogenetic history, and (10) the medical history.

In order to explore these regions effectively, one must become familiar with their intricacies. In later sections of this book we will look at these regions in more detail. At present it is only important to emphasize that most topics of discussion occurring during an interview can be categorized within one of these 10 regions.

In order to ensure a common, initial understanding of these critical informational regions, they will be briefly summarized here.

1. *History of the Present Illness:* This region examines the chronologic development of symptoms. It emphasizes the types, characteristics, and severity of the symptoms and their duration. Naturally, the history of the present illness frequently includes one or more of the diagnostic regions as well.
2. *Diagnostic Regions:* The diagnostic regions are defined by the DSM-IV criteria. As a rule of thumb, a diagnostic region has been well explored if one can state whether or not the diagnostic criteria for a particular entity are fulfilled.
3. *Interviewee's Perspective:* The interviewee's perspective was discussed earlier, when dealing with the scouting period. It generally includes an attempt to understand the interviewee's views on his or her problems and how help can be utilized, as well as the fears, pains, and expectations uncovered in the interview. This region remains the cornerstone of crisis intervention.
4. *Formal Mental Status Examination:* This section represents observations concerning the following broad topics: appearance and behavior, speech and language, thought process and content, mood and affect, and cognitive functioning (including such processes as orientation, concentration, memory, and intellectual functioning). Naturally, many elements of the mental status are evaluated simultaneously with the exploration of the other regions. The more specialized cognitive mental status, in which a

clinician examines orientation, attention span, memory functions, and general intellect, tends to form a more discrete region that is easily identifiable during an interview.

5. *Social History:* Broadly speaking, the social history includes both interpersonal and environmental information. With regard to interpersonal history, one is interested in interaction with family, friends, employers, and even strangers in both the past and the present. Concerning environmental history, a clinician is interested in factors such as living conditions, neighborhood, economic status, and availability of food and shelter. This region often includes current and past stressors. A careful examination of possible alcohol or drug abuse can also be included here.

6. *Family History:* This region includes an exploration of psychiatric and other medical illnesses in the patient's blood-related family. It commonly includes a survey of entities such as schizophrenia, affective disorders, suicide, alcoholism/drug abuse, mental retardation, and seizure disorders, as well as any other major medical illnesses such as diabetes, cancer, and hypertension.

7. *Determination of Suicidal/Homicidal Potential:* This lethality region requires a careful and sensitive expansion by the interviewer and should never be omitted.

8. *Past Psychiatric History:* This region explores previous mental health problems, as well as previous interventions, such as forms of treatment (e.g., medication, psychotherapy, counseling, hospitalization).

9. *Developmental and Psychogenetic History:* This region traces the development of the individual from birth onwards, and it includes topics such as birth trauma, developmental milestones, toilet training, schooling, and early object relationships.

10. *Medical History:* This region includes past and present illnesses as well as a medical review of systems. Other areas, including allergies, medications, and current physicians, are also examined.

This brief survey illustrates that despite the immensity of an initial database, the contents tend to fall into relatively discrete regions. Many of these regions tend to overlap. In general, however, a given section of an interview tends to focus on a single region, much as a conversation tends to focus on a single topic at a time. In the following excerpt the general region concerning drug and alcohol abuse is readily apparent.

Clin.:   . . . So right now you haven't been using alcohol?

Pt.:   No.

Clin.: You talked about using drugs in the past. I'm wondering what kinds of things you used then and now.

Pt.: Right now I'm only using pot. I don't mess around with anything else.

Clin.: Are you using it every day?

Pt.: Almost every day.

Clin.: How many joints might you have in a day?

Pt.: Maybe split two; me and Jack might split two.

Clin.: Uh, huh.

Pt.: Because it really does calm me down. It doesn't make you sick like alcohol can make you sick, or give you a bad head the next day. It just relaxes you.

Clin.: Any type of pills you're taking now?

Pt.: No.

Clin.: Nothing but the marijuana . . . What kinds of drugs were you using in the past?

Pt.: Well, I never got into any one drug real heavy.

Clin.: Uh, huh.

Pt.: But I have taken LSD, speed, different goofballs, and stuff . . . but I never injected any drugs like dope.

PROCESS REGIONS

In addition to focusing on content, thereby gathering factual data, the interviewer may opt to focus on the process of the interview itself. Three such "process regions" include the following:

1. Free Facilitation Regions. This region remains one of the foundations of all interviewing. It is the traditional method of nondirective listening. In it, the interviewer invests effort in creating an atmosphere that is optimally conducive for the interviewee to feel safe enough to begin sharing his or her problems. The interviewee is able to wander freely to whatever topics chosen, while the interviewer maintains a nondirective attitude. The major interventions of the interviewer are usually facilitating head nods, uh-huhs, and simple facilitatory statements.

These facilitation regions can appear anywhere in an interview and are often a very useful method of enhancing engagement. As noted earlier, during the opening phase of the interview the clinician frequently utilizes a free facilitation region. In actuality, the scouting phase is a combination of content regions intermixed with facilitatory activities. Furthermore, a psychotherapeutic interview may consist almost entirely of free facilitation regions strung together. Naturally, most content regions have many attributes in common with free facilitation regions; but a facilitation region differs in the goal of its use, which remains the uncovering of information that the patient reveals spontaneously without direction from the interviewer.

A brief example may help to clarify when a section of an interview can be labeled as a free facilitation region.

> **Pt.:** I don't know what's coming over me . . . I just feel sort of crazy.
>
> **Clin.:** What do you mean?
>
> **Pt.:** All my thoughts seem to be mixing like a wet rainbow; distinctions are blurred, people distorted . . . (pause) I feel this way when I'm with my mother. She . . . (pause).
>
> **Clin.:** Go on.
>
> **Pt.:** She seems so oppressive, so large, like a giant machine always pushing, always pulling. Honestly, I don't know where to go with her.
>
> **Clin:** In what sense?
>
> **Pt.:** She wants me to be a success, lord knows what *that* means. I think she wants me to be a college professor or some dean of this or that. But she's not interested in what I need, never was. A baby without a bottle, that's what I am . . .

A free facilitation region often helps to lower the defenses of the interviewee so that his or her major concerns will surface. It can also be utilized to foster the uncovering of psychotic process, as will be described later.

2. Resistance Regions. In a resistance region the interviewer actively attempts to decrease a specific resistance to the engagement process. Such resistances may arise from any number of factors, including the interviewee's fears, expectations, or other ramifications of the self-system. Without a resolution of these resistances, the validity of subsequent data and the power of the therapeutic alliance may be greatly reduced. In any case, the defining characteristic remains that in a resistance region, the interviewer consciously attempts to resolve a resistance shown by the patient.

In the following selection we see an interviewer in the midst of a resistance region:

Pt.: My boss was really into my work and thinks I may be a little . . . you know . . . I don't really think I ought to go on. Do you have a supervisor around?

Clin.: You seem concerned about something . . .

Pt.: Well, I'd just feel a little better if I were talking to someone a little older.

Clin.: What do you think an older clinician would be able to do to help you?

Pt.: He'd understand what I've gone through better.

Clin.: You know, it's true I'm younger than you and, consequently, I haven't experienced the same things, but I can try to gain some understanding of what you're experiencing. You could help me by telling me a little more about how people have been pressuring you about your age.

Pt.: It all started with my wife. She left me about 3 years ago . . .

3. Psychodynamic Regions. In a psychodynamic region the interviewer asks questions in which the clinician is more interested in how and why the patient responds, as opposed to the content of what the patient says. In general, the clinician attempts to answer questions such as the following: How reflective is the patient? Does the patient have much insight? How does the patient respond to interpretive questions? How good is the patient's observing ego? Answers to these questions may help determine the suitability of the patient for time-limited psychotherapy, as well as provide insight into the patient's intellectual development, ego strength, defense mechanisms, and self-concept. To answer questions in a psychodynamic region the patient must reflect and offer an opinion.

The following excerpt may clarify when a psychodynamic region is occurring:

Pt.: My father always kept a strangle hold on me. He wanted to know my every move. God pity the boy who wanted to take me out. It was like a gestapo interview for the guy.

> **Clin.:** What kind of impact do you think your father's behavior has had on you?
>
> **Pt.:** He's made me scared. I'm afraid of him, and who knows, maybe I keep my distance from him because of it . . . Sort of strange though, 'cause when I was a kid I always wanted to be around him. I even would wait for him when he was at work.
>
> **Clin.:** Go on.
>
> **Pt.:** Oh, it's sort of silly, but I wondered if he had a toy or something for me . . . I remember a small doll he brought home once, with big black eyes. Just a little doll, but important to me.
>
> **Clin.:** Go on.
>
> **Pt.:** Not too much more to say, except that it's sort of sad the way things have turned out between us.
>
> **Clin.:** What are you feeling as you talk about your father right now?

Here, content is clearly taking a second place to process. The interviewee's responses suggest a willingness and a certain degree of proficiency at self-exploration. This type of region can occur anywhere in an interview, often appearing frequently between. content regions.

Thus far, three types of process regions have been illustrated: (1) the free facilitation region, (2) the resistance region, and (3) the psychodynamic region. In actuality, other types of process regions are common, including regions focusing on interviewee ventilation of emotions, interviewee education, or phenomenological regions of questioning as discussed in Chapter 1. These process regions often provide windows through which an understanding of the patient gradually emerges.

Equipped with a facility to move freely among both content regions and process regions, the clinician possesses a powerful flexibility with which to approach any given interviewing task. It is not a matter of learning to interview only in a fairly structured fashion (emphasizing content) or learning to interview in a nondirective style (emphasizing process regions). One needs to master both styles, at times delicately interweaving them. There does not exist a single "correct style" of interweaving these regions. Instead, one finds styles that may be more or less useful for any given clinical situation. Too frequently students learn only one approach, while building an unfounded bias that other styles of interviewing are inferior. No surer method of handicapping one's clinical flexibility can be found.

Having reviewed the type of database needed in a full intake interview, the focus can be shifted towards a discussion of techniques for exploring these numerous regions in a fruitful fashion.

In the first place, many interviews are made or broken before a word is spoken, because the preinterview planning frequently determines the success of the subsequent interaction. As discussed above, the clinician needs to ascertain what demands on information gathering are needed by the clinical situation. In an intake interview situation, most, if not all, of the content regions discussed earlier may need to be addressed, many of them thoroughly. In contrast, an emergency room evaluation of a patient well known to the system may require a significantly different strategy. In this emergency room situation the clinician may have only 20 to 30 minutes available. Consequently, a conscious decision will need to be made as to which content regions to decrease or eliminate.

One of the most common complaints voiced by supervisees can be summarized as, "I didn't have enough time to gather the information I wanted!" This complaint is often paralleled by harried clinic directors mumbling phrases such as, "My god, how much longer is he going to take with that patient!" Both exclamations represent the end product of a poorly structured interview.

To counteract this problem, an understanding of facilics provides the clinician with an awareness of "where he or she is at" with regard to the thoroughness of the database during the interview itself. From this heightened awareness, the clinician develops an ability to control the pace and flow of the interview.

When discussing the scouting period we examined the problem of the wandering interview in which a patient with a loquacious manner encounters an interviewer incapable of focusing the flow of the dialogue. The result can be a disappointing experience for both participants. But many times a patient with a normal verbal output, who could be easily directed, meets an interviewer with poor focusing abilities. Even in this case, the interview may become quite unproductive, because the patient does not know which information is most needed. The resultant hodgepodge of dialogue can best be called an "unguided interview."

One may wonder why unguided interviews are so common. The answer is relatively simple and hinges upon the concept called "tracking." Tracking refers to a clinician's ability to sensitively follow up the statements of a patient with questions pertinent to the area discussed. At a more sophisticated level, good tracking also requires the ability to follow up with questions pertinent to the patient's immediate emotional state. This ability to track well is one of the main attributes of a good listener. Indeed, the ability to track well is a prerequisite if one is to become a good interviewer.

And here lies the catch, for good tracking must be accompanied by an equally good ability to focus the patient sensitively. Many mental health trainees have developed good techniques for tracking through the process of attentively listening to family and friends. However, few have learned equally effective methods of focusing. Fortunately, this crucial ability to focus sensitively can be learned.

Generally speaking, once within a content region, it is frequently best to expand that region relatively fully, because the patient will generally find such expansions natural, the topics of discussion being essentially related. If one leaves a specific content region prematurely, one will have to return to that region, sometimes many times. Obviously, if the interviewer makes a habit of approaching most content regions in this haphazard manner, it becomes very difficult to monitor what information has been adequately gathered. Consequently, mistakes of omission occur more frequently. This haphazard approach also tends to decrease the sense of conversational flow.

Considering these pitfalls, one can begin to delineate a general approach to the body of the interview that will decrease the frequency of both wandering and unguided interviews. During the scouting period the clinician should formulate a tentative plan for the interview, utilizing the data gained from PACE. From this analysis, an initial content or process region will be chosen as an entrance into the main body of the interview. Frequently, the patient's own spontaneous discussion will have naturally led into a specific content region, such as the history of the present illness, or a diagnostic area, such as the depression region. If so, the clinician can expand this region fully and then proceed to the next pertinent region as desired. Wandering patients are gently refocused if they prematurely leave regions.

To the degree that the clinician determines which content regions are pertinent for a particular patient in a particular clinical situation, subsequent regions are successfully entered and expanded as the main body of the interview unfolds. Naturally, as deemed necessary, the clinician may pepper the content expansions with process areas such as psychodynamic regions or facilitation regions. Slowly the patient's story emerges and with it an increasing sense of understanding.

Problems tend to arise when clinicians lose awareness of the pacing of the data collection. One of the most frequent problems occurs during the second 15 minutes of the interview. In this critical region, "the dead quarter," clinicians often utilize too many free facilitation regions instead of focusing upon appropriate content regions.

When this approach is used, the clinician often finds that in 30 minutes very little of the needed information for a sound triage decision has been gathered. This early mistake in the structuring of the interview begets a second error. In reaction to the first misjudgement the clinician will proceed to force a rigid structure into the remaining part of the interview in an effort to catch up. Phrases such as "Let me ask just a few other questions here" or "Oh, I forgot to ask this" frequently appear en masse, as the scramble for needed information takes over. The result may be a patient who begins to perceive that the clinician is more interested in data gathering than in listening.

This vicious circle of disengagement can be eliminated if the interviewer begins gently structuring as soon as he or she emerges from the scouting period somewhere around 7 to 8 minutes into the interview. As the second 15 minutes closes, the clinician should be nearing the completion of the eight to ten content regions that seem most pertinent to a particular patient. When such a gradual approach is utilized, rapid focusing is seldom required, and the pace of the interview seems appropriately unrushed to the patient.

If this has been accomplished, the third 15 minutes can be utilized for expanding content regions deemed more important than originally expected, as well as for gathering data from the remaining content regions felt to be pertinent for treatment planning and triage. It is in this third 15 minutes that regions such as family history, medical history, social history, and the more formal mental status are often explored.

During the last 15 minutes, these regional explorations are continued, and new questions, generated by the unfolding information, may be asked. Psychodynamic regions may be explored more intensively and clarifications of previous points may be pursued. The last 5 to 10 minutes are generally utilized for the closing and terminating phases.

As can be seen, the body of the interview represents a delicate organism, whose growth and development warrant careful attention by the interviewer. Perhaps a review of the basic facilic principle utilized to move gracefully through this area of the interview would be useful.

1. Before beginning the interview, make a tentative determination of which content regions are most appropriate considering time constraints, the needs of the patient, and the goals of the interview.
2. During the interview, occasionally (at least every 5 to 10 min-

utes) monitor the progress of your data gathering and adjust your pace as needed.

3. Avoid the overuse of facilitation regions during the body of the interview.

4. Begin gently but persistently structuring as soon as you leave the scouting period and during the second 15 minutes.

5. Keep in mind that an inadequately structured second 15 minutes often forces a more rigid and potentially disengaging structuring later in the interview as a means of catching up.

6. Generally speaking, once within an appropriate content region, it is often useful to expand it thoroughly. If the patient pivots into a new area, it is usually best to gently pull the patient back to the current region until it is completed. The exception to this principle occurs if the patient pivots into a highly charged or sensitive area such as suicidal ideation or incest.

Thus far we have focused on the general strategy needed to determine and monitor the regions of dialogue encountered in an interview. Next we will examine the actual process of exploring a given region once it has been entered.

Expansion of Regions

The process of exploring a given content region is referred to as the expansion of the region. Different interviewers may approach this expansion in radically different ways.

Speaking broadly, two methods, forming somewhat opposing extremes, can be defined as "stilted expansions" and "blended expansions." In stilted expansions the expansion lacks a feeling of conversational flow. Instead, the interviewee is asked a series of questions that appear somewhat forced, because the interviewer is rigidly attempting to ask specific questions. This type of expansion may cause interviewees to experience the unpleasant feeling that they are "being interviewed," as opposed to talking *with* someone. I suppose one could call this process a "Meet the Press" type of expansion. Rigidly structured interviews sometimes foster this style of expansion such as illustrated below:

> **Pt.:** The pressures at home have really reached a crisis point. I'm not certain where it will all lead; I only know I'm feeling the heat.
>
> **Clin.:** What's your appetite like?
>
> **Pt.:** I guess it's okay . . .
>
> **Clin.:** What's your sleep like?

Pt.: Not too good. I have a hard time falling asleep. My days are such a blur. I never feel balanced, even when I try to fall asleep. I can't concentrate enough to even read.

Clin.: What about your sexual drive?

Pt.: What do you mean?

Clin.: Have you noticed any changes in how interested you are in sex?

Pt.: Maybe a little.

Clin.: In what direction?

Pt.: I guess I'm not as interested in sex as I used to be.

Clin.: And what about your energy level? How has it been?

Pt.: Fairly uneven. It's hard to explain; but sometimes I don't feel like doing anything.

This particular interviewer seems decidedly intent on expanding the depression region, specifically the neurovegetative symptoms of depression. This style of expansion exhibits a mechanical quality, as if the interviewer has a list of questions to reel off. Such rigidity characterizes stilted expansions.

As a study in contrasts, in a blended expansion the interviewer once again focuses on a specific region. However, in this expansion the interviewer attempts to blend the questions into the natural flow of the conversation. Rather than feeling like they are "being interviewed," this type of expansion creates in interviewees a sense of gentle flow, which tends to foster the engagement process. Moreover, this type of interviewing, by decreasing the anxiety of the patient, may enhance both the quantity and validity of the database as well.

In the following excerpt, a blended expansion unfolds, once again exploring the depression region:

Pt.: The pressures at home have really reached a crisis point. I'm not certain where it will all lead; I only know I'm feeling the heat.

Clin.: Sounds like you've been going through a lot. How has it affected the way you feel in general?

Pt.: I always feel drained. I'm simply tired. Life seems like one giant chore.

Clin.: What about your sleep? Has that been affected as well?

Pt.: Absolutely. Perhaps that's the reason I'm drained. I just can't rest. My sleep is horrible.

Clin.: Tell me about it.

Pt.: I can't fall asleep. It takes several hours just to get to sleep. I'm wired. I'm wired even in the day. And I'm so agitated I can't concentrate, even enough to read to put me to sleep.

Clin.: Once you're asleep, do you stay asleep?

Pt.: Never, I bet I wake up four or five times a night. And about 5:00 A.M. I'm awake, as if someone slapped me.

Clin.: How do you mean?

Pt.: It's like an alarm went off, and no matter how hard I try, I can't get back to sleep.

Clin.: What do you do instead?

Pt.: Worry . . . I'm not kidding . . . My mind fills with all sorts of worthless junk.

Clin.: You mentioned earlier that you have problems with concentration. Tell me a little more about that.

Pt.: Just simply can't function like I used to. Dictating letters, reading, writing notes, all those things take much longer than usual. It really disturbs me. My system seems out of whack.

Clin.: Do you think your appetite has been affected as well?

Pt.: No question. My appetite is way down. Food tastes like paste; really very little taste at all. I've even lost weight.

Clin.: About how much and over how long a time?

Pt.: Oh, about 5 pounds, maybe over a month or two . . .

In the above process the same region as before was expanded, but this time the questioning appeared to flow naturally, generating an increasing flow of information. The interviewer's questions seemed to relate directly to what the interviewee was saying, thus creating a sense that the interviewer was "with" the interviewee.

This example also illustrates an important point. While expanding the content region, one continuously attends to the engagement process. For instance, early in the above selection the inter-viewer sensitively utilized a complex empathic statement, "Sounds like you've been going through a lot." And later, facilitative open-ended techniques were used, such as the gentle command, "Tell me about it," and the open-ended question, "How do you mean?" Such a consistent and effective use of engagement techniques coalesces to create a feeling in patients that the interviewer is moving with them in a relatively unstructured fashion, while, in actuality, the clinician is gently structuring the interview, harvesting an ever more mean-ingful field of information.

A further point to consider concerning the expansion of regions is the usefulness of brief excursions out of a region. For instance, while expanding the anxiety disorder region, the patient may men-tion the use of Valium (diazepam). At this point, the clinician may choose to expand the medication history briefly, after which he or she can return to the anxiety disorder region to complete its expan-sion. Such short excursions offer yet another flexible option for the clinician. Humor can also be utilized to further the natural feeling of the interview.

The clinician may also choose to utilize split expansions, with a single region expanded at several different locations during the interview. Although useful, these split expansions can lead to serious omissions if the clinician does not keep track of what information has been gathered. But on a limited basis, split expansions further increase the interviewer's adaptability.

The over-riding point remains the clinician's need to develop an active and conscious awareness of the data flow while simultane-ously creating the sensation of the natural flow of conversation. Perhaps a few facilic principles warrant review at this point:

1. Generally speaking, an effort should be made to achieve blended expansions as opposed to stilted expansions; such blended expan-sions move with the patient.
2. As long as one remembers to monitor the completeness of his or her database, then techniques such as split expansions and brief excursions can be useful, but need to be used judiciously.
3. Always attend to engagement during the expansion of content regions both on a verbal and nonverbal level.

Before ending our discussion of the various methods of expanding regions, one more point warrants attention. Although stilted expan-sions generally tend to disengage patients, some patients may, ironi-cally, prefer them. This peculiar preference may surface in the case of a patient suffering from hypochondriacal concerns, associated with the belief that, "Nothing is wrong with my head." Some of these patients may actually prefer the check-list flavor of a stilted expansion, because it parallels the feeling generated by a medical review of systems. Hence, the patient feels more at home with an interaction more redolent of a medical examination than of a psychiatric assessment. Once again, the art consists of adapting one's style to the needs of the patient.

At this time, we can move to the third and last major concern of facilics, the transition utilized between regions. The ability to master these transitions will determine the clinician's ultimate ability to create a smoothly flowing dialogue.

Gates: The Pathways of Transition

As a conversation or an interview passes from one topic to another, different types of transitions occur. We will refer to the actual statements joining two regions as "gates." Although there exist numerous types of gates, five major forms are most common: (1) the spontaneous gate, (2) the natural gate, (3) the referred gate, (4) the implied gate, and (5) the phantom gate. An understanding of the use of these gates provides interviewers with a simple but elegant method of gracefully maneuvering an interview.

Spontaneous Gate. The spontaneous gate, as its name suggests, initially unfolds without any effort by the interviewer. Instead, the gate results from a change in course unilaterally taken by the interviewee. These gates occur when the patient spontaneously moves into a new region (called a "pivot point") and the clinician proceeds to ask a follow-up question in this new region. The patient does the shifting here. The clinician merely follows, sometimes with phrases as simple as "Tell me more about that," or "How do you mean?" In the following example, a spontaneous gate provides an essentially unnoticeable movement into a new region:

> Pt.: The past 2 months have been so horrible. I think it's the worst time of my life. I just can't get away from the feeling.
>
> Clin.: Which feelings are you referring to?
>
> Pt.: The sadness; the heaviness.
>
> Clin.: Earlier you had mentioned that you've lost your appetite and always feel tired. What else have you noticed when you're feeling sad and heavy?
>
> Pt.: Nothing seems worth doing. It's late November and my yard is covered with leaves. Usually they'd all be gone into neat little piles, like a little farm, but not now . . .

Clin.: Besides not having energy for chores, do you find you can still enjoy your bridge club or other hobbies?

Pt.: Not really. Things seem so bland. I haven't even gone to bridge club for several months. It is all so different from before. In fact, there were times in the past when I could barely keep still, I was so active.

*Clin.: How do you mean?

Pt.: Oh, I used to be super active, into bridge, tennis, golf, and everything. I was a real dynamo.

Clin.: Did you ever move too fast?

Pt.: In what sense?

Clin.: Oh, sometimes one can get so energized that it gets difficult to get things done.

Pt.: Actually, there were a couple of odd times when people kept telling me to "slow down, slow down."

Clin.: Tell me a little about one of those times.

Pt.: About a year ago I got so wound up I hardly slept for almost a week. I'd stay up most of the night cleaning the house, washing the car, and writing furiously. I didn't seem to need sleep.

Clin.: Did you notice if your thoughts seemed slowed down or speeded up then?

Pt.: Speeded up. I was flying. Everything seemed crystal clear and moved like lightning. It was strange . . .

In this example, two topics are being discussed sequentially. In the first region, the interviewee's symptoms of depression are being explored. In the course of this exploration, the interviewee brings up a statement that suggests a different diagnostic region dealing with mania. The transition statement was, "In fact, there were times in the past when I could barely keep still, I was so active."

The interviewer then followed this movement into a region exploring manic symptoms by simply asking, "How do you mean?" (indicated by an asterisk). Once within the diagnostic region of mania, a blended expansion was begun. This movement into a new topic was practically imperceptible.

Spontaneous gates create movement that seems unblemished by effort or resistance. In this sense, a clever interviewer will frequently make use of such gates whenever transitions into new regions are desirable. But herein lies a potential pitfall mentioned earlier, because it is frequently not desirable to leave a region before it is fully expanded.

In this light pivot points represent critical areas in which the interviewer should consciously decide whether to stay within an expansion or move to a new one. If the clinician can gain conscious awareness of such pivot points, then the clinician will gain considerable control over the flow of questioning. One does not and should not follow every spontaneous cue with a transition into a new region.

Indeed, the concept of spontaneous gates and pivot points provides us with a new way of conceptualizing both the wandering interview and the unguided interview. These interviews occur when pivot points are followed by the clinician whenever they appear, resulting in a consistent pattern of incomplete expansions. To prevent this wandering process, the clinician must apply the refocusing techniques described earlier. Nine times out of ten, in the body of the interview, pivot points should not be followed into spontaneous gates. There are exceptions to this principle.

As alluded to earlier, at times the clinician may wisely decide to follow a pivot point into a spontaneous gate even in the middle of an incomplete expansion. Such times include situations such as the following: (1) the patient may have unexpectedly related highly emotionally charged material that needs to be ventilated; (2) the patient may have spontaneously mentioned highly sensitive material that may best be approached immediately; and (3) specific memories may warrant immediate follow-up, such as screen memories, dreams, or traumatic events.

Of course, during process regions, such as psychodynamic regions or free facilitation regions, the clinician generally follows most spontaneous gates as they appear, utilizing an occasional restraint. The scouting period is also often filled with spontaneous gates. Along these same lines, during periods of free association, as may appear in therapy itself, spontaneous gates are essentially always followed; indeed, they are nurtured. But no matter what the facilic situation, we return to the all-important realization that clinicians can exercise significant choice as to the pattern any given interview will pursue as long as they recognize pivot points and consciously decide whether or not to follow them.

Natural Gate. The natural gate consists of two parts: the cue statement and the transitional question. The cue statement represents a comment made by the interviewee that contains content material that can be creatively related to a new region by the interviewer. If the interviewer cues off from this statement to enter a new region, the interviewee will feel that the conversation is flowing from his own speech, as, indeed, it is. Such a transition seems both natural and caring to the interviewee.

The transitional question represents the actual question made by the interviewer, which made a bridge from the cue statement into the new region. As opposed to the spontaneous gate, the clinician, not the patient, is entering a new region.

In the following excerpt we will see a transition made from the region covering depressive symptoms into the drug and alcohol region. This smooth transformation will be made via a natural gate.

> **Clin.:** Have you been able to enjoy your poker games or your shop work?
>
> **Pt.:** No, I just don't feel like doing anything since I've been feeling depressed. It's a really ugly feeling.
>
> **Clin.:** Tell me more about what it feels like.
>
> **Pt.:** Really pretty miserable. Life doesn't seem the same. I'm tired all the time; no sleep.
>
> **Clin.:** How do you mean?
>
> **Pt.:** Over the past several months sleep has almost become a chore. I'm always having trouble getting to sleep, and then I wake up all night. I must wake up five times and it took me 2 hours to fall asleep in the first place.
>
> ***Clin.:** Have you ever used anything like a nightcap to sort of knock yourself out?
>
> **Pt.:** Yeah, sometimes a good belt really relaxes me.
>
> **Clin.:** How much do you need to drink to make yourself sleepy?
>
> **Pt.:** Oh, not too terribly much. Maybe a couple of beers. Sometimes more than a couple of beers.
>
> **Clin.:** Just, in general, how many drinks do you have in a given day?
>
> **Pt.:** Probably . . . Now, I'm just guessing, but probably a six-pack or two, maybe three. I hold liquor pretty well. I don't get drunk or nothing.
>
> **Clin.:** What other kinds of drugs do you like to take to relax?
>
> **Pt.:** Well, I might smoke a joint here or there.

In this excerpt, the cue statement was, "I must wake up five times and it took me 2 hours to fall asleep in the first place." Note that

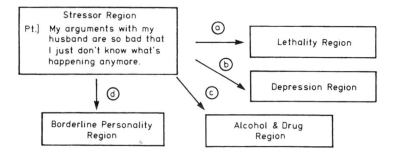

Transition Questions:

a) With all these tensions mounting, have you had any thoughts of wanting
   to kill yourself?

b) How have all these stresses affected your mood?

c) With all these stresses, have you been drinking at all
   in an effort to calm yourself?

d) Some people hold all their anger in and others really let it out,
   maybe even throwing things like glasses or plates. How do you
   handle your anger?

F i g u r e   **2**

Natural gates utilized as smooth transitions.

the patient's cue statement is still within the region of depression. But the clinician, wanting to change content regions, sensed that this statement could be used as a springboard into a new topic. The succeeding transition question (indicated by an asterisk) imperceptibly achieved this desired transition into the drug and alcohol region with the phrase, "Have you ever used anything like a nightcap to sort of knock yourself out?"

Transitions of this sort are seldom perceived as focusing mechanisms, because the patient generally feels as if he or she brought up the new topic. This type of smooth transition can greatly enhance a conversational feeling in the interview, slowly bringing the patient into a more powerful sense of safety and spontaneity. The interview begins to take on a self-perpetuating momentum, unique to its own nature.

In Figure 2, the immense power of the natural gate is demonstrated. We shall assume that the expansion of the stressor region has been winding down. The patient then provides a cue statement, which can be utilized by the clinician to enter one of any number of new content regions as illustrated. The flexibility of the natural gate is essentially only limited by the awareness and creativity of the clinician.

One helpful device, with regard to the use of natural gates, consists of the so-called "manufactured gate." Suppose the clinician has reason to suspect potential homicidal ideation in the patient. In order to get to this delicate topic, the interviewer can set up or manufacture a natural gate as follows:

Pt.: I've really been feeling out of sorts. Frankly, I don't know if I'm coming or going.

Clin.: Does it ever help you to relax by drinking?

Pt.: . . . Uh, that's hard to say. Sometimes a few calm me down, like after a good Steelers game with Terry Bradshaw (professional football quarterback) throwing passes all over the place. The beer just goes well with it. But at other times it just upsets me more.

Clin.: Sometimes when people drink they notice an increased desire to just let off steam, you know, let out the anger, maybe have a good time with a barroom brawl.

Pt.: Oh, yeah. I've been in my share of brawls. Won a few, too.

Clin.: Has that ever carried over into other areas? Like getting mad at your wife and wanting to hit her?

Pt.: Yeah. Just a few weeks ago I wanted to beat the hell out of my wife. She can be such a royal pain in the ass.

Clin.: Have you ever really wanted to hurt her, in a more serious way?

Pt.: (pause) Once in a while I guess I have. And sometimes I still think she deserves it.

Clin.: Deserves what?

Pt.: To be killed. It's crossed my mind, I have to admit it.

Clin.: What have you thought of doing?

Pt.: Cracking her upside the head with a hammer. One real quick snap, like Terry Bradshaw releasing a long pass.

In this excerpt, the clinician was expanding the depression region and wanted to get unobtrusively into the homicidal region. This appears at first glance to be quite a task. It is not exactly easy to ask people if they are murderers. But this clinician makes the difficult seem surprisingly easy. From previous experience, he knew that the homicide region could be frequently entered by a natural gate from the drug and alcohol region, by relating the homidical thoughts to the poor impulse control commonly associated with drinking.

Consequently, the clinician steered the conversation into the drug and alcohol region, thus setting up a natural gate through which he entered the region of homicidal ideation with barely a hint of structuring.

Referred Gate. A referred gate occurs when the interviewer enters a new region by referring back to an earlier statement made by the interviewee. To the interviewee, a referred gate suggests that the interviewer has been carefully registering what is being said. It is a wonderful example of a structuring tool that is also an engagement technique. Also, it allows the interviewer to enter a fresh region smoothly at almost any place in an interview. It remains extremely useful for re-entering a region that was not fully expanded earlier. Structurally, a referred gate lacks an immediate cue statement, because the cue has been taken from a previous area of the interview.

In the following illustration we will enter the interview at the end of a psychodynamic process region in which the patient's feelings concerning his siblings have been explored. As this process region winds down, the interviewer will enter the content region dealing with psychotic phenomena by using a referred gate.

Clin.: What was it like for you when your brother would come home from college?

Pt.: Sort of odd; a little bit like a trespass. You see, when he was gone I had the room all to myself, even the phone was mine alone. As soon as he came back, boom, the room was his again.

Clin.: What other feelings did you have?

Pt.: Some excitement. I really did look up to him, and when he'd come home he'd tell me all about college, frat parties, smoking grass; and it was exciting.

*Clin.: Earlier you had told me that sometimes when you were alone you'd have scary thoughts. Tell me a little more about those moments.

Pt.: O.K. It's sort of like this. I might be sitting late at night listening to some music and things seem sort of weird, almost like something bad is going to happen. And then I have thoughts that keep coming at me and they tell me to do things.

Clin.: Do the thoughts ever get so intense they sound almost like a voice?

Pt.: They *are* voices. They seem very real. In fact,

sometimes I try to cover my ears. I just don't know. I don't know . . .

Referred gates, such as the one illustrated above (indicated by asterisk), are unobtrusively powerful. They can be used for entering new regions essentially at will as well as for re-entering incompletely expanded regions. Moreover, when combined with a creative sensitivity, the clinician can utilize referred gates to enter potentially disengaging regions gracefully. One of these awkward regions, which frequently poses problems for clinicians, remains the formal mental status examination, or cognitive examination as it is frequently called. While asking questions about orientation and checking digit spans or serial sevens, clinicians frequently worry that patients will feel insulted by the simple nature of the questions. To this end, clinicians may utter phrases such as, "I'm going to ask you some silly questions now, I hope you don't mind," or "Now I have to ask you some routine questions that I have to ask everybody." These phrases are usually accompanied by an apologetic tone of voice or an insecure rustling of the clinician in his or her chair.

The irony of such introductions lies in the fact that rather than dispelling anxiety in the patient, they sometimes create it. The patient can sense that the clinician feels insecure with the subsequent material. All that remains for the patient to wonder is why the clinician needs to apologize. What do these *routine* questions mean and why does a professional ask questions if they are silly? In short, the clinician's sudden obsequiousness serves to signal the patient that something odd is underfoot.

It is here that one of the many uses of the referred gate becomes apparent. By referring to earlier statements of the patient concerning problems of concentration or thinking, the interviewer can enter the cognitive examination smoothly and without a need to apologize. Quite to the contrary, the interviewer's interest indicates a sincere concern to the patient as well as a display of professional knowledge in the sense that these cognitive questions are serving a specific function, a joint undertaking between the patient and the clinician. Let us take a look at such an approach in action. The patient is suffering from an agitated depression and had complained earlier in the interview of "problems concentrating":

Pt.: Overall, I know it's all my fault. I should never have retired, it's ruined everything. But life goes on. I only hope I feel better some day.

Clin.: Earlier, you had mentioned the one thing that was bothering you most was your lack of concentration. Tell me a little more about that.

Pt.: It's a big problem. I have problems even reading the newspapers, which I used to love to do. Now I read a paragraph and I might as well have my eyes closed. I don't register any of it.

Clin.: Has this affected your memory as well?

Pt.: Yes, I think so, simple things, just don't remember them well, like names and telephone numbers or even paying my bills.

Clin.: It sounds like you are having some significant problems. I'd like to get a clearer idea of exactly how your thinking has been affected. To do this I'd like to ask you a series of questions that can help us sort out some of the specific problems with concentration and memory you have been having. Some of the questions will be very simple while some of them may get fairly challenging. Why don't we start with some of the simple ones first.

Pt.: Sure.

Clin.: What day of the week is this?

Pt.: I think it's Wednesday.

Clin.: That's correct. What city is this?

Pt.: Pittsburgh.

This interview dyad moved into the cognitive mental status examination with a sense of purpose and no hint of uneasiness on the part of the clinician. Even if the patient does not "pick up" on the referred gate, an easy transition can be made as follows:

Clin.: Earlier you had mentioned how depressed and out of it you sometimes feel at dusk. I am wondering if during this period of the day you notice any problems with concentration or your memory.

Pt.: No, I don't think so. No problems with my concentration.

Clin.: That's very fortunate, because frequently when people feel depressed, they have problems with concentration or organizing their thoughts. In fact, I would like to ask some questions designed to pick up even subtle problems with concentration, because if we find some subtle problems, it may give us some idea of how we can best help you. Does that sound okay to you?

Pt.:   Yes. I don't think I've got any problems here, but I guess it's worth taking a look.

Clin.:   Good, we'll start with some very simple questions and move towards some harder ones. To start with, what is today's date?

Once again the mental status examination has been entered unobtrusively. Perhaps at this time a few other comments concerning the formal mental status examination are in order. Some authors will state that the formal cognitive examination should not be done unless the clinician strongly suspects a true cognitive deficit, because the questions may be disengaging. I disagree with this point of view for a variety of reasons. First, as we have just seen, when approached with a referred gate the cognitive examination is seldom significantly disengaging. Second, one cannot effectively learn the implication of answers to these questions until one has learned, through experience, the range of answers that normally functioning people make. For instance, it is not at all unusual for normal people to make a mistake on serial sevens. In short, to interpret abnormal answers well, one must first become familiar with normal replies. The only way to achieve this familiarity is to perform a brief cognitive examination frequently on patients. Moreover, one may also actually uncover early signs of a true cognitive deficit, as seen in the first stages of dementia or in a simmering delirium.

And the third reason, one of the most important justifications, remains the fact that these questions are not asked solely to check cognitive functioning. To the contrary, they represent one of the few areas in the interview in which the clinician receives an opportunity to observe the patient directly solving problems and coping with a potentially anxiety-arousing situation. In short, the clinician gets a first-hand look at the patient dealing with a challenge. This glimpse can be revealing with regard to the patient's psychodynamic defenses.

This psychodynamic window provided by the formal cognitive exam was highlighted to me during an initial interview with an honor student in physiology from a prestigious university. Bruce, as we shall call him, walked into my office with a mildly hesitant step. He was conservatively dressed with an alligator riding his chest. Short-cropped hair framed a reasonably handsome face. Not only was he an honor student; he was also a star athlete. At first, Bruce seemed ill at ease and tended to avoid eye contact. During the preceding months, he had grown increasingly stressed, relating, "I've never been happy, this has been eating at me my whole life." As would be expected, during the main body of the interview he demonstrated no evidence of cognitive dysfunction. He was articulate and reflective. But as the cognitive examination proceeded, an interesting change occurred. More specifically, an interpersonal process emerged, a process that apparently plagued him practically on a daily basis. In order to observe this process we will enter the dialogue a short time after the cognitive examination was begun:

Clin.: I am going to ask you to remember four items and I'll ask you to repeat them in about 5 minutes. Do you understand?

Pt.: Yes. (He looked anxious and sat up in his chair.)

Clin.: Purple, football, oak tree, and hope. Can you say these words back to me?

Pt.: Purple, football, oak tree, and hope (said quickly and assertively).

Clin.: Now I'd like to check your concentration by asking you to repeat some numbers for me. I will say a line of digits and when I nod you say them back . . . 8–6–1–5.

Pt.: 8–6–1–5 (looking even more intense).

Clin.: 7–9–5–6–3.

Pt.: 7–9–5, uh, uh, 6–3.

Clin.: 2–1–4–5–3–8.

Pt.: 2–1–4–3, uh, 5–8.

Clin.: Not quite right. Let's try another one.

Pt.: (looking very intense) I'm going to beat you at this.

Clin.: (pause) Bruce, you seem like you're sort of feeling uptight about this. What are you actually feeling at this time?

Pt.: You're not going to beat me on this—that's what I'm feeling—I'm going to get this right.

Clin.: You seem very competitive right now.

Pt.: I am. I get this way anytime I take a test.

Clin.: Does that ever interfere with your performance?

Pt.: Oh yeah, sometimes I get so upset I almost feel like I'm going to run from the room. It's one of the problems I need help with. I'm very competitive.

Clin.: Just now, it seemed like that feeling was making you feel very uptight with me. What kind of effect does it have on you with other people, if any?

Pt.: I feel it very frequently. Any time I meet new people, I wonder if the new guy is a threat, somebody who can beat me. It's rough out there. Everybody wants to get ahead of you. And they'll cheat if they have to . . . (pause) but I even feel this with Jennifer, my girlfriend, not much, but it's there, like a sharp stick in my gut.

This interchange generated by the cognitive examination revealed several striking characterologic traits in this young college student. His world was one brimming with enemies created in large part by his own mind. Besides uncovering these processes, this exchange provided a reference topic for many of the following psychotherapy sessions. With time, he began to perceive a less threatening environment, one not overrun with hostile figures. In any case, it was the mental status examination that led into this rich vein of psychopathology, while allowing me to watch the patient's reaction to the task at hand.

Perhaps it would be expedient to return to the main topic of referred gates at this time. We have just seen the usefulness of the referred gate in guiding the discussion into a cognitive examination. In a similar way, referred gates can frequently decrease the awkwardness of entering sensitive regions of discussion such as the drug or sexual history. This effectiveness probably results from the fact that relating the sensitive material to previous statements by the patient decreases the perceived social inappropriateness of the question. This principle may seem a bit abstract at present, but the following illustration will clarify the concept.

In this interview, the patient was an attractive woman of about 30 years of age. She had her blonde hair pulled back in a bun, giving an impression of a young professional. Her hands punctuated her words like a well-struck typewriter key. She described her various plights in a dramatic and telling manner. After 30 minutes, numerous soap opera vignettes had been laid out on the table, including many years of heavy drug abuse in the past, a striking lack of any stable relationships, five abortions, over 200 sexual encounters, and a current investigation by the FBI of her old friends.

She emphasized her sexual freedom early during the interview stating, "I'm not hung up on having to like the person I have sex with. Sex is something I can easily divorce from my feelings." Later in the interview, as the facts of her life became clearer, I began to wonder if I was talking with someone who one might call a "slick sociopath." To this end I wanted to expand the antisocial personality region in more detail.

I wondered if she might be involved in prostitution. Needless to say, asking a person during the initial interview if she may be a prostitute can be a delicate matter. In this case a referred gate provided a smooth entry into this sensitive topic.

> **Pt.:** All of my men have ended up leaving me. None of them want to be fathers. We always fight. I'm bored by it all now.
>
> **Clin.:** Earlier you had mentioned that you have been able to successfully separate your sexual feelings from your emotional ones as you've matured. I'm wondering if, because of this ability, you've been able to use your own body in a more practical sense, for instance, by selling sexual favors.
>
> **Pt.:** Yeah, I've done that too. Back in New York I used to be a prostitute for about 4 or 5 months, not much longer though.
>
> **Clin.:** What was that like for you?
>
> **Pt.:** Not really that tough. It's a dirty business though and I'm glad I'm out of it. But it helped when I needed it and believe me I needed the money.
>
> **Clin.:** Did you ever sell drugs back then to help pay the rent and other needs?
>
> **Pt.:** No. I never really sold drugs, I would use them like crazy, my life has been a wild one. In fact, someone ought to write a novel about me. I've seen it all, but I never got into pushing drugs.

This referred gate, voiced matter of factly, seemed to flow quite naturally. She did not appear particularly flustered, and the blending remained high. Once again, to the interviewee, referred gates suggest that the clinician has been listening carefully in an effort to piece together the patient's story. One can imagine how differently the above situation may have unfolded if the clinician had abruptly asked without a referred gate, "By the way, are you a prostitute?" This method of transition certainly needs a little more polish. Such abrupt gates are the next topic of discussion.

Phantom Gate. A phantom gate appears to come from nowhere. It lacks a cue statement and also lacks previous referential points, as seen in referred or natural gates. In short, it jolts the spontaneous flow, as the following example will show:

Pt.: I haven't felt the same for months. I'm always down and I'm sick of it.

Clin.: What does it feel like to be down?

Pt.: Very unsettling. I'm like a slab. I don't want to do anything. I miss doing things with my best friend, silly as that may sound. I really haven't been the same since she died.

*Clin.: Was your father an alcoholic?

Pt.: No . . . (pause) I don't think he was. He drank every once in a while.

Clin.: What about your brothers, sisters, or blood relatives? Have any of them had drinking problems?

Pt.: Not that I know of.

Clin.: What about depression? Have any of your relatives been depressed?

This interviewer's sudden leap into the family history region certainly appeared abrupt and ill-timed. Obviously, if such phantom gates (indicated by an asterisk) occur frequently throughout the interview, engagement can be seriously hampered. Even in milder forms, they can quickly produce the "Meet the Press" feeling discussed earlier. They often pop up toward the end of interviews, when interviewers suddenly realize several things they forgot to ask. If important regions have been incompletely expanded, then referred gates, as opposed to phantom gates, can often return the interviewee to these unanswered questions without substantially interrupting the flow of the interview.

In the meantime, a phantom gate placed here and there will probably not cause much of a problem, especially if the blending appears high and the content of the question is not sensitive in nature. In general though, one should avoid phantom gates, because it seems senseless to risk damaging the flow of the interview by their use.

With regard to the utility of phantom gates, two instances come to mind. First, when dealing with a wandering interview, phantom gates may be useful in focusing the patient, especially if milder forms of focusing have been unsuccessful. A second use of phantom gates arises during the exploration of certain psychodynamic regions. Specifically, if one wants to catch a patient off guard in order to observe the patient's spontaneously occurring defenses, then an unexpected phantom gate may be very effective. Phantom gates may also help one break through the resistance caused by a patient bent on manipulating the interviewer or during a rehearsed interview.

In a less antagonistic sense, phantom gates may also be utilized when attempting to help patients reflect upon themselves through the use of interpretive questions. Interpretive questions may assume more bite if asked at an unexpected moment. These latter uses of phantom gates find minimal applicability during initial interviews, but they are more commonplace during psychotherapy interviews, once the therapeutic alliance has been solidified.

Implied Gate. To complete our summary of transitions used during the body of the interview we can turn our attention to implied gates. These gates are frequently used during chit-chat between friends and may have been the predominant gate overheard as we listened in upon the café conversation mentioned earlier.

In an implied gate, the movement into a new region is characterized by asking a question that seems to be generally related to the region already under expansion. Thus, it is somewhat "implied" that the interviewer is simply expanding a topic already germane to the interviewee. Similar to the referred gate, an implied gate lacks a true immediate cue statement. In the following example, movement is made from the region dealing with immediate stressors into past social history. The transition (indicated by an asterisk) seems smooth, an effect that is probably secondary to the similarity in content between these two regions.

> **Pt.:** We're living in a fairly nice house now. It has three bedrooms and a couple of acres. Believe me, we need the space with our four kids.
>
> **Clin.:** How are the kids getting along?
>
> **Pt.:** The two oldest, Sharon and Jim, get along pretty well, on different tracks. They stay out of each other's way. But the two little ones—oh my! They live to torture each other . . . Pulling each other's hair, yelling, screaming. It's a zoo.
>
> **Clin.:** I'm wondering if, with all those mouths to feed, money is a problem?
>
> **Pt.:** In some respects, yes; but my husband is a lawyer and is doing well. In fact, if anything, our income has increased recently.

*Clin.: Tell me a little bit about what it was like for you when you grew up back in Arkansas.

Pt.: First of all, I came from a large family of eight children. So we sometimes, many times, had to do without. I remember all the hand-me-down's and, believe me, I appreciated them. My mother was a loving woman, but beaten down by life. She was tough, but her pain showed through.

Clin.: Do you remember a specific time when her pain showed through?

Pt.: Oh, yes. I was about 5, I think, and . . .

It may be of value to spend a few moments comparing implied gates to the gates previously discussed. As mentioned earlier, unlike a natural gate, an implied gate does not cue directly off the preceding statement. Furthermore, unlike a referred gate, the interviewer does not directly refer back to earlier statements. And, in contrast to the phantom gate, the implied gate seems to fit in fairly naturally with the current flow of the dialogue. Indeed, when the newly entered region appears very similar to the preceding one, an implied gate is practically imperceptible and rivals a natural gate for smoothness of transition (as in this example).

As the regions connected increase in disparity, the implied gate becomes increasingly more abrupt. Thus, with regard to smoothness, implied gates range on a continuum between natural gates and phantom gates. When the two regions are closely related, implied gates approach the gracefulness of natural gates. On the other hand, if the topics are poorly related, an implied gate may approach the awkwardness of a phantom gate.

Implied gates can frequently be used to enter new regions smoothly. In fact, not infrequently, the clinician may simultaneously expand two regions whose contents are similar in nature. For instance, one can easily expand the anxiety disorder region and the affective disorder region in a parallel fashion, because the symptoms in these disorders frequently overlap.

At this junction, we are nearing the end of our discussion of the various methods by which one can structure the body of the interview. Some of these principles are summarized below:

a. When the patient spontaneously moves into a new region, the clinician always has the choice of whether to follow it or not. These decision moments are called pivot points.
b. If a premium is put upon efficient data gathering, then it is often best not to follow these pivots into new regions. Instead, the

clinician can gently continue the expansion of the region currently being explored.

c. If a premium is put upon a dynamic understanding of the patient, then these pivots into new regions are frequently completed by the use of simple follow-up questions, creating a spontaneous gate. These wanderings of the patient can provide valuable insights into the patient's psychodynamics. These pivot points are also followed if it appears that the patient has begun spontaneously discussing sensitive areas or seems to need to ventilate disturbing emotions.

d. Natural gates, in which the clinician enters a new region by cueing directly off the patient's preceding statement, offer another method of smooth transition and should be employed frequently.

e. These natural gates offer a means of effectively structuring an interview while conveying an unstructured feeling to the interviewee.

f. Referred gates, in which the clinician literally refers back to earlier statements by the patient, offer effective methods of re-entering poorly expanded regions or bringing up new regions.

g. Referred gates are particularly useful for tying in sensitive or awkward regions such as the mental status examination, for once again the patient feels that this "new topic" appears to relate naturally to the spontaneous dialogue.

h. Implied gates allow one to join similar regions and can also provide parallel expansions of related regions.

i. Phantom gates should be generally avoided unless used for a specific purpose such as focusing a persistent wanderer.

Facilics provides a simple language with which to follow the complex structuring techniques of both ourselves and those we supervise. To enhance this system, a supervisor's "shorthand" has been designed in which easily learned symbols are used to represent regions and gates. These facilic schematics allow the supervisor to quickly make a permanent record of the supervisee's interview, while providing a concrete and visual springboard for immediate feedback or group discussion. For those readers who supervise interviewing, I think you will find this system to be very valuable. In the research done on our interviewing training program, course participants chose facilics, as one of the most valuable tools for their growth, more often than any other tool including videotape, role-playing, and didactics.[22] The interested reader can find an introduction to the use of facilic schematics in Appendix I on page 622.

Once a clinician understands the principles of facilics, then the body of the interview can be developed and altered almost at the whim of the interviewer. These tricks of the trade can greatly increase the engagement with the patient, the effectiveness of the data gathering, and ultimately the validity of the database itself.

In short, initiated by the conscious decisions of the interviewer, the clinical dialogue unfolds. With each unfolding, the initial resistance of the interviewee gradually recedes, for the interviewer, instead of opposing this resistance, moves with it. The natural gates and blended expansions discussed in this section generate interviews that move with the gentle dynamics of a conversation. The patient feels more relaxed, defenses drop, and the interviewer finds a rich field of pertinent information opening before him.

This section on the body of the interview began with a quotation concerning a master artist of China, Wang Hsia, who painted in the 8th century A.D. He worked in a different time and in a different medium than we have discussed. Yet, he, too, was a student of movement. Like ours, his work was based on a few simple principles, practiced until discipline had transformed them into art. Our "painting" is the clinical dialogue we leave behind us. We, too, strive for sensitivity and subtlety. Perhaps, with work, fellow students of interviewing will study one of our future transcripts and find, to their admiration, that "when one looks carefully, one cannot find any marks of demarcation in the ink."

CLOSING OF THE INTERVIEW: PHASE 4

As the interview steadily moves towards its closure, certain tensions may arise in the interviewee. These tensions arise from the patient's concern as to whether or not help is at hand. From the patient's perspective, the question becomes one of "What have we accomplished here?" or "Was this worth my time?" A variety of questions may be formulating in the patient's mind, either consciously or unconsciously. Not every patient will have all of these concerns, but many patients will be seeking answers to a significant number of them, such as:

1. What is wrong with me?
2. Am I crazy?
3. Did I tell the interviewer what he or she needed to know?
4. Does this interviewer understand my problems?
5. Did this interviewer like me as a person?
6. Do I have a diagnosis?
7. Will I get better?

8. Can I be helped?
9. What are my treatment options?
10. What will happen to me next, and will I see this clinician again?

All of these questions are appropriate and natural. Indeed, the patient, in a sense, has a right to a discussion of these issues with the clinician. The clinician will possess only tentative answers to many of these questions, and the patient should be made aware of this fact, but even tentative answers may provide a powerfully reassuring experience for the patient. If answered sensitively, the clinician can help decrease the patient's fear of the unknown, including the plaguing question of "What's happening to me?"

Addressing this point, Sullivan has stated that a patient should gain something from the assessment process itself.[23] He emphasizes that patients frequently gain a considerable sense of relief merely by exploring their problems in an orderly fashion with a concerned listener. An orderly inquiry frequently begets a more orderly and calming perspective. Over and above this benefit patients may literally come away with tentative answers to some of the disturbing questions raised above.

It should be kept in mind that one of the major goals, perhaps the major goal, of the clinician during the closing phase of the interview consists of solidifying the patient's desire to return for a second appointment or to follow the clinician's referral. Indeed, if the patient decides not to comply with the clinician's recommendations, then the interview has in many respects failed. The clinician may have an extremely accurate diagnosis, but if no patient returns, the utility of the diagnosis is certainly of dubious value.

Towards achieving a better understanding of compliance it is valuable to look at some of the reasons that would motivate a patient to return. Although many reasons exist, the following seem to be most telling:

a. The patient feels that something was gained from the interview.
b. The patient feels comfortable with the interviewer.
c. The patient feels that the interviewer also feels comfortable with the interaction.
d. The patient trusts the clinician.
e. The patient feels that the clinician may be able to help in the future.
f. The patient feels that the clinician appears to be down to earth and accessible.
g. The patient feels that the clinician appears balanced and calm.

To a significant extent, the presence of such favorable "compliance feelings" will at least partially be determined by the manner in which the clinician has handled the introduction, the opening, and the body of the interview. But it remains the closing phase in which many of these compliance feelings can be significantly enhanced. One of the major methods of enhancing these favorable feelings consists of taking the time to carefully address the questions mentioned earlier.

The very fact that the clinician addresses these issues may convey to the patient that the clinician can be trusted and seems to understand the patient's needs. Indeed, the clinician's actions represent a direct acknowledgment of the patient's needs at the moment.

One could discuss the issues concerning the closing phase in great detail, but I think it may be of more value to look at a closing phase as it unfolds. This dialogue will represent only one approach to the closing, but it illustrates many of the principles discussed earlier.

In the following illustration, the clinician has been interviewing a middle-aged woman at a local mental health center. The clinician is functioning as an assessment clinician and has decided that the patient is most likely suffering from a major depression. We will pick up the dialogue near the end of the body of the interview. In order to highlight the various aspects of this interview phase, the entire closing phase is included.

> **Pt.:** I don't think any other members of my family . . . let me see . . . no, I don't think anyone else besides my sister and my uncle have been depressed like this. My mother certainly never went through anything like this, perhaps that's why she doesn't seem to understand.

> **Clin.:** Well, it doesn't seem like too many people in your family have been depressed, but at least two people have. We've covered a lot of ground so far. At this point, we are coming to the close of our interview today. I'd like to spend some time summarizing what we've talked about and discussing some ways of possibly helping you to help yourself. But first, you mentioned that your mother doesn't seem to understand. I'm wondering how you put together what is happening to you?

> **Pt.:** Hmmm . . . it all seems so complicated. I think I may have reached a time of life when my bad qualities are catching up with me. Certainly I'm becoming a burden for my husband and I'm not really doing my share.

Clin.: Why do you think it's happening now?

Pt.: Maybe because I deserve it, I don't know. Or maybe because the kids are starting to leave the nest as they say.

Clin.: Do you think there is anything you might want to add as we close that we haven't covered, that might help us to understand what is going on?

Pt.: No, not really, we've covered an awful lot . . . well, one thing though, I didn't mention this because it was so long ago, but in college I had one semester in which I did very poorly in school. Now that I think about it, maybe I was suffering from the same type of thing.

Clin.: What were you feeling back then, that makes you feel these experiences were similar?

Pt.: Many of the same things. I couldn't sleep well and I was constantly worried, I was so worried about flunking out I almost did.

Clin.: Did you seek help back then?

Pt.: Are you kidding! My parents didn't think anything was wrong except I was lazy. It never even crossed my mind to get help.

Clin.: But you've come for help today and I'm wondering what kinds of ways you thought we might be able to help you?

Pt.: I'm not really certain. Maybe I thought you might have some magic pill that would take all this away (patient smiles and begins a subdued chuckle). I'll tell you one thing though, it was hard to come here.

Clin.: I'll bet it was . . . tell me a little about what it was like actually coming here today.

Pt.: Oh, I felt very self-conscious walking in off the street. In fact, I looked around first to see if anybody I knew was around. When the coast was clear, I shot in like a dive bomber . . . while I was waiting to see you, I felt very awkward. I didn't know what I was getting into. I almost left.

Clin.: What made you stay?

Pt.: I think I realized I needed help of some sort. I really am at a loss. What do you actually think is happening?

Clin.: First, let me reassure you, most everyone who comes for a first appointment feels much as you have. That's totally normal. It's difficult to share with a stranger. You've done an excellent job of helping me to get a good picture of what you've been experiencing. From what you said I have some ideas of what might be going on. I agree with you that you seem to be dealing with a lot of stresses within your home, including a changing relationship with your children as they leave, and a fair amount of tension with your husband.

Pt.: Yes, I really didn't emphasize the problems with Jack but they are there and have been for years. It's not just the kids.

Clin.: These problems are certainly worth trying to understand so that you can cope with them more effectively. And sometimes some of the pains we feel from the past, like your leaving home at an early age, may also be contributing to the present. Because of this, I think it would benefit you to talk with one of our clinicians perhaps on a weekly basis for a while, to try to sort things out. But, I think there is more to the picture as well. You described a variety of symptoms such as an inability to sleep, a loss of energy, decreased enthusiasm, and a loss of sexual drive. All these symptoms suggest that you may be suffering from a major depression.

Pt.: How do you mean?

Clin.: Over the past 10 or so years, we have made tremendous advances in understanding various forms of depression. It used to be thought that depression was only caused by psychological problems, but now we have discovered that some forms of depression are caused, or at least partially caused, by chemical imbalances in the brain. No one thinks about how incredibly complicated the brain is, it is no wonder that sometimes minor chemical imbalances arise. In any case, the symptoms you have are commonly seen in these forms of depression. Another item pointing that way is the fact that two members of your family seem to have also suffered from a very similar depression, and we have found that the biological forms of depression are frequently seen among family members.

Pt.:   What does all this mean?

Clin.: Well, some of these depressive symptoms, perhaps caused by your biology, make it difficult for people to effectively work on the psychological problems and even to cope with daily chores. Fortunately, we have found a variety of medications that frequently help to get rid of these depressive symptoms. There are no magic pills though, nor are there promises for success, but these antidepressant medications can be very effective with some people. Because your symptoms do suggest that you may also have a biological depression, I'm going to make a referral to our mood disorders clinic. If you are interested in going there, you'll find the therapists are very skilled in both talking therapy and medications. After they get to know you better, they will let you know exactly which therapy may help you the most. (Pause) I've given you a lot of information, I'm wondering if this is making any sense?

Pt.:   Yes, yeah, I think so at least.

Clin.: Try to tell me in your own words what I've been explaining to make sure that I'm being clear.

Pt.:   Let me see, you think that there may be something wrong with the chemistry in my brain and that's making me feel depressed. And you think some medications may help.

Clin.: That's right. Now this doesn't mean you don't want to look at the psychological stresses as well. This means that there may be more than one way to help you feel better. Do you think you'd be interested in seeing our therapist, I think it could really help.

Pt.:   Yes, I think I would like to give it a try, at least. I'd read about depression being caused by chemical problems, I just really never recognized myself as being depressed.

Clin.: Sometimes depression is hard to recognize. Perhaps back in college your parents didn't recognize it in you just as you didn't recognize it yourself today.

Pt.:   I never thought of it that way, but I guess it's actually possible.

Clin.:   In any case, as we wrap up here, I'm wondering what this interview has been like for you, was it what you were expecting?

Pt.:   For the most part, yes. I really didn't know exactly what to expect. I really felt we covered a lot of important ground. It seemed very thorough.

Clin.:   Is there anything I could have done differently that might have made you feel more comfortable?

Pt.:   No, no . . . I felt, I feel very comfortable with you. I do think you could use more magazines out in the lobby though. It really gets uncomfortable sitting out there.

Clin.:   Hmmm . . . that might be a good idea.

Pt.:   Will I be working with you again?

Clin.:   No, I only work over here in the Assessment Clinic, but I think you'll find the therapists in the Mood Disorders Clinic very knowledgeable and also very nice. Like myself, they will try to gain a broad knowledge of how things have been going for you over the years, in an effort to understand you better.

Pt.:   Good, do I call them or what?

Clin.:   I'll give you a card here (hands card to patient). This has their number on it, and you can call later today for an appointment. This card also has our number on it, if there are any other unexpected problems before your appointment. I think you made a very good decision coming here today. I think they'll be able to help you to help yourself.

Pt.:   Well, thank you. I actually feel a little better.

Clin.:   Good, I hope things go well. Give us a call if there's a problem.

Pt.:   Thank you very much (patient exits).

This was a nice example of a straightforward closing phase. The first thing to note is that the closing phase takes time. To have this time available, the clinician must leave appropriate time for the closing to occur. One of the most frequent problems I see in supervision remains the over-extension of the main body of the interview, thus forcing the clinician to rush through the closing phase.

This rushed closing can leave the patient feeling disjointed and uncertain as to what just happened. To the contrary, during this phase, where engagement looms so critical for compliance purposes, the clinician should appear unhurried, concerned, and calm. There is a give-and-take element to the closing phase. The clinician is truly interested in the patient's opinions, and this respect helps the patient to feel a sense of trust and control.

If one looks through this dialogue, most of the questions listed earlier as being pertinent to the closing phase were addressed. The clinician added a nice touch by asking for comments about his own performance. I frequently ask this type of question for several reasons. Sometimes patients literally provide very good constructive criticism. Second, the metacommunication of the clinician to the patient is reassuring, for the clinician is stating, "I care about how I come across to you and am aware that I make mistakes and can improve as well." This type of metacommunication can help the patient to feel that he or she will be listened to and not just ordered about.

Before leaving the topic of the closing phase, two areas that may be part of the closing phase are worthy of note. The first area concerns the psychiatrist or nurse clinician, who is expected to prescribe a medication, if appropriate, at the end of the first session. Introducing a medication is a fine art and it requires time, probably at least 7 to 10 minutes. In such cases the clinician must cut back on the body of the interview by about 10 minutes or simply run overtime. I have certainly done both. Sometimes one has the option of introducing the medication at the next session, which can provide a more leisurely approach.

In any case, it is critical that this education about medication be done in a sensitive and engaging fashion, optimizing the patient's comfort and interest in the medication. Here are a few tips:

a. Ask the patient what his or her previous experiences with medications have been like.
b. Ask the patient if he or she feels particularly sensitive to meds. If the patient states that this is a concern, it is important to listen and convey that this concerns you too. Often such a patient feels better if the physician subsequently starts off with a lower than normal dose. This is a powerful metacommunication that you are listening to the patient carefully.
c. Ask the patient if he or she has heard anything about the medication or knows someone who is taking it. If a close friend has had horrible experiences, this might not be the smart med to choose.

Consider using an equivalent medication. If none are available, addressing the patient's fears directly may alleviate the patient's hesitancy to take the med. Not eliciting this information is almost a sure fire method of guaranteeing that the med will soon be stopped.

d. Be very open about side effects, and explain common side effects clearly. Any more serious dangers regarding the med should be discussed in a calm and reassuring manner, which accurately reflects any risks.

e. Alert the patient that side effects sometimes occur before benefits and that if the patient knows what the side effects are, he or she will not be frightened by them. This is the reason it is important to explain side effects in detail.

f. Emphasize to the patient that you need his or her help regarding side effects. Only the patient knows what he or she is feeling. Ensure that the patient knows that your goal is not to keep him or her on a medication but to help the patient to find a medication that he or she genuinely wants to be on because it helps.

g. Emphasize that you are the patient's consultant. Ultimately, the patient makes the final decision regarding whether to take a medication or not (this might not be the case in an involuntary commitment), and you are there to help by providing the best possible medical advice.

h. Carefully delineate the benefits of the medication and point out specific areas of relief that you are expecting to see.

i. Emphasize the effectiveness of the medication and describe successes you've had with it and how much better people felt.

There are many other considerations in this area, bridging into the topic of ongoing efforts to increase patient understanding and interest in medications, which are beyond the scope of the initial interview. However, the above principles provide a starting point.

The second area that sometimes becomes a component of the closing phase of the initial interview is asking permission to contact corroborative informants such as significant others and friends. Most of the time, I find that this is not a problem. If the patient does have concerns, the wisest course is to explore these concerns in detail. By the way, sometimes the concerns are good ones, and the patient is correct that the person should not be contacted.

Many times the patient's main concern deals with confidentiality. Once reassurances are made on this point, the patient feels comfortable with the contact. Clinicians seem to vary regarding when they talk about confidentiality. Some therapists discuss it routinely in the introduction phase of the interview, and others discuss it in the closing phase. Some do not discuss it at all unless it appears to be an issue. You can find out what style seems most comfortable to you. This is also an excellent topic to raise with supervisors.

If the patient still seems a little edgy, Morrison has a nice way of phrasing the reasons for contacting a corroborative source:

*W*hat you've told me is confidential, and I'll respect that confidence. You have that right. But you also have a right to the best help I can give. For that I need to know more about you. That's why I'd like to talk with your wife. Of course, she'll want to know what's wrong and what we plan to do about it. I think I should tell her, but I'll only tell what you and I have already agreed upon. I won't tell her anything else we've discussed, unless you give me permission in advance.[24]

Such a reassuring approach often transforms the patient's hesitancies.

Naturally, each closing phase will be different, but the basic principles outlined above offer at least one practical approach. The reader may discover many others. The important thing remains the realization that the closing phase is different from other sections of the interview, its character being formed by the changing needs of the two co-participants.

Before ending our discussion of the dynamic structure of the interview, one short phase of the interview warrants some attention.

TERMINATION OF THE INTERVIEW: PHASE 5

The termination phase consists of the actual closing words and gestures of the interviewer and interviewee. As with the introduction, the clinician frequently shakes hands and smiles appropriately. It is not uncommon, if the clinician is functioning as a triage agent and will not be seeing the patient again, to wish the patient good luck with a simple phrase such as, "I hope things go well for you."

The only problems that tend to arise here occur when the clinician feels, for some odd reason, the need to be overly formal and cool. Once again, such pseudo-professionalism runs the risk only of creating alienation in the patient. Instead, a quiet warmness seems more appropriate, a warmness generated by two people who have worked together in an attempt to increase understanding.

I would like to add only that if the clinician will be seeing the patient again, perhaps as the patient's therapist, then increased attention to the actions of the patient at termination may be valuable. Indeed, termination functions as a mini-loss to the patient. In responding to such a loss phenomenon, the patient may betray behaviors suggesting dependent feelings and difficulties with separation. These behaviors may offer early clues to more far-reaching psychodynamic processes.

For instance, some patients may dawdle at the door, looking anxiously back at the clinician for one more sign of approval or acceptance. Other patients may suddenly become cooler, as if they resent the ending of their hour. Such a display may be an early sign of narcissistic entitlement or borderline rage. In any case, a sensitive clinician can gain some insight from even a small piece of patient behavior, ranging from a peculiarly soft knock on the door to an unusually rapid series of departing footsteps.

Reader Note: After finishing this chapter, the reader may find it useful to read Appendix II, a completely annotated initial interview. The interview provides an illustration of all of the key principles from this chapter, as well as offering some peeks at concepts from the remaining chapters.

CONCLUSION

In this chapter we have studied the subtle transformations that evolve as the clinical interview proceeds. The interview was described as a dynamic process, an event born from the immediate needs of the clinician and the person seeking help. At times the agenda of these two people appear vastly different, and the art becomes one of moving through this world of opposites in such a manner that the agenda seem less antagonistic or even become unified.

In this chapter we have seen two quotations from Eastern disciplines, ink brush painting and the graceful martial art of T'ai Chi. These references were not chosen simply to produce a more literary work, but because the similarity between interviewing and these other highly skilled activities stands as a striking one. An understanding of this similarity lies at the center of mastering the art of interviewing.

One will find that in order to master these Eastern disciplines, the dedicated student may spend months or years practicing the basic brush strokes and body movements from which these arts were born. Through rigorous emphasis upon learning basic principles, mastery gradually occurs. At first these movements may appear artificial and somewhat limiting, but through intensive practice the pupil eventually develops a creative intuition not possible without first learning the basic maneuvers. One need only watch a T'ai Chi master sparring in order to comprehend the immense creativity cultivated through years of discipline.

In a similar fashion, this chapter has presented a highly analytical approach to interviewing, as if studying the process through a microscope. The use of these techniques may seem awkward at first, but with practice they become a natural and integral part of the clinician's style. A new and more penetrating intuition emerges from the balance, poise, and confidence that characterize an interviewer who understands not only patients but the interview process itself. Moreover, patients sense this internal balance and are powerfully attracted to it. As we pointed out in Chapter 1, talented interviewers are neither solely intuitive nor solely analytic. They are both.

With interviewing one is reminded of a fictional art form described by the writer Herman Hesse in his novel *The Glass Bead Game*. This so-called game was, in reality, the most highly evolved of all art forms. In it, an artist attempts to synthesize two totally opposing views into a unified statement. The more graceful the metamorphosis, the more brilliant the artist. One cannot help but see the parallel between this fictional art form and the craft of clinical interviewing. In this context the reward is not artistic adulation but increased understanding of the patient and a more powerful sense of caring.

I mention Hesse's game because the following excerpt, depicting the qualities sought for in a glass bead player, illustrates the very essence of a talented and flexible interviewer.

*R*emember this: One can be a strict logician or grammarian, and at the same time full of imagination and music. One can be a musician or Glass Bead Player and at the same time wholly devoted to rule and order. The kind of person we aim to produce, would at any time be able to exchange his discipline or art for any other. He would infuse the *Glass Bead Game* with crystalline logic, and grammar with creative imagination. That is how we ought to be. We should be so constituted that we can at any time be placed in a different position without offering resistance or losing our heads.[25]

And so it is with interviewing: flexibility and creativity are born from understanding and discipline.

References

1. Storr, A.: *The Art of Psychotherapy*, New York, Methuen, 1980, p. 9.
2. Lazare, A.: *Outpatient Psychiatry Diagnosis and Treatment*. Baltimore, Williams & Wilkins, 1979.

3. Morrison, J.: *The First Interview: A Guide for Clinicians*, New York, Guilford Press, 1993, p. 176.
4. Campbell, A. A.: Two problems in the use of the open question. *Journal of Abnormal and Social Psychology* 40:340–343, 1945.
5. Converse, J. M.: Strong arguments and weak evidence: the open/closed questioning controversy of the 1940s. *Public Opinion Quarterly* 48:267–282, 1984.
6. Dohrenwend, B. S.: Some effects of open and closed questions on respondents' answers. *Human Organization* 24:175–184, 1965.
7. Elliot, R., Hill, C. E., Stiles, W. B., et al.: Primary therapist response modes: Comparison of six rating systems. *Journal of Consulting and Clinical Psychology* 55:212–223, 1987.
8. Friedlander, M. L.: Counseling discourse as a speech event: Revision and extension of the Hill counselor verbal response category system. *Journal of Counseling Psychology* 29:425–429, 1982.
9. Hill, C. E.: Development of a counselor verbal response category system. *Journal of Counseling Psychology* 25:461–468, 1978.
10. Lazarsfeld, P. F.: The controversy over detailed interviews—An offer for negotiation. *Public Opinion Quarterly* 8:38–60, 1944.
11. Marquis, K. H., Marshall, J., and Oskamp, S.: Testimony validity as a function of question form, atmosphere, and item difficulty. *Journal of Applied Social Psychology.* 2:167–186, 1972.
12. Metzner, H., and Mann, F.: A limited comparison of two methods of data collection: The fixed alternative questionnaire and the open-ended interview. *American Sociological Review* 17:486–491, 1952.
13. Naik, R. D. Responses to open and closed questions: An analysis. *Indian Journal of Social Work,* 44, 1984.
14. Rockers, O. S. F. Dolore: The effects of open and closed inquiry modes used by counselors and physicians in an initial interview on interviewee perceptions and self-disclosure. Ph.D. dissertation, 1976.
15. Rugg, D., and Cantril, H.: The wording of questions. *Journal of Abnormal and Social Psychology* 37:469–495, 1942.
16. Schuman, H.: The random probe: A technique for evaluating the validity of closed questions. *American Sociological Review* 21:218–222, 1966.
17. Schuman, H., and Presser, S.: The open and closed question. *American Sociological Review* 44:692–712, 1979.
18. Singelman, C. K.: Evaluating alternative techniques of questioning mentally retarded persons. *American Journal of Mental Deficiency* 86:511–518, 1982.
19. Singleman, C. K., Schoenrock, C. J., Spanhel, C. L., et al.: Surveying mentally retarded persons: Responsiveness and response validity in three samples. *American Journal of Mental Deficiency* 84:479–486, 1980.
20. Benjamin, A.: *The Helping Interview,* 2nd ed. Boston, Houghton Mifflin Company, 1974.
21. Chung-yuang, C.: *Creativity and Taoism: A Study of Chinese Philosophy, Art, and Poetry.* New York, Harper Torchbooks, 1963.
22. Shea, S. C., Mezzich, J. E., Bohon, S., and Zeiders, A.: A comprehensive and individualized psychiatric training program. *Academic Psychiatry* 13:61–72, 1989.
23. Sullivan, H. S.: *The Psychiatric Interview.* New York, W. W. Norton, 1970, p. 219.
24. Morrison, J., 1993, p. 166.
25. Hesse, H.: *The Glass Bead Game.* New York, Holt, Rinehart and Winston, 1970, p. 68.

CHAPTER 3

Nonverbal Behavior: The Interview as Mime

And now a dark cloud of seriousness spread over her face. It was indeed like a magic mirror to me. Of a sudden her face bespoke seriousness and tragedy and it looked as fathomless as the hollow eyes of a mask.

Herman Hesse
Steppenwolf

I n this chapter we will explore the intricate processes known as nonverbal behavior. Few studies are more intriguing or more pertinent for the clinician. Our study will include not only body movements but also those elements of verbal communication that are concerned not with the content of spoken word but with how the words are spoken. Indeed, the noted social scientist Edward T. Hall has commented that communication is roughly 10% words and 90% a "hidden cultural grammar." He continues, "In that 90% is an amalgam of feelings, feedback, local wisdom, cultural rhythms, ways to avoid confrontation, and unconscious views of how the world works. When we try to communicate only in words, the results range from the humorous to the destructive."[1]

The practical relevance of Hall's words can be readily seen in the following clinical vignette. During an afternoon of supervision, I had the opportunity to watch two interviewers interact with the same patient in back-to-back interviews. The patient, a male in his early twenties, sat with a slumped posture, his head seemingly pulled to his chest by an invisible chain. His legs were open, and his hands lay resting quietly on his lap. The interviewer was a young woman, who spoke in a quiet but persistent voice. The blending between the two was weak at best, provoking an occasional upward nod from the patient, rewarding the starved interviewer with a momentary scrap of interest.

When the second interviewer entered the room, an intriguing process unfolded. Within 5 minutes the patient sat more alertly in his chair. Eye contact improved significantly and was accompanied by actual animation, albeit mild, in his voice. By the end of the interview, the conversation was proceeding naturally, and a reasonably good therapeutic alliance had been formed. Both interviewers were relatively young women, both of whom conveyed a caring attitude. One wonders what factors resulted in the clearly more powerful blending of the second interview.

Some of the answers may lie in the communication channels each of these interviewers used in an effort to engage the patient. The first interviewer spoke in a quiet tone of voice intermixed with numerous nods of her head. Such head nodding frequently appears to facilitate interaction. Unfortunately, visual cues lose their impact if the patient refuses to look at the clinician. In short, her facilitatory efforts were on the wrong sensory channel. To the contrary, the second interviewer spoke in a more lively tone of voice, which appeared to perk the patient's attention. More important, her words were frequently punctuated with auditory facilitators such as, "uh huh" and "go on." In contrast, the first interviewer verbalized few such auditory facilitators. The patient had been stranded in the room, responding with detachment to the clinician's monotone voice. Like the first clinician, the second interviewer also utilized head nodding, but her nods became progressively more effective as the patient met her eyes more frequently.

This example demonstrates the usefulness of flexibly employing different communication channels depending on the receptiveness of the patient. If the patient's head is down, one can increase the number of facilitatory vocalizations. With a deaf patient, one can increase head nodding. Perhaps more important this example emphasizes the overall influence of the interviewer's nonverbal communication on the patient. It suggests that we may be able to consciously alter our nonverbal style in an effort to create a specific impact on the patient.

This fact brings us to one of the most important challenges of this chapter. In order to flexibly alter their styles, interviewers must become familiar with the baseline characteristics defining their own styles. From such a self-understanding, flexibility emerges.

Thus a study of nonverbal behavior provides two distinct avenues of exploration. First, as the opening quotation from *Steppenwolf* suggests, one can learn an immense amount about the patient by studying nonverbal cues. This aspect of nonverbal behavior is the most commonly acknowledged. Hesse's protagonist quickly perceives his companion's change of affect as "a dark cloud of seriousness spread over her face." Second, as our clinical vignette illustrates, one can discover the impact of one's own nonverbal behavior on the patient and subsequently alter it as deemed appropriate.

Before proceeding it may be expedient to examine the definition of nonverbal behavior, for this term can have different meanings. In their excellent book, *Nonverbal Communication: The State of the Art*, Harper, Wiens, and Matarazzo explore some of the ramifications of defining this term.[2] In the first place, it is of value to make a distinction between the terms nonverbal communication and nonverbal sign. Nonverbal communication consists of an actual attempt to communicate a message using an accepted code between an encoder and a decoder.[3] A nonverbal sign does not involve an attempt at communication but represents a nonverbal behavior to which the observer infers a meaning.

Although developed as a refinement of research theory, this distinction between nonverbal communications and nonverbal signs can be adapted to provide a sound background through which to discuss clinical work. Specifically, in this book nonverbal behavior is viewed as the general category of all behaviors displayed by an individual other than the actual content of speech. In this context, tone of voice and the pacing of speech are also considered as examples of nonverbal behavior.

This broad category of nonverbal behavior can then be split into two subcategories, nonverbal communications and nonverbal activities. In the first category, nonverbal communications, the patient is using a commonly accepted symbol associated with a specific meaning. An irate football fan "throwing the finger" to the quarterback of the visiting team is displaying a piece of rather vivid nonverbal communication. In the second category, nonverbal activities, the overt behavior does not have a single commonly agreed upon meaning, and the sender may not be consciously trying to convey a message. The act of chain smoking cigarettes would represent a nonverbal activity. This activity may indeed be usefully interpreted by the observer as having a meaning, perhaps indicating anxiety; however, this interpretation is inferred and may be wrong. In short, nonverbal activities may have numerous meanings.

As clinicians we are interested in attempting to understand the significance of both nonverbal communications and nonverbal activities. It is important to keep in mind that nonverbal activities are generally multiply determined. It seems unwise to begin assuming that one "knows" exactly what any given activity means. In this regard Wiener and associates criticized some psychoanalytically oriented researchers as immediately positing unwarranted unconscious meanings to nonverbal activities.

Considering this context one is reminded of the old psychoanalytic saw in which the astute clinician observes that the patient is experiencing severe marital discord because the patient is playing with her wedding band. Such interpretations of nonverbal activities are invaluable if kept in perspective. The clinician needs to think about other possible causes of the stated activity. For instance, this patient may be playing with her wedding band because she feels intimidated by the interviewer. She releases her anxiety by playing with objects in her hands. Normally she rolls a pencil back and forth, but because no pencil is available, she twists her ring. Other interpretations may be equally correct. To ignore these other possibilities while assuming the marriage is troubled is to ignore sound clinical judgment. On the other hand, having considered the various possibilities, the experienced clinician may gently probe to sort out which is correct and may indeed uncover marital discord.

From this discussion, the following general principle emerges. Nonverbal communications are relatively easily deciphered, whereas nonverbal activities should be cautiously interpreted, because more than one process may be responsible for the behavior. This point deserves emphasis because both clinical literature and popular literature sometimes read as if the authors felt that they knew the exact meanings of nonverbal activities. They imply that one can read a person like a book. In a similar vein, the concept of "body language" suggests that nonverbal activities are more codified than behavior actually is.

A similar element of caution emerges as one surveys the research concerning nonverbal behavior. The body of research appears both vast and promising, but there exist many limitations. Nonverbal interactions are so complex that it remains difficult to successfully isolate variables to study. For instance, suppose research was designed to prove that it was the paralanguage (how the words were said) of the second interviewer in our clinical vignette that directly increased blending. An attempt to isolate this single variable would prove difficult, for a variety of other variables could have had an impact, such as the interviewer's physical attractiveness, the distance between seats, and even the fact that there were two interviews.

Even when one successfully isolates the relevant variables, the very act of isolation poses serious problems. Nonverbal elements seldom function as isolated units.[4] Instead, the various nonverbal elements exert their influences jointly, making the findings of research based on single channels such as paralanguage or eye gaze somewhat artificial. A different approach, the functional approach, attempts to study the various nonverbal elements as they function in unison.

These research issues are worth mentioning because it is important for the clinician to realize that little knowledge exists on nonverbal activity that can be called "factual." It is safe to say that this body of exciting research is in its childhood. In this regard the material of this chapter is best viewed as opinion concerning an evolving craft or art. The subsequent material is culled from a variety of sources, including clinical work, supervision, research literature, personal communications, and even popular literature[5] if it seems to shed light on clinical issues.

The following chapter is divided into two sections. In the first section three of the main categories of nonverbal behavior are briefly surveyed. As with the previous chapter, we shall develop a practical language through which to study the phenomena in question. Specifically, the following three areas are addressed: (1) proxemics (the study of the use of space), (2) kinesics (the study of body movement), and (3) paralanguage (the study of how things are said).

In the second section we shall adopt a functional perspective, carefully investigating the interplay of these three areas as applied to clinical practice. The broad clinical tasks studied include assessing the nonverbal behaviors of patients, actively engaging patients, persuading and focusing patients, and calming hostile patients.

BASIC PRINCIPLES OF NONVERBAL BEHAVIOR

Proxemics

Edward T. Hall was quoted at the beginning of the chapter. Few people would be more suitable for introducing the topic of nonverbal behavior, because Hall literally coined the term "proxemics." It was in his book *The Hidden Dimension* that he defined proxemics as "the inter-related observations and theories of man's use of space as a specialized elaboration of culture."[6]

Proxemics deals with the manner in which people are affected by the distances set between themselves and objects in the environment, including other people. As Hall notes, humans, like other animals, tend to protect their interpersonal territories. As humans move progressively closer to one another, new feelings are generated and new behaviors are anticipated. Hall postulates that people learn specific "situational personalities" that interact with the core traits of the individual, depending on the proximity of other individuals. This set of expected behaviors and feelings can be used by the clinician to improve blending. By observing the patient's use of space, the clinician may even uncover certain diagnostic clues.

Hall delineated four interpersonal distances: (1) intimate distance, (2) personal distance, (3) social distance, and (4) public distance. With each of these distances different sensory channels assume various levels of importance.

At the intimate distance (zero to 18 inches), the primary sensory channels tend to be tactile and olfactory. People feel at home with the specific scents they associate with lovers and children. At these close distances, thermal sensations also play a role, especially when making love or cuddling. Visual cues are of diminished importance. In fact, at the intimate distance, most objects become blurred unless specific small areas are focused upon. Voice is used sparingly. Even whispered words can sometimes create the sensation of more distance.

As one moves to the personal distance (1½ feet to 4 feet), kinesthetic cues continue to be used but olfactory and thermal sensations diminish in importance. With their decline the sense of sight begins to assume more importance, especially at the further ranges of this interpersonal space.

Upon arriving at the social distance (4 to 12 feet), we have reached the region where most face-to-face social interchange occurs. Touch is less important, and olfactory sensations are markedly less common. This region is the playland of the voice and the eyes. Most conversations and interviews unfold within the range of 4 to 7 feet.

At the public distance (12 feet or more), vision and audition remain the main channels of communication. Most important, as people move further and further away, they tend to lose their individuality and are perceived more as part of their surroundings.

A respect for these spaces is of immediate value to the initial interviewer. In general, people seem to feel awkward or resentful when strangers, such as initial interviewers, encroach upon their intimate or personal space. With this idea in mind it is probably generally best to begin interviews roughly 4 to 6 feet away from the patient. If an interviewer is by nature extroverted, by habit the interviewer may sit inappropriately close to the patient, intruding upon the patient's personal space. Obviously such a practice can interfere with blending and should be monitored.

It should be kept in mind that patients do not determine a sense of interpersonal space by slapping yardsticks down between themselves and clinicians. As observed by Hall, it is the intensity of input from various sensory channels that creates the sensation of distance. An interviewer with a loud speaking voice may be invading a patient's personal space even when seated at 6 feet. Once again clinicians must examine their own tendencies in order to determine how they come across to patients.

To emphasize the point that it is sensory input, not geographic distance, that determines interpersonal space, one need only consider the impact of a patient who seldom bathes. Such patients frequently create a sense of resentment, because, in essence, olfactory sensations are supposed to occur only at intimate and personal distances. These patients invade the intimate space of those around them even when seated at a distance. The same principle can explain why even pleasant odors such as perfume can also be resented if they are too strong.

If a clinician intrudes into a patient's personal space, the clinician can set into motion the same awkward feelings and defenses commonly encountered in elevators. The artificial intimacy created by invading the patient's space results in a shutdown of interactive channels, so as not to further the intimate contact. Like a person in an elevator the patient will avoid eye contact and move as little as possible. The patient's uneasiness may even predispose the patient to decreased conversation. In effect, the clinician might just as well be conducting the interview on an elevator, hardly the image of an ideal office. This "elevator effect" can also occur if the clinician ignores cultural differences.

Hall's distances were determined primarily for white Americans. These distances may vary from culture to culture. One piece of research found that Arab students spoke louder, stood closer, touched more frequently, and met the eyes of fellow conversants more frequently.[7] Sue and Sue relate that Latin-Americans, Africans, and Indonesians like to converse at closer distances than do most Anglos.[8] They go on to describe that when interviewing a Latin-American, an interviewer may push away, because the situation may feel crowded. Unfortunately this need for distance by the clinician could be perceived as an element of coolness or indifference by the client. In a similar light, the clinician may make the mistake of immediately feeling that the client is socially invasive, when in reality the client is merely interacting at the appropriate distance for Latin-American culture.

Race may also play a role during the interview. Research suggests that African-Americans may prefer greater distances than Caucasians.[9] Moreover, Wiens discusses the finding that the sexes of the participants can affect the preference for interpersonal distance.[10] One study demonstrated that male-female pairs sat the closest, followed by female-female pairs. Male-male pairs sat the furthest apart.

Kinesics

Kinesics is the study of the body in movement. It includes "gestures, movements of the body, limbs, hands, head, feet, and legs, facial expressions (smiles), eye behavior (blinking, direction and length of gaze, and pupil dilation) and posture."[11] In short, kinesics is the study of how people move their body parts through space with an added attempt to understand why such movements are made. As a field, it is a natural companion to proxemics. Like proxemics, it had its own avatar of sorts, Ray T. Birdwhistell, who first elaborated his work in 1952 with the book *Introduction to Kinesics: An Annotation System for Analysis of Body Motion and Gesture.*[12]

Birdwhistell is an anthropologist and emphasized understanding body movements in the context of their occurrence. He also pioneered the study of videotapes in an effort to decipher the subtle nuances of movement. Through his microanalysis he attempted to define the basic identifiable units of movement. For instance, he coined the word "kine" to represent the basic kinesic unit with a discernible meaning.[13]

Albert Scheflen, a student of Birdwhistell's, expanded these notions to the study of broad patterns of kinesic exchange between people. In this context Scheflen postulated that kinesic behavior frequently functions as a method of controlling the actions of others.[14] By way of example, hand gestures and eye contact may be used to determine who should be speaking at any given moment in a conversation.

Kinesics plays a role in all interviews. Specific activities may shut down or facilitate the verbal output of any given patient. Besides yielding information that may help the clinician to foster engagement, the study of kinesics can provide valuable insights into the feelings and thoughts of patients. Freud phrased it nicely when he stated, "He that has eyes to see and ears to hear may convince himself that no mortal can keep a secret. If his lips are silent, he chatters with his finger-tips; betrayal oozes out of him at every pore."[15]

Paralanguage

The study of paralanguage focuses on how messages are delivered. It may include elements such as tone of voice, loudness of voice, pitch of voice, and fluency of speech.[16] The power of paralanguage is immense and popularly acknowledged. Phrases such as, "It's not what you said, but the way you said it that I don't like," are considered legitimate complaints in our society. One can easily picture John Wayne snarling out such a phrase to some unruly bandit. Moreover, actors and comedians are well aware of the power of timing and tone of voice as it impacts upon the meaning of a statement.

By way of illustration, the phrase "that was a real nice job in there" appears complimentary at first glance. But one cannot determine its meaning unless one hears the tone of voice used in its conveyance. It could be far from pleasant if it was said with a sarcastic sneer by a displeased supervisor following an interview observed via a one-way mirror.

Besides the tone of the voice, speech is characterized by a number of other vocalizations. Although not words per se, vocalizations can play an important role in communication. One set of vocalizations consists of "speech disturbances."[17] Under the heading of flustered or confused speech, these disturbances include entities such as stutters, slips of the tongue, repetitions, word omissions, and sentence incompletions, as well as familiar vocalizations such as "ah" or "uhm." Such disturbances occur roughly one time for every 16 spoken words. As would be expected, under stressful conditions these disturbances increase significantly. Thus they can serve to warn the clinician of patient anxiety as the interview proceeds.

There is more to vocalizations than just their appearance or lack of it. Some vocalizations serve to enhance blending, as seen with the frequently used facilitatory statements "uh-huh" and "go on." But once again the way in which these vocalizations are used can significantly alter their effectiveness, as shown in the following vignette.

The interviewer in question possessed a pleasant and upbeat personality. He was a caring clinician, but he found patients shutting down at times during his interviews. Videotape analysis revealed an interesting phenomenon. As he listened to patients, he frequently interspersed his silences with the vocalization "uh-huh." His "uh-huhs" were said quickly with a mild sharpness to his voice as if chopping off sausages. He also used vocalizations such as "yep" and "yea," also stated with a curt tone of voice.

The net result was the creation of the feeling that he was in a hurry, wanting just the facts. And that is exactly what his patients gave him. This habit, combined with a tendency to overutilize note-taking, fostered a business-like persona, despite his natural warmness in daily conversation. It was a habit well worth breaking and once again highlights the power of paralanguage.

Cross-cultural differences also affect paralanguage. Sue and Sue describe the variations in paralanguage that can interfere with the blending or assessment process when working with people outside the clinician's culture. For instance, silences are frequently interpreted as moments when the patient, for conscious or unconscious reasons, is holding back. Silence may also signal that the patient is ready for a new question. At other moments, silence can create a feeling of uneasiness in both interviewer and interviewee.

But as Sue and Sue clearly state, the obvious may be too obvious.

*A*lthough silence may be viewed negatively by Americans, other cultures interpret and use silence much differently. The English and Arabs use silence for privacy, whereas the Russians, French, and Spanish read it as agreement among parties. In Asian culture silence is traditionally a sign of respect for elders. Furthermore, silence by many Chinese and Japanese is not a floor-yielding signal inviting others to pick up the conversation. Rather, it may indicate a desire to continue speaking after making a particular point. Oftentimes, silence is a sign of politeness and respect rather than lack of desire to continue speaking. A counselor uncomfortable with silence may fill in and prevent the client from elaborating further. An even greater danger is to impute false motives to the client's apparent reticence.[18]

Many other cultural subleties exist, but they are beyond the scope of this text. Clinicians frequently working with other cultures should make it a point to understand the cultural characteristics of their clients.

CLINICAL APPLICATION OF NONVERBAL BEHAVIOR

Assessment of the Patient

Sir Denis Hill made the following observations during the 47th Maudsley Lecture in 1972:

*M*any experienced psychiatrists of an earlier generation believed that they could predict the likely mental state of the majority of the patients they met by observations within the first few minutes of contact before verbal interchange had begun. They did this from observation of nonverbal behavior—the appearance, bodily posture, facial expression, spontaneous movements and the initial bodily responses to forthcoming verbal interaction.[19]

Sir Denis Hill was concerned that the ability to observe nonverbal behavior astutely represented a skill that had fallen by the wayside. Let us hope this demise is not the case, because experienced clinicians today as much as yesterday need to utilize nonverbal clues throughout their clinical work. The knowledge available today concerning nonverbal behaviors is significantly more advanced than 40 or 50 years ago. It is to this knowledge that we now turn our attention.

To begin our discussion we will look at another statement by Sir Denis Hill: "An important difference between the disturbed mental states which we term 'neurotic' and those we term 'psychotic' is that in the latter, but not in the former, those aspects of nonverbal behavior which maintain social interactional processes tend to be lost."[20]

An awareness of these potential deficits in the psychotic patient can alert the clinician to carefully probe for more explicit psychotic material in a patient whose psychotic process is subtle.

Perhaps an example will be useful at this time. I was observing an initial assessment between a talented trainee and a woman in her mid-20s. The patient had been urged to the assessment by her sister and a close friend. Apparently the patient's mother was currently hospitalized with major depression.

By the end of the interview, the clinician seemed aware that the patient was probably also suffering from major depression or some form of an affective illness. But the severity of the patient's condition did not seem to have registered. Instead the clinician was about to recommend outpatient follow-up. The patient's nonverbal behavior was telling the clinician to take another look. In the second interview, which I performed, the patient disclosed a recent weekend brimming with psychotic terror. She had felt that her long-dead father had returned to the house to murder her. She was so convinced of this delusion that she had shared her secret with several young siblings, not a good idea if one is trying to get baby brother and sister to sleep. Eventually she ran from her house to escape her father's wrath. Even in the interview she could not clearly state that her father's return was an impossibility, although she hesitatingly said she thought it was.

Let us return to the interview in order to uncover the nonverbal cues that suggested the possibility of an underlying psychotic process. The patient, whom we shall call Mary, answered honestly and appeared cooperative. She displayed no loosening of associations or other overt evidence of thought process disorganization, but she demonstrated some oddities in her communicational style. With regard to paralanguage, she demonstrated long pauses (about 4 to 8 seconds) before beginning many of her responses. This gave her a somewhat distracted appearance as if muddled by her thinking. This effect was heightened by a mild slowing of her speech and a flattening of the tone of her speech as well.

As we have seen, silences, especially of this length, are generally avoided in daily conversation. Everyday social protocol would ordinarily pressure Mary to answer more quickly. This breakdown in normal communicational interaction was one suggestion that all was not well and represents a disruption of the empathy cycle. Her body also spoke to her internal turmoil.

Although for the most part she had reasonably good eye contact, there existed protracted periods of time when she looked slightly away from the interviewer in a distracted fashion, whether she was talking or listening. This lack of "visual touching" during conversation is unusual.[21, 22]

Frequently, before beginning to speak, the intended speaker glances away briefly. As he or she looks back, speech will begin. While talking the speaker will frequently look away. But as the end of the speaker's statement is reached, the speaker will look towards the listener. This glance signals the listener that the speaker's message is over. The speaker and the listener glance at each other's eye regions in varying lengths, usually between 1 and 7 seconds, the listener giving longer contact. This complex eye duet was frequently missing with Mary. In depression the eyes are frequently cast downward, but it is the peculiar manner in which Mary tended to stare past the clinician that hinted at the possible presence of psychotic process. As Sir Denis Hill had suggested, Mary had lost some of the nonverbal cues that maintain social interaction.

Other kinesic indicators of speech pattern have been called "markers of speech."[23] For instance, hand gestures are generally made as one initiates words or phrases. As the speaker finishes commenting, the hands may tend to assume a position of rest. To keep one's hands upwards, in front of oneself, can indicate that one is not done speaking or will soon interrupt.

In Mary these markers of speech were generally diminished. She sat stiffly with her feet flat on the floor. Her head seemed to weigh her body down as she sat slightly hunched over with her fingers interlocked. She displayed little hand gesturing, leaving the interviewer with the odd sensation that it was not clear when Mary was going to start or stop speaking. Most likely, Mary's lack of movement was an associated aspect of her major depression, but it may also have been a ramification of her psychotic process.

A more striking nonverbal clue to the degree of Mary's psychopathology lay in her method of dealing with unwanted environmental input, in this instance the questions of the interviewer. Apparently Mary had been concerned for some time that she might be "just like her mother," who was currently in the hospital. In addition, her sister had undergone a psychotic depression approximately 6 months earlier. Mary had been attempting to hide from herself the evidence of her own psychotic process, while the fear of an impending breakdown nagged at her daily. During the interview, as questions directed her back into her paranoid fears, she began to realize the extent of her problems. At this moment she did something out of the ordinary.

Mary leaned forward slowly, her elbows perched upon the tops of her knees with her head cupped between her hands. In this position her hands literally covered her ears, as if keeping out unwanted questions or thoughts. All eye contact was disrupted. Mary remained in this position for a good 5 minutes, answering questions slowly but cooperatively. She appeared detached from the world around her. This type of behavior has been studied under the rubric of "cut-offs."[24] Cut-offs represent nonverbal behaviors made to dampen out environmental stress. When exaggerated to the degree of appearing socially inappropriate, as was the case with Mary, they may be indicators of psychotic process. Indeed, catatonic withdrawal represents a prolonged and drastic cut-off.

One must also attempt to compare nonverbal activities to the patient's baseline behavior. Mary was normally a high-functioning secretary and most likely possessed better than average social skills. In this light, her preoccupied conversational attitude, and in particular her prolonged cut-off, represents very deviant behavior for her. A subsequent interview with Mary's friend revealed that Mary had been observed at work sitting and staring at the phone for hours.

For a moment I would like to elaborate on the issue of cut-offs. We have been discussing dramatic forms of cut-off behavior, which may indicate underlying psychotic activity, but mild forms of cut-off behavior occur routinely in our work with nonpsychotic individuals. These more subtle forms of cut-off are not without meaning and warrant some discussion. Morris[25] described four such visual cut-offs, to which he attaches some descriptively poetic names.

With the "Evasive Eye," the patient shuns eye contact by looking distractedly towards the ground, as if studying some invisible object. It can create the feeling that the patient is purposely not attending to the conversation and may frequently accompany the speech of disinterested adolescents. In the so-called "Shifty Eye," the patient repeatedly glances away and back again. With the "Stuttering Eye," the patient now faces the interviewer directly, but the eyelids rapidly waver up and down as if swatting away the clinician's glance. Finally, in the "Stammering Eye" the patient once again faces the clinician but shuts the eyes with an exaggerated blink.

These four eye maneuvers represent nonverbal activities whose meaning may be multiple. They may indicate that the patient at some level no longer wants to communicate. Perhaps a specific topic has been raised that is disturbing to the patient, resulting in a nonverbal resistance. At such moments a simple question such as, "I am wondering what is passing through your mind right now," may uncover pertinent material. Such cut-offs may also represent objective signs of decreased blending and movement into a shut-down interview. Exaggerated examples of these cut-offs can also be part of a histrionic presentation and in this sense could also be seen in both wandering and rehearsed interviews.

Investigators have also looked at the promising possibility that nonverbal activities could provide even more specific diagnostic clues, but at this point the research results remain tentative.[26, 27] Moreover, the results appear to be in accordance with what common clinical sense would predict.

Concerning the diagnoses found on Axis I, schizophrenia appears to be accompanied by some distinctive nonverbal behaviors. Studies show that schizophrenic presentations are marked by a tendency for gaze aversion. A flattening of affect with decreased movement of the eyebrows was noted (which could alternatively be secondary to antipsychotic medication). Patients' postures were slumped, and they had a tendency to lean away from the interviewer. Naturally the type of schizophrenia and the stage of the process could significantly affect the type of nonverbal behavior present, emphasizing a cautionary note to these generalizations.

Depression has also been investigated. Researchers have noted that nonverbal behaviors vary depending on whether one is observing an agitated depression or a retarded depression. In the agitated depression, patients demonstrated "a puzzled expression, grimacing and frowning, gaze aversion, agitated movements, a crouched posture, and body leaning towards the interviewer. Subgroup 2 (retarded depressives) showed some increase in gaze, slowed movements, self-touching, an emotionally blank expression, and a backward lean away from the interviewer."[28] In many respects, these findings have limited usefulness, because they simply seem to confirm the obvious.

But at a different level, especially with depressive patients, these findings emphasize the importance of nonverbal behaviors as clinical indicators of improvement.[29] The return of routine hand gesturing may herald an oncoming remission even before the patient admits to much subjective improvement. As the clinician becomes more aware of such behaviors as spontaneity of facial expression, smiling behavior, and eye contact, the informal monitoring of such cues to improvement can become a routine element of clinical follow-up.

With regard to Axis II, less research is available. Consequently, we will emphasize principles derived from clinical observations. Observations made during the first 5 minutes of the scouting period may provide important diagnostic clues. In this sense, these cues can help determine which diagnostic regions to emphasize in the body of the interview, for in the limited time available, it is generally not feasible to explore all areas of Axis II pathology. The following three clinical vignettes illustrate the usefulness of nonverbal activities in suggesting the presence of possible character pathology.

In the first example, I was observing an interview performed by a psychiatric resident during morning rounds on an inpatient unit. The patient was an adolescent girl with a head of curly light-reddish hair. The interviewer was sitting on a couch in a group activity room. The patient pertly entered the room and promptly plunked down beside the clinician. At first she leaned towards him with her right arm straddling the back of the couch behind his shoulder, but she quickly withdrew the arm. Her final perch was with her right knee up on the couch resting a few inches from the clinician's body.

In a proxemic sense, she had positioned herself well within the personal distance zone and actually very close to being within the clinician's intimate zone. Her speech was bright and snappy, percolating from a face rich with expressions and playful eyes. All this activity occurred in a matter of a few seconds. The clinician immediately responded by leaning away from the patient and crossing his legs by placing his left ankle over his right knee. This brief territorial excursion by this patient is not a typical initial interaction, even with adolescents who frequently feel more comfortable with "chummier" interpersonal distances. Instead, this type of interpersonal game may be seen in people with underlying histrionic personality traits or borderline personality traits.

The second patient was a woman in late middle age, with graying hair pulled back in a bun. Before the interview, she had had to wait longer than usual before entering the room. Initially, the clinician gently apologized for the inconvenience with a warm smile on his face. She made cool eye contact. Her lips did not so much as consider returning his smile. She fluctuated between a baseline of mildly cooperative answers, with a reasonably lengthy duration of utterance (DOU), to brusque shut-down remarks.

A peculiar piece of body movement gradually evolved as she continued with her acerbic tone of voice. She tended to lean back in her chair and gradually proceeded to stretch her legs out in front of her towards the interviewer. The movement was ingeniously slow but as steady as a barge pulling into a dock. As usually happens, the dock was gently bumped by her feet, at which point she did not pull away. Instead, the dock recoiled, with the interviewer quickly tucking his feet beneath his chair.

Her nonverbal activities may be multiply determined, but one possibility well worth exploring would be underlying passive-

160 Fundamentals of Interviewing

aggressive traits. Later historical information from the interview tended to further substantiate this diagnostic hunch.

The third and final patient carefully orchestrated a relatively unappealing opening gambit. She was a tall woman in her mid-20s with long black hair hanging limply about her body. She was dressed in jeans and a black pullover sweater. Her first noticeably unusual action consisted of reaching over to pull up a chair, which she promptly used as a footstool. She stretched her body out, making herself conspicuously at home. This settling in did not signify the beginning of an easy engagement, because she proceeded to visually cut the female interviewer off throughout most of the interview. She would look down at her hands, frequently using the Evasive Eye movement described earlier.

All of this display was topped with a convincingly dour facial expression. Concerning paralanguage, she managed to push through her disinterested facial mask an equally disinterested and mumbling voice. Her attitude visibly disturbed the interviewer. She also demonstrated one other nonverbal communication with a set meaning. Specifically, she held her coat on her lap throughout the interview, perhaps communicating an eagerness to leave.

Her collection of behaviors, all present during the first few minutes of the interview, suggested a variety of personality traits worth exploring later. Her lack of concern for making the interviewer feel more at ease could suggest a possible hint of antisocial leanings. Along similar lines her obvious attempt to display disinterest could be part of the manipulative trappings of a borderline personality or perhaps of a narcissistic personality. And as we saw with our previous example, some passive-aggressive tendencies may be present. Her behaviors in no way prove that she has any of these disorders, but they do provide suggestions of which disorders warrant additional consideration, further highlighting the importance of noting nonverbal behavior.

Let us now move from away from diagnostic issues, and look at some of the nonverbal clues that may suggest that patients are feeling uncomfortable or anxious.

One of the most well-known indicators of increased anxiety remains the activation of the sympathetic nervous system, the system geared to prepare the organism for fight or flight. During the activation of this system a variety of physiologic adaptations occur that can serve as hallmarks of anxiety. The heart will beat faster and blood will be shunted away from the skin and gut to be preferentially directed towards the muscle tissue that is being prepared for action. This shunting accounts for the paleness so frequently seen in acutely anxious people, who look like they have seen a ghost. Saliva production decreases, and the bowels and bladder are slower to eliminate. Breathing rate increases, as does the production of sweat.

This last sign, increased sweating, reminds me of one of the more striking and humorous examples of autonomic discharge I have encountered. A medical student was doing one of his first physical examinations on a real patient, which can truly be an upsetting experience, as the student frequently feels painfully inept. In this case, the patient was a child about 9 years old, who could be generally classified under the label "brat." As the exam labored onward, with the worried mother looking increasingly fretful, the student began to sweat profusely. As the student leaned over to listen to the child's heart, a bead of sweat fell from his forehead directly onto the child's chest. Being a subtle kid, he immediately looked the student in the eye and in a loud voice said, "What's a matter with you, you're sweatin' all over me!"

If the poor student was not already uptight, that little proclamation did it. He sheepishly turned to the increasingly upset mother and produced a quick-witted white lie, "Don't worry, I've got a thyroid condition." I know this story all too well because I was the poor panic-stricken medical student. It clearly shows the truth that the autonomic system does not lie. With our patients, subtle signs of anxiety such as sweating, damp palms, and increased breathing rate can help us detect anxiety. If the anxiety represents evidence of poor blending, we may be able to purposely attend to the patient's fears. If it represents the presence of unsettling thoughts, we may be inclined to probe deeper.

If the sympathetic system is not presented with a chance to actually get the organism into action soon enough, the parasympathetic system may try to counterbalance with a discharge of its own. In these cases, one may find a sudden urge to urinate or defecate, as people frequently feel before public performances or job interviews. If a patient begins a session by immediately requesting the need for a restroom, this may represent a clue to a higher anxiety level than the patient may verbally admit.

Other good indicators of anxiety are described by Morris under the rubric of "displacement activities."[30] These activities are those body movements that release underlying tension. I recently watched a businessman waiting for a meeting. As he sat in the lobby, he nervously tugged at his tie and picked at his clothes. He then hoisted his briefcase onto his lap and meticulously unloaded it piece by piece, after which he gingerly repacked the case, carefully feeling each object as he delicately reassembled his "peripheral brain."

These behaviors were accomplishing very little in the way of needed physical functions, but they offered a calming effect of some sort for the businessman. Other typical displacement activities include smoking, twirling one's hair, picking at one's fingers, nailbiting, playing with rings, twitching one's feet, tugging at the ear lobe, self-grooming activities, tearing at paper cups, and twirling and biting pens. The list could certainly be extended. For instance, Morris points out that serving drinks and holding them in one's hands at cocktail parties probably serve to decrease people's anxiety, as they "have something to do."[31]

Clinically speaking, displacement activities are worth noting during both the initial interview and subsequent psychotherapy. Each patient seems to display a unique set of displacement activities. Once decoded by the clinician, these activities can be usually reliable indicators of patient anxiety. When suddenly increased, they may represent a more reliable indicator than the patient's facial expression or verbal response that an interpretation was on the mark.

It is also of interest that anxiety will sometimes display itself not through the appearance of displacement activities but in their conspicuous absence. When engaged in an active conversation, most people will display a normal amount of periodic displacement activities. If these suddenly stop or are not present from the beginning, then the person may be experiencing anxiety. In a sense the person may be trying to avoid mistakes by doing nothing.

This "still-life response" frequently appears when people are videotaped or interviewed in public. It seems to afflict interviewers even more than patients. Supervisors need to be aware that this response may be more of an artifact than a stylistic marker.

Another area of interest revolves around facial clues that the patient is visibly shaken or on the verge of tears. I am sure the reader is well aware of the faint quiverings of the chin and glazed quality of the eyes that frequently indicate that a patient is close to tears. But a fact not as well publicized is the tendency for people to demonstrate extremely fine muscle twitches across their faces when stressed. These frequently occur beside the nostrils and on the cheek. In people who demonstrate this tendency, these fine twitches can be extremely accurate indicators of tension.

By way of example, I was working with a young businesswoman during an initial interview. She had been referred to me for psychotherapy. She was attractively dressed with a bright disposition and her speech was accompanied by a collection of animated gestures. When asked to talk about her history, she launched into a detailed review of her life since age 16. Of note was her striking avoidance of any events prior to age 16.

When asked why she had done this, she responded that she did not know and had not noticed it. I asked her if any aspects of her life seemed different before the age of 16. She commented, "Not really, although I spent more time with my father back then." At that point a few muscle twitches appeared by her left nostril. I commented that I had a feeling she was feeling upset, and she burst into tears. Subsequent therapy revealed a complex and ambivalent relationship with her father and other male figures. Throughout therapy, these faint twitches were a sure sign of tension.

This issue of tension leads directly to another important aspect of nonverbal behavior, the detection of deception. In one piece of research a group of nursing students were asked to participate in a study in which they would be asked to deceive a person.[32] They were told that gentle deceptions were sometimes needed in clinical work, as when comforting frightened patients. Thus the nurses felt a need to perform well in the testing situation.

In the research itself the nurses were exposed to two different types of films. Some films were pleasant in nature, such as an ocean scene, and other films depicted unpleasant scenes such as a burn victim and a limb amputation. After seeing the pleasant film segments, the nurses were asked to describe their feelings to the listener. This task was obviously not problematic. But after viewing the unsettling film, in one experimental design, the nurse had to convince the listener that the gory film was pleasant and enjoyable to watch. This task was not so easy. Indeed, it so reproduced the sensation of lying that some nurses dropped out of the study.

All of these interactions were videotaped. Segments of these videotapes were then shown to subjects, who were supposed to determine from the visual images who was indeed lying. It was an ingenious experiment and represents the foundation work upon which further research on deception proceeded.

The original researchers, Ekman and Friesen, predicted that subjects would state that while lying they would focus on making their faces "look natural." This prediction proved to be true. The deceivers did attend to their faces more, which suggested that nonverbal activities from the neck down may provide a better lead concerning deception. Interestingly, trained observers could pick up clues of deception from videotaped facial expressions. These microexpressions represent accurate clues but are too difficult to pick up routinely.

On the other hand, the body of the deceiver had a tendency to betray its own head, so to speak, and further research has substantiated many of these initial findings as described in Ekman's fascinating book *Telling Lies*.[33] Apparently, changes in below-the-neck movements may be of the most practical significance for accurately detecting deception. Direct communications or emblems, as Ekman refers to them, can sometimes be useful indicators of deceit. Emblems represent nonverbal behaviors that carry a distinct meaning, such as a yes or no head nod or pointing to an object. Just as slips of the tongue may betray hidden feelings, slips of the body can occur. With the nursing students in the above study, many felt a helpless sensation that they were not hiding their feelings well. This feeling of helplessness was sometimes inadvertently conveyed by a shrugging movement.

When representing indicators of nonverbal leakage, emblems usually appear in part. Thus only one shoulder may partially rise or one palm may turn up during a shrug. Another good indicator that an emblem represents a deceitful mannerism is the display of the emblem in an unusual placement. An angry fist will not be raised towards an antagonist but will quietly appear by the side of the patient.

Hand gestures, which people make while speaking, have been called illustrators by Ekman, and they tend to decrease when deceit is under way. This decrease is particularly true if the patient has not had time to rehearse the lie and must carefully attend to what is being said. The clinician can monitor behaviors such as those described above while exploring regions in which resistance and deceit may be high. For example, when eliciting a drug and alcohol history from a typically active interviewee, a sudden decrease in associated hand movements may suggest that deception is occurring. Several other studies have also found supportive evidence for the idea that below-the-neck clues are best for detecting deceit on a practical level.[34, 35]

Besides kinesic indicators of deception, the clinician can look for paralanguage clues that deceit is occurring.[36] For instance, a higher pitch to the voice has been associated with deception as well as emotions such as fear. In a complementary sense, lower pitches have been associated with judgments by observers that the subject is more relaxed and sociable. Another possible clue to deception involves the response time latency (RTL). Deceptive subjects were found to demonstrate a longer RTL and to give longer answers when in the act of deceiving.

It should be kept in mind that most of the kinesic and paralanguage clues to deception mentioned so far represent nonverbal activities, not nonverbal communications. Thus these behaviors may be multiply determined and do not in any way ensure that the patient is being deceitful. In many cases, they may simply indicate that the patient is feeling more anxious. Each activity must be interpreted in the interpersonal matrix in which it was born. By way of example, one researcher found that an increased latency of response could be interpreted in different fashions. If it was followed by a self-promoting comment, then it was often interpreted as being an indication of deception. On the other hand, if the pause was followed by a self-deprecating comment, it was often registered in the opposite direction as evidence of a truthful remark.[37]

It is probably best to conclude the discussion of cues of deception at this point. Clearly the research is somewhat tentative, but it suggests that some changes in the baseline behavior of the patient may provide useful hints that deception may be at hand. Two practical points warrant mentioning. First, as the interview proceeds, it is generally a good idea to ascertain the baseline body movements that are typical of the patient. Second, during sensitive inquiries, it is best to avoid notetaking. Notetaking can completely eliminate the ability of the interviewer to observe the subtle nonverbal clues that may be the only warnings of deception.

In the same sense that nonverbal activities may indicate that the patient may be deceiving the clinician, a variety of important mixed nonverbal messages may be sent to an interviewer. These mixed messages are not necessarily deceptions. Instead, they may represent hallmarks of patient ambivalence and confusion.

In order to explore this fascinating area, the work of Grinder and Bandler[38] offers a wellspring of practical and sound clinical observation. Although controversy has arisen over their later work, their first two books provide some pioneering insights into engagement techniques.

Their work follows naturally from the principles we have been discussing thus far. Put simplistically, they state that as a person communicates a message, the message is transferred through a variety of communicational channels simultaneously. The patient's message may be conveyed through the content of the spoken words, the tone of voice, the rate of speech, the amount and type of hand gesturing, the posture, and the facial expression. These messages are termed paramessages. When all paramessages have the same meaning, the paramessages are said to be congruent. But if some of the channels convey discordant information, then the paramessages are said to be incongruent.

The underlying theory is simple; perhaps that is why it proves to be so powerful therapeutically. People who consistently communicate with an incongruent style can frequently create a confusing impression. Their incongruence may make the people around them feel ill at ease and uncomfortable. If the clinician can detect this self-defeating interpersonal style, he or she may be able to help the patient modify it. In a more immediate sense, incongruent paramessages may indicate underlying mixed feelings of which the patient is unaware. Once again, the therapist may be able to cue off this incongruence, leading the patient into an exploration of the uncovered mixed feelings.

More germane to the topic of the initial diagnostic interview, episodes of incongruent communication may alert the clinician to areas worthy of more immediate investigation or perhaps regions pertinent to explore in later sessions.

I am reminded of a woman in her early 30s who I was evaluating for possible psychotherapy or medication. Ms. Davis, as we shall call her, was coping with a variety of stresses, not the least of which was the loss of her mother several months earlier. For years she had been her mother's caretaker and verbal whipping post. Ms. Davis was mildly overweight with stocky legs, offset by a face embraced by a full head of black hair. As she spoke, her conversation turned to her bitter relationship with her boyfriend, who apparently enjoyed her sexually but found marital ceremonies not to his liking. She commented, "I hate him, I'll never go back to him. He's not worth it."

Harsh words, but one should be wary of taking them too seriously, for Ms. Davis' body spoke differently. The words were spoken with a tone of pained resignation, not biting anger. They had the quality of the child-like pout, "Daddy's not bringing home a present from his vacation." Not only did her voice lack self-indignation, but her hands played a martyr's role. Rather than the more typical pointing and jerking movements of an angry accusation, they were held low towards her lap with the palms upwards. This type of hand positioning is frequently associated with a tone of supplication and need.

Put more precisely, Ms. Davis was communicating with an incongruent set of paramessages. As Grinder and Bandler point out, all of these messages may have elements of truth to them. In Ms. Davis' case, she certainly did have angry feelings towards her boyfriend, as suggested by the content of her words. But she also had extremely powerful needs to be accepted by him; indeed, these needs bordered on a masochistic willingness to be verbally beaten by him. Her tone of voice and hand gestures suggested her strong need for acceptance. Even her breathing rate did not increase or become more spurt-like, as is frequently seen as someone becomes increasingly angered. This set of incongruent messages was one of the first clues to her deeply rooted problems concerning hostile dependence, which became central working issues in the remaining therapy. Indeed, her relationship with her mother was in reality no different from her relationship with her boyfriend.

In any given initial interview, periods of incongruent communication may occur. If noted, they can serve as road signs that effectively guide the interviewer towards a deeper understanding of the patient.

In a similar fashion the work of Scheflen, whom I mentioned earlier, deserves more detailed examination, because it too focuses on the nonverbal interactions that serve as communication scripts for people.[39] Scheflen discusses the idea that humans, like other animals, engage in certain shared behaviors that tend to escalate into specific actions. Such actions include fighting behavior, mating behavior, and parenting behavior. Frequently, these mutually arousing actions serve to eliminate the actual need to engage in the final activity. In such a manner animals will frequently avoid actual combat by undergoing a territorial display of sorts. Scheflen calls such escalating patterns of behavior "kinesic reciprocals."

Kinesic reciprocals can frequently be seen in clinical interactions. If the patient begins the reciprocal, the clinician may inadvertently continue the process. I have certainly seen this process occur within the realm of the courting or mating reciprocal. I remember watching a videotape of a session of psychotherapy. The patient was a young woman interacting with her therapist, who was a relatively young man with about 7 years of clinical experience. The patient sat pertly forward, cigarette hanging aesthetically from her fingers. The therapist, who was dressed casually in a sport shirt, sat rakishly back, also with a cigarette in hand. Their voices possessed a spritely coyness.

It was unclear whether I was watching the beginning moments of a therapy session or the opening sequences of a grade B movie. In any case, the therapist and his patient were engaging in the courting reciprocal, otherwise known as flirting. Inadvertent participation in such reciprocals can create a variety of problems. Obviously it can stimulate an erotic transference. Moreover, if initiated unconsciously by the therapist and then reciprocated by the patient, it can lead the therapist towards the inappropriate perception that the patient is histrionic.

I am reminded of one clinician who tended to be pleasantly flirtatious and buoyant with staff. She was surprised when male patients, following initial evaluations, would ask her out. On videotape the answer was obvious in that some of her flirtatious qualities appeared in her clinical work, albeit in a much toned down fashion.

Scheflen provides a good description of kinesic behaviors utilized by both sexes in the courting reciprocal:

*T*he full-blown picture of the female courting posture is well known to us, for models and actresses simulate it continually in being seductive or attractive. The head is held high and cocked. The "mark" is looked at from the corners of the eyes. The chest is brought out so that the breasts protrude. And the legs appear "sexy" as the foot is extended and the calf musculature is tightened. . . . An actively courting woman may present her palm, a highly affiliative act, in many ways; e.g., when she pushes back her hair, when she smokes, or when she covers her mouth while coughing.

. . . The man's state of high tonus is evident most clearly in the thoracic-abdominal behavior. He moves from a slump, with abdominal protrusion to thoracic display by sucking in his belly and squaring his shoulders. A man may use some of the same behavior in courting that he uses in dominance. He may draw up to full height, protrude his jaw, stand in close, and display what is generally regarded as a masculine stance.[40]

Other reciprocal behaviors besides the courting reciprocal can occur in an initial interview. A striking example was provided by a videotape made of an initial interview for use in supervision.

The interviewer was a young woman. Across from her the patient sat with eyes occasionally cast downwards. As the interview unfolded, the patient produced a folded piece of paper, and she asked the clinician to read the paper before proceeding. Her voice seemed to step meekly away from her lips. In the meantime the patient began fumbling with the microphone. She had correctly wrapped it around her neck but had problems attaching it to her blouse. Noticing her problems the clinician looked over and asked if she needed help. The patient did not look up for a moment as she continued to fumble. Then with her head cocked downwards, she innocently glanced upwards shaking her head "yes." She gazed with the helpless eyes of a little girl and said not a word. The clinician promptly leaned over and fixed the microphone.

The parenting reciprocal had emerged as naturally as if enacted between a true mother and her child. In this brief vignette, the power of the first few minutes of the scouting period to provide clues for further diagnostic probing is once again amply demonstrated. This patient's manipulative style and dependent behavior suggested the possibility of some form of character pathology. Indeed, further interviewing revealed a mixed personality disorder with histrionic, passive-aggressive, and dependent characteristics. Apparently this patient had perfected the art of eliciting parental responses as a method of garnering attention.

This patient also displayed another type of nonverbal activity, auto-contact behavior. Auto-contact behavior consists of movements involving self-touching.[41] Such behaviors may consist of grooming behaviors, defensive-covering behaviors, and self-intimacies.

Self-intimacies are defined as, "movements that provide comfort because they are unconsciously mimed acts of being touched by someone else."[42] These self-intimacies appear frequently during interviews. Patients may hold their own hands or sit with their knees pulled up to their faces, arms literally hugging their own legs. In regressed patients, one can see even more extreme forms of self-hugging as patients lay in tightly curled fetal positions.

With regard to frequency, the most common self-intimacies in order of most to least frequent are as follows: (1) the jaw support,

(2) the chin support, (3) the hair clasp, (4) the cheek support, (5) the mouth touch, and (6) the temple support. With hair touching there is a 3:1 bias in favor of women. Temple touching demonstrates the opposite bias with a preference in men of 2:1. Sometimes these kinesthetic comforters can be tied into other sensory modalities as well. I remember one patient who would pull her hair across her cheek. She would simultaneously gently sniff at her hair, which she related as being very comforting. Such activity was a sure sign of her underlying anxiety, much like a displacement activity.

In this manner these behaviors may serve to alert the interviewer that the patient is feeling pained or anxious. It can cue the interviewer that the patient may need some verbal comforting, perhaps prompting an empathic statement. It can also alert the clinician that powerful affective material is being approached, possibly suggesting the need for further exploration.

In summary, in the above material the focus has been on the power of the patient's body to convey information to the perceptive clinician. It is now time to explore the reverse situation, those moments when the clinician uses his or her body to affect the patient.

Utilization of Nonverbal Behavior to Engage the Patient

SEATING ARRANGEMENT AND PROXEMICS

One of the exercises undertaken in our interviewing class concerns the use of seating arrangement. Two of the trainees sit in the middle of the room on easily rolled chairs. They are given a simple task, to situate themselves so that they feel the most comfortable with regard to conversing with one another. In about 90% of the cases, the participants choose a similar position.

They sit roughly 4 to 5 feet apart. They are turned towards each other but do not quite directly face one another. Instead, they are turned about a 5 to 10-degree angle off the line directly between them, both in the same direction, as shown in Figure 3A. Only about 10% choose to face each other directly.

If the participants are asked to turn directly towards each other, they complain of feeling significantly less comfortable. Some will even push their chairs back a bit. The discomfort is related as feeling "too close." More specifically, many of the trainees complain that the head-on position forces eye contact, making it difficult to break eye contact without undertaking a significant head movement. This head-on position fosters a sensation of confrontation.

On the other hand, the preferred position readily allows for good eye contact but also makes it easy to break contact in an unawkward fashion. In my own practice, I have certainly found this position to be the most comfortable and the most flexible inter-

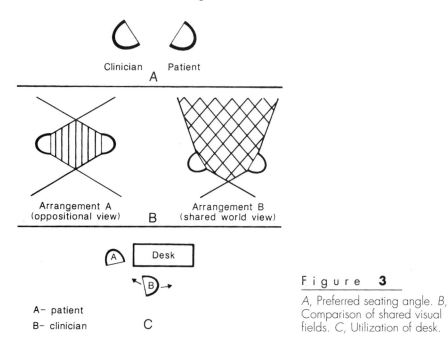

Clinician   Patient

A

Arrangement A
(oppositional view)   B   Arrangement B
(shared world view)

Desk

A— patient
B— clinician   C

F i g u r e   **3**

A, Preferred seating angle. B,
Comparison of shared visual
fields. C, Utilization of desk.

viewing position for me. This last statement is important, because it emphasizes that the most comfortable position may be different for each interviewer and indeed for each interviewing dyad. Each clinician needs to discover a comfortable position, keeping in mind that the clinician must also be willing to alter this position depending on the needs of the patient.

In addition to the nonconfrontational feeling provided by the position described above, another phenomenon may be enhancing its comfortableness. As discussed before, one of the key processes that enhances blending is the ability of the clinician to convey a sense of seeing the world through a shared perspective.

If one looks at the actual fields of vision available to each participant in the interview, an important relationship readily becomes apparent. When two people are directly facing each other, the fields of vision exhibit little overlap. What overlap exists lies directly between the two participants. This situation tends to foster the sensation that "You are over there, and I am here." It seems to work against the sensation of "We are here together." On the other hand, when the two participants are turned slightly away from each other, so that they are subtly facing the same direction, then the feeling that "We are here, and the rest of the world is out there" naturally emerges.

Thus, in a phenomenological sense, the feeling of confrontation is decreased, while the sense of blending is given a gentle boost, as illustrated in Figure 3B. It should be noted that the directly opposi-tional position may be preferred by some people. Indeed, some clinicians recommend it,[43] but I myself do not, for the reasons pro-vided above.

The concept of seating raises the more general issue of furniture arrangement. Some clinicians prefer setting, away from their desk, two large comfortable chairs. Another alternative is to utilize the desk creatively. In general, I believe a desk should not sit between the clinician and the patient, because this creates an authoritarian distance appropriate for chief executive officers, not therapists.

On the other hand, the desk can be placed as shown in Figure 3C with only a corner protruding between the clinician and the patient. If the clinician's chair rides on wheels, the clinician can move the chair and alter the resultant interpersonal distance either by increasing or decreasing the amount of desk between the partici-pants. A paranoid patient may require more distance from the clinician, which can easily be accomplished by moving only a short way, because the desk quickly provides a protective barrier. On the other hand, the clinician can easily move to a point where essentially no desk intervenes.

The overall concept of the clinical setting warrants attention. When designing a private office, an effort should be made to provide a comfortable and professional atmosphere. The office represents an extension of the clinician's persona, and the patient's first impression in the scouting period may be significantly affected by the decor of the clinician's waiting area or office. Calming prints or photographs, accompanied by several diplomas and shelves of books, provide a reassuring and pleasant environment.

Trainees are faced with limited financial resources. But three or four unframed art posters and a few plants can be bought very reasonably, producing a sometimes startling change in the atmo-sphere of the room. There is no need for a trainee's room to look like a prison cell. On the contrary, part of the training experience is learning to consider the principles behind creating an appropriate private office.

Outside the office, situations can be a bit more difficult, because the clinician faces crowded hospital rooms and disorganized emer-gency rooms. It remains important in these situations to consider the comfort of both the patient and the clinician. While performing a consultation in a crowded hospital room, there is nothing wrong with saying, "Before we start, would you mind if I slide your bed over, so both of us can have more room to talk."

This discussion of seating arrangements leads to the issue of determining an optimum distance between the clinician and the patient, which will vary for each interviewing dyad. There does seem to exist a small region in which the clinician's presence respects the patient's sense of personal space while still allowing the movements of the clinician to have an immediate impact on the patient. This zone of effective interpersonal space may be referred to as the "responsive zone" (RZ). If the clinician moves out of the RZ towards the patient, then the interviewer risks frightening the patient or creating a sense of discomfort. On the other hand, if the interviewer leaves the RZ by moving too far away from the patient, then the movements of the clinician may have little impact on the patient. For instance, the act of gently leaning forward towards a patient, which can enhance communication during particularly sensitive moments of an interview, may have no effect if done outside the RZ.

Two examples may help clarify the importance of establishing an RZ that seems most comfortable for each patient. First, if one intuits that a patient may be feeling paranoid, it is useful to remember that such patients may require a larger space around them in order to feel more comfortable. In these cases the RZ is larger and it may be wise to begin such interviews sitting further from the patient than one normally would sit or perhaps using a desk or table to help provide a safety barrier as mentioned earlier. As the interchange proceeds the clinician may find that the distance can be gradually decreased; hence the RZ frequently may change as the blending waxes or wanes.

In the second example, one looks at the problem of accurately eliciting a formal cognitive examination in elderly patients who are seriously depressed and withdrawn. To attract and maintain their attention, the interviewer might need to sit considerably closer than normal. This more intimate RZ may help decrease the likelihood of obtaining poor cognitive results secondary to the patient's lack of attention or interest. If a patient is not interested in answering, then the risk of getting artificially low scores becomes very real indeed. In such cases the tendency to suspect a real dementia when only a pseudodementia is present can become a true dilemma.

Another way of obtaining the withdrawn patient's attention during the cognitive examination is to speak more loudly, effectively moving closer but not moving one's chair. At times it is also important to ensure attention by literally asking the patient to look at the clinician as the questions are asked. For instance, the interviewer can gently but firmly make statements such as, "It may help you to do well on these questions if you watch me as I actually say the digits to you." In the last analysis, if a withdrawn patient is looking down at the floor as the clinician performs the cognitive mental status, the validity of the results are certainly questionable.

The concept of increasing the validity of the cognitive examination also raises the issue of touching patients. Some clinicians seem to have a block against the idea of touching a patient. Although it is not frequent for me to touch a patient during an initial interview (except for handshakes), I sometimes find touching useful and poignant. With regard to the cognitive examination, some depressed and withdrawn patients may ignore the clinician's attempts to make eye contact and attend to the task at hand. In such instances, one can touch the arm of the patient, offering comments such as, "I know it is difficult for you to concentrate right now, but it really is important." At such points, the patient may glance up at the interviewer and more effective contact will have begun.

Of course, touching, a method of entering the patient's intimate space, as described by Hall, may also be used at points at which the patient may benefit from some simple comforting. I am reminded of a sad, middle-aged man who I interviewed as he was entering the hospital. For all of his life he had been a kind and hard-working mill worker. Unbeknownst to himself he was being exposed to an extremely toxic industrial poison. Over the years he experienced gradual changes in his behavior, including irritability and occasional violent outbursts, which frightened him and produced extreme guilt. Simultaneously he underwent marked changes in his intellectual functioning, to the point that he had problems dealing with everyday activities. Only recently had he learned that his problems were secondary to brain damage.

As we neared the end of the interview, he told me that he was afraid of the hospitalization because "people say mean things to me, they think I'm stupid. Please let me come in, I promise I won't hurt anybody, I promise, and I'm not that stupid." At which point he began to weep. It seemed only natural to reach over and grasp his arm while reassuring him that I believed what he said and that we would help him make the transition to the hospital.

Outside of the types of situations described above, touching patients is not common during initial interviews, because touch is a powerful communication, that may carry numerous connotations, not all of which are appropriate. Patients may misinterpret touch as an erotic gesture or at a minimum as a sign of implied intimacy. Although the clinician may intend the gesture as a sign of caring, a psychotic patient or a patient with a histrionic personality may distort the message considerably. Indeed, if a clinician finds a routine need to touch patients during initial interviews, it would be wise for the clinician to determine why such a need is arising. Usually it is not from clinical considerations. Such clinicians frequently have a desire to be perceived as "comforting angels." Ironically, this drive to be perceived as "comforting" may get in the way of effective care giving. Such self-exploration may also reveal flirtatious traits or histrionic qualities in the therapist.

At this point we can turn our attention to another aspect of nonverbal behavior, which frequently emerges if the clinician has effectively determined the appropriate RZ for the patient. At such times the appearance of certain nonverbal behaviors can suggest that the blending process is proceeding well. As mentioned in Chapter 1, several verbal signs, such as an increased DOU, may indicate the presence of improved engagement. In a similar fashion nonverbal activities may also be used routinely to monitor the blending process.

For instance, as blending increases, the patient may begin to make progressively better eye contact, while spontaneous arm gestures and "talking with one's hands" may increase. Along similar lines, if a patient in a shut-down interview begins to talk more with his or her hands, this may be a hint to pursue the present topic more fully in order to further strengthen the engagement process. The clinician can also frequently see the patient turn more towards him or her as blending increases. Relaxation is also shown by an asymmetry in posture, while tense posture is frequently seen with a person who feels threatened.[44]

We have been discussing the nonverbal activities that may suggest powerful levels of blending. It is important to return to a topic approached earlier, namely, the differences seen cross-culturally. With regard to the African-American culture, eye contact is not considered as important in conveying attention to a listener.[45] Just being in the room or close to the speaker may be considered enough to convey that attention is being given.

Direct eye contact may be considered disrespectful in certain cultures, such as with Mexican-Americans and with the Japanese. In this context, a clinician could be making a serious error in judgment by interpreting poor eye contact with members of these ethnic groups as an indication of rudeness, boredom, lack of assertiveness, or poor blending.

Another process that may emerge more frequently when one has successfully found the RZ is the surprising phenomenon of postural echoing.[46] In postural echoing one finds that two people who are communicating effectively tend to adopt similar postures and hand gestures. At a cafe, two lovers may sit across from each other, both heads perched in their hands, as they animatedly stare into each other's eyes.

A frequent phenomenon seen in interviewing occurs when one member suddenly shifts positions and relaxes. Simultaneously the other person will also shift and relax. Moreover microanalysis of videotapes has suggested that as blending increases, the minute movements of the interviewer and the interviewee tend to parallel each other as if a miniature minuet were being performed. During moments of discordant interchange this reciprocity decreased.

At one level these findings suggest that the appearance of postural echoing may serve as a clue to the clinician that the blending process is on the right track. In a slightly different vein, the clinician can subtly match some of the patient's postures in an effort to actively increase blending. For example, if a male clinician is interviewing a steel worker who is crossing his legs with his ankle over one knee, the therapist may cross his leg in the same manner, as opposed to crossing his leg at the knees. The latter method could be misconstrued by the interviewee as "feminine." By adopting a style similar to that of the patient, the metacommunication is passed that "we do certain things similarly and we may not be as different as one might first suppose." This discussion of the use of postural echoing, in an effort to actively engage the patient, leads to a consideration of other methods of nonverbally increasing the blending process.

BASIC FACILITATIVE TECHNIQUES

One collection of nonverbal behaviors potentially useful in the art of engagement consists of the so-called affiliative behaviors. Such behaviors include eye contact, smiles, and gesticulations. It has been shown that counselors who demonstrate these behaviors are viewed as significantly more persuasive than counselors who do not.[47] Another commonly encountered affiliative behavior consists of a body lean of about 20 degrees towards the patient.[48]

One of the most well-recognized affiliative gestures is the simple head nod. Morris makes the interesting observation that the vertical head nod indicates a "yes" or "positive" response in all cultures and groups in which it has been observed, including Caucasians, African-Americans, Balinese, Japanese, and Eskimos. It has been observed in deaf and blind individuals as well as in microcephalic people incapable of speech. He relates that the head nod may convey different types of "yes" messages, such as the following:

The Acknowledgment Nod: "Yes, I am still listening."
The Encouraging Nod: "Yes, how fascinating."
The Understanding Nod: "Yes, I see what you mean."
The Agreement Nod: "Yes, I will."
The Factual Nod: "Yes, that is correct."[49]

Interviewers should make an attempt to learn the frequency with which they typically head nod. This frequency can vary significantly among interviews. From my own observations it appears that interviewers who are particularly adept at engaging patients tend to head nod numerous times during any several minutes of an interview. As obvious as the utility of the head nod may appear, I have found that approximately 20% of professionals I supervise tend to underuse it. A few barely head nod at all.

The power of the head nod became apparent to me in an unexpected fashion during a session of psychotherapy. I had been working with a middle-aged male patient for several months. I decided to try a brief exercise in which I would purposely stop my typical head nodding for several minutes, in order to see what this practice would feel like to me. To my surprise I found it difficult to do, because it had become habitual. But more to my surprise, the patient broke off his spontaneous conversation after about 2 minutes and asked, "What's wrong? Somehow I feel that you don't like what I'm saying." This vignette emphasizes the power of nonverbal cues during clinical interaction.

ENGAGING GUARDED OR PARANOID PATIENTS

In Chapter 1 we discovered that with guarded or paranoid patients, certain changes in approach could enhance engagement. In particular, certain verbal approaches that were effective with most patients could be potentially disengaging with guarded patients. For instance, guarded patients frequently respond better to basic empathic statements rather than to complex empathic statements. In a similar fashion, with certain patients, the clinician's nonverbal behavior may be too empathic or intimate.

As mentioned earlier when discussing proxemics, guarded and paranoid patients may appreciate being provided with more space than most other patients. Along these lines, some of the affiliative gestures, when done too frequently, may prove disruptive to the guarded patient. I have heard paranoid patients comment that they have disliked frequent eye contact, perhaps twisting the attentive gaze of the "good listener" into the stark gaze of a potential persecutor. In this context, one may purposely break eye contact more frequently with paranoid patients, providing them with visual space.

Even head nodding and arm gestures can be unsettling when done too frequently with guarded or paranoid patients. I vividly remember one patient whom I interviewed in an emergency room. He was an intoxicated male about 30 years old, who wore a frequent sneer. He challenged me frequently with not-so-subtle sniper's remarks such as, "I bet you think you're a good listener Doc." And at one point he suddenly began mocking my head nodding by aping it, with his jaw jutting outwards while grunting out loud "Uh-huhs." This was not one of my more rewarding interviews. He was the patient who later, while waiting for his disposition, spontaneously attacked one of our safety guards.

This patient also illustrates the point that if the clinician finds a patient giving negative responses to typically engaging nonverbal behavior, then the interviewer should consider the idea that the patient may be guarded, hostile, or potentially violent.

CLINICIAN'S SELF-AWARENESS OF PARALANGUAGE

Each clinician has a unique personality. In particular, clinicians will vary on parameters such as tone of voice, rate of speech, and loudness of voice. It is important for clinicians to discover their own typical way of coming across. This knowledge is of value, because certain patients may respond better to different approaches. An understanding one's own natural style offers the clinician the chance to modify it, if necessary, to enhance the blending process.

With this idea in mind, it is useful for clinicians to practice exercises such as speaking more gently and slowing down their rate of speech. If an interviewer tends to speak loudly and quickly, a toning down of these parameters may prove more effective with a frightened or guarded patient. By way of example, my own personality is somewhat upbeat, with a mild pressure to my speech and a slightly louder voice than many people. When beginning interviews, I purposely adjust to a calmer middle ground until I understand the specific needs of the patient. Adjustments can then be made as deemed necessary. In instances when I have not made this adjustment, I have certainly come on too strongly for certain patients.

There exists another area in which tone of voice can frequently disengage a patient. Specifically, when talking with geriatric patients, clinicians often unconsciously adopt a rather distinctive tone of voice. They talk as if they were speaking to a helpless child. This tone of voice, which is often mildly slowed, can easily be perceived as condescending. It is an extremely frequent phenomenon, and clinicians must guard against it carefully. It is sometimes even done with psychotic patients and adolescents. In both cases the clinician is flirting with trouble.

NONVERBAL CUES OF THE CLINICIAN

We are generally well trained to observe the behavior of others, but the value of self-observation is frequently underplayed. As we have seen, the interview represents a dyadic process in which an understanding of one component depends on an understanding of the impact of the other component. The clinician's nonverbal activity always has the potential to significantly alter the behavior of the patient, as we have seen in our discussion of reciprocal behaviors.

With regard to gestures, as with paralanguage, clinicians need to develop a sound sense of their natural nonverbal style. One exercise that helps clinicians in developing self-awareness consists of repeatedly picturing a mirror descending during the interview itself. This mirror is to drop into place between the clinician and the patient. Such a visualization exercise rather rudely awakens clinicians to the fact that their every move is potentially an object of scrutiny to an inquisitive patient. As a complement to this visualization exercise, videotaping provides invaluable objective self-observation.

In any case the clinician should foster an awareness of those nonverbal activities that may inadvertently decrease blending. I am reminded of an interview, which I supervised, of an adolescent boy. The patient sat in a pool of brooding preoccupation. He wore a worrisome expression more suited to a 60-year-old man coping with an agitated depression than to a boy beginning adolescence. Curiously he had referred himself to the evaluation center and did not want his mother to be contacted.

During the interview he moved about anxiously in his chair and had considerable difficulty looking at the interviewer. He had a rounded face framed by a bowl of sandy hair, which was neatly clipped around his ears. It was about one of these ears that his discussion soon focused. Apparently he had the misfortune of watching a television documentary on cancer several days earlier. Since then he had become fixated on a small bump on his right ear, to which he gingerly pointed. He was convinced that he had developed a malignant tumor. This gnawing obsession, which may very well have reached delusional proportions, was nestled amidst a variety of depressive symptoms and difficult life circumstances.

As the interview proceeded the boy became progressively more ill at ease. At several points he stopped talking, asking the interviewer, "You don't understand, do you?" To which the interviewer responded in a reassuring fashion that he was trying to understand and wanted to hear more. This type of response generally might have decreased the tension, but in this case it seemed of no avail.

What the interviewer did not realize was the message conveyed by his own face. Each time the boy discussed his "tumor" the clinician furrowed his brow in a not-so-subtle fashion, forming two small vertical lines between his eyebrows. Apparently the patient interpreted this facial gesture as a look of disbelief or condemnation. The clinician had no conscious awareness of this particular expression, which frequently cropped up as a habit during his interviews. It is just this type of habit that can lead to recurrent problems with poor blending.

These habits are difficult to recognize unless the clinician is directly supervised or videotaped. They are also sometimes hard to accept. The clinician above seemed unimpressed with my explanation for the poor engagement until several weeks later. He then approached me sheepishly and said, "You'll never believe what a patient just did. In the middle of the interview he cut me off and asked me why I was frowning. My God, I must actually do it!"

One of my own habits illustrates another category of clinician movement that can become problematic. As I become anxious, I begin to twist my hair behind my ears. This nonverbal activity represents what we have discussed earlier as a displacement activity. These displacement activities can be used to monitor patient anxiety, but on the flip side, they can be a useful self-monitor, indicating anxiety in the clinician.

The clinician may not even have been aware of the presence of stress, but the appearance of numerous displacement activities warns that anxiety is present. At such points of self-awareness in the interview the clinician can explore the origins of the tension. Sometimes the interviewer is concerned about personal matters not related to the interview, including countertransference tensions. At other times the clinician may be intuitively registering patient hostility or even well-hidden psychotic process. In any case, the recognition of clinician displacement activities can provide yet another avenue for understanding.

Another good reason for studying displacement activities concerns the eradication of potentially disengaging gestures. For the most part, displacement activities are natural and help to create a feeling of spontaneous communication. As such there is no need to eliminate them; indeed, they may actually foster good blending. But there exist certain displacement gestures that are probably best eliminated. We can return to my own habit of twisting my hair. This displacement activity has the potential to be disengaging. To some patients it may appear effeminate, because as mentioned earlier women touch their hair three times more frequently than do men. To others it may simply be distracting. In either case it serves no purpose and is probably best discarded.

Similarly, certain categories of patients may not respond well to demonstrations of increased anxiety in the clinician. The immediate category that comes to mind includes patients escalating towards violence. These patients are frequently frightened that they are about to lose control. If they see the clinician becoming progressively more tense as well, they may become even more agitated. The same holds true for paranoid patients, who may appear almost ludicrously hyperattentive to their environments. I remember an older man with marked paranoid process who once asked me why I had just scratched my head. When I said I had an itch, he did not seem particularly reassured.

Two other clinician displacement activities warrant discussion. The first activity is smoking. I personally do not believe that clinicians should smoke cigarettes or even the proverbial "Freudian pipe" while interviewing patients. My bias evolves from the feeling that smoking, at the very least, represents a possible distraction to the patient. More likely, it may sometimes actually function as an irritant. Even if one asks permission from the patient, many patients who do not like smoking may find it difficult to convey such concerns. Pipe smoking is so stereotypic of "a shrink" that it may bias transference or simply turn some patients off.

The second displacement activity is much more of a mixed blessing, because it clearly serves some useful purposes. I had never even viewed it as a displacement activity until I had asked one student what his most common displacement activities were, and he replied, "That's easy, I'm constantly scribbling notes."

There exist many good reasons for taking detailed notes, such as making process notes to be shared with a psychotherapy supervisor. On the other hand, in initial interviews I have become more and more convinced that much of notetaking represents a displacement activity that frequently distracts both the clinician and the patient. No matter how one views it, a clinician looking down at his or her clipboard while actively composing sentences cannot possibly be attending to the fine nuances of patient behavior available to the clinician with undivided attention.

Once again I am sharing a bias that some clinicians would disagree with, but I feel that notetaking should be minimized in the initial interview. It should be utilized to jot down hard-to-remember details such as dates, medication dosages, and family trees. Instead of meticulously making a transcription of the patient's words, the clinician can carefully attend to the patient directly. In particular, during the early scouting period, I believe it is much better to do little, if any, notetaking. At this early stage the emphasis should be on actively engaging the patient. To this end, I find that patients are more responsive to clinicians who seem more interested in them than in the clinician's clipboard.

I frequently do not even pick up a clipboard until well into the interview. When I do begin to write, as a sign of respect, I often say to the patient, "I'm going to jot down a few notes to make sure I'm remembering everything correctly. Is that all right with you?" Patients seem to respond very nicely to this simple sign of courtesy. This statement of purpose also tends to decrease the paranoia that patients sometimes project onto notetaking, as they wonder if the clinician is madly analyzing their every thought and action. Along these lines, notetaking should be avoided with actively paranoid patients.

NONVERBAL ASPECTS OF CALMING POTENTIALLY VIOLENT PATIENTS

Interacting with a patient who is escalating towards violence presents the clinician with one of the most difficult of clinical situations. Although it would be nice to think that violent interactions are rare, the facts speak otherwise. Tardiff reports that approximately 17% of patients reporting to an emergency room are violent. He further reports that roughly 40% of psychiatrists have reported being assaulted at least once in their careers.[50]

Obviously, it is to the clinician's benefit to review the various approaches that may de-escalate an angry patient. In particular, the nonverbal characteristics of potentially violent dyads are of considerable importance, because issues concerning proxemics, kinesics, and paralanguage can all be of value in handling these situations. The interaction with the potentially violent patient provides an excellent topic with which to close this chapter, for the craft of utilizing nonverbal behavior is seldom put to a more critical test.

I would also like to emphasize that violence is frequently a dyadic process. The clinician and the patient represent a two-person system, and it is this system that becomes violent. Clinicians may inadvertently, with their nonverbal behavior, further escalate an already agitated patient. Fortunately this cycle, representing a violence reciprocal, can frequently be broken.

To begin with I am reminded of a curious story related by an anthropology professor during my undergraduate education. He described an interspecies encounter in which violence was averted by the quick thinking of a field anthropologist. This anthropologist had been extensively studying the behaviors of a baboon troop. One day he accidentally startled a mother baboon and her baby. Within seconds the squawkings of the alarmed mother attracted a swarming bevy of guard males. One can assume their intent was not of a social variety. Indeed, baboons are both intelligent and ferocious when provoked. The appearance of an ugly white ape with a mustache and safari hat was more than ample stimulus to prompt a display of their virility. Indeed, the baboons could have quickly disposed of the anthropologist.

Having observed baboons demonstrating submissive behavior within the troop, he purposely replicated their submissive gestures, which apparently involved lowering oneself and making certain jaw movements. To his relief, the baboons grunted and snarled but waved off their attack.

Besides representing a delightful tale for college professors to relate to wide-eyed undergraduates, the above story has a valuable message. A group of animals were about to interact violently. The violence was prevented by the use of specific nonverbal behaviors, which functioned as actual nonverbal communications. Similar to these baboons the human animal possesses a repertoire of nonverbal activities and communications that signal the intent to attack and the intent to submit.

For the clinician, the signals of impending attack, when recognized in a patient, can quickly alert the clinician that something needs to be altered in the interpersonal dyad before a violence reciprocal ensues. Through a knowledge of the signals of submission, the clinician may alter behavior in a fashion that appears less threatening to the paranoid or intoxicated patient. In many instances these alterations can break the dyadic cycle of violence, as effectively as the anthropologist supplicating the baboon warriors. It should be kept in mind that in some instances no matter what preventive actions are undertaken, violence will erupt. The goal is not to eliminate violence but to decrease its likelihood.

Towards this endeavor the clinician should consider whether the clinical environment suggests that violence may be a possibility. In the first place, diagnosis can alert the clinician to an increased likelihood of aggression. Most psychotic patients are not violent, but psychotic process as manifested in schizophrenia, bipolar disorder, paranoid disorder, and other atypical psychoses may predispose the patient towards aggression, especially when paranoid delusions are simmering beneath the patient's social facade. If frightened, these paranoid patients may go to great extremes to protect themselves, as we would if we shared their vision of the world. It is always important to remember that such patients may believe that they are literally fighting for their lives.

Other types of psychosis or poor impulse control may present problems. For instance, patients suffering from organic brain disease, as seen in frontal lobe syndromes, deliriums, and various dementias, may be predisposed towards aggression. A particular red flag should arise in the clinician's mind when interacting with people under the influence of various drugs, including speed, Quaaludes, and PCP. Alcohol intoxication remains a major area in which violence erupts, especially in settings such as emergency rooms. Because we frequently deal with alcohol intoxication in social settings in our culture, it is easy to be lulled into underestimating the potential for violence when dealing with an intoxicated patient. Such patients can quickly move from jovial jesting into a fit of rage.

Diagnoses do not tell the clinician that any specific patient is about to be violent. Most people suffering from schizophrenia are not violent, but the diagnosis does alert the clinician to the possibility of aggression. This consideration may represent the first step in preventing violence. In addition, the clinician may note that a patient has a history of assaultive behavior. In such instances, the clinician is well advised to take appropriate precautions, such as having safety officers unobtrusively nearby and aware of the situation.

Besides diagnostic and historical factors, the clinician may be part of a situation in which violence is more likely. If the clinician has been asked to participate in the evaluation of a patient who is being committed involuntarily, then caution is always advised. There are probably few life situations more frightening than to have one's freedom taken away. In this situation patients should always be considered as potentially violent.

I remember one instance in our emergency room late at night. The patient, an agitated woman of about 30 years of age, was being committed. Safety officers had been called down and were appropriately nearby. The patient appeared to have calmed and was quietly sitting with family members by her side. Everything seemed in control. The clinician began to move away from the patient and turned her back as she headed for the staff room. In a matter of seconds the patient was ferociously choking the clinician, for no apparent reason. I mention this vignette because it highlights the need to think cautiously while evaluating committed patients. It also reminds one of the old adage that one should never turn one's back on a patient, an adage as true today as when it was first coined.

One other clinical situation to keep in mind arises when patients are agitated and accompanied by family members. In such situations the clinician should attempt to determine quickly whether the family member is calming or upsetting the patient. In emergency rooms a common mistake is to not separate feuding family members until it is too late. It is often best to separate the antagonistic family members quickly, while allowing different staff members to attempt to calm and understand the perspectives of both parties.

I have strayed from the topic of nonverbal behavior. However in a practical sense, the first step in utilizing nonverbal behavior with violent patients consists of recognizing the violent situation in its infancy, not its adolescence. If the clinician is aware of the potential for violence, then the following nonverbal techniques can be brought into play.

We will first look at various nonverbal activities that may alert the clinician that violence may be incubating. Subsequently we will look at ways in which to change our own behaviors in an effort to avoid confrontation.

The signs of impending aggression can be loosely grouped into two categories—early warning signs and late warning signs. Although it is extremely difficult to predict whether a patient will engage in violence in the future, it is not particularly difficult to tell when a patient may be headed towards immediate violence.

The early warning signs consist of behaviors that suggest emerging agitation. In the simplest examples, one may notice the patient beginning to speak more quickly with a subtly angry tone of voice. These paralanguage clues may be augmented by a display of sarcastic statements or challenges, such as, "You think you're a big shot, don't you!"

These types of early warning signs may appear obvious, which is the exact reason why they warrant mentioning. As clinicians we may inadvertently ignore these signs, in the process unintentionally escalating the patient. This seems to occur during periods of intense time pressure or when the clinical situation has become increasingly hectic, as in a busy emergency room. Such obstinacy can unfortunately return as an unwanted gremlin. When these early warning signs are present, it is very important to crystallize in one's mind what the patient's needs may be. If the clinician can move with the patient's needs, hostility will frequently decrease.

Kinesic early-warning signs consist of actual evidence of agitation, such as pacing and refusing to sit down. If patients refuse to sit, it is frequently useful to gently request them to return to their seat. One can use phrases such as, "It might help you to relax some if you sit over here," or "Let's sit down and see if we can sort some things out." If comments such as these fail to elicit compliance, one can more firmly state, "I'd like you to sit over here so we can talk." Some clinicians might quietly add, "It's difficult to have to keep staring up. I think we'll both be more comfortable if we sit." If these maneuvers fail, then it is probably best to let the patient walk around freely, while recognizing that this patient may be seriously impaired with regard to impulse control. In short, the patient may be on the way towards violence, and appropriate steps should be taken. If no one is aware that the clinician is alone with such a patient, it is generally best to let someone know what is going on. It is relatively easy for a clinician to make an excuse for leaving the room at such points. It may not be so easy 10 minutes later. Along these lines, if the clinician is at all suspicious of possible violence, the clinician should carry a "safety button" or know where the safety button is located in the interview room, so that other staff can be alerted if problems arise.

Other kinesic early warning clues include rapid and jerky gesturing. Of particular note is the action of vigorously pointing one's finger at the clinician to "make a point." Such a gesture may be a harbinger of impending hostility. Increased and intense staring may also suggest anger. Finally, the appearance of suspiciousness or other increases in psychotic process, such as an increasing disorganization, should alert the clinician to the possibility of violence.

As a person comes closer to overt violence, specific behaviors may serve as reliable indicators that aggression is imminent. Just like the charging guard baboons with their bared teeth, humans have evolved symbolic signs of threat.

Morris has described behaviors known as intention movements.[51] These intention movements consist of those small gestures that suggest impending movement. For instance, as persons intend to rise from a chair, they frequently lean forward grasping the arms of the chair. This is a clear signal that they want to rise, signaling that the conversation is about to end. The intention movements suggesting possible violence include activities such as clenching of the fists, whitening of the knuckles as one tightly grasps an inanimate object, and even a snarling as the lips are pulled back from the teeth. People may not be as different from baboons as we would like to think.

Perhaps the most common intention movement of attack is the raising of a closed fist over the head. Overhand blows delivered from this position are the most frequent blows seen in street brawls and riots despite the unlikelihood of hurting one's opponent in this manner. This behavior may be instinctual in nature, because it is frequently seen in children who are fighting.

Morris also describes vacuum gestures, which represent completed actions but are not actually carried out on the enemy. Frequent vacuum gestures include shaking the fist, assuming a boxing stance, gesturing as if strangling the opponent, and the pounding of the fist into the opposite palm. All of these intention movements and vacuum gestures serve as late warning signals that violence is near at hand.

It should also be noted that verbal threats or statements that one is about to strike out often accompany the nonverbal behaviors described above. When the above late warning signs are present, violence is a distinct possibility. At this point an application of nonverbal skills may help to prevent aggression.

Earlier, reciprocal behaviors were discussed, such as the mating reciprocal, in which two organisms engage in an orderly sequence of events leading to a final outcome. Scheflen describes dominance and submission reciprocals.[52] In our story of the baboons, the anthropologist refused to participate in the dominance reciprocal. If he had, he might very well have been killed. Instead he chose to begin the submission reciprocal, which his would-be attackers fortunately agreed to follow. In a similar fashion, humans can engage in either of these reciprocals.

When faced with a hostile patient, the trick is to avoid engaging in the dominance reciprocal while utilizing some submissive behavior. One avoids the dominance reciprocal by not demonstrating any of the early or late warning signs of aggression. Although this appears to make an obvious point, it is striking to watch the maladaptive behavior of clinicians when faced with an agitated patient. The fear generated by the patient's hostility frequently results in unconscious behaviors that may threaten the patient. The clinician's voice may be raised. At times, the actual movements of the clinician speed up as the waiting area is hurriedly cleared of furniture and other patients. Even frankly antagonistic remarks may emerge. In this respect, it is not an exaggeration to say that clinicians can actually precipitate violence.

There exist no absolute rules for interacting with a patient on the verge of violence, but some principles seem relevant. In the first place, the clinician should appear calm. The speaking voice should appear normal and unharried. It is particularly important to avoid speaking loudly or in an authoritarian manner. With regard to kinesics, the clinician wants to avoid an excessive display of displacement activities, which may be misinterpreted as aggressive displays. Moreover, exaggerated displacement activities may create an increasing atmosphere of fear, stoking the patient's own fears of an impending loss of control.

Eye contact should probably be decreased, and the hands should not be raised in any gesture that may signify an intent to attack or defend oneself. Curiously, some clinicians will place their hands behind their backs, a situation that may raise fears in the patient that a weapon is being hidden. With regard to posture, one can purposely stoop one's shoulders slightly in an effort to appear smaller, because humans, when about to attack, frequently raise their shoulders and chests, a bit of gorilla-like display. It is probably also wise to remain in front of the patient, because an approach from behind or from the side may startle the agitated patient.

One of the most important points concerns an issue mentioned earlier when discussing proxemics. At least one study has suggested that potentially violent patients may have significantly altered buffer zones.[53] Specifically, they will feel that their intimate body space is being invaded at distances much further away than for most people. These patients may feel that the interviewer is "in my face" while standing a full 6 feet away. In general, the agitated patient needs more room and interpersonal space. This can be a tough principle to remember, because some good-hearted clinicians feel a desire to calm the angry patient by touching them. This desire usually goes away after a few unfortunate encounters with feet or fists.

If these principles are followed, accompanied by an intelligent use of safety officers and medication as needed, many violent encounters can be avoided. With regard to avoiding dangerous situations, another point warrants mentioning. When sitting in a room with a patient who one does not know, it is probably wise to arrange the chairs so that the clinician is closer to the doorway, while not obstructing the patient's pathway to the doorway. With this arrangement one can always get away if the patient becomes threatening or produces a weapon. It is naive to think that these situations do not arise, especially in emergency rooms. To pretend that they do not probably represents a defensive denial that prevents the clinician from fully thinking about these situations in a manner that could help prevent them in the first place.

In conclusion, nonverbal processes are core elements of human communication during violent interactions. A sound knowledge of these processes can help the clinician to calm the angry or frightened patient. Helping patients to regain a sense of internal control remains one of the fine points of the art of interviewing. It also increases the chances that the clinician will be around to practice his or her art.

CONCLUSION

In this chapter we have reviewed the basic principles of proxemics, kinesics, and paralanguage. It can readily be seen that these processes are at the very root of communication. As such integral parts of human interaction, they remain pivotal in bringing the initial interview to a successful conclusion.

In these first three chapters, we have reviewed many of the basic principles of both verbal and nonverbal behaviors as they apply to the initial interview. Before proceeding much further, the important topic of gathering and organizing information for treatment planning warrants a thorough discussion. Such a discussion will quickly move us into some of the most complex and fascinating aspects of assessment interviewing.

References

1. Hall, E. T.: Excerpts from an interview conducted by Carol Travis. *GEO* 25(3):12, 1983.
2. Harper, R. G., Wiens, A. N., and Matarazzo, J. D.: *Nonverbal Communication: The State of the Art.* New York, John Wiley, 1978.
3. Wiener, M., Devoe, S., Rubinow, S., and Geller, J.: Nonverbal behavior and nonverbal communication. *Psychological Review* 79:185–214, 1972.
4. Edinger, J. A., and Patterson, M. L.: Nonverbal involvement and social control. *Psychology Bulletin* 93(1):30–56, 1983.

5. Morris, D.: *Manwatching: A Field Guide to Human Behavior.* New York, Harry N. Abrams, 1977.
6. Hall, E. T.: *The Hidden Dimension.* New York, Doubleday, 1966.
7. Watson, O. M., and Graves, T. D.: Quantitative research in proxemic behavior. *American Anthropologist* 68:971–985, 1966.
8. Sue, D. W., and Sue, D.: Barrier to effective cross-cultural counseling. *Journal of Counseling Psychology* 24(5):420–429, 1977.
9. Baxter, J. C.: Interpersonal spacing in natural settings. *Sociometry* 33:444–456, 1970.
10. Wiens, A. N.: The assessment interview. In *Clinical Methods in Psychology,* edited by Irving Weiner. New York, John Wiley, 1976.
11. Knapp, M. L.: *Nonverbal Communication in Human Interaction.* New York, Holt, Rinehart, and Winston, 1972.
12. Birdwhistell, M. L.: *Introduction to Kinesis: An Annotation System for Analysis of Body Motion and Gesture.* Louisville, KY, University of Louisville Press, 1952.
13. Harper, R. G., 1978, p. 123.
14. Scheflen, A. E.: *Body Language and Social Order.* Englewood Cliffs, NJ, Prentice-Hall, 1972.
15. Freud, S.: Fragment of an analysis of a case of hysteria. In *Collected Papers,* Vol. 3. New York, Barri Books, 1959 (originally published in 1925).
16. Carmier, W. H., and Carmier, L. A.: *Interviewing Strategies for Helpers: A Guide to Assessment, Treatment and Evaluation.* California, Brooks/Cole Publishing Company, 1979.
17. Wiens, A. N., 1976, p. 27.
18. Sue, D. W., 1977, p. 427.
19. Hill, Sir Denis: Non-verbal behavior in mental illness. *British Journal of Psychiatry* 24:221–230, 1974.
20. Hill, Sir Denis, 1974, p. 227.
21. Wiens, A. N., 1976, p. 33.
22. Morris, D., 1977, p. 75.
23. Scheflen, A. E., 1972, p. 46.
24. Morris, D., 1977, p. 164.
25. Morris, D., 1977, p. 165.
26. Pansa-Hendersen, M., De L'Horne, D. J., and Jones, I. H.: Nonverbal behavior as a supplement to psychiatric diagnosis in schizophrenia, depression, and anxiety neurosis. *Journal of Psychiatric Treatment and Evaluation* 43:489–496, 1982.
27. Jones, I. H., and Pansa, M.: Some nonverbal aspects of depression and schizophrenia during the interview. *Journal of Nervous and Mental Disease* 167(7):402–409, 1979.
28. Pansa-Henderson, 1982, p. 495.
29. Jones, I. H., 1979, pp. 402–409.
30. Morris, D., 1977, p. 181.
31. Morris, D., 1977, p. 109.
32. Ekman, P., and Friesen, W. V.: Detecting deception from the body or face. *Journal of Personality and Social Psychology* 29(3):288–298, 1974.
33. Ekman, P.: *Telling Lies: Clues to Deceit in the Marketplace, Politics, and Marriage.* New York, W. W. Norton, 1985.
34. Littlepage, G. E., and Pineault, M. A.: Detection of deceptive factual statements from the body and face. *Personality and Social Psychology Bulletin* 53(5):325–328, 1979.
35. McClintock, C. C., and Hung, R. G.: Nonverbal indicators of affect and deception in an interview setting. *Journal of Applied Social Psychology* 5:54–67, 1975.
36. Edinger, J. A., 1983, pp. 42–43.

37. Kraut, R. E.: Verbal and nonverbal cues in the perception of lying. *Journal of Personality and Social Psychology* 36:380–391, 1978.
38. Grinder, J., and Bandler, R.: *The Structure of Magic II.* Palo Alto, California, Science and Behavior Books, 1976.
39. Scheflen, A. E.: *Body Language and Social Order.* Englewood Cliffs, NJ, Prentice-Hall, 1972.
40. Scheflen, A. E., 1972, p. 16.
41. Morris, D., 1977, p. 102.
42. Morris, D., 1977, p. 102.
43. Egan, G.: *The Skilled Helper: A Model for Systematic Helping and Interpersonal Relating.* California, Brooks/Cole Publishing Company.
44. Wiens, A. N., 1976, p. 35.
45. Sue, D. W., 1977, pp. 420–429.
46. Morris, D., 1977, p. 83.
47. La Crosse, M. B.: Nonverbal behavior and perceived counselor attractiveness and persuasiveness. *Journal of Counseling Psychology* 19:417–424, 1972.
48. Hasse, R. F., and Tepper, D.: Nonverbal component of empathetic communication. *Journal of Counseling Psychology* 19:417–424, 1972.
49. Morris, D., 1977, p. 68.
50. Tardiff, K.: The violent patient. In *Manual of Psychiatric Consultation and Emergency Care,* edited by F. Guggenheim and M. Weiner. New York, Jason Aronson, 1984.
51. Morris, D., 1977, p. 173.
52. Scheflen, A. E., 1977, p. 173.
53. Wiens, A. N., 1976, p. 28.

CHAPTER 4

Assessment Perspectives: Pathways to Effective Treatment Planning

*W*e shall not cease from exploration
And the end of all our exploring
Will be to arrive where we started
And know the place for the first time.

T. S. Eliot
Little Gidding

I n the first three chapters we examined a variety of principles fundamental to the development of the verbal tapestry we call an assessment interview. We focused on both verbal and non-verbal skills, exploring proxemics, kinesics, facilics, and blending techniques. The interviewer is now faced with the challenging task of "listening" to the database, of resourcefully utilizing the carefully procured information.

I must emphasize that this is not a chapter about how to choose specific therapies and design concrete treatment plans. Such a topic as treatment planning is both complex and vast, well beyond the scope of a book focused on the interviewing process. Instead, this is a chapter about the decisions that a clinician must make, during the interview itself, about what data to gather in the first place. It is also about how, both during and immediately after the interview, to organize this information so that the resultant databases can be fashioned into legible signposts that point towards effective treatment options.

Frequently I have seen clinicians falter, not because they lack adequate knowledge about the use of specific treatment modalities, but because the use of certain modalities never comes to mind. They become lost in the database, emphasizing certain information while ignoring, or not even obtaining, other pertinent data. We are dealing with an information processing problem, a not unexpected dilemma considering the vastness of the information involved in understanding another person's problems.

By way of example, one such instance that comes to mind concerns a clinician who might select an antipsychotic medication for a person suffering from an acute psychotic breakdown. Suppose for a moment that the clinician has not involved the patient's family in the reasoning behind the use of such a medication. Suppose further that the family has a deep-rooted bias that drugs are not good for people. When this patient returns home, there exists a significant chance that the patient's family will support or even instigate noncompliance with the medication. In this instance the family system was ignored during the development of the treatment plan. The result is both disappointing and predictable. More important, it is potentially preventable.

In this chapter we will study a common-sense approach to creating a realistic list of viable treatment options. No attempt is made to suggest the pros and cons of any specific treatment; rather, the focus is upon making the transition from the interview itself to the initial stage of treatment planning. This is a chapter devoted to a discussion of the process of determining what data need to be gathered for treatment planning purposes and how to effectively organize this material. The chapter is based on the idea that one cannot truly understand how to interview if one does not understand the reason for the interview.

This chapter also demonstrates that the treatment opportunities that come to mind for the clinician appear to be directly related to both the data collected and the method of organizing these data. For example, a clinician who does not learn to ask questions concerning symptoms suggestive of a drug-responsive depression will most likely not think to utilize such a medication. Likewise, a clinician is less likely to think of intervening via social work channels if current stressors are ignored.

To avoid such tunnel vision, clinicians can organize their data into schemata that emphasize conceptualization from multiple viewpoints. In this chapter we will look at three such systems. Through them the power of a well-organized database to lead to effective treatment planning will become apparent. In an ironic sense, the art of treatment planning returns us to our original starting point, the data gleaned from the initial interview itself. As T. S. Eliot suggested in our opening quotation, significant insight can be gained by learning to listen more openly to what is already familiar.

We shall look at the following three assessment perspectives: (1) the diagnostic perspective provided by the fourth edition of the Diagnostic and Statistical Manual of Mental Disorders (DSM-IV),[2] (2) the systems analysis perspective, and (3) the perspective provided by understanding the "core pains" of the patient. Although overlapping at their interfaces, each of these perspectives generates unique clues for treatment planning. Consequently it is expedient to create an initial treatment plan utilizing all three perspectives. I have found single-perspective treatment planning unsatisfactory, akin to beginning a watercolor with only half of the necessary paints.

Each of the three assessment perspectives provides the following approaches for usefully organizing clinical information:

1. An easy and rapid method of checking, during the interview itself, whether pertinent data regions have been explored
2. A reliable method of reminding the clinician to borrow from different data perspectives when formulating a treatment plan
3. A flexible approach to actually delineating a list of potential treatment modalities
4. A method that the therapist can use during the ongoing treatment of the patient in order to review treatment planning, as well as generating new ideas when treatment has reached a setback or an impasse

The chapter will begin by reviewing a database gleaned from an actual initial interview. Following this presentation the information from each of the three perspectives mentioned above will be examined, observing the utility provided by each viewpoint.

CASE PRESENTATION

When I first saw Miss Baker she was sitting in the waiting room. Her eyes were hiding behind a pair of large, pink-framed sun glasses. These frames were rimmed by her shortly bobbed brown hair. She had a round face and a rather short frame. She was wearing a T-shirt and a pair of freshly washed jeans. Around her left wrist a wide leather band was wrapped with the name Paul tooled into it.

When I asked if she was Miss Baker she pertly looked up, smiled and replied, "Yes, I'm Miss Baker but not for long." I asked what she meant, and she replied, "Oh, I'm getting married in a month to another woman."

Once in my office she related a story of a longstanding problem with fluctuating moods. She spoke in a quiet voice, frequently casting her eyes to the floor, as if to avoid seeing the impact of her words upon my face. She displayed no evidence of loose associations, thought blocking, pressured speech, or flight of ideas. She gave no evidence of responding to hallucinations and denied both auditory and visual hallucinations.

With regard to her moodiness, she stated that her moods frequently changed throughout the day. It was not at all unusual for her to feel various moods, including anger and rejection, during the course of a single day. Although she reported intermittent periods of feeling decreased energy, decreased interest in activities, decreased libido, and difficulty falling asleep, she denied any periods of 2 weeks or more in which these symptoms were persistent. She denied manic or hypomanic symptoms past or present.

She lived in a world of imagined fear, persistently worried that she would be abandoned. At nights she would become angered if her partner fell asleep first, because she would quickly become engulfed by her fear of being alone. These fears fostered an intense dependency, which she readily admitted was a major handicap. She went out of her way to please her partner, allowing all major decisions to be made by her, including the upcoming wedding plans. This dependency also surfaced with the string of therapists lying in her wake. Her most recent therapist had had her forcibly removed from his office by the police, an act marking the end of their contact.

As one might have surmised, impulse control was not a strong point. For instance, several years earlier she had managed to toss a picnic table bench through a friend's picture window while enraged. Moreover, she had a history of popping pills in small suicidal gestures about every 2 to 3 months over the past 3 years.

Her relationship with her parents was very strained, and she felt she had always been marked as the black sheep of the family. She had one sister 2 years older than she who was employed as an accountant and was reported as happily married. One of her earliest memories was of standing behind the front door weeping as her father walked away down the stone path. As she cried her mother shook her violently, pulling her away from the doorway.

To my surprise, the wristband bearing the name Paul had nothing to do with past or present friends or lovers. Instead it referred to herself, for she often fantasized that she was Paul Newman. This vivid fantasy game was fostered by her partner, who would call her Paul, relating to her in this pseudoidentity. At no time did Miss Baker lose sight that this was merely a fantasy, although she longed to be anyone but herself. When talking of her fantasy identities, she would occasionally cry softly, as if punctuating her story with tears.

DIAGNOSTIC PERSPECTIVE OF THE DSM-IV

General Diagnostic Principles

For clinicians diagnosis serves one major purpose—to discover information that may lead to more effective methods of helping the patient. A diagnostic schema provides this avenue by allowing clinicians and researchers the opportunity to share their experiences in a common language. For example, when a clinician discovers a treatment plan that is useful in relieving a resistant major depression, these findings may be applicable to a patient being treated by a fellow clinician, who might benefit from the shared knowledge. Diagnosis should not be an intellectual game or a pastime used to placate insurance companies. It is a practical passport to the knowledge housed in journals, books, and the minds of our fellow clinicians.

Like the common language we have developed for discussing the interviewing process, diagnosis allows one to conceptualize more clearly. In particular, diagnosis can provide valuable information concerning prognosis, possible treatment modalities, and pitfalls to be avoided in dealing with certain syndromes. For these reasons the art of diagnostic formulation remains of pivotal importance to the initial interviewer. Basic triage decisions may be dependent upon the diagnostic assessment.

In particular, diagnoses can be valuable in suggesting possible treatment modalities. For instance, major depressions frequently respond to antidepressants. Bipolar disorder (manic phase) is usually approached with lithium, antipsychotic medications, or antiseizure medications such as carbamazepine and valproic acid. Phobias are frequently alleviated by using behavioral techniques. Milder forms of major depression can be approached using dynamic and cognitive psychotherapies, behavioral approaches, or numerous counseling techniques. The above list merely represents a terse survey, but it nevertheless highlights the power of a diagnostic system to help in developing a diverse treatment approach.

A clinical vignette will make this abstract discussion more concrete. I was working with a couple whose marriage was riddled with a nasty streak of passive aggression and strained communication. After several sessions the marital therapy seemed to be bogging down. The husband, a rather narcissistic man, kept insisting that nothing was being done for him. In reviewing my notes I discovered that the referring clinician had diagnosed the husband as suffering from a dysthymic disorder. To my surprise I had recently read an article in which certain types of dysthymic disorders responded well to antidepressant medication. My patient fit one of these descriptions and consequently was begun on an appropriate antidepressant. He quickly found significant relief. Moreover, to the chagrin of both the patient and his spouse, their marital friction remained painfully present. Up to this point he had balked at couples therapy, because he felt that it was his depression that was causing all the problems. Now he realized the relationship itself needed attention. He no longer had an excuse for avoiding the work of therapy, thanks to the antidepressant, and suddenly the marital therapy could move ahead more effectively.

This vignette illustrates the power of a common diagnostic language to provide a clinician with knowledge discovered by others. Without the diagnostic label, this learning would have been unavailable.

Before proceeding it seems expedient to review some of the important limitations of diagnostic approaches, such as the DSM-IV. Only through a knowledge of a system's weaknesses can its strengths be utilized safely.

One of the most obvious limitations remains the fact that diagnoses are labels. As labels they can be abused. One such abuse occurs when clinicians fall into the trap of using diagnoses as stereotypical explanations for human behavior. It should be remembered that a diagnosis provides no particular knowledge about any given patient. It merely suggests possible characteristics that may or may not be generalizable to the patient in question.

Moreover, diagnostic formulations are evolving processes and as such should be periodically re-examined. There is a realistic danger that patients can become stuck with inappropriate diagnoses, a problem that can only be avoided through persistent reappraisal. In a similar fashion the clinician should remain healthily aware of the potential ramifications of certain diagnostic labels with regard to the patient's culture and family. By way of example, the label schizophrenia can result in the loss of a job or in the development of a scapegoating process within a given family. Considerations of these problematic aspects of diagnosis should be integral parts of sound clinical care.

The issue of the significance of a specific diagnostic label to the patient himself or herself can be of marked importance. For this reason I frequently ask patients if anyone has given them a diagnosis in the past. If the answer is a "yes," one can follow with questions such as, "What is your understanding of the word schizophrenia?" or "Do you think that diagnosis is right?" The answers to these questions can provide valuable insights into the patient's self-image, intellectual level, and previous care.

One of the most important considerations remains the necessity of reminding oneself that a correct diagnosis does not necessarily give one much information about the patient as a unique individual. Other conceptualizations must be used to provide this critical understanding, as we shall discuss later in this chapter and throughout the remainder of this book.

With these ideas in mind we can now explore the DSM-IV in more detail. In 1980, the DSM-III system introduced many of the innovations, such as multiaxial formulation, that formed the foundation of the DSM-IV system. A bridge between the two systems, called the DSM-III-R,[3] appeared in 1987, and added its own new ideas and refinements. The DSM-IV itself was published in 1994, and it is to this system that we will now turn. We will not attempt to review diagnostic criteria, because these are discussed in subsequent chapters. Instead we will look at the principles that help make diagnostic formulation possible in the first sixty minutes.

Multiaxial Formulation

One of the most useful aspects of the DSM-IV is the fact that the system pushes the clinician to consider various perspectives while formulating a diagnostic picture. Each perspective is placed upon one of five axes, which in a simplified version appear as follows in the DSM-IV*:

> Axis I: All clinical disorders and other conditions that may be a focus of clinical attention (except for Personality Disorders and Mental Retardation)
> Axis II: Personality Disorders and Mental Retardation
> Axis III: General Medical Conditions
> Axis IV: Psychosocial and Environmental Problems
> Axis V: Global Assessment of Functioning

Axis I

At first glance Axis I may appear confusing because of the large number of diagnostic entities that it contains. But there is little need for concern. The craft lies in approaching the task by first uncovering the general diagnostic probabilities and then delineating the specific diagnoses (Fig. 4).

As the initial interviewer listens during the opening phase and the body of the interview, the symptoms of the patient will suggest diagnostic regions worthy of more elaborate expansion. This primary delineation will lead the clinician to one or more of the following easily remembered regions:

---

*Reprinted with permission from the Diagnostic and Statistical Manual of Mental Disorders, 4th ed. Copyright 1994 American Psychiatric Association.

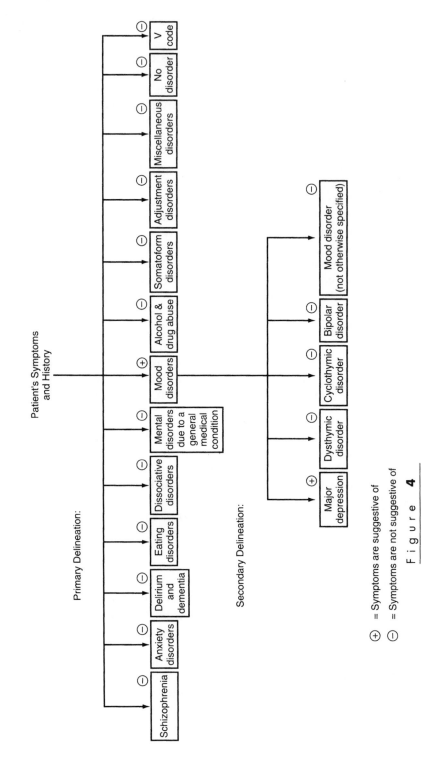

Patient's Symptoms and History

Primary Delineation:

Schizophrenia (–) | Anxiety disorders (–) | Delirium and dementia (–) | Eating disorders (–) | Dissociative disorders (–) | Mental disorders due to a general medical condition (–) | Mood disorders (+) | Alcohol & drug abuse (–) | Somatoform disorders (–) | Adjustment disorders (–) | Miscellaneous disorders (–) | No disorder (–) | V code (–)

Secondary Delineation:

Major depression (+) | Dysthymic disorder (–) | Cyclothymic disorder (–) | Bipolar disorder (–) | Mood disorder (not otherwise specified) (–)

⊕ = Symptoms are suggestive of
⊖ = Symptoms are not suggestive of

Figure 4

Basic approach to diagnostic utilization (patient with a major depression).

1. Mood disorders
2. Schizophrenia and related disorders
3. Anxiety disorders
4. Delirium, dementia, and other cognitive disorders
5. Alcohol and drug abuse disorders
6. Somatoform disorders (e.g., hypochondriasis, somatization disorder, etc.)
7. Eating disorders
8. Dissociative disorders
9. Adjustment disorders
10. Other miscellaneous disorders (e.g., sexual and gender identity disorders, factitious disorders, impulse control disorders, and sleep disorders)
11. Mental disorders due to a general medical condition (e.g., personality change secondary to a frontal lobe tumor, etc.)
12. No disorder
13. V codes and other conditions that may be a focus of clinical attention

Looked at in this simplified fashion the first step in utilizing the DSM-IV appears considerably more manageable than at first glance. In order to succeed, the clinician must be well grounded in psychopathology, as will be discussed in the following chapters. This knowledge base will allow the interviewer to quickly determine which of the thirteen areas are most pertinent. As the interview proceeds the clinician can reflect upon whether each of these broad areas has at least been considered, thus avoiding errors of omission.

Once the primary delineation has been made, the interviewer can proceed with the secondary delineation, in which the specific diagnoses subsumed under the broad diagnostic areas are explored and the more exact DSM-IV differential diagnosis is determined. Thus, if the clinician suspects a mood disorder, the clinician will eventually hunt for criteria substantiating specific mood diagnoses such as major depression, bipolar disorder, dysthymic disorder, cyclothymic disorder, bipolar disorder not otherwise specified, and depressive disorder not otherwise specified. This secondary delineation would be performed in each broad diagnostic area deemed pertinent.

As already described in Chapter 2, these explorations occur during the main body of the interview. Most important, they are done in a highly flexible fashion, always patterning the questioning in the fashion most compatible with the needs of the patient and the clinical situation. Consequently the clinician expands these diagnostic regions in a unique fashion with each patient, mixing them with various other content regions and process regions. When done well, the result is an interview that feels unstructured to the patient, yet delineates an accurate diagnosis.

The No Disorder category serves as a timely reminder to the clinician to always look for the strengths and normal coping mechanisms of the patient. Too many clinicians fall into the biasing perspective of only "seeing with the eyes of psychopathology" as opposed to the equally important "eyes of health."

V codes represent conditions not attributable to a mental disorder that have nevertheless become a focus of therapeutic intervention. Examples include academic problems, occupational problems, uncomplicated bereavement, noncompliance with medical treatment, marital problems, parent-child problems, and others. Sometimes these codes are used because no mental disorder is present, and the patient is coping with one of the stresses just listed. They can also be used if the clinician feels that not enough information is available to rule out a psychiatric syndrome, but, in the meantime, an area for specific intervention is being highlighted. Finally, these V codes can be used with a patient who carries a specific psychiatric syndrome but for whom that syndrome is not the immediate problem or the focus of intervention. For example, an individual with chronic schizophrenia in remission may present with marital distress.

Axis II

Axis II emphasizes the realization that all of the Axis I diagnoses exist in the unique psychological milieu we call personality. Indeed, many mental health problems are primarily related to the vicissitudes of personality development. Moreover, the underlying personality of the patient can greatly affect the manner in which we choose to relate to the patient both in the initial interview and in subsequent therapy. Consequently it is expedient to conceptualize which personality characteristics have evolved in any given interviewee.

The basic approach to diagnosis follows the same two-step delineation discussed for Axis I. In the first delineation one asks whether the interviewee's story suggests evidence of long-term interpersonal dysfunction that has remained relatively consistent from adolescence onwards. If so, the patient may very well fulfill the criteria for a personality disorder or disorders.

After determining that a personality disorder may very well be present, the clinician proceeds with the secondary delineation in which specific regions of personality diagnoses are expanded. This secondary delineation will result in the generation of a differential from the following list:

1. Paranoid personality disorder
2. Schizoid personality disorder
3. Schizotypal personality disorder
4. Histrionic personality disorder
5. Narcissistic personality disorder
6. Antisocial personality disorder
7. Borderline personality disorder
8. Avoidant personality disorder
9. Dependent personality disorder
10. Obsessive-compulsive personality disorder
11. Personality disorder, not otherwise specified (NOS)

In Chapter 7 we will examine in great detail the many fascinating subtleties involved in exploring personality structure during an initial interview. However, at this point I would like to mention an often forgotten point. In many cases the interviewee will not demonstrate psychopathology warranting the diagnosis of a personality disorder. Instead, he or she will possess traits found in these disorders in smaller degrees. The DSM-IV is very flexible in such cases, allowing the clinician to simply list the traits that are present. One might simply write on Axis II that "the patient displayed some histrionic and paranoid traits."

Besides personality traits, on Axis II the clinician may also list specific defense mechanisms, which may be pertinent with regard to future treatment. These defense mechanisms range from those commonly seen in neurotic disorders such as rationalization and intellectualization to those seen in more severe disorders such as denial, projection, and splitting. These defense mechanisms are defined in Appendix B of the DSM-IV.

It should be noted that Axis II was further revised in the DSM-IV to include mental retardation.

Axis III

On this axis the clinician considers the role of physical disorders and conditions. Stated differently, this axis reminds the clinician to adopt a holistic approach to the patient, one in which both the patient's mind and the patient's body are considered as parts of the same organism.

I do not think that this axis can be emphasized too much. In my opinion all patients who exhibit psychological complaints for an extended time period should be evaluated by a physician to rule out any underlying physiologic condition or causative agent. To not perform this examination is to risk a real disservice to the patient, because entities such as endocrine disorders and malignancies can easily present with psychological symptoms.

In this same light a medical review of systems and a past medical history should become a standard part of an initial assessment. Other physical conditions that are not diseases may also provide important information concerning the holistic state of the interviewee. For instance, it is relevant to know if the interviewee is pregnant or a trained athlete, because these conditions may point towards germane biologic and psychological issues.

Axis IV

This axis concerns itself with an examination of the current stresses affecting the interviewee. It examines the crucial interaction between the patient and the environment in which he or she lives. All too often interviewers are swept away by diagnostic intrigues and fail to uncover the reality-based problems confronting the patient. These reality-based concerns frequently suggest avenues for therapeutic intervention.

By way of illustration, on this axis the interviewer may discover that secondary to a job layoff, the home of the patient is about to be foreclosed. Such information may suggest the need to help the patient make contact with a specific social agency or may suggest the utility of a referral to a social worker.

This axis also remains of paramount importance in crisis intervention, time-limited therapies, and solution-focused therapies, as are commonly utilized in managed care settings. Any time a patient presents in crisis, it is generally useful to determine what perceived stressors have brought the patient to the point of seeking professional help. A question such as the following is often useful: "What stresses have you been coping with recently?" or "What thoughts made you decide to actually come here tonight as opposed to coming tomorrow or some other time?" In any case the fourth axis provides another pathway for both understanding and treatment planning.

Axis V

A variety of changes were made in Axis V when the DSM-III was revised into the DSM-III-R. In DSM-III this axis solely differentiated the highest functioning of the patient over a 2-month period in the preceding year. This relatively narrow perspective did not provide an abundance of practical information. Consequently, in DSM-III-R this axis was broadened. It included not only a rating of the highest functioning in the past year but also a rating of the current functioning, which provides immediate data pertinent to treatment planning and the decision as to whether hospitalization is warranted. These ratings were to be made by combining both symptoms and occupational and interpersonal functioning on a 90-point scale, the Global Assessment Functioning (GAF) Scale.

In the DSM-IV the same procedure and scale are used, except the scale range is now 0 to 100 and only "current functioning" is required to be rated. Other time frames can be added, in which case the additional time frame is indicated in parentheses after the additional score. Examples would be as follows: 45 (highest level in the past year) or 70 (at discharge from hospital).

The following inquiries, including both open- and closed-ended questions, can help the clinician uncover coping skills possessed by the patient:

a. When you are functioning well, what do you do to help yourself relax?
b. What kinds of things do you like to do in your spare time?
c. How do you go about making important decisions in your life?
d. What are some of your hobbies?
e. How many people have you shared your problems with? (This question may indirectly give the clinician some views on the patient's communication skills and his or her support systems.)
f. Do you enjoy sports or dancing?
g. Do you enjoy reading or the arts?
h. Have you ever kept a journal?
i. If someone asked you to list two of your best skills or talents, what would you say?

These types of questions may uncover important coping skills of a patient in crisis. For instance, one might discover that a patient has frequently kept a journal or diary as a method of sorting out problems. The clinician might use this information to remind the patient of past successes in dealing with problems, thus helping the patient to regain confidence. The clinician may also choose to have the patient solve problems, using his or her journal, before the next session, a therapeutic technique that will utilize the patient's natural skills while rekindling feelings of mastery during a time of crisis.

The assessment of actual current functioning pushes the clinician to carefully review evidence of immediate coping skills as affected by symptomatology. It is important to utilize behavioral incidents in this exploration, for patients, if asked for opinions, may give very misleading answers. By way of example, an acutely psychotic patient, who does not want to enter the hospital, may reply with a simple "not often" when asked, "Are the voices bothering you frequently?" Utilizing a behavioral incident approach, the clinician may find that the dialogue develops more along the following lines:

> **Clin.:** Looking at the last 2 days, how many times have you heard the voices per day, 100 times, 10 times?
>
> **Pt.:** (pausing and glancing away for a moment) Probably, well ... maybe a good 50 times a day.
>
> **Clin.:** What types of things do they say?
>
> **Pt.:** (pause) They tell me I'm ugly.
>
> **Clin.:** What do you feel when the voices say mean things like that to you?
>
> **Pt.:** It hurts, but I try to push them out of mind.
>
> **Clin.:** Do they ever tell you to hurt yourself?
>
> **Pt.:** You could say that.
>
> **Clin.:** What exactly do they tell you?

Using the behavioral incident technique, the clinician has found not only that the voices are bothersome but also that they are quite frequent.

Also keep in mind with regard to current functioning that sources outside the patient, such as family and friends, frequently provide more valid information than the patient. Once again, when questioning corroborative sources, behavioral incidents should be elicited to ensure validity.

Case Application of DSM-IV

To begin using our first assessment perspective, the DSM-IV, we must first organize our data axis by axis. We will then ask ourselves what if any treatment modalities are suggested by the diagnoses we have generated. With regard to the first axis, Miss Baker's presentation suggests several diagnostic entities. The primary delineation suggests that her symptoms are those of some type of mood disorder. Regarding the secondary delineation into the specific mood disorders present, she does not appear to currently fit the criteria for a major depression, but she may represent a variant of dysthymic disorder. As mentioned earlier, the presence of this disorder might suggest the use of an antidepressant. Dysthymic Disorder can also be approached using a variety of psychotherapeutic modalities, including behavioral techniques.

Her history suggests no strong evidence for entities such as schizophrenia or other psychotic processes, although the clinician may want to explore her vivid fantasy productions in more detail to rule out the possibility of delusional material. There is no evidence on Axis I of delirium or dementia. Two areas not well explored are the areas of anxiety disorders and dissociative disorders, and in a later interview these omissions should be corrected.

Along Axis II several possibilities are emerging, which may provide important clues as to how to proceed. Many of her symptoms, such as her deep fears of abandonment and being alone, suggest the possibility of the diagnosis of a borderline personality and perhaps a dependent personality. Both of these diagnoses serve to warn the clinician that Miss Baker may be predisposed to becoming overly dependent upon the clinician. Dependency issues may be important areas for focus in the upcoming therapy. Also of importance is the fact that a large body of literature exists concerning the treatment of the borderline personality, a literature that can be easily tapped by the clinician. As a triage agent, the diagnostic label of a borderline personality may also suggest the wisdom of not assigning this patient to a newly trained or poorly skilled therapist, because such patients are frequently difficult to manage. On this axis one might further explore entities such as a histrionic personality, a schizotypal personality, or an antisocial personality.

An exploration of Axis III brings many important points to mind. In the first place Miss Baker's depressive symptoms suggest the possibility of a mood disorder due to a general medical condition. She needs a medical examination. If the initial clinician is a psychiatrist, then this clinician has omitted a good medical review of systems. This omission, brought to our attention by the use of Axis III, will need to be rectified. Pertinent laboratory work will be ordered, and a physical examination may be indicated.

But the value of Axis III does not end here. The history of episodic violence may suggest an underlying seizure disorder that has been routinely missed by previous clinicians. Once again the interviewer will want to ask questions pertinent to this diagnosis and may consider ordering an electroencephalogram (EEG). Her worsening of symptoms near her menstrual periods also adds the possibility of a premenstrual syndrome, which may suggest the use of medications such as Motrin (ibuprofen) to relieve cramping and an antianxiety agent used for a day or two near her periods to decrease her premenstrual tension or the addition of an SSRI (selective serotonin reuptake inhibitor) antidepressant.

A final consideration on Axis III concerns Miss Baker's obesity. One wonders whether there may be an organic etiology for her obesity as well as whether her weight represents a powerful psychological concern, which she was hesitant to discuss.

Axis IV provides further pertinent information. In particular, one questions what the impact of the upcoming wedding will be. Even for the most stable of people, weddings are far from unstressful. A review of this axis also indicates that the interviewer has not explored stressors very well yet. With regard to triage and the determination of when this patient should be seen next, it would be useful for the interviewer to have a much clearer picture of the current stressors.

As we end our survey of this perspective, we come to the global assessment of adaptive functioning as delineated on Axis V. The information is sparse here, reflecting a weakness in the database thus far collected. A more thorough examination of current functioning would be of value in determining disposition. One also wonders what skills she may possess, which may be utilized in her treatment. For instance, her overactive fantasy life, if toned down, may represent a fertile imagination, which could be an asset in her development as an individual. This axis clearly warrants further exploration.

The above discussion illustrates the immense power the DSM-IV represents as a method of organizing data in a fashion that generates treatment options and also "pointing out" areas of important clinical information that have been overlooked. But this assessment perspective alone yields an incomplete picture. It is now time to move to a different assessment perspective with which to understand the problems facing Miss Baker.

SYSTEMS ANALYSIS

Nothing exists in isolation. Whether a cell or a person, every system is influenced by the configuration of the systems of which each is a part, that is, by its environment.

George L. Engel

Basic Paradigm

Systems analysis provides a stimulating method of organizing and utilizing the data gained from the initial interview. In this perspective one conceptualizes the patient not as a static "thing" with permanent characteristics but rather as an intertwining series of processes. Each process or system offers a potential wedge for therapeutic intervention.

George Engel, an internist with many interests in psychosomatic medicine, has been an elegant proponent of utilizing the systems approach.[3] Many of the following ideas parallel his thinking, although the subsequent paradigm is simpler, having been developed specifically for use in conceptualizing data for mental health assessments.

In this approach each person is viewed as representing the conjunction of seven progressively larger systems. These seven systems include: (1) the physiologic system, (2) the psychological system, (3) the dyadic system, (4) the family system, (5) the group system, (6) the societal system, and (7) the existential system: the patient's framework for meaning. Each smaller system is subsumed by the system above it. Like the axes of the DSM-IV, each of these systems can be used as a level at which to organize data and subsequently develop a list of potential treatment modalities, each system providing a clarifying lens through which to understand the patient. These seven systems are illustrated in Figure 5.

As the interview proceeds, the clinician asks himself or herself whether enough information, if any, has been gathered in each of these seven systems. Such self-reflection ensures that errors of omission are not being made and that a powerful database for treatment planning is evolving. Even as the information from a given system is revealed, treatment options may "pop into the mind" of the interviewer. Just as was the case with the diagnostic assessment perspective of the DSM-IV, if the clinician carefully listens to the

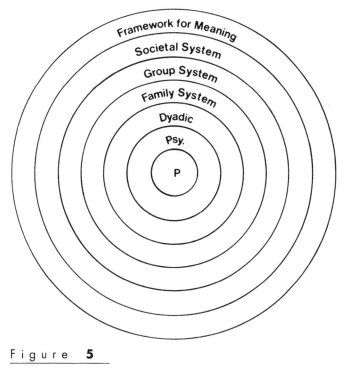

F i g u r e **5**

Systems analysis. (P = physiologic system; Psy = psychological system.)

patient's problems, the problems begin to suggest their own solutions. It is the organization of the data that provides this momentum.

Physiologic System

On the first level, the interviewer focuses on the physiologic make-up of the patient. This system is identical to the third axis of DSM-IV. In it the clinician hunts for evidence of medical illness as well as the presence of symptoms suggesting that somatic treatments may be of value. The clinician reviews whether any investigations or interventions can be made at the physiologic level. Investigations may include entities such as laboratory tests, computed tomography (CT) scans, EEGs, or a physical examination. Physiologic interventions could include antidepressants, antipsychotics, other medications, relaxation techniques, meditational techniques, or electroconvulsive therapy (ECT). The main point centers upon an active inquiry into the workings of the patient's body as well as the patient's mind.

With regard to the physiologic system, an analysis of Miss Baker remains essentially unchanged from our discussion with regards to Axis III. In this case there exists a direct overlap between the DSM-IV and systems analysis.

Psychological System

In the second system, the psychological system, one enters an area that only partially overlaps the DSM-IV as reflected by considerations of personality development on Axis II. Consequently, it is an exploration ripe with implications. At this level the clinician attempts to understand the patient both in a phenomenological sense as a unique human and in a psychodynamic sense as a product of past development. Each interviewer will have preferences for which psychological theories seem relevant, whether they be Freudian, Jungian, Rogerian, or some combination of the numerous viewpoints available. But the important point remains that the clinician attempts to understand the patient in a human context and not merely as a diagnostic entity. In this system perspective interviewers expand their lists of treatment options by considering the use of individual psychotherapies or counseling techniques.

As the psychological system is reviewed, a more personalized view of Miss Baker emerges as she becomes at once more complicated and more human. Several conflictual issues are readily apparent, including: (1) fears of abandonment, (2) problems with anger and impulse control, (3) ongoing problems with low self-esteem, (4) suicidal gestures, and (5) problems with identity and a sense of self. By delineating these areas the clinician can begin to generate further options for treatment. For example, her problems with anger and impulse control could be approached using behavioral modification, perhaps training her to self-monitor behaviors suggesting that an angry outburst is imminent, at which point alternative ways of relieving her hostile tension could be implemented. From a different perspective, an analytic viewpoint, one could look at her disturbances in her sense of self as indicating the need for specific psychotherapeutic approaches developed by clinicians such as Kohut, Kernberg, or Masterson.

Furthermore, a survey of the information known at this level reveals that not much psychogenetic data have been garnered yet, a deficit that can be tended to in future sessions. The important point remains that by conceptualizing in the psychological system interviewers prompt themselves to consider areas of intervention utilizing individual psychotherapy, as well as checking to see if this region of highly pertinent information has been adequately tapped.

Dyadic System

When we move to the third level, the dyadic system, the patient is viewed as one component of the numerous two-person interactions that fill the patient's daily interactions. The patient's interpersonal skills are assessed. For instance, does the patient have adequate verbal skills and social skills? Some patients suffering from schizophrenia may act oddly or may share their delusions with others without realizing the disengaging impact of these activities. Such patients may benefit from social skills training. In a similar vein, people with mental retardation represent another category of patients with whom social skills training may yield gratifying results. The interviewer should also bear in mind that the patient's interaction with the interviewer provides direct and immediate information concerning this system. Unfortunately, this arena is frequently overlooked by clinicians. Utilizing the systems approach helps to prevent this important omission.

In the case of Miss Baker the dyadic system focuses attention on her style of relating to other individuals. One wonders if her angry outbursts may be reactions to a chronic style of passively deferring to the needs of others. Such a situation may suggest the utility of self-assertiveness training.

This system refocuses attention on the impact of the patient's physical appearance and behavior. Miss Baker's loud sunglasses and old T-shirt, coupled with her obesity, may indeed strike an unappreciative chord upon first contact. Miss Baker may be unaware of the ramifications of her behavior, and social skills training may be useful at some point. In the end all of these interpersonal issues are of relevance to her relationship with her significant other, an appropriate invitation to the next level of analysis, the family.

Family System

As we look at the fourth system, the family, we come upon one of the most powerful systems affecting all humans. To conceptualize patients without considering the dynamics of their family is to see half a picture at best. To plan treatment without considering the needs and opinions of the patient's family may represent an invitation to treatment failure.

Moreover, whether interviewers like to admit it or not, the patient's family is psychologically present in any interview, representing a powerful determining force on the patient's behavior. The interviewer should always consider the utility of a family assessment or eventual employment of family therapy.

Ideally, a clinician may actually be presented with an opportunity to interact with the family as a unit in a joint interview. For example, in an emergency room situation, the patient is frequently accompanied by family members. On these occasions the clinician can directly observe the process of family interaction.

But even within the confines of an individual assessment, an enormous amount of information can be gained concerning family dynamics by gently probing. Pertinent data will emerge simply by learning some of the background facts and pieces of demographic information. The clinician can begin a familiarization with the family matrix by inquiring into where various family members have chosen to live. It is probably not merely chance that leads to a situation in which all the children have moved thousands of miles away from mom and dad. Nor should one ignore the implications of a family in which most members have chosen to live on the same block.

I remember a young woman seeking help for severe marital discord, who complained that she could not get her mother "to mind her own business." Later in the interview I was surprised to find that the patient had recently moved back into the same apartment complex where her parents lived, ostensibly for convenience. The issue of inappropriate attachment to her parents appeared as a psychodynamic theme throughout the remaining therapy.

Another important area reveals itself when one inquires about which people are living under the same roof with the patient. Such questioning may uncover unexpected findings, such as a domineering grandparent whose ideas of discipline clash with the concepts of the parents.

On a more specific level, further questioning may directly begin to unravel the complexities of the family, such as:

a. What were holidays like at your house?
b. What kinds of things did your brothers or sisters like to do? (often yields clues to sibling rivalry)
c. Describe the physical appearance of your brother (another nice gate through which to explore sibling rivalry).
d. Whom do you share secrets with in your family?
e. Who makes the decisions in your family?
f. Who do you think you are most like in your family?
g. Tell me a little about what kinds of things your parents used to argue about.
h. Did you go to the same schools as your brother? (and if so, what was that like?)
i. Did you share a room with any siblings? (and if so, what was that like?)

With questions such as the above the initial interviewer can begin to determine whether a family assessment may be indicated.

An analysis of the family system is not emphasized in the DSM-IV except as an aspect of the stressors on Axis IV, once again highlighting the utility of applying several assessment grids when planning treatment. Some authors have suggested creating a new axis in the next DSM revision upon which to conceptualize family pathology. Further discussion of this critical area of assessment would take us out of the topic of the book, but the interested reader may find the writings of Stephen Fleck useful in building a foundation for a more specific approach to family assessment.[4, 5]

With regard to Miss Baker, the importance of her relationship with her significant other immediately emerges as she boldly announces her upcoming wedding. It is as if she can hardly wait to shed her identity, washing her hands of her own name with a brisk shrug as she meets the clinician. As the interview progresses the additional information that her significant other also indulges the patient's fantasy identities is further evidence of a powerful bond between the two, perhaps a bond laced with pathology. This relationship, on the other hand, has endured for several years and may represent a potentially powerful resource in therapy. To increase the light on this relationship, the clinician may consider the use of a joint assessment session with the couple.

Turning towards the impact of her nuclear family, Miss Baker's poignant early memory of being tugged away from the door as her father vanishes conveys the sense of a deeply troubled childhood. Clearly, more information in this region will be enlightening, and the clinician is reminded once again of the potential utility of family assessment or therapy.

Group System

In the fifth system, the group system, the interviewer investigates the patient's ability to function within groups outside of the family. In particular one looks at the patient's relationships at work and with networks of friends. A pivotal issue concerns the patient's abilities to handle authority figures such as employers. The clinician keeps an eye open for evidence that the patient is generalizing feelings from family members onto other relationships, such as sibling rivalry reappearing as intense competitiveness at the workplace. It is also valuable to search for subcultures to which the patient may look for values and support. Such cultures could include the drug culture, the bar culture, the jock culture, or ideologic entities such as the Ku Klux Klan. An ignorance of a patient's cultural subgroup can lead to major errors in treatment planning. Alcohol detoxification will probably serve little purpose if the patient immediately returns to the bar scene for a rendezvous with drinking buddies. While contemplating this system, the interviewer should consider whether group therapy may be of value. Moreover one is also reminded of utilizing subcultures for therapeutic effect, such as recommending Alcoholics Anonymous.

Little is known about the functioning of Miss Baker at a group level. Indeed, the absence of her mentioning friends perks our attention, perhaps suggesting problematic relationships or none at all. There also seems to be a conspicuous absence of support groups or outside activities. A potentially important subculture worth exploring with Miss Baker remains the impact of the gay culture upon herself and her significant other. While reviewing the information gathered at this level concerning Miss Baker, the clinician is reminded of the possible advantages of group therapy. On a behavioral level, as therapy progresses, it may be beneficial to steer her towards rewarding group activities such as volunteer work.

Societal System

The sixth level represents the societal system. This system can be viewed as consisting of the various social forces shaping the patient's functioning within the community. These forces include economic, political, institutional, and social class factors. As Engel's quotation suggests at the beginning of this section, the patient's environment should always be considered. In particular, an investigation of the patient's financial status, housing, and food availability remains an important area for inquiry. All of these conditions are intimately related to the political climate of the patient's county, state, and federal governments. It is also possible that a patient's society is problematic, disabling the patient through prejudice or violence. Once again the interviewer must remember not to focus solely on individual dynamics, because the patient is part of many different systems, any one of which may be malfunctioning. It remains a basic tenet of assessment interviewing that one must understand the patient's culture in order to understand the patient's behavior.

In this light the issue of Miss Baker's sexual preference warrants an understanding of her culture. Further interviewing revealed that she and her significant other had been forced to deal with considerable ostracism. At first glance this ostracism seems totally at odds with the further development of Miss Baker, but there may be a curious catch here. In essence this easily identified enemy has served as a common threat around which Miss Baker and her significant other have mobilized, thus stabilizing their relationship.

Perhaps a digression is warranted at this point. Thus far we have been using the systems perspective to help organize data into distinct regions, which provide potential approaches to treatment. For the initial interviewer this aspect of systems thinking is very productive. But as therapy progresses, a different characteristic of systems thinking becomes increasingly important, namely, the actual interaction among the seven systems.

A change in any one system may have a potential impact, not always a beneficial one, on all other systems. The clinician needs to weigh the potential impact of intervention at one level upon the overall development of the patient. This ever-changing web of relationships stands at the very heart of therapy. Many a therapist has rued the day he or she blindly intervened at one level without considering potential ramifications at other levels.

By way of clarification, suppose Miss Baker and her significant other lived in a community that was overtly hostile towards homosexuality, as was the case. A clinician might suggest that moving to another neighborhood could be beneficial, but such a suggestion could be a serious miscalculation. One of the most powerful glues for this relationship could be their unified need to protect each other from this community's attacks. If placed in a new and benign community, the relationship itself could begin to collapse, fulfilling Miss Baker's frightening fear of abandonment. In this example it might be better to stabilize the relationship upon more solid ground before suggesting such a move.

It is well beyond the scope of this book to explore the interactional aspect of systems theory further, but I think it is important, even in a discussion of an initial interview, to keep it in mind.

It also reminds us, at the societal level, to consider one other crucial system when planning treatment, namely, the mental health system itself. The clinician needs to be aware of the actual resources available for follow-up. It is useless to recommend behavioral therapy to a patient if there is no behavioral therapist available to the patient. Indeed, such "pie in the sky" thinking can frustrate patients, hanging false hopes before their eyes. Similarly, a common error at academic centers is the tendency to generate complex treatment plans for patients referred from community centers that these centers cannot implement when the patient returns to them. Such state-of-the-art treatment planning is in reality an example of poor assessment formulation, because its impracticality breeds frustration in the patient and anger in the treating clinician.

To finish our discussion of the societal system, an important mental health resource for Miss Baker was uncovered by further interviewing. An excellent day clinic had been providing intermittent support for Miss Baker over the past year or so. This community system suggested a future area for support.

Existential System: The Framework for Meaning

On the seventh level, the interviewer examines the patient's framework for meaning. Although in actuality this system could be conceived of as part of the psychological system already discussed, it is so important that it is best viewed separately. To understand the patient more fully it becomes necessary to understand his or her religious beliefs, philosophical beliefs, and ethical standards. At times the patient's symptoms may be related to unrest within these basic existential areas. It is important to remember that in addition to religious beliefs, patients may find meaning in processes such as patriotism, community activity, and the care of their families. Information gained in this system may suggest the utility of individual psychotherapy slanted towards existential issues. A review of this system also serves to remind the clinician of the availability of clergy and pastoral counselors in the treatment of the patient.

In the initial interview this region was left relatively poorly explored in the case of Miss Baker. Later interviews revealed a paucity of religious and philosophical supports at this level, suggesting avenues for intervention such as augmenting the patient's participation in community or religious groups.

We have now concluded a brief survey of the seven levels used in a systems analysis. Although there exists some obvious overlap with the DSM-IV, a systems analysis provides several new areas in which to deepen an understanding of the patient and suggests as well new areas of intervention. Systems analysis also provides a more realistic picture of the patient as one process inextricably woven among the other systems of the world at large.

ASSESSMENT OF CORE PAINS

I can see behind everyone's masks. Peacefully smiling faces, pale corpses who endlessly wend their tortuous way down the road that leads to the grave.

Edvard Munch, 19th century expressionist painter

Although Munch depicts a somewhat grim picture of human existence, he was a man keenly aware of the pains that all of us endure by our very nature of being human. His ability to intuitively sense underlying pain represents a gift that all clinicians hope to possess. Indeed this ability to understand pain provides a major gateway through which therapeutic trust is born.

Throughout this book an emphasis has been placed on combining intuition and analysis. Many times the clinician will be able to intuitively sense the pains of the interviewee, but this intuition is enhanced when guided by an increased awareness of underlying themes. One of the more fascinating themes is the coexistence of the complexity of human nature with the simplicity of that same nature. Nowhere is this curious juxtaposition more prominent than with the issue of psychological pain. Patients frequently present with complicated histories and concerns, sometimes even involving bizarre delusions and idiosyncratic perceptions. But the underlying pains from which these patients are fleeing are few in number.

Skilled clinicians possess the knack of cutting through the complexities until the bare wounds, the core pains, are understood. An understanding of these core pains is a powerful clinical tool. This empathic understanding can suggest avenues for treatment planning. Even more important, it can also guide the interviewer towards methods of navigating the resistances that develop during the interview itself, because the seeds of resistance are generally attempts to avoid these core pains by the patient. We have already had a glimpse of this process when we discussed methods of handling resistance in the opening phase of the interview in Chapter 2. Later we will use the same concepts as the cornerstone of our approach to resistance as explored in Chapter 10.

In any case, an understanding of core pains and the increased sensitivity such an understanding can bring provides an assessment perspective that complements both the DSM-IV and systems analysis. It is based on the principle that clinicians should intermittently ask themselves, "What are the core pains that are hurting this patient at this time?" Or as Edvard Munch would have it, what is behind the mask?

The relevance of the concept of core pains was made plain to me by a psychotic patient when I was least expecting it. The patient was a young woman in her mid-20s who presented violently and was riddled with terrifying delusions. During the initial interview she described her sincere belief that aliens were speaking directly into her mind, taunting her sanity. Her world was convulsed with a pricking sensation of paranoia. She had become convinced that the aliens were about to kidnap her to a distant world. Her affect was intense, and she spoke in a disorganized fashion with a loosening of associations.

At this point I asked her why she felt the aliens were coming for her. To my surprise she looked at me as if I had not been listening. Her affect calmed; her speech became coherent; and she said, "Don't you understand? I am alone here. No one cares for me. I have no family, no friends. And I have no reason to be here. Wouldn't you want to leave this horrid place if you were me?" At which point she promptly popped back into her psychotic language and refuge.

In a sense she was right concerning my inadequate listening, because I had become overly involved in diagnosis and systems analysis. A balancing perspective was needed, a sense of her pathos on a human level. She provided me with a lesson that led me to think more carefully about the presence of core pains and methods of conceptualizing them more clearly even as the interview itself proceeds.

Towards this goal one can generate a list of core pains that singly or in combination appear to be driving any given individual. Each clinician may have a unique list; the following serve only as a platform for discussion. To me the core pains are as follows:

1. Fear of being alone
2. Fear of worthlessness
3. Fear of impending rejection
4. Fear of failure
5. Fear of loss of external control
6. Fear of loss of internal control
7. Fear of the unknown

With Miss Baker in mind one can survey these pains, examining their usefulness in both treatment planning and in understanding the dynamics of the interview itself.

The fear of being ultimately alone remains one of the most powerful and common pains. In the case of Miss Baker it appears to be surfacing in one of its frequent guises, intense dependency. As such it serves to remind the interviewer that some patients may seek an unhealthy dependency on the clinician even during the initial interview. Miss Baker would be one such person in whom this process could occur, as reflected by her intense feelings of abandonment when her significant other goes to sleep.

Her dependency needs may be intimately related to the second core pain, the fear of worthlessness. Miss Baker may be convinced of her ultimate inability to cope with life. In this sense she probably avoids situations in which she could modestly succeed, thus depriving herself of the positive reinforcement needed to gain a sense of mastery. With these factors in mind the clinician might consider assigning Miss Baker small easily accomplished tasks, resulting in a gradually increasing sense of worth. A cognitive therapy approach might reveal that Miss Baker has a distorted self-image maintained by tendencies for negative thinking and inappropriate self-blame. In this light, techniques such as cognitive restructuring might be of use.

Like its predecessor this core pain appears to lead naturally into a discussion of the next core pain, an impending sense of rejection. This fear reared its head throughout the interviewing process. Miss Baker demonstrated poor eye contact and frequently commented, "That's a stupid thing for me to say." Such anxieties can hamper the progress of the initial interview as the patient expends inordinate amounts of attention attempting to please the interviewer. Alert to this situation, the interviewer may purposely reassure the patient. For instance, the clinician might choose to say to Miss Baker, "You are doing a very good job of discussing difficult material. It's really helping me to get a clearer picture of what has been going on." Even such a simple statement can make a patient such as Miss Baker feel considerably more comfortable, decreasing her fear of imminent rejection.

The fourth pain, the fear of failure, overlaps with a sense of worthlessness but has an intensity all its own. The initial interviewer needs to attend to this particular pain, because the patient may bring it into the initial interview itself. Specifically, the patient may predict an impending failure in therapy and consequently decide not to appear for follow-up. If left as a hidden issue, the risk of losing the patient is real. In the closing phase of the interview, the clinician may opt to bring this fear to the surface with questions such as, "Now that we have talked about possible therapies, I'm wondering what you think about their usefulness for you?" or "If you tried outpatient therapy, how do you think it would go?" The interviewer may be able to cite the patient's success in handling the initial interview as evidence that the patient has the necessary abilities to succeed in therapy.

The fear of losing external control, the fifth pain, can be extremely frightening to patients, because suddenly it seems as if nothing they can do will alter their situation. This combination of fear and anger can present a fertile field for suicidal ideation. If one listens to the steelworker laid off indefinitely, the roar of this pain can certainly be heard. While interviewing elderly patients one should bear in mind that they may be dealing with a sense of the ultimate loss of external control, death itself. When this core pain appears particularly prominent, the initial interviewer can make an effort to consciously increase the patient's sense of control within the interview itself by using statements such as, "At this point what do you think would be the most important area we should focus our discussion on?" Such modest yet timely intervention can significantly return some feeling of control to the patient.

The sixth core pain, the fear of loss of internal control, surfaces in patients who are becoming increasingly frightened of their own impulses, such as drives towards suicide or violence. I doubt that this pain could be more vividly portrayed than in patients who are moving into progressively more psychotic or manic behavior. In Miss Baker's case her history of episodic violence, as evidenced by her throwing a picnic table bench through a picture window, suggests that this core pain may be a frequent motivator of her behaviors. Fortunately, in her initial interview she appeared to be in good control.

But in other situations the interviewer may find a patient who reports feeling imminently unstable. In such cases it is generally, if not always, sound to attend to these fears on the spot. If the interviewer chooses to ignore these feelings, the interviewer risks driving the patient into an act of violence. Ironically, the patient's own increasing fears of losing control may act to spur further anxiety, perhaps pushing the patient even closer to a loss of control. The clinician can gently probe to see what the patient is afraid may happen and ask the patient if indeed he or she feels in control. The appearance of this core pain may suggest the usefulness of an antipsychotic medication.

We now come to the last and seventh element in the assessment of core pains, the fear of the unknown. As described in Chapter 2, most patients are probably experiencing this pain during the interview itself, because they are frightened of what the results of the interview will be. As mentioned earlier a few minutes spent performing a sound introduction can greatly relieve the patient's unnecessary fears. In Miss Baker's case, her fear of the unknown may add to her dependent patterns, making her reluctant to try things on her own. With regard to treatment planning, one sometimes finds that patients such as Miss Baker do not have the communication skills or the assertiveness to find out what the future may hold, thus locking them into the paralysis of the moment. Their lack of assertiveness may prevent them from asking appropriate questions, even of the interviewer. The presence of this core pain should alert the clinician to the potential use of assertiveness training and social skills work as well as to the need to address unasked questions.

We have now reviewed our third assessment schema. I have not explored the use of this system in detail; we will do this in upcoming chapters. Instead I have tried to survey this assessment system, which provides yet another set of pathways toward treatment planning. This particular schema provides more on-the-spot information pertinent to altering the course of the interview itself than either the DSM-IV or systems analysis. Together, these three assessment perspectives complement each other, helping the interviewer change a potentially impotent mass of data into a crisp and practical formulation, bridging directly into the treatment planning process itself.

As the clinician becomes familiar with using these three systems, one of their most appealing aspects surfaces—their speed. Once familiar with their use the clinician can assess the known database while generating a powerful list of treatment options in about 5 to 10 minutes. This rapid integration of a large database can be a godsend in a busy clinic or private practice. Furthermore the clinician can review the ongoing treatment plan quickly and with a fresh perspective as time passes.

Before wrapping up this chapter it may be gratifying to review the actual progress of Miss Baker in therapy, while also looking at the actual selections that were made from the lists of potential treatments generated by the above perspectives.

REVIEW OF THE CLINICAL COURSE OF MISS BAKER

In the first place, despite her chaotic history, Miss Baker brought to therapy a variety of healthy coping skills. Viewed in the light of Axis V, she displayed motivation, intelligence, and a keen ability at self-reflection. She also possessed the often too rare quality of compassion. Indeed, it was her apparent inability to recognize and accept her strengths that stood as one of the major obstacles to her development. In a large measure, therapy consisted of an attempt to help Miss Baker develop the attributes hinted at during her moments of high functioning.

The rest of her eventual treatment plan evolved directly from the data gathered in the initial interview. On Axis I she did not fulfill the criteria for a major depression. She did appear to meet the criteria for dysthymia, which, as mentioned earlier, may respond to antidepressant medication. In her case I opted to forgo an antidepressant at first, hoping that psychotherapeutic measures would be more effective. In particular, because of her long-established pattern of self-debasement and a sense of worthlessness, I was concerned that she would immediately deny any credit for improvement if an antidepressant could be pointed to as the curative agent. If she had developed a major depression or if the chosen treatment track would have failed, I would most likely have promptly added an antidepressant. In the long run, the goal was to enable her to gain an increasing sense of self-worth and mastery over her environment.

Her problems with the development of a stable self were reflected by her primary Axis II diagnosis of a borderline personality disorder. She would probably have also met the criteria for a dependent personality. In any case, these diagnoses suggested the need to attend to her dependency issues quickly, a generalization extrapolated from the diagnosis and borne out by her long history of dependent relations. Consequently, in the closing phase of the initial interview, the issues of possible dependency upon me were discussed openly and mutually decided upon as a major concern to be avoided.

To sidestep a maladaptive dependency upon myself, she was seen only on a weekly basis. Moreover we agreed to adopt a long-term treatment plan built around the concept of meeting for 3-month periods in which we focused on a specific problem list generated by her. At the end of each 3-month period, we would break from therapy for progressively longer periods of time as she began functioning more and more independently.

During her 3-month period of active therapy, specific tasks were assigned as homework, which she mastered easily, increasing her sense of worth. She also became adept at utilizing cognitive restructuring, which helped her to decrease her tendency for overgeneralization, splitting, and inappropriate self-blame. These cognitive techniques were implemented while simultaneously considering the psychodynamic issues of the development of her self.

Miss Baker began to make strides in her bewildering battle to discover her own identity. Her successes in this regard were poignantly illustrated by the fact that she began signing her real name to pieces of artwork instead of her fantasy name of "Paul." Furthermore, as therapy proceeded she stopped wearing her wristband with the false identity, a behavioral change paralleled by a significant decrease in her fantasy activity.

This treatment approach characterized by intermittent stretches of therapist-free time was only possible because of considerations made with regard to the societal system. Specifically, it was discovered that a day clinic was available that could offer appropriate support when needed, as she underwent the pangs of separating from me. Thus she received enough support to gain the additional sense of independence offered by successfully navigating her loss of me. Only through the cooperation received by this agency of the mental health system could the treatment plan be made operational.

To help her with impulse control during her premenstrual unrest, small doses of the antianxiety agent Xanax (alprazolam) were used as deemed necessary by Miss Baker and carefully monitored by me. A behavioral system, on which she played a major role in developing, was employed to help her to prevent suicidal and violent activity. The emphasis remained on her to help herself, using her decreased need for my "parenting" as reinforcing evidence of her ability to manage independently.

A further area for intervention appeared in the family assessment. To this end a session was arranged for Miss Baker and her partner. By explaining to her partner certain aspects of the overall plan for increasing Miss Baker's independence, her partner was better able to support progress. It was also discovered that her partner appeared to be a loving and dependable support system. This session also served to decrease her partner's anxieties concerning the therapy itself, thus decreasing the risk of resistance generated by her partner.

Two and one-half years later Miss Baker had been involved in three 3-month therapy courses separated by increasingly large interludes. Her mood shifts have stabilized markedly as has her relationship with her partner. She has had only two minor suicidal gestures in this time period. She reports a significant sense of increased self-worth. Naturally much work lies ahead, but the progress so far has been very satisfying.

CONCLUSION

In this chapter we have looked at the process of effectively organizing the information gained from an initial interview. It has become apparent that the methods chosen for conceptualizing data can greatly affect the ultimate usefulness of the data. The three organizational methods discussed here provide a reliable method of generating a practical list of treatment options. These three assessment systems also establish a reliable method of noting pertinent gaps in the database.

In the long run, the major reason for performing an assessment interview remains the generation of a sound treatment plan. As we have seen, this treatment plan arises from a thorough attempt to understand the patient and the systems of which the patient is an integral part. This understanding evolves directly from our abilities to sensibly organize data. At such times it almost seems as if the database speaks for itself. Our task becomes one of learning to listen.

References

1. American Psychiatric Association: *Diagnostic and Statistical Manual of Mental Disorders*, 3rd ed. Washington, DC, APA, 1980.
2. American Psychiatric Association: *Diagnostic and Statistical Manual of Mental Disorders*, 4th ed. Washington, DC, APA, 1994.
3. American Psychiatric Association: *Diagnostic and Statistical Manual of Mental Disorders*, 3rd ed., revised. Washington, DC, APA, 1987.
4. Fleck, S.: Family functioning and family psychopathology. *Psychiatric Annuals* 10:17–35, 1980.
5. Fleck, S.: A holistic approach to family typology and the axes of DSM-III. *Archives of General Psychiatry* 40:901–906, 1983.

PART 2

The Interview and Psychopathology

CHAPTER 5

Interviewing Techniques in Depression and Other Mood Disorders

I wander thro' each charter'd street,
Near where the charter'd Thames does flow
And mark in every face I meet
Marks of weakness, marks of woe.

William Blake
London

I n the early 1800s as Blake wandered the drab lanes of London, his eyes met the face of depression at every corner. Depression stalked among merchants, seamen, and prostitutes alike, because depression impolitely ignored the proper boundaries of social class. Today, whether on Fifth Avenue in New York or at a community mental health center in rural Pennsylvania, mental health professionals encounter faces strongly reminiscent of those that William Blake described centuries ago. As in Blake's time, depression masquerades in many costumes and clinical presentations.

As an illustration of this diversity, I remember working with a woman of about 40, who had been a successful interior designer. In the economic depression of the early 1980s, she found herself jobless. Her confidence and self-esteem were affronted with each passing day. Her belief in herself insidiously weakened as if she were an invalid who decided that there was no hope. Anxiety attacks punctuated her daily routine. Despite her pain she continued her frantic job search, terrified by each job interview. Her days be-

225

came compacted cells of anxiety neatly delineated by bars of self-doubt.

How differently this woman's presentation appears when contrasted with a strikingly white-haired woman I met in North Carolina. Although only 50 years old, this woman's face was branded by thick wrinkles. She had been extremely dependent on her father, a caricature of "daddy's little girl." Following his death 4 months earlier, she had felt as if her skin had emptied. She was no longer whole. The sight of his face could not comfort her. His touch could not reassure her. She was brought into the hospital on an involuntary commitment. According to the police she had been found wandering a local cemetery with a butcher knife in hand. She related that her father's voice was pleading with her to join him.

These people were obviously experiencing life very differently, yet both were suffering from depressive symptoms. I highlight this diversity of presentation to emphasize that depression is not a "thing." It is a constantly evolving process. As a process, depression becomes a way of living. It is unique for each individual and for each environment that the individual encounters. On the other hand, there are many similarities in the presentations of depression that enable the clinician to recognize depression despite atypical patterns. This dual capacity of depression to appear both foreign and familiar provides the interviewer with the first inkling that depression requires many levels of understanding. In the initial interview the interviewer attempts to integrate diagnosis and understanding with each question, continually probing deeper. Only when the patient feels this drive for understanding is it likely that the clinician's help will be accepted, whether it exists in the form of psychotherapy or medication.

In the two sections of this chapter, two areas of major importance to the first interview will be explored: (1) diagnosis by DSM-IV criteria, and (2) understanding of the person and the personal ramifications of the depression.

These two processes occur simultaneously, but for clarity they will be discussed in separate sections. With regard to understanding the patient, one of the more expedient routes to understanding, systems analysis, has been described in Chapter 4. In section two of this chapter we will study the ramifications of depression using this systems paradigm. It is beyond the scope of this chapter to be either a complete guide to the use of diagnosis or an all-encompassing review of the ramifications of depression. Instead I hope to offer a view of various ideas that may stimulate clinicians to develop their own methods of exploring depression in an initial interview. At this time I would like to describe four people who sought help for depression. These four presentations will provide a clinical base for entry into section I, Diagnosis of Depression.

SECTION I: DIAGNOSIS OF DEPRESSION

Four Case Presentations

CASE 1: MR. WHITE

Mr. White is a 61-year-old white single man who retired from a prestigious job at the police department 1 year ago. He is accompanied by his fiancée. With her help he hopes to open a bar in the next 6 months, if they can get a liquor license. Mr. White is well groomed and dressed in a simple flannel work shirt and corduroy trousers. He appears very sad and relates, "It seems strange, but I can't really cry." He speaks softly and slowly, taking a while before answering questions as if thought required immense effort. On occasion, he tries to manage a smile. His eyes study the floor, seldom meeting the eyes of the interviewer. He complains of severe depression, of not being able to enjoy anything, sleep disturbance, loss of appetite and libido, and severe loss of energy. In the past 3 weeks he had held a loaded revolver to his head on several occasions. He spontaneously reports seeing no future. His fiancée, although obviously concerned, seems agitated and a bit cool. "He just won't help himself," she comments, "no matter how much I try to help him. Now I've got to meet with the Liquor Control Board agent alone next week."

CASE 2: MR. WHITSTONE

Mr. Whitstone was admitted to a general hospital for evaluation of bizarre behavior described by his family as paranoid. He is a distinguished appearing 62-year-old white man who has been a prominent businessman. At the time of the interview he is refusing all hospital care, including intravenous lines and medication. The interviewer has been called in as an emergency consultant. During the interview Mr. Whitstone appears guarded, thoroughly grilling the interviewer about his training and his purpose. Outside of his suspiciousness Mr. Whitstone is cooperative. During the first 10 minutes of the interview he appears tense, complaining, "I'm really having trouble with my thinking. I can't concentrate anymore. But they don't understand." When asked whether he feels depressed, he answers, "No, I don't feel particularly depressed." He reports problems with appetite and sleep. But of all his concerns, he is most upset about his business company, since he feels "someone in the company, and I'm not quite sure who, is out to get me." He has not returned to work since his triple bypass heart surgery in January, 6 months earlier. He is alert and oriented times three with a stable level of consciousness. Three members of his family are at bedside when the interviewer first enters the room.

CASE 3: MS. WILKINS

Ms. Wilkins entered the outpatient office with hesitant steps. Her patterned blue dress was faded and wrinkled. She is a 21-year-old white single woman who reports, "I feel horrible. I am so very depressed. Last night I was thinking of maybe (pause—tearfulness) killing myself." She reports numerous neurovegetative symptoms of depression such as sleep disturbance, decreased energy, decreased libido, and decreased appetite. She reports, "I've been depressed for years." She truly appears very sad. As the interview proceeds, the interviewer feels a deepening desire to help as well as an increasing concern. There is also an angry quality to Ms. Wilkins as she relates, "My best friend is really a bastard. I can't believe I trusted her." Ms. Wilkins denies concrete suicidal or homicidal ideation at the time of the interview, stating, "I'm feeling in control now." She wishes to have both medication and psychotherapy.

CASE 4: MR. COLLIER

Mr. Collier and his wife presented at the psychiatric emergency room. Mr. Collier is a 26-year-old white man who is casually but nicely dressed. He has dark brown hair and a strong jaw. His voice is rich with a vigorous, almost aggressive tone. He answers quickly with authority. While he interacts with his wife, the interviewer finds it easy to picture Mr. Collier giving his wife "the third degree." Mr. Collier complains bitterly of severe depression "ever since I was a teenager." He continues, "I remind myself of my father." He reports a tendency to sleep during the day and always feels tired. His appetite and libido are good. He complains of feeling worthless and lazy. He is upset that he has been sharp with his kids. In the week preceding their emergency room visit he slapped his 10-year-old daughter, Jackie, on the face. This incident frightened him and prompted the emergency room visit. He occasionally has fleeting suicidal ideation, remarking, "I'd jump in front of a car or bus . . . you know, to make sure my wife gets the insurance." He denies current suicidal ideation. He states "I'm the problem here. Help me and you'll help my family."

Discussion of Case Material

For the sake of discussion, let us assume that the above material had been elicited after roughly 15 minutes of interviewing. As one reviews this material two points are obvious: (1) all of these people are in significant psychological pain, and (2) all of them appear depressed. The next question facing the clinician deals with whether all of these people should be diagnosed as having a true major depression. The following case discussions will focus on the various lines of questioning that an interviewer might use to sort out this difficult differential.

In the first place, in order to diagnose accurately, the clinician needs to be thoroughly familiar with the basic criteria of DSM-IV. This familiarization does not mean that the clinician should obsessively memorize hundreds of criteria. On the contrary, this suggests a working knowledge of what material is necessary to clarify the major diagnoses. This diagnostic familiarization allows the clinician to focus on the art of eliciting the necessary material while successfully engaging the interviewee. The establishment of therapeutic alliance, as usual, remains of paramount importance. The diagnostic criteria for two of the common mood disorders in the DSM-IV are reviewed below. Before proceeding the reader might also find it useful to review the DSM-IV criteria for other common mood disorders, such as Bipolar I Disorder, Bipolar II Disorder, Cyclothymic Disorder, bipolor disorder not otherwise specified, and depressive disorder not otherwise specified. The DSM-IV defines major depression and dysthymic disorder as follows.

Criteria for Major Depressive Episode*

A. Five (or more) of the following symptoms have been present during the same 2-week period and represent a change from previous functioning; at least one of the symptoms is either: (1) depressed mood, or (2) loss of interest or pleasure.

Note: Do not include symptoms that are clearly due to a general medical condition, or mood-incongruent delusions or hallucinations.

1. Depressed mood most of the day, nearly every day, as indicated by either subjective report (e.g., feels sad or empty) or observation made by others (e.g., appears tearful). **Note:** In children and adolescents, can be irritable mood.
2. Markedly diminished interest or pleasure in all, or almost all, activities most of the day, nearly every day (as indicated by either subjective account or observation made by others)
3. Significant weight loss when not dieting or weight gain (e.g., a change of more than 5% of body weight in a month), or decrease or increase in appetite nearly every day. **Note:** In children, consider failure to make expected weight gains.
4. Insomnia or hypersomnia nearly every day

5. Psychomotor agitation or retardation nearly every day (observable by others, not merely subjective feelings of restlessness or being slowed down)
6. Fatigue or loss of energy nearly every day
7. Feelings of worthlessness or excessive or inappropriate guilt (which may be delusional) nearly every day (not merely self-reproach or guilt about being sick)
8. Diminished ability to think or concentrate, or indecisiveness, nearly every day (either by subjective account or as observed by others)
9. Recurrent thoughts of death (not just fear of dying), recurrent suicidal ideation without a specific plan, or a suicide attempt or a specific plan for committing suicide

B. The symptoms do not meet criteria for a Mixed Episode (see p. 335).
C. The symptoms cause clinically significant distress or impairment in social, occupational, or other important areas of functioning.
D. The symptoms are not due to the direct physiological effects of a substance (e.g., a drug of abuse, a medication) or a general medical condition (e.g., hypothyroidism).
E. The symptoms are not better accounted for by Bereavement; that is, after the loss of a loved one, the symptoms persist for longer than 2 months or are characterized by marked functional impairment, morbid preoccupation with worthlessness, suicidal ideation, psychotic symptoms, or psychomotor retardation.

---

*Reprinted with permission from the Diagnostic and Statistical Manual of Mental Disorders, 4th ed., p. 327. Copyright 1994 American Psychiatric Association.

Diagnostic Criteria for 296.2x Major Depressive Disorder, Single Episode†

A. Presence of a single Major Depressive Episode (see p. 327).
B. The Major Depressive Episode is not better accounted for by Schizoaffective Disorder and is not superimposed on Schizophrenia, Schizophreniform Disorder, Delusional Disorder, or Psychotic Disorder Not Otherwise Specified.
C. There has never been a Manic Episode (see p. 332), a Mixed Episode (see p. 335), or a Hypomanic Episode (see p. 338). **Note:** This exclusion does not apply if all of the manic-like, mixed-like, or hypomanic-like episodes are substance or treatment induced or are due to the direct physiologic effects of a general medical condition.

Specify
(for current or most recent episode):
    Severity/Psychotic/Remission Specifiers (see p. 376)

Chronic (see p. 382)
With Catatonic Features (see p. 382)
With Melancholic Features (see p. 383)
With Atypical Features (see p. 384)
With Postpartum Onset (see p. 386)

†Reprinted with permission from the Diagnostic and Statistical Manual of Mental Disorders, 4th ed., p. 344. Copyright 1994 American Psychiatric Association.

Diagnostic Criteria for 296.3x Major Depressive Disorder, Recurrent‡

A. Presence of two or more Major Depressive Episodes (see p. 327).

Note: To be considered separate episodes, there must be an interval of at least 2 consecutive months in which criteria are not met for a Major Depressive Episode.

B. The Major Depressive Episodes are not better accounted for by Schizoaffective Disorder and are not superimposed on Schizophrenia, Schizophreniform Disorder, Delusional Disorder, or Psychotic Disorder Not Otherwise Specified.
C. There has never been a Manic Episode (see p. 332), a Mixed Episode (see p. 335), or a Hypomanic Episode (see p. 338). **Note:** This exclusion does not apply if all of the manic-like, mixed-like, or hypomanic-like episodes are substance or treatment induced or are due to the direct physiologic effects of a general medical condition.

Specify
(for current or most recent episode):
Severity/Psychotic/Remission Specifiers (see p. 376)
Chronic (see p. 382)
With Catatonic Features (see p. 382)
With Melancholic Features (see p. 383)
With Atypical Features (see p. 384)
With Postpartum Onset (see p. 386)

Specify:
Longitudinal Course Specifiers (With and Without Interepisode Recovery) (see p. 387)
With Seasonal Pattern (see p. 389)

‡Reprinted with permission from the Diagnostic and Statistical Manual of Mental Disorders, 4th ed., p. 345. Copyright 1994 American Psychiatric Association.

Diagnostic Criteria for 300.4 Dysthymic Disorder§

A. Depressed mood for most of the day, for more days than not, as indicated either by subjective account or observation by others, for at least 2 years. **Note:** In children and adolescents, mood can be irritable and duration must be at least 1 year.
B. Presence, while depressed, of two (or more) of the following:
   1. Poor appetite or overeating
   2. Insomnia or hypersomnia
   3. Low energy or fatigue
   4. Low self-esteem
   5. Poor concentration or difficulty making decisions
   6. Feelings of hopelessness
C. During the 2-year period (1 year for children or adolescents) of the disturbance, the person has never been without the symptoms in Criteria A and B for more than 2 months at a time.
D. No Major Depressive Episode (see p. 327) has been present during the first 2 years of the disturbance (1 year for children and adolescents); that is, the disturbance is not better accounted for by chronic Major Depressive Disorder, or Major Depressive Disorder, In Partial Remission.

   Note: There may have been a previous Major Depressive Episode provided there was a full remission (no significant signs or symptoms for 2 months) before development of the Dysthymic Disorder. In addition, after the initial 2 years (1 year in children or adolescents) of Dysthymic Disorder, there may be superimposed episodes of Major Depressive Disorder, in which case both diagnoses may be given when the criteria are met for a Major Depressive Episode.

E. There has never been a Manic Episode (see p. 332), a Mixed Episode (see p. 335), or a Hypomanic Episode (see p. 338), and criteria have never been met for Cyclothymic Disorder.
F. The disturbance does not occur exclusively during the course of a chronic Psychotic Disorder, such as Schizophrenia or Delusional Disorder.
G. The symptoms are not due to the direct physiologic effects of a substance (e.g., a drug of abuse, a medication) or a general medical condition (e.g., hypothyroidism).
H. The symptoms cause clinically significant distress or impairment in social, occupational, or other important areas of functioning.

Specify if:
   Early Onset: if onset is before age 21 years
   Late Onset: if onset is age 21 years or older

Specify
(for most recent 2 years of Dysthymic Disorder):
With Atypical Features (see p. 384)

---

§Reprinted with permission from the Diagnostic and Statistical Manual of Mental Disorders, 4th ed., p. 349. Copyright 1994 American Psychiatric Association.

DISCUSSION OF MR. WHITE

Mr. White was the 61-year-old retired police officer who had held a loaded revolver to his head. Of all the cases presented, Mr. White appears to be showing some of the most classic symptoms of a major depression. The craft of eliciting such symptoms deserves further examination. In the first place, Mr. White states clearly that he has a persistently dysphoric mood, thus fulfilling one of the first two symptoms of criterion A needed for a diagnosis of major depression in the DSM-IV. It is important to note that one does not need to feel "depressed" to fulfill criterion A, because one needs the presence of either symptom 1 or symptom 2 for making a diagnosis of a major depression. Symptom 2 reads "markedly diminished interest or pleasure in all, or almost all, activities most of the day, nearly every day." Symptom 2 is essentially an undeclared definition of anhedonia. The word "anhedonia" is a derivative of the Greek word "hēdonē," referring to pleasure, as also seen in the English "hedonism." In anhedonia, one demonstrates a decreased ability to experience pleasure or to develop interest. This alteration in the experience of pleasure is a common symptom of depression, warranting a careful search in the initial interview.

One of the ways in which to explore anhedonia smoothly is to discover first what types of activities the interviewee enjoys in general. Questions such as the following may be fruitful for setting up such an exploration:

a. What kinds of things do you like to do when you're away from work?
b. In the past, have you generally enjoyed your work?
c. Do you have any types of hobbies or sports you enjoy?
d. Do you enjoy reading or watching television?
e. In the past have you enjoyed socializing?

Often I will spend considerable time exploring these interests further, because they can provide important insights to the clinician about the person's viewpoints and psychological integration, as seen, for instance, in the following:

Clin.: Do you enjoy reading or listening to music?

> **Pt.:**   I used to enjoy reading quite a bit . . . sort of odd stuff . . . (tiny smile) . . . like St. Augustine, Thomas Aquinas, and other theological books.
>
> **Clin.:**   Sounds like pretty heavy reading?
>
> **Pt.:**   Yeah, it is. But I used to enjoy it (pause). I used to be fairly religious . . . used to be (said with a trailing off of the voice).

From this dialogue it appears that religious themes may be important issues for this patient, perhaps contributing to his depressive anxiety. This questioning has not only laid the groundwork for a discussion of anhedonia, but it has also served the dual function of gathering pertinent intrapsychic material about the patient's framework for meaning, while further engaging the patient. At this point one may continue the search for anhedonia with questions referring to the groundwork laid above.

a. Over the past several weeks have you felt like doing these activities?
b. Do you find it as enjoyable to do these things as you used to, or has there been a change?
c. Have you been feeling interested in your hobbies over the past several weeks?

At times interpersonal questions can uncover anhedonic complaints, as evidenced by the following:

> **Clin.:**   You mentioned your grandchildren. Do you have a good time when you're around them now?
>
> **Pt.:**   (sigh) Sort of . . . Don't get me wrong, I love my grandchildren, but I just can't seem to enjoy anything any more, even them.

Along with anhedonia, Mr. White appears to be suffering from many of the neurovegetative symptoms of depression. Although it is difficult to find a standard definition of neurovegetative symptoms, I view them as symptoms suggesting that basic regulatory physiology has been disturbed. With such a definition in mind, the neurovegetative symptoms can be listed as follows: change in appetite, change in weight, sleep disturbance, change in energy, change in libido, altered concentration, and retarded or agitated motor activity. Although not always labeled as neurovegetative symptoms, other common physiologic correlates of depression exist, including constipation, dry mouth, and cold extremities.

Sleep disturbance warrants a more thorough discussion. Part of the lore of psychiatry has been that people suffering from major depressions often display early morning awakening. The exact frequency of this phenomenon is not entirely clear yet, although there is good evidence that feeling worse in the morning is a reasonably reliable indicator of a major depression. In any case it seems expedient to understand the extent and pattern of the sleep disturbance in the patient for the following reasons.

Thorough questioning of such a topic conveys to the patient that the interviewer is sensitively interested in the day-to-day disturbances of the patient's life caused by the depression. Furthermore, sleep disturbances can also provide early clues to other diagnostic possibilities. For instance, sleep continuity disturbances (e.g., waking up during the night) are common in depression, psychosis, drug and alcohol abuse, and in the elderly. Difficulty falling asleep can also be seen in a variety of disturbances, including depression, mania, anxiety disorders, adjustment disorders, and various psychotic processes. Besides decreased sleep, one should also search for evidence of increased sleep or a tendency for daytime sleeping. A reversed diurnal pattern of sleep, whereby the patient sleeps during the day and remains awake at night, can be seen in entities such as depression, bipolar disorder, and schizophrenia. By eliciting a detailed sleep history, one may also stumble upon an unsuspected primary sleep disturbance such as sleep apnea, narcolepsy, or nocturnal myoclonus.

With regard to neurovegetative symptoms, such as decreased energy, mention should also be made concerning the investigation of libido. At times interviewers feel shy about asking about libido. Seldom should this present a problem in engaging a patient if approached appropriately. In the first place, the topic should be broached smoothly while in a natural context. For example, if the clinician has been discussing the neurovegetative symptoms at length one might ask:

a. It sounds like your depression has really upset your system. Do you think it has also affected your sexual drive?

Alternatively, if the patient has been talking at length about the disruption of a romantic relationship one might query:

a. From what you are saying, it sounds as if there has been a lot of tension between you and your husband. Do you think it has also affected your sexual relationship?

I would like to add several points about questions concerning libido. I have found many patients relieved to know that decreased libido is a common feature of depression. Consequently, after asking about libido, I might add, "I ask about sexual drive because basic drives such as appetite and sexual desire are commonly decreased by depression." To such a statement, patients sometimes respond with sentiments such as "Thank God. I thought my loss of desire was just another one of my failures. "

Another important issue is the tone of voice. If interviewers ask their questions matter-of-factly, without hesitation, it greatly decreases the risk that the patient will feel put off. In a different light, if the patient does react unusually strongly, then one may have incidentally learned something about the patient's views on sex or their bodies or their views on what is proper for them to disclose. Such information is grist for the mill in later sessions. As a final note, some people confuse sexual drive with actual intercourse. It sometimes helps to clarify this issue with remarks such as "By sexual drive, I mean your interest in having sex, not whether you are actually having it or not." If this point is not clarified, a patient who is not dating may quickly state that libido is absent, "since I'm not seeing anyone," when in actuality a strong libido may be present.

The neurovegetative symptoms are classic hallmarks of a major depression, fulfilling many of the criteria of the A section of the DSM-IV. If they are not elicited spontaneously, they should always be actively sought. When done properly, such questioning powerfully engages the interviewee. It shows the interviewee two reassuring characteristics: (1) that the interviewer is interested in the individual as a person whose depression affects every aspect of his or her life, and (2) that the interviewer is knowledgeable as witnessed by the fact that the questions seem right on the mark.

Questions dealing with neurovegetative symptoms should seldom be asked in a checklist fashion with statements such as, "I need to ask a few questions now," or "Let me just go over a few things here." Instead, they should be imperceptibly woven into the fabric of the conversation, as shown below:

> **Pt.:** I don't know how to keep coping with all this strain, what with my unemployment and now my wife on my back.
>
> **Clin.:** You're going through some tough times. Is this affecting your sleep at all?
>
> **Pt.:** Hell, yes. I can't sleep at all.
>
> **Clin.:** Tell me more about it?
>
> **Pt.:** I'm waking up a couple of times a night. I just toss

and turn thinking about Janet and whether she'll leave me. I don't know why she stays, except I think she needs the money.

Clin.: How many times do you think you actually wake up?

Pt.: Maybe four or five, it's really bad. I feel horrible in the morning, no rest.

Clin.: Roughly what time are you waking up in the morning?

Pt.: Around 5:00 A.M.

Clin.: Do you wake up naturally or are you sort of jolted out of your sleep by worries?

Pt.: Oh no, I feel horrible. I can't get back to sleep no matter how hard I try. It ruins the whole rest of my day.

Clin.: It sounds like mornings are really a rough time for you. Are you having any problems falling asleep too?

Pt.: Nope, and I never have. Oh, maybe a little bit years ago, but not much now.

Clin.: Well, it sounds like your sleep has been pretty disturbed. I'm wondering whether all the loss of sleep has affected your energy at all?

Pt.: None. Everything is an effort. Just getting up is an effort. Trying to cut the grass is like trying to swim the English Channel. I have no energy, no desire to do anything.

Clin.: What about your golf, or your dancing?

Pt.: Sometimes I get a little satisfaction, but I really just don't enjoy them anymore. I haven't golfed in four weeks, and I used to golf three times a week. When I was a young man, I golfed five times a week.

Clin.: That must be an upsetting feeling, not wanting to do anything.

Pt.: Yes it is (pause) everybody just thinks I'm lazy . . . who knows.

Clin.: It's not uncommon for people with depression to lose their interest in things. Sometimes it even affects their appetite. Have you noticed any change in your appetite?

Pt.:   As a matter of fact, food doesn't taste very good. I only eat two meals a day, and sometimes I don't even eat at all.

Clin.:   Have you lost any weight?

Pt.:   A little, I think.

Clin.:   Are your clothes getting too big or loose?

Pt.:   Actually, they are. I probably lost at least 5 lb.

Clin.:   Over how long a time did it take to lose that weight?

Pt.:   Oh, about 2 months.

Clin.:   So your appetite has decreased, your energy is low, and your interest in things has decreased. What about your concentration? [And so on.]

In summary, anhedonia and the neurovegetative symptoms are critical areas to explore when considering any mood syndrome such as a major depression or dysthymic disorder. Furthermore, by asking such questions, one can gain a vivid picture of what depression feels like to the interviewee. To the interviewee, the interviewer will appear one step closer to understanding.

At this point I would like to look at some further, revealing dialogue with Mr. White.

Clin.:   Mr. White, you've been explaining how very depressed you feel. I'm wondering if there has been a time in your life when you felt just the opposite?

Pt.:   I'm not sure I know what you mean.

Clin.:   Well, have there ever been several days or even weeks when you felt really super energized?

Pt.:   (very faint smile) Hmm, yeah, about 15 years ago, I was really on the go.

Clin.:   Tell me a little about that time.

Pt.:   I was working real hard and suddenly it all became so easy. It seemed like I just didn't need sleep. I went for days with only a couple of hours of sleep. I was like Mighty Mouse.

Clin.: Did you start to speak rapidly or did any of your friends remark that you were talking too fast?

Pt.: Yeah. They began calling me motor mouth. At first I thought that was funny. God, it all seems so foreign to me now. I'd give my right arm for one tenth of that energy right now.

Clin.: Certainly it would be nice for you to have some of that energy now, but do you think that you might have had too much energy back then?

Pt.: Oh yeah, things got crazy back then.

Clin.: How do you mean?

Pt.: Well I didn't really know what I was doing. I couldn't get anything done well. Oh I started plenty of stuff, but I didn't finish anything.

Clin.: Did you start to do anything you were embarrassed about, like spending too much money or giving your money away?

Pt.: Yes I did. I wanted to help everybody. I wanted to help the prisoners. That's why I tried to let a couple of them go . . . (pause) and that's when the Chief called me in and told me I needed a rest, and they put me in a hospital.

Clin.: So things got so upsetting you needed a hospital?

Pt.: Oh yeah.

Clin.: What hospital was that?

Pt.: Saint Anthony's. It was a tolerable place.

Clin.: Have you ever had any other episodes like that one?

Pt.: Yeah, one other time but just for a couple of days. I didn't think anything of it.

The above dialogue strongly suggests that Mr. White is not suffering only from a major depression. On the contrary he is probably best viewed as having bipolar disorder in a depressed phase. He illustrates one of the easiest traps to fall prey to when interviewing a severely depressed person. As both the interviewer and the interviewee become empathically absorbed by the depression, contextual clues suggesting mania do not appear. Without such clues the interviewer may forget to ask about current or past manic behavior. The depressed patient may be too preoccupied with depressive thought content to spontaneously bring up manic history if not asked. Therefore, one should always inquire about manic symptoms. The DSM-IV criteria for mania and hypomania are as follows.

Criteria for Manic Episode*

A. A distinct period of abnormally and persistently elevated, expansive, or irritable mood, lasting at least 1 week (or any duration if hospitalization is necessary).

B. During the period of mood disturbance, three (or more) of the following symptoms have persisted (four if the mood is only irritable) and have been present to a significant degree:
   1. Inflated self-esteem or grandiosity
   2. Decreased need for sleep (e.g., feels rested after only 3 hours of sleep)
   3. More talkative than usual or pressure to keep talking
   4. Flight of ideas or subjective experience that thoughts are racing
   5. Distractibility (i.e., attention too easily drawn to unimportant or irrelevant external stimuli)
   6. Increase in goal-directed activity (either socially, at work or school, or sexually) or psychomotor agitation
   7. Excessive involvement in pleasurable activities that have a high potential for painful consequences (e.g., engaging in unrestrained buying sprees, sexual indiscretions, or foolish business investments)

C. The symptoms do not meet criteria for a Mixed Episode (see p. 335).

D. The mood disturbance is sufficiently severe to cause marked impairment in occupational functioning or in usual social activities or relationships with others, or to necessitate hospitalization to prevent harm to self or others, or there are psychotic features.

E. The symptoms are not due to the direct physiologic effects of a substance (e.g., a drug of abuse, a medication, or other treatment) or a general medical condition (e.g., hyperthyroidism).

Note: Manic-like episodes that are clearly caused by somatic antidepressant treatment (e.g., medication, electroconvulsive therapy, light therapy) should not count toward a diagnosis of Bipolar I Disorder.

---

*Reprinted with permission from the Diagnostic and Statistical Manual of Mental Disorders, 4th ed., p. 332. Copyright 1994 American Psychiatric Association.

Criteria for Mixed Episode†

A. The criteria are met both for a Manic Episode (see p. 332) and for a Major Depressive Episode (see p. 327) (except for duration) nearly every day during at least a 1-week period.
B. The mood disturbance is sufficiently severe to cause marked impairment in occupational functioning or in usual social activities or relationships with others, or to necessitate hospitalization to prevent harm to self or others, or there are psychotic features.
C. The symptoms are not due to the direct physiologic effects of a substance (e.g., a drug of abuse, a medication, or other treatment) or a general medical condition (e.g., hyperthyroidism).

Note: Mixed-like episodes that are clearly caused by somatic antidepressant treatment (e.g., medication, electroconvulsive therapy, light therapy) should not count toward a diagnosis of Bipolar I Disorder.

---

†Reprinted with permission from the Diagnostic and Statistical Manual of Mental Disorders, 4th ed., p. 335. Copyright 1994 American Psychiatric Association.

Criteria for Hypomanic Episode‡

A. A distinct period of persistently elevated, expansive, or irritable mood, lasting throughout at least 4 days, that is clearly different from the usual nondepressed mood.
B. During the period of mood disturbance, three (or more) of the following symptoms have persisted (four if the mood is only irritable) and have been present to a significant degree:
   1. Inflated self-esteem or grandiosity
   2. Decreased need for sleep (e.g., feels rested after only 3 hours of sleep)
   3. More talkative than usual or pressure to keep talking
   4. Flight of ideas or subjective experience that thoughts are racing
   5. Distractibility (i.e., attention too easily drawn to unimportant or irrelevant external stimuli)
   6. Increase in goal-directed activity (either socially, at work or school, or sexually) or psychomotor agitation
   7. Excessive involvement in pleasurable activities that have a high potential for painful consequences (e.g., the person engages in unrestrained buying sprees, sexual indiscretions, or foolish business investments)
C. The episode is associated with an unequivocal change in functioning that is uncharacteristic of the person when not symptomatic.

D. The disturbance in mood and the change in functioning are observable by others.

E. The episode is not severe enough to cause marked impairment in social or occupational functioning, or to necessitate hospitalization, and there are no psychotic features.

F. The symptoms are not due to the direct physiologic effects of a substance (e.g., a drug of abuse, a medication, or other treatment) or a general medical condition (e.g., hyperthyroidism).

Note: Hypomanic-like episodes that are clearly caused by somatic antidepressant treatment (e.g., medication, electroconvulsive therapy, light therapy) should not count toward a diagnosis of Bipolar II Disorder.

---

‡Reprinted with permission from the Diagnostic and Statistical Manual of Mental Disorders, 4th ed., p. 338. Copyright 1994 American Psychiatric Association.

Another important issue to remember about bipolar disorders concerns the fact that they may demonstrate a mixed presentation. "Mixed presentation" suggests that simultaneously (or in extremely rapid alternation) the person exhibits the full symptomatic picture of both mania and depression. The first time I encountered this phenomenon, I was stunned by its apparent oddness. The patient, an x-ray technician, was in his mid-30s. He had a scraggly beard and a pair of wild eyes. He could barely sit still. He kept leaning forward as if about ready to bolt from his chair. His speech was extremely rapid and pressured with a tangential quality, suggesting mania. Yet the content of his speech was markedly depressive, with guilty ruminations, self-derogatory exclamations, and suicidal ideation. Within a split second his eyes would fill with tears, which would soon transform into laughter. Such incongruities of behavior, affect, and thought content should alert the interviewer to a possible mixed state.

Another important consideration with regard to bipolar process is the need to search for periods of hypomania. Hypomania presents as bursts of low-grade manic-like symptoms that last for at least four days. The patient may experience an inflated sense of self-importance or increased energy with less need to sleep; or the patient may feel more talkative and unusually social (perhaps having an increased sex drive as well). The patient's thoughts may seem to be racing, and there may be a significant increase in his or her irritability. These changes will be noticeable to those who know the patient well. Sometimes patients feel pretty good during these periods and will relate that they are more productive, witty, and creative, which is sometimes true. Indeed, if we could all be programmed to have a consistent low-grade hypomania, the world might be a better place. It would certainly be a happier one.

However, the problem is that these episodes are often more disruptive and unpleasant than they are valuable. During the hypomanic episodes, the patients may often report feeling scattered, unproductive, and bothered by an unsettling sensation that he or she is just "not myself." They may be more likely to do things impulsively (e.g., initiate inappropriate drinking or a regretted sexual liaison). Such episodes are also an indication of an underlying instability of mood regulation in the brain, which frequently trip off into depressed mood swings that are sometimes severe. In fact, this syndrome represents an actual form of bipolar disorder in which the patient experiences major depression interspersed with hypomanic bursts that never reach the severity of a manic episode by DSM-IV criteria. This form of bipolar disorder is called Bipolar II Disorder. These patients sometimes go on to develop a full-blown Bipolar I Disorder.

With any person who presents with depression, it is critical to look for episodes of hypomania, because this can influence which medicines may be of value. The addition of a mood stabilizer, in the case of a patient who has a Bipolar II Disorder, sometimes dramatically improves the quality of the patient's life. This diagnosis is routinely missed. The clinician should be on the look-out for it.

The clinician should also be aware that a few patients with depression develop a hypomanic presentation (occasionally an overt manic episode) in response to the use of an antidepressant. I believe that some of these people actually had a Bipolar II process. If this process had been diagnosed beforehand, the use of a mood stabilizer prophylactically with the antidepressant may have prevented such an unpleasant outcome. This represents yet another reason to search for this entity aggressively. Note that a patient who presents for the first time with major depressive episodes and a hypomanic or manic episode, which is clearly triggered by an antidepressant, should be given the diagnosis of Bipolar Disorder, Not Otherwise Specified.

One other diagnosis, which is a variation of the above disorders, should be mentioned. In a cyclothymic disorder the patient, over a 2-year time frame, has intermittent and frequent bouts of low-grade depression and hypomania, neither of which reach the proportions of a full-grade depressive or manic episode. If the clinician discovers this disorder, he or she can once again change a patient's life in a very positive fashion by prescribing a mood stabilizing agent. But let's return to the case involving Mr. White.

Mr. White's case underscores another important point. Past psychiatric history may be very valuable. In particular, the following material should be actively elicited:

a. Previous hospitalizations (names and dates of hospitalizations)
b. Previous outpatient treatment (including names of mental health professionals)
c. Previous medications (names, dosages, and length of time on medications). I also often ask if the patient liked the drugs, or if he or she experienced side effects.
d. Previous psychotherapy (name of clinician and when). I often ask the patient's opinion of the psychotherapy as well as a brief description of what he or she did in therapy.
e. Any history of electroconvulsive therapy (ECT)
f. Past diagnosis
g. Current therapy
h. Periods of time when the patient feels that he or she could have benefited from mental health care but did not seek it

The information from the first 10 minutes of Mr. White's interview highlights another important issue. He relates that he hopes to open a bar with his fiancée. Further questioning revealed that Mr. White had had severe problems with drinking in the past, including evidence of both dependence and significant social dysfunction. He has not been drinking for over 1 year. Drinking, drug abuse, and depression often go hand in hand. Drinking itself can actually be an organic cause of depression. According to Renner, most alcoholics complain of depression and anxiety.[4] In most cases these depressive symptoms clear after detoxification. But depressive symptoms can continue up to 2 months after detoxification, with sleep disturbances lasting as long as 6 months. Consequently, when heavy drinking appears, the validity of the diagnosis of a major depression is somewhat suspect and may best be viewed as a tentative diagnosis or a rule-out diagnosis. Many clinicians would wait to see if the depressive symptoms remained after detoxification, before considering the use of antidepressants. In actuality, depressive symptoms, triggered by the alcohol abuse, could actually remain for many months after detoxification.

As opposed to being caused by the drinking, the depression may antecede the drinking or coincide. In a sense these patients may be self-medicating with either alcohol or drugs as opposed to antidepressants. A true major depression is more likely if there is clear-cut evidence of depressive symptoms before the onset of sustained drinking. In any case no survey of depressive symptoms is complete until a thorough drug and alcohol history has been taken.

With regard to Mr. White, a summary of his diagnostic formulation seems in order. There was no evidence of a personality disorder upon further interviewing. Concerning Axis III and physical disorders, Mr. White complained of chronic and painful osteoarthritis in his knees. His formulation might appear as follows:

> *Axis I:* Bipolar I Disorder, Depressed 296.53
> Alcohol Dependence (in remission) 303.90
> *Axis II:* None V71.09
> *Axis III:* Chronic Osteoarthritis

Before leaving the discussion of Mr. White, some key points are worth reiterating.

1. A major depression may present with anhedonia as the major complaint instead of a dysphoric mood.
2. Neurovegetative symptoms should be artfully woven into the fabric of the interview and seldom used in a checklist fashion.
3. Manic and hypomanic symptoms should always be actively sought.
4. Past psychiatric history may not be spontaneously stated and should always be elicited.
5. Alcohol and drug abuse are commonly associated with depression. What may appear as a major depression may actually be primarily related to alcohol or street drugs.

DISCUSSION OF MR. WHITSTONE

Mr. Whitstone was the distinguished appearing 62-year-old man admitted to the medical hospital because of paranoia. He had had heart surgery 6 months earlier. Currently he was refusing all medical help. One of the curious facets of Mr. Whitstone's presentation remains the fact that when asked directly about depression he stated, "No, I don't feel particularly depressed." Further questioning suggested differently. Since his bypass surgery in January, he had been experiencing many neurovegetative symptoms of depression, including difficulty falling asleep, sleep continuity disturbance, loss of appetite, weight loss, poor concentration, and anhedonia. Corroborative information from his wife and children pointed towards depression. They felt that he appeared withdrawn, sad, and not himself. Mr. Whitstone appeared to be depressed, and yet he denied it. Such a denial of depression is common. Donald Klein estimates that approximately 30% of people fulfilling the criteria of major depression will deny being depressed.[5] Consequently the following series of questions may be useful in determining whether dysphoric mood may be present:

a. How would you describe your mood over the past several weeks?
b. Tell me a little bit about how you've been feeling recently.
c. Would you say that you've been feeling depressed?

If they deny depression, the interviewer can then switch to a different word than "depressed," which, for whatever reason, patients may identify with more, such as:

a. Have you been feeling sad at all?
b. Have you been feeling unhappy?

It is not uncommon for a person suffering from depression to deny depression while admitting to sadness. Another useful question for uncovering dysphoric mood remains, "When was the last time you felt like crying?" The phrasing of this question automatically conveys that the interviewer feels it is both normal and acceptable to cry. Certain patients, especially males, feel hesitant to admit tearfulness. This question helps to skirt this resistance by asking only if they felt like crying. Such sensitive phrasing allows the self-conscious patient many avenues for saving face. The direct question, "Have you been crying?" may yield false negatives, since it does not offer any avenue for the patient except denial or admission of tearfulness.

Finally, if the patient denies both depression and sadness (Mr. Whitstone actually vigorously denied both), the following question may unearth material suggesting dysphoric mood:

a. Have you been feeling yourself recently? or,
b. Have you been feeling up to par over the past several weeks?

Upon such questioning, Mr. Whitstone pensively yet openly discussed his concerns over inadequacy and his fears about his thinking:

Clin.: In what ways haven't you felt yourself?

Pt.: My concentration is shot. It's been very upsetting, let me tell you. I'm a fairly intelligent man, I've gone far. But about a month ago, I called my secretary to dictate a memo. I had to hang up, because I couldn't do it. (Mr. Whitstone was dismally nodding his head from side to side.) It took me 2 days to write that memo (pause). I could normally do it in 20 minutes.

Other useful questions concerning cognitive processes include:

a. Have you noticed if your thinking appears to have speeded up or slowed down?
b. Are you finding it more difficult to make decisions recently?
c. Do you find yourself feeling frustrated when you are trying to make a decision?
d. Does it ever seem like your thoughts are getting disconnected or confused?
e. Has it been difficult for you to hold a train of thought?
f. Are you finding it difficult to read or to follow people as they talk?

The above discussion illustrates that a seriously depressed person may not always complain of depression. In line with this thinking, the possibility of an atypical depression naturally comes to mind. With an atypical presentation, the patient often finds that his or her mood can brighten in response to actual or potential positive events, a phenomenon known as "mood reactivity."

This mood reactivity is often accompanied by an exquisite rejection sensitivity, which can play havoc with interpersonal relationships. In addition these patients frequently find that they are combatting problems with overeating and weight gain. Hypersomnia is sometimes present, including feelings of needing to sleep during the day and being just too tired to work, although the patient may feel suddenly more perky if pleasant activities are available. Patients with an atypical presentation sometimes experience a peculiar sensation of heaviness of "leadenness" in their limbs. If a person meets the criteria for a major depression and also has mood reactivity, accompanied by at least two of the other symptoms described above, then he or she is given the diagnosis of major depression further qualified with the specifier "With Atypical Features."

Another feature that can sometimes confuse the picture, in everyday practice, is the tendency for some patients to present with pain or numerous somatic complaints, presentations that are quite common in the primary care setting. In such patients, if the interviewer vigorously pursues the neurovegetative symptoms, he or she will often uncover a depression lurking below the surface.

Mr. Whitstone's case also emphasizes the critical importance of sources of information other than the patient. A hallmark of shrewd interviewers remains the ability to know when their interview was inadequate. In the case of Mr. Whitstone, both his wife and other family members felt that he had been pervasively depressed for at least 2 months.

Mr. Whitstone also demonstrates that psychotic process often emerges in severely depressed patients. The DSM-IV refers to such psychotic material as either mood-congruent or mood-incongruent. Mood-congruent material concerns itself with depressive ideation or themes of decay. According to the DSM-IV, such themes include personal inadequacy, guilt, disease, poverty, nihilism, or deserved punishment. Mood-incongruent delusions or hallucinations do not revolve about the above themes. They are more bizarre or peculiar and include phenomena such as paranoid delusions, thought insertion, delusions of control, and other themes not necessarily related to depressive ideation. Mr. Whitstone would fulfill the criteria for mood incongruent psychotic features.

Finally, I have saved perhaps the most important point for last. When confronted with an affective presentation, one should always "think organic." Further investigation revealed that Mr. Whitstone had qualities suggestive of delirium, including auditory hallucinations, rapid fluctuations in affect, and a few periods of a fluctuating level of consciousness according to the nursing notes. Besides the standard clues hinting at an organic state, Mr. Whitstone's history was suggestive of an organic etiology for several reasons: (1) He had not seemed normal since his bypass surgery; (2) he had been on anticoagulants, raising the possibility of emboli (blood clots) having been previously dislodged from his heart and passed to his brain or of a hemorrhage in his brain related to his anticoagulants; and (3) he was significantly dehydrated.

In relation to organic precipitants of depression, it is important to stress the need for asking questions about both over-the-counter medications and prescription medications. A brief list of medications that commonly affect mood includes cimetidine, propranolol, methyldopa, reserpine, amantadine, steroids, birth control pills, and opiates. Even thiazide diuretics can cause depression by altering electrolyte balance.[6] When considering an organic cause of depression besides medications and intracranial disease, one should keep in mind extracranial diseases such as hypothyroidism, hyperparathyroidism, lupus, hepatitis, and carcinoma. Pancreatic carcinoma is notorious for initially presenting with depressive complaints. Looked at more systematically, Anderson has separated the organic causes of depression into six categories, including: (1) drugs and poisons, (2) metabolic and endocrine disturbances, (3) infectious diseases, (4) degenerative diseases such as multiple sclerosis, (5) neoplasm, and (6) miscellaneous conditions such as chronic pyelonephritis or Meniere's disease.[7] It is well beyond the scope of this chapter to discuss a thorough differential of the organic causes of depression, but I heartily urge the reader to review this material.

Naturally, even the best clinician will sometimes miss organic causes of depression despite a search for them. This failure is to be expected. But in the last analysis, there is probably no excuse for not having thought of looking for an organic cause of depression. In particular, one situation presents itself in which I unfortunately find it very easy to forget about possible organic factors. This situation arises when the patient presents complaining of a significant life stress such as unemployment, housing problems, divorce, or a death in the family. In such instances it is easy to assume psychological causality, but this assumption is patently misleading. Simply because a person has ample reason to be depressed does not mean that a depression does not also have a concurrent organic cause. Quite to the contrary, physical and psychological disability often go hand in hand. For instance, Schmale has reported a high incidence of separation events preceding the onset of medical illnesses.[8] The clinician should think holistically, checking for both psychological and physiologic roots of depression. One can often be fooled by what appears obvious. Thus, apparent adjustment reactions may be hiding something more ominous. On the other hand, the obvious endogenous depression may actually be triggered or sustained by some not so obvious psychological factor or family dynamic.

In closing the discussion of Mr. Whitstone, let me diagnostically summarize his situation at the end of the initial interview.

> *Axis I:* Psychotic disorder due to a medical condition, condition unknown (provisional) 293.81
> Rule out delirium 293.00
> Rule out major depression with mood incongruent psychotic features 296.24
> *Axis II:* Deferred
> Possible paranoid or compulsive traits (derived from data elicited from the family)
> *Axis III:* Significant dehydration
> Status post-bypass cardiac surgery
> Rule out embolism to brain or hemorrhage

By way of follow-up, a rigorous organic evaluation, including delirium/dementia chemistry screen, electroencephalogram (EEG), computed tomography (CT) scan of head, lumbar puncture, and echocardiogram (checking for clots in the heart which could have embolized to the brain), was without abnormality. Moreover, once Mr. Whitstone was rehydrated he continued to be symptomatic. Apparently he was most likely suffering from a major depression with psychotic features, although there may have been some brief periods of mild delirium, possibly secondary to dehydration, as well.

At this point I would like to summarize the major issues under-scored by Mr. Whitstone's interview:

1. People suffering from depression often deny that they are de-pressed.
2. Specific questions should be asked in an effort to uncover dys-phoric mood not readily described by the patient.
3. Atypical depression often presents with mood reactivity accom-panied by symptoms such as increased appetite, hypersomnia, "leadenness" of the limbs, and rejection sensitivity.
4. Outside information from family and significant others may be needed to delineate the diagnosis.
5. Even mood-incongruent psychotic features such as paranoia or thought insertion can occur during severe depression.
6. It is imperative to ask questions that help rule out possible organic causes of depression.

DISCUSSION OF MS. WILKINS

Ms. Wilkins was the tearful, 21-year-old woman recently contem-plating suicide who remarked, "My best friend is really a bastard." She was requesting medication and psychotherapy. Despite her sad affect, further questioning revealed some intriguing differences when comparing her with both previous individuals:

> Pt.: I'm really feeling horrible. My whole world is collapsing. I don't know who to trust.

> Clin.: How long have you been feeling this way?

> Pt.: Years, for years. I can't think of a time when my life went smoothly. It's all a big mess.

> Clin.: When you say "for years" do you mean your depression never lifts?

> Pt.: Well, not really, I mean, I have my good days. Even a bad apple has its good parts . . . so . . . sometimes I feel fine.

> Clin.: When looking back over the past several weeks, did you have some of those good days?

> Pt.: Oh, I actually had a couple of good days last week, right before the big blow-up with Janet, but I knew Janet would blow it.

Clin.: Tell me how you felt on those days.

Pt.: Fine. In fact, I was having a great day on Friday until Janet had to open her mouth.

Clin.: You say you've been feeling depressed for years, but it sounds like your mood changes a lot. Have you ever had a period of at least 2 weeks, where for the entire 2 weeks, you felt down and depressed?

Pt.: That's a little hard to answer. I haven't felt that way for a long time . . . back home though, yeah, back home I was about 19, I was depressed for almost 4 months straight.

Clin.: Tell me more about it.

From this dialogue it becomes apparent that Ms. Wilkins is probably not experiencing a sustained depression. She would later describe a history of intermittent, low-grade depressive symptoms for many years, meeting the criteria for having a dysthymic disorder. Without a sustained alteration in mood or marked anhedonia lasting for 2 weeks, she will not fulfill criteria for a major depression. On the other hand, she appears to have undergone a 4-month major depression in her teens. Further interviewing revealed that this episode was accompanied by persistent neurovegetative symptoms. From her history she appears to have had a major depression, which is currently in remission. This previous depression had responded to paroxetine successfully.

The above dialogue emphasizes two points: (1) A detailed history of the present illness should be carefully elicited. In this exploration, the interviewer pays particular attention to both the time course and the duration of the symptoms. The foundation of a good diagnostic interview remains a good history of present illness. (2) One should rigorously evaluate whether the depressive symptoms are sustained or whether they fluctuate towards normal. Many people whose depressed feelings come and go will describe their symptoms as unrelenting unless questioned carefully, perhaps related to the fact that most depressive feelings tend to be experienced as intolerable, thus overshadowing the moments of normal mood. The DSM-IV criteria suggest that the depressive symptoms need to have each been present nearly every day for a period of at least 2 weeks. Consequently if the interviewer uncovers a significant fluctuation of symptoms, then he or she must look elsewhere than a major depression for a diagnosis.

Incidentally, I have found that statements such as, "I've been depressed for years," are, curiously enough, often indications that a classic major depression is not present. When questioned in more detail such people often do not describe a sustained depression. Instead, they relate histories of depressive symptoms that fluctuate in response to environmental rewards or pleasures as is commonly seen in some personality disorders, with a dysthymic disorder, and in some atypical depressions. The following questions may be of value concerning the exploration of mood fluctuation:

a. Do you find that your mood can shift during a single day?
b. Would you describe yourself as a moody person?
c. When you are feeling down, do you ever find that a friend or "something to do" can perk you up quickly?

If the patient answers "yes," then the interviewer asks the person to describe some examples of such experiences. Another very useful question for determining whether a depression is persistent or not is, "Some people tell me that, when they are depressed, their symptoms stay with them day after day. Others tell me that their symptoms come and go almost like a roller-coaster. Where on that continuum would you place yourself?"

The lack of sustained depressive symptoms suggests other diagnoses such as a dysthymic disorder, cyclothymic disorder, certain personality disorders, or drug abuse. Upon further interviewing, Ms. Wilkins described a long-standing history of angry outbursts (e.g., throwing a hammer through a window), severe loneliness, intense feelings of boredom and emptiness, confusion over homosexual versus heterosexual relationships, and a series of overdoses. Later in the interview, Ms. Wilkins would provide further information, suggesting personality dysfunction and would go on to fulfill the criteria for a diagnosis of borderline personality disorder. Her presentation emphasizes the following simple but easily forgotten principle: No matter how severely depressed a person looks, the diagnosis is not always that of a major depression. In fact, when it comes to looking severely upset, individuals with borderline personality disorder have a knack for such a dramatic presentation. With these ideas in mind, when the interviewee complains of sadness or depression, the following diagnoses should be considered in addition to a major depression or a bipolar disorder:

a. Borderline personality disorder
b. Other personality disorders such as the histrionic personality, dependent personality, or compulsive personality
c. Dysthymic disorder
d. Cyclothymic disorder

e. Alcohol or drug abuse
f. Adjustment disorders with depressed mood
g. Medical etiologies of depression such as hypothyroidism
h. V codes such as marital problem or a phase of life problem

Far from being a complete differential, this list represents the common entities that are often misdiagnosed as a major depression. As opposed to a major depression, these entities tend to show significant fluctuation in both mood and symptomatology. To mislabel these disorders as a major depression can lead to rather serious errors in triage or medication prescription. For instance, it could be a fatal mistake to prematurely prescribe antidepressants for Ms. Wilkins because one has mistakenly diagnosed her as having a major depression. Indeed, Ms. Wilkin's psychiatric trail is littered with empty bottles signifying her suicidal gestures by overdosage.

Delineating the history of the present illness and determining the consistency of the symptoms are not tasks as easily accomplished as one might think. The process is greatly complicated by a variety of factors, including: (1) patient difficulties with memory, (2) unconscious distortion of the facts by the patient, (3) conscious or histrionic distortions by the patient, and (4) misunderstandings by the patient of the questions asked. These problems are only compounded when the clinician becomes lost in the facts and has no general approach to eliciting the history of the present illness.

Consequently it is worth spending some time examining some approaches to gathering a valid history of the present illness for Axis I disorders in general. This history can be broken down into three contiguous phases: the early phase, the mid-phase, and the recent phase of the illness (the 2 months directly preceding the interview). All three phases are important, but because of the time constraints facing the intake clinician, an emphasis should be placed on the early phase and the recent phase.

The early phase may provide critical diagnostic information, because it allows the clinician to see the natural unfolding of the pathologic process. A patient may present with striking hallucinations while also reporting depressive feelings. If the patient has a major depression, then the early phase will generally demonstrate the appearance of depressed symptoms first, subsequently followed by psychotic symptoms. On the other hand, the schizophrenic patient will generally demonstrate psychotic symptoms and agitation first with depressive symptoms appearing later. Unless the clinician asks the patient or corroborative sources for this information, it can easily remain buried in the history.

A careful delineation of the recent history is an absolute necessity, because it provides the information needed to determine the patient's immediate level of functioning and the present diagnostic reality of the patient. This immediate diagnostic picture can be confusing if the patient is currently taking medications, because the patient's symptom picture may be incomplete, since partial remission may be present. As obvious as this point may seem, it is surprisingly easy in a busy clinic setting to be trapped into thinking that a patient does not have a major depression when, in actuality, it is hiding beneath the facade created by partial treatment. In such circumstances it is important to explore the symptom picture at the time directly preceding the use of medications.

With the understanding that it may be valuable to emphasize the early phase and the recent phase, two rather different approaches can be utilized when eliciting the history of the present illness. Both are effective. Clinicians must learn which seems best suited to their styles and the needs of the specific patient.

In the first technique, as the patient discusses the history of the present illness, an effort is made to quickly direct the patient to the early phase of the illness. The history is then taken chronologically from past to present with less emphasis upon the middle phase. Stressors and responses to stressors are frequently elicited as the history naturally unfolds. The strength of this approach is the detailed and well-ordered history that results. The weakness is the fact that because patient histories are frequently both complex and fascinating the clinician can easily spend too much time on the early and middle phase, coming away with a hazier picture of the immediate problems and current presentation.

A brief piece of dialogue will demonstrate two important features concerning the delineation of the onset of the illness.

Clin.:   When did this depression first begin for you?

Pt.:   Uh . . . a couple weeks after Thanksgiving . . . yeah, after Thanksgiving everything began to fall apart.

Clin.:   Think carefully, in the months before Thanksgiving were you feeling totally normal or were you already feeling not quite yourself?

Pt.:   Huh . . . actually I had been feeling somewhat depressed shortly after Patty, my daughter, went away to college.

Clin.:   What were the first symptoms you noticed?

Pt.:   I felt tearful at times and unusually tired, yes, yes I remember being struck at how little I wanted to get out of bed in the morning. But I'm not really certain when that feeling began . . . no, now that I think of it, that might have happened much later, I'm just not certain (looking frustrated).

Clin.: It's hard to remember details like this and you're doing an excellent job. Let's focus upon Thanksgiving. Did you have a hard time getting out of bed then?

Pt.: Oh yes, that I do remember. I didn't want to clean the house either or even cook the turkey.

Clin.: What was your appetite like over Thanksgiving?

Pt.: Very poor.

As illustrated in the preceding, when first asked to date the onset of the illness, patients frequently give an inaccurately late date, because it is easiest to remember when they began to feel really bad, a period after several weeks or months of the illness. Consequently they should be gently pushed by asking a second time, as shown in the example. Another useful method of increasing the validity of the data, as illustrated in the dialogue, is to prime the memory of the patient by giving specific holidays or personal events that can function as a trigger for increased memory production.[9]

The second approach to elicit the history of the present illness consists of focusing the patient upon the recent and current phase of the illness first. The clinician then skips to the early phase and delineates the remainder of the history chronologically, with less emphasis upon the middle phase. This method provides the clinician with a sound understanding of current symptoms, stresses, and level of functioning, ensuring that these critical areas do not get short shrift because of time constraints. Patients also frequently like talking about recent symptoms first. Generally, this method also provides the early generation of a good diagnostic differential, which can help guide the subsequent questioning concerning the earlier phases of the history of the present illness.

When delineating the recent history, it is often useful to frame the time period with comments such as, "Let's look for a moment at just the last 3 weeks. All of the following questions deal only with the last 3 weeks. During that time how has your energy been?" Because the patient has been coping with large amounts of psychological pain and confusion, even with the above framing, it is easy for that person to eventually begin discussing earlier symptoms without letting the clinician know that this is the case. Consequently, it is useful to remind the patient several times of the time frame with statements such as, "Once again, just looking at the past 3 weeks, what has your sleep been like?"

Let us now return to the presentation of Ms. Wilkins, because her history provides one more practical interviewing point.

With further questioning she denied the recent death of any close friends or family. This point is mentioned because her initial symptoms would have been consistent with an uncomplicated bereavement. In fact, the full major depressive syndrome often appears in an uncomplicated bereavement. If the full major depressive syndrome appears during grief, it is labeled simply as an uncomplicated bereavement. On the other hand, if the depression lasts for too long a time (the DSM-IV suggests roughly around 2 months, but I feel that one should be flexible about this time frame, remembering that the length of time for a normal grief may vary from one culture to another), then the diagnosis of a major depression should be made instead of an uncomplicated bereavement. In a similar light, if the bereavement begins to present with atypical qualities, then a diagnosis of major depression should be made. Atypical qualities include morbid preoccupation with worthlessness, prolonged and marked functional impairment, marked psychomotor retardation, or any psychotic features.

As a final note, like an uncomplicated bereavement, an adjustment disorder can present some confusion with regard to the diagnosis of a major depression. For purposes of clarification, an adjustment disorder must have a clear-cut psychosocial stressor within 3 months of the depression. But even if there is a clear-cut stressor, once the criteria for a major depression are fulfilled, then the diagnosis adjustment disorder is no longer applicable. If the criteria for a major depression are present, then the diagnosis should be a major depression and the diagnosis of an adjustment disorder should be dropped. As we close, a diagnostic summary for Ms. Wilkins seems in order.

> *Axis I:* Dysthymic disorder 300.4
> *Axis II:* Borderline personality (principal diagnosis) 301.83
> *Axis III:* None

Notice that if an Axis II disorder is the main presenting problem (often becoming the focus of care) or the reason for a hospital admission, it should be identified as the "principal diagnosis."

By way of summary Ms. Wilkins' presentation illustrates the following points:

1. A careful history of present illness is the foundation of a diagnostic interview.

2. The duration of the depressive mood should be thoroughly discussed. To fulfill a major depression it must last at least 2 weeks with little fluctuation in symptoms.
3. Many other diagnoses may present with depression. In particular, one should be careful to check for a borderline personality disorder, dysthymic disorder, drug or alcohol abuse, or an adjustment disorder.
4. The clinician should develop a well thought out approach to the history of the present illness. Otherwise, it is easy to become lost in the database.
5. Patients frequently date the onset of their illness later than it was in reality. Once a date is given, ask the patient to carefully consider whether he or she had felt completely normal in the month or two before that date.
6. One can prime the patient's memory by referring to holidays or to special events in the patient's life.
7. When gathering the recent history, it is useful to frame the time period for the patient and intermittently remind him or her of the time frame being discussed.
8. Uncomplicated bereavement may fulfill the criteria for a major depression. If this occurs, the process is still labeled an uncomplicated bereavement. The diagnosis of a major depression is not made, unless the serious symptoms last longer than 2 months or are uncharacteristic of a normal grief response.

DISCUSSION OF MR. COLLIER

Mr. Collier was the 26-year-old man with dark brown hair and a strong jaw. He had an authoritarian air and had recently slapped his 10-year-old daughter. In some respects, Mr. Collier's interview sounds reminiscent of Ms. Wilkins' presentation. Further questioning revealed that, like Ms. Wilkins, his mood tends to fluctuate. He has never had a period of pervasively depressed mood lasting for 2 weeks or more. Questions pertaining to the history of the present illness revealed that he had felt intermittently depressed for over 10 years. He had had no periods of good mood lasting consistently longer than a month or two. Mr. Collier did not relate further symptoms consistent with a borderline personality or any other personality disorder. The above information once again suggests a diagnosis of dysthymic disorder, a relatively common psychiatric syndrome.

Mr. Collier's comment that "I remind myself of my father," warrants further follow-up. This statement may be the first indication that mood disorders run in his family. The clinician should carefully probe for evidence of such a genetic predisposition when dealing with a depressed or manic patient. Genetic studies by Rudin indicated that the incidence of manic depressive psychosis is 25 times as high among the siblings of bipolar patients compared with the normal population. Furthermore, monozygotic twins will be affected in more than half the cases.[10] In a similar fashion, patients with a major depression show a higher prevalence of relatives with major depression and depressive personalities. Other studies have suggested some correlation between affective disorders and alcoholism. For instance, Winokur studied 259 alcoholics and 507 of their relatives. In this study, female relatives appeared to have an increased incidence of unipolar depression.[11] In any case, such material emphasizes the importance of taking a thorough family history.

Elaborating a valid family history in the first 50 minutes is no easy task. A variety of variables can get in the way, including: (1) the patient's lack of information about his family history; (2) the patient's decreased concentration and other cognitive impairments, decreasing the accuracy of his statements; (3) the patient's protection of other family members; and (4) the interviewer's ineffective exploration of the patient's family history. This last variable is the only one that we have direct control over.

Frequently, vague questions, such as "Does anyone in your family have a mental illness?" can often lead to blanket negatives. The interviewee may have no idea that the interviewer is including blood relatives such as aunts, uncles, or cousins in such a question. Along the same lines, the interviewee may have no idea that the interviewer is including alcoholism as a mental illness. To anticipate these problems, it may be of value to help the patient understand the reason for obtaining a family history. Such an approach also "focuses" patients, increasing their willingness to jog their memories. Just one of many lead-ins is illustrated below:

Clin.: Carl, you mentioned earlier that you sometimes remind yourself of your father. In what ways is this true?

Pt.: Hmm . . . Well, my father often seemed upset to me as a kid. He got irritable and would yell at us, all of us, even Annie, the baby. He just seemed troubled.

Clin.: Do you think he was depressed?

Pt.: Yeah, I do.

Clin.: Had he ever received help from a therapist or psychiatrist?

> **Pt.:** Oh, no! He would never do that. He didn't believe in that sort of thing; even so, I think he needed help.

> **Clin.:** While we are talking about your father's depression, I would like to touch upon other family members. Sometimes we can gain clues from psychiatric problems in relatives, that may give us better ideas of how to help you.

Following such an introduction to the topic, the clinician can proceed to discuss each member of Carl's nuclear family, inquiring specifically about drinking, schizophrenia, and other affective disorders. With regard to more distant family members, it is important to state whom you are interested in.

> **Clin.:** The rest of these questions concern any of your blood relatives, including grandparents, aunts, uncles, and cousins. Have any of your father's blood relatives had depression or schizophrenia? (Repeat questions later from other side of family.)

> **Pt.:** Well, I'm not really sure. I had an aunt who was sort of crazy.

> **Clin.:** How do you mean?

> **Pt.:** They put her away for a while because she had a nervous breakdown.

The preceding exchange illustrates several points. First, one needs to be careful of technical words like "schizophrenia" or "bipolar disorder." Many patients do not know what these terms mean and will consequently deny their presence. A brief definition may help clarify the issue. Second, it can be of use to ask the question, "Has anybody in your family been hospitalized or institutionalized for a mental disorder?" People may remember a concrete hospitalization concerning a distant relative much easier than a nebulous process like depression. Third, terms such as "bad nerves" or "nervous breakdown" are common labels for serious disorders such as schizophrenia or an agitated depression. Such terms warrant further inquiry. Another helpful question is simple and to the point, "Has anybody in your family ever tried to hurt themselves or actually kill themselves?" Surprisingly, after having denied any serious psychiatric illnesses in their family, interviewees will suddenly recall a suicide following this question. This phenomenon parallels the finding that later interviewing will often reveal positive family history that the initial interview missed.

Before leaving the issue of family history, I would like to add a few points. The family history may provide even more information than indicated by the genetic findings of such an inquiry. The tone of voice and the manner in which the patient talks about family members may provide subtle clues concerning family relations themselves. At times it pays to take a brief excursion into interpersonal and dynamic issues during this part of the interview, as illustrated below.

Clin.: Do you feel your brother had problems with depression or drugs?

Pt.: Him (said with an astonished and sarcastic tone)! No. He's lily white. He's never had any problems.

Clin.: You sound almost surprised by my question.

Pt.: Oh, it's just that he has always been everybody's favorite.

Clin.: How have you noticed that?

Pt.: He always made better grades. Report card day was a real pain in the ass for me. I used to . . .

In this example, "family history" has taken on a richer meaning.

Mr. Collier's presentation also raises some issues concerning medication. One wonders whether certain symptoms suggest responsiveness to antidepressants. It is generally believed that neurovegetative symptoms and those seen with melancholia will often predict a good response to antidepressants. With regard to anhedonia, Klein feels that persistent anhedonia (as well as autonomous depressive symptoms) may indicate drug responsiveness. By "autonomous mood" he refers to the idea that a biochemical depression will not abate even if good or pleasant stimuli occur to the person. The underlying pathophysiology prevents the normal responsiveness to pleasurable stimuli such as friends or changes in luck.[12] Aesthetically this idea appears pleasing but is not yet fully substantiated. A review article by Nelson and Charney addresses some of these issues directly.[13]

Nelson and Charney reviewed 13 research papers that performed factor analytic studies of depressed patients. The studies were searching for evidence of symptom clusters suggestive of an endogenous or drug-responsive depression. According to Nelson and Charney motor retardation remains the most valid indication of treatment response. Other moderate indicators were agitation, severe depressed mood, depressive delusions, self-reproach, and loss of interest. They also feel there is some indication—but with less supporting evidence—that endogenous depressions are associated with a distinct quality of mood, diurnal morning worsening, and difficulty concentrating. Some symptoms commonly assumed to indicate an endogenous depression were also supported but not as strongly, such as early morning awakening, other sleep difficulties, and appetite and weight loss. Obviously the answers are not completely available at present. In the meantime, the first two clusters of symptoms mentioned, as well as the presence of other neurovegetative symptoms, should arouse the clinician's suspicion of possible medication responsiveness.

Mr. Collier demonstrated several of these symptoms, including motor retardation, intermittently depressed mood, self-reproach, and a sporadic loss of interest. A growing body of evidence reviewed by Akiskal suggests that certain forms of dysthymic disorder may respond to antidepressants.[14] It is beyond the scope of this chapter to discuss this material thoroughly; however, I feel it is important for the initial interviewer to keep in mind the symptoms suggesting drug responsiveness. Such diligence may result in more appropriate triage.

At this juncture, a diagnostic summary of Mr. Collier's presentation seems in order. Two points should be added. First, with regard to medical problems, Mr. Collier related having bronchitis secondary to smoking. Second, on an interpersonal level, further interviewing indicated significant marital distress. Couples therapy was recommended. This interpersonal problem represented a core issue with regard to Mr. Collier's depression. The next part of this chapter will more fully investigate the importance of such issues in the initial interview. Mr. Collier's diagnostic summary is as follows:

Axis I: Dysthymic Disorder (early onset) 300.4
              Partner Relational Problem V61.1
   Axis II: None V71.09
  Axis III: Chronic bronchitis secondary to smoking

In conclusion Mr. Collier's presentation emphasizes several points:

1. Individuals with dysthymic disorder commonly experience many neurovegetative symptoms of depression, but the symptoms do not last in a sustained manner for over 2 weeks.
2. The depressive symptoms of a dysthymic disorder can often rapidly shift towards normal if there is something "fun" to do.
3. Family history should be an integral component of any interview where depression is suspected.
4. Blanket questions such as "Does anybody in your family have a mental illness?" will often yield false negatives.

5. A detailed family history provides a nice take-off point for exploring family dynamics.
6. Certain syndromes, such as various subtypes of dysthymic disorder, may respond to tricyclics, SSRIs, and "third-generation antidepressants."
7. Certain symptoms such as motor retardation, agitation, severely depressed mood, depressive delusions, self-reproach, and loss of interest may be positively correlated with medication responsiveness.

The above four case discussions are not intended to be an exhaustive review of the diagnostic subtleties associated with mood disorders. I have attempted to present a sound introduction to the process of diagnostic evaluation during an initial interview. The "art of diagnosis," of learning about the person as one delineates the diagnosis, will always present the clinician with a challenge. In the next section of this chapter, an attempt will be made to explore some of the phenomena that help the interviewer reach a deeper understanding of depression as a human experience, because this understanding is the path to both compassion and more sensitive interviewing.

SECTION II: THE UNDERSTANDING OF DEPRESSION

*W*hen the low heavy sky weighs like a lid
Upon the spirit aching for the light,
And all the wide horizon's line is hid
By a black day sadder than any night; . . .

When like grim prison bars stretch down the thin,
Straight, rigid pillars of the endless rain,
And the dumb throngs of infamous spiders spin
Their meshes in the cavern of the brain, . . .

    Charles Baudelaire
    Spleen

Diagnosis represents a powerful and rigorous instrument for conceptualizing depression, often laying the critical foundation for effective treatment planning. But, as shown in the previous section, the search for a diagnosis provides even more. It represents one step in the process of understanding the person in the manner in which that individual experiences the world. In this section, emphasis will be upon the search for an understanding of depressive phenomena, exploring more fully the impact of such a search on the initial interview.

To begin with, depression is not a static thing that occurs in isolated items called people. Depression is a process. As a process, it constantly unfolds, manifesting itself in phenomena that affect numerous systems outside the individual identified as depressed. Depression exists as an impact that can be identified, and perhaps treated, through any number of systems. The more the interviewer understands this concept, the more open the interviewer becomes to the subtle clues suggesting depression and the harsh realities of the destruction left in its wake. From this understanding, interviewers enhance their sensitivity, their clinical acumen, and their ultimate engagement with patients. The interview is, at once, both more human and more clarifying.

In Section II an effort will be made to explore the ramifications of depression throughout various systems. The discussion will begin with the very smallest system of interaction, physiologic, and move outwards, through progressively larger systems, as was discussed in Chapter 4.

To understand depression more fully in the initial interview, the clinician must understand its reflection in each system. Ultimately, the knowledge gathered may suggest possible interventions within that system, as described in detail in Chapter 4. A good interview immediately suggests possible avenues of intervention. By understanding the depressive process, treatment planning suggests itself.

At another level, the following approach emphasizes the fact that interviewers, whether they want to or not, will by their very presence become a subsystem touched by the patient's depression. The interviewer will both affect and be affected by the depressive processes explored. Awareness of this fact can lead to important insights in intervention. Blindness to this fact can lead to dismally short-sighted conclusions and mislaid interventions. With these ideas in mind the exploration begins. At its conclusion we will have a better understanding of what it is like to be at a place where:

. . . all the wide horizon's line is hid
By a black day sadder than any night.

Fields of Interaction

I: PHYSIOLOGIC SYSTEM

As one enters the room occupied by a person experiencing depression, the physiologic ravages of the process are often disturbingly apparent. In a severely depressed person the initial glance may reveal unkempt hair, ragged or mismatched clothes, dirty nails, untied shoes, and a vacant look to the eyes. More striking may be the slowness of movement and the person's lack of responsiveness. It may take a few seconds or much longer for the depressed person to acknowledge the interviewer, if such acknowledgment occurs at all. In a similar manner, more subtle decrements in responsiveness may be the first clues of a milder depressive state. Thus, the interview begins with the first look, before any words are uttered.

The slowness of movement probably parallels the disquieting sensation of heaviness often reported by depressed people. Depression, as Baudelaire suggested with his line "When the low heavy sky weighs like a lid . . . ," often feels like a heavy shawl descending on leaden shoulders. The arms and limbs may literally feel weighted down. This abnormal sensation may be related to the powerfully intense sense of inertia that can accompany depression. It becomes distressing for the depressed person to initiate movement; it seems so much easier to simply rest. A young woman with a dysthymic disorder vividly describes this phenomenon:

*I*t is so strange. Depression is exhausting in a physical sense. You know, most people have chores they have to do just to keep their lives going. And if the chores are waiting for you, and you sit there and look at them, they just seem overwhelming. And I could easily sit for 2 hours in a chair just looking at some clothes I left on the bedroom floor and not be able to motivate myself to pick them up. My body just feels heavy, as if it wouldn't want to respond unless I absolutely forced it to . . . Hmm . . . You know it is actually almost as if your brain lost half of its ability to control your body in the sense that even making a decision to pick something up required so much energy that you don't want to make it. You feel like it couldn't possibly be worth it. I just want to vegetate.

This sensitive excerpt brings up another important point with the opening comment, "It is so strange." Depressed patients, at times, present a peculiar dichotomy in the manner in which they cognitively and affectively experience their profound condition. On a cognitive level, they often feel they are the root of their problem, their speech becoming an entangled web of self-recrimination and belittlement. They cognitively experience their depression as being actively caused by their own flaws. Simultaneously, they affectively experience the depression as coming on them or over them from an outside source. In a sense, they feel invaded and violated. They feel they are the passive recipients of a phenomenon that they do not understand or control. This incipient "loss of control" presents a terrifying threat to their sense of ideal self. Jaspers with a single word captures the pith of this process when he describes depressed patients as experiencing a physical and emotional "ossification."[15]

At present the etiologic meaning of such radical changes in movement and body perception remains unclear. Such changes may represent psychological defenses, biologic attempts to withdraw a malfunctioning organism from a potentially dangerous environment, social indicators that an organism needs help, or direct results of primary biochemical imbalance. Any combination of the preceding is possible. No matter what the etiology of these phenomena, they can create a frightening experience for the depressed person. In essence, even their bodies become strangers to them, one more step toward their intense sense of isolation.

The other neurovegetative symptoms also represent an array of physiologic markers of depression. Baseline energy withers. Appetite and libido dry up, as if parched by the intensity of the process. These feelings of altered functioning can become immensely disturbing to patients, sometimes being perceived as further evidence of their personal failure. With these phenomena in mind, questions such as the following may add depth to the interview:

a. What has your body felt like to you recently?
b. What does it feel like to you to have lost your energy and drive?
c. You mention that you have lost your energy, your appetite, and your ability to sleep. How have all these changes made you feel about yourself?

As well as allowing patients the chance to ventilate, these questions emphasize that the interviewer is interested in them as unique people whose depression they alone can explain.

Before leaving the physiologic field, I would like to briefly describe some of the biologic ramifications of an agitated depression. Here too there exists a peculiar dichotomy, as described by an elderly male patient in response to a question about losing energy, "I don't know exactly what you mean, but yeah, I've got energy all over the place, driving me constantly, but no, I don't have any sustained energy to do anything." In the agitated state there exists a nagging need to move. The energy is unbridled and disobedient. Consequently, the body tends to assume an incessant display of "bad nerves." Hands wring each other in a frenzy of confusion. Fingers pick at the body or pluck the clothes. Sitting becomes an act of will power. From deep inside the legs, there erupts a need to move. Pacing becomes a necessary method of release as natural as breathing. In many instances, this agitated state appears worse in the morning. In the interview it can be revealing to ask, "What part of the day seems worse to you?" It is important to remind oneself that a relatively calm patient interviewed at 4:00 P.M. may have

looked remarkably more agitated at 8:00 A.M. Depression nags the
body with an intermittent voice.

II: PSYCHOLOGICAL SYSTEM

Depression has a calling card. This calling card consists of a distinct
set of changes that occur within the mind of those experiencing the
depression. Not all depressed people experience these feelings, but
many do in one combination or another. Four broad areas are
touched by depression and will be the focus of this discussion: (1)
perception of the world, (2) cognitive processes, (3) thought content,
and (4) psychodynamic defenses. An understanding of the above
processes can increase the ability of the interviewer to recognize
the subtle clues of depression and can increase empathic abilities,
as well.

Concerning the perception of the world, depression alters both
the sense of time and the size of the world actively engaged. To the
depressed person the concept of current or future change appears
conspicuously absent. A mantle of flatness suffocates spontaneity.
Moment-by-moment existence seems void of any chance of alteration. Without this feeling of possible change, time passes arrogantly
slowly. In a literal sense, time passes painfully. Such a state of
psychic monotony can have a curious effect on the interviewee's
perception of the future. In effect, if change does not exist, then the
future is essentially meaningless. All days are merely replicas. Our
sense of the future is partially dependent upon our sense that the
future may be different. To the depressed interviewee, the future is
draped in a radically bland light. This perception may be one reason
why depressed people often appear unmotivated. Without a perceived future why should they attempt change? This phenomenon
has been described by the phenomenologist Eugene Minkowski as
a "blocking of the future."[16]

The second alteration in world perception does not involve
time. It revolves about space. The "active world" of the depressed
person undergoes a profound alteration. By active world I refer to
the area of the environment that a person remains interested in
engaging. In depression the active world shrinks. The patient's sense
of space gradually vanishes, creating a cataract of the mind. This
shrinking of the active world can powerfully short circuit environmental reinforcement and reward. The depressed person becomes a
behavioral isolate. The dysthymic woman quoted before elegantly
depicts this process.

I'm so focused inward . . . When I feel depressed it is such a great pain,
and I am paying so much attention to it trying to control it, that I walk down the

street and really don't see much at all . . . I screen out other people because I don't want to interact with others . . . I probably miss a lot. Even in the sense that I can walk down the street where I work and there can be roses blooming. And if I am really depressed, I don't even see them. And I love roses. Whereas, if I am feeling better, even despite the smell of the buses running around, I will still smell the roses. And I will admire them. . . .

It can come as quite a shock to the interviewer to realize that the interviewer may not be a feature of the interviewee's active world. To engage such patients, the clinician needs to enter their world as best as possible. Consequently, the interview with a severely depressed patient may require a change in style. At times the clinician must be more active while also accepting, with patience, the interviewee's difficulty in responding.

A second broad area of alteration concerns changes in the cognitive processes of the depressed person. In a retarded depression, the thought process slows as if the stream of thought were frozen by an unexpected drop in temperature. In contrast, in an agitated depression thought races as if the same stream had sustained a turbulent boil. In both cases, the thought process becomes disjointed. Concentration becomes annoyingly elusive.

Besides these alterations in the speed and flow of thought, depression creates an ideational caging. The term "caging" suggests that the mind becomes trapped within a small network of limiting themes. Such depressive rumination can lock the depressed person into worries about the past, the present, or the future. Once within the cage, the depressed patient has great difficulty attending to new and perhaps therapeutic influences. In the interview, caging may demonstrate itself as a frustrating tendency for the patient to return to a specific topic. Or the patient may, alternatively, repeatedly ask the same question, despite the interviewer's reasonable reassurances. Such caging can seriously block an interview. One method of trying to circumvent it consists of attempting to acknowledge it while simultaneously refocusing the patient, as illustrated below. In this interview more than enough time had been spent helping the patient to ventilate. When more direct questions were asked, the patient would not move on.

Clin.: Mrs. Jones, can you tell me a little bit about the effect of all these troubles on your sleep?

Pt.: Sleep, can't sleep . . . (pause) can't sleep because of the bills. I just know we won't be able to pay the bills. Oh God, my children, we'll be ruined.

Clin.:   I understand your concern, Mrs. Jones, but I need to know about your sleep, it will help me to understand your depression. For instance, how long has it been taking you to fall asleep?

Pt.:   I don't know, all I think about are the bills. I know that somehow I'm to blame. What will we do? What will we do! Somebody has got to help.

Clin.:   Mrs. Jones, it seems very hard for you to stop talking about your finances. I understand your concern, but in order to help you, I must learn more about what has happened to you. I will ask you some important questions and if you get side-tracked, I will pull you back to the question. I want to help, but I need your help as well. Once again think carefully, how long is it taking you to fall asleep? (The preceding is said with a calm but firmer tone.)

With proper timing, such an intervention may open a cage. At other times, the caging of the patient will not yield despite the interviewer's best intentions.

Aaron Beck, one of the founders of cognitive psychotherapy, has delineated many specific cognitive impairments in depression. Beck has pointed out that depressed patients may overgeneralize with statements such as "Everything has fallen apart" or "No one cares about me." They can exaggerate, in essence creating the proverbial mountain out of a mole hill with a statement such as, "My boss Mr. Henry looked angry. He's dissatisfied with me. I'm sure it is only a matter of time until I'm fired." They also have a tendency to ignore the positive. For instance, a businesswoman confused me with the following statement which illustrates this principle, "It's the best Christmas season we've ever had. We're really selling books all over the place. I set myself a remarkably high quota. If we don't meet it, I will have failed miserably as a manager."

Beck has also described a trio of distortions, the cognitive triad, that frequently appears in depression.[17] The patient relates a negative view of the world, a negative concept of the self, and a negative appraisal of the future. This negative view of the world is partially generated by the tendency of the depressed patient to continually validate his or her depression. The patient speaks as if he or she had placed a negative filter over the eyes, as witnessed by the following taped comments:

*W*hen I'm really depressed every negative, every unpleasant thing that I could possibly think of that might be happening to another person like someone being hit by a car or someone getting cancer or a dog being injured will trigger personal fear and worry that the world is bad. And so the depression has no justification to ever lift because everything about life is horrible. It's all just proof that depression is reality just looking itself in the face . . .

With regard to negative self-concept, the tendency to assume self-blame may be a major contributing factor. I do not think I have ever seen this quality as strikingly portrayed as in the original Bob Newhart Show. In this show, Newhart plays a psychologist with a client named Mr. Herd who epitomizes the self-blamer. A typical exchange might be as follows:

Newhart: (After entering the office) I can't believe it, I left my wallet at home.

Mr. Herd: I did it . . . You were worried about me and forgot your wallet over me . . . I'm sorry, I'm really sorry. I won't let it happen again.

Although funny in the Newhart Show, the process of self-blame stands as a vicious cognitive trap. In a sense, it may represent a milder variant of the much more ominous symptom known as delusional guilt.

Another jarring twist in cognitive process comes to mind at this point. Depressed patients sometimes exhibit a trait that I prefer to call "an immunity to logic," which can be very frustrating to the family, therapist, or initial interviewer. This immunity to logic was brilliantly depicted by Minkowski while at the same time he illustrated the blocking of the future mentioned earlier. Minkowski spent several months living with a man experiencing a psychotic depression. The following excerpt refers to Minkowski's vain efforts to convince him that he would not be horribly mutilated and subsequently executed:

$\mathcal{F}$rom the first day of my life with the patient, my attention was drawn to the following point. When I arrived, he stated that his execution would certainly take place that night; in his terror, unable to sleep, he also kept me awake all that night. I comforted myself with the thought that, come the morning, he would see that all his fears had been in vain. However, the same scene was repeated the next day and the next, until after 3 or 4 days I had given up hope, whereas his attitude had not budged one iota. What had happened? It was simply that I, as a normal human being, had rapidly drawn from the observed facts my conclusions about the future. He, on the other hand, had let the same facts go by him, totally unable to draw any profit from them for relating himself to the same future. I now knew that he would continue to go on, day after day, swearing that he was to be tortured to death that night, and so he did, giving no thought to the present or the past. Our thinking is essentially empirical; we are interested in facts only in so far as we can use them as basis for planning the future. This carry-over from past and present into the future was completely lacking in him; he did not show the slightest tendency to generalize or to arrive at any empirical rules.[18]

Although this is a description of a psychotically depressed man, a similar, albeit milder, process commonly accompanies nonpsychotic depression.

All of these disturbances in cognitive process may be encountered by the initial interviewer. By training themselves to listen for such abnormalities, interviewers may increase their ability to detect depression. For instance, people with atypical depressions may initially betray their underlying depression by the use of such pathologic processes. Of course, the presence of such processes, in a less severely disturbed patient, may also alert the interviewer to the possible use of cognitive psychotherapy as a future treatment modality. At this juncture, I would like to turn attention to the third major psychological area affected by depression, thought content itself.

The distinction between cognitive process and cognitive content is sometimes a blurred one, but I would like to focus briefly on four content themes: loneliness, self-loathing, helplessness, and hopelessness. These factors blend with one another, reinforcing their mutual perpetuation. The loneliness of the depressed person can become practically insurmountable. As shown earlier, processes such as caging and the shrinking of the active world separate depressed patients from friends, family, and even the clinician. Their loneliness reaches such a magnitude of intensity that it may begin to assume a qualitative difference from the more common loneliness encountered in daily living. Put differently, they are not only lonely, they feel alone. The loneliness assumes an irrefutable realization that they are isolated, somehow cut off permanently from others. Such isolation does indeed diminish social reinforcement and therapeutic intervention.

Combined with this alienation from others, depressed patients may encounter a profound alienation from and hatred of their selves. Such a self-loathing only intensifies their feeling of loneliness because they are repulsed by their own company. To the seriously depressed patient, it seems as if he or she lacks any real existence or purpose at all, except for his or her pain. These feelings can shift imperceptibly into the potentially lethal thought that, "I am truly a burden to those I love." These ideas may emerge in the interview in a more oblique fashion as in, "Don't bother with me. Talk with someone you can help." The initial interviewer needs to probe beneath such comments, hunting for the more dangerous logic that "others would be better off if I were dead."

From their social isolation and their repugnance toward their selves, feelings of helplessness emerge naturally. This profound sense of helplessness can contribute to the inertia that effectively prevents therapeutic encounters. Phrased succinctly, they wonder "Why bother?" The interviewer can easily estimate the role of this factor by simply asking, "Have you been feeling helpless?" A more sophisticated gauge may emerge with the question, "At this time, what kinds of ways of getting help do you see for yourself?" A blank negative or dismal shake of the head in response to this question should alert the interviewer to the potential seriousness of the depression.

Finally, all of the above depressive themes may lead to hopelessness. Beck has demonstrated that hopelessness represents a more specific and sensitive predictor of suicide potential than depressive mood itself.[19] As such, the interviewer should always try to measure the degree of hopelessness with either oblique questions, such as "What do you see for yourself in the future?," or more simply, "Are you feeling hopeless?"

The above discussion has examined the critical role of depressive thought content in the initial interview. It is time to examine the fourth major area of psychological disturbance in depression, dynamic defenses.

I have found the discussion by MacKinnon and Michels in their book, *The Psychiatric Interview in Clinical Practice*[20] to be particularly illuminating in this area. I shall summarize some of these points, focusing on those defenses that can most easily confuse the interviewer.

In the first place, some people seem incapable of admitting depression into cognitive awareness. They tend to verbally deny depression. In fact, they may be truly unaware that they are depressed. Such an ironic state may be the result of dynamic defenses such as denial and repression. Despite these defenses careful questioning will often uncover the depression by eliciting neurovegetative symptoms or evidence of depressive cognitive functioning such as caging or generalization. Other common defenses include isolation and rationalization. The patient may isolate all his or her depressive rumination onto one symptom complex. The patient too may deny depression, as illustrated by "I've got no real problems other than the fact that I can't sleep at night and I've got daily headaches."

The patient's anger can provide the interviewer with the first glimpse of the depressive phenomenon. Analytic theorists such as Abraham and Freud have stressed the idea that depression may represent anger turned inward.[21] This anger may originate in a variety of situations, including perceived abandonment, rejection, frustration, direct or indirect attacks on oneself, or feelings of betrayal or injustice. In line with this thinking, anger often pierces the sadness of the person experiencing an agitated depression. Thus a patient who quickly verbally attacks the interviewer may be betraying his or her depression to that same interviewer. I have even been surprised to see anger unexpectedly shooting through the apathy of the supposed "retarded depression," as evidenced by vicious diatribes against past doctors or relatives. Anger also routinely disrupts the existence of people displaying borderline personality disorders or dysthymic disorder. Anger and depression can form a damaging positive feedback loop, as follows. The patient lashes out at a close friend. From this angry display, the patient develops guilt for having such inappropriate feelings. This guilt triggers further depression. As the depression deepens, the patient becomes increasingly irritable. Soon enough, the patient lashes out again, thus completing and fueling the cycle.

A third confusing clinical picture, resulting from dynamic defenses, involves the defense of projection with resultant paranoia. MacKinnon emphasizes that depression and paranoia may alternate with each other. The person's intense self-incrimination can become too painful. Deflection of this pain occurs through projection. Instead of hating himself or herself, the person finds that "other people hate me," or "others want to punish me." This last statement demonstrates the projection of suicidal ideation outwards. The need to consider paranoia as a defense against depression dramatically demonstrates itself in the following vignette provided by one of my colleagues.

Apparently he had consulted on a patient who presented as psychotically paranoid in a medical hospital. This patient denied all suicidal ideation; furthermore, he related few neurovegetative symptoms. Transfer to the psychiatric hospital was recommended in the morning. The patient was checked throughout the night but was not placed on a one-to-one observation. During a period of nonsurveillance, the patient quickly and efficiently hanged himself. Little more need be said.

A final dynamic mechanism that can easily fool the interviewer exhibits itself in the process of hypomanic or manic defenses against depression. One needs to be wary of anybody who appears "too happy" while describing numerous unsettling stressors. If watched carefully, the surprisingly buoyant person may betray sadness by a minute quivering of the chin or a hesitancy to the voice. At these moments a quiet statement, such as "You know, as you are talking you seem sort of sad to me" may open a floodgate of tears. This hypomanic defense is very apparent in bipolar patients with a mixed presentation. In fact, in my own experience I have seldom found a purely elated mania. Usually, patients with mania have some elements of anger or sadness that linger just beneath the surface of their laughter.

Perhaps it is best to end the exploration of the psychological field at this time. Much more could be said, but it seems an opportune time to move to the next larger system in which depression manifests itself—the realm of the interpersonal system.

III: DYADIC SYSTEM

When two people interact, a dyadic system is born. Depression often first shows itself through its impact on the flow of communication and affection within this dyadic system. In this sense depression exists as an interpersonal phenomenon, seldom, if ever, restricted to the world of a single individual. Perhaps the following description by a patient will illustrate the power of depression to alter the interpersonal field:

*I*t makes it harder to interact with people. It decreases your motivation for talking . . . first of all because you are so acutely aware of how depressed you are that you are convinced that other people are going to recognize it immediately, and it is very embarrassing to think that. So it makes you feel as if any interaction with other people will make you feel as if you will need to put on a front. It requires a lot of energy to do that. And that makes you very tired. It is sort of a circular motion . . . you see how much energy it will take to relate so you avoid doing it. I have even noticed that if I enter a store or see a Burger King and I want coffee I tend to speak softer and not really smile like I normally do. When I am depressed I want to limit the interaction as much as possible so I don't smile and I don't really look at them. I just want to get it over with and pretend it is all over . . . .

This excerpt illustrates several subtle facets of interpersonal disruption. At one level, the depressed person feels withdrawn and consequently attempts to decrease interaction. This decrease in interaction robs the depressed person of the chance to gain positive reinforcement from others, as mentioned earlier. But, perhaps more important, depression decreases the quality of the remaining interactions as evidenced in the above excerpt. The decreased smiling, decreased spontaneity, and curtness of interaction displayed by the patient can be perceived by others as coolness or aloofness. Once perceived in this manner, people may treat the depressed person with increased reserve. For instance, a hamburger-stand attendant may snap at the person, thus further creating a hostile environment.

Setting into motion a self-fulfilling prophecy, the patient creates a hostile world, a world lacking rewards for interactions with others.

This destructive cycle can be one of the forerunners of the learned helplessness sometimes seen in depression and postulated by Seligman as an etiology of depression.[22] Seligman discovered that if you experimentally expose an animal, such as a dog, to inescapable aversive stimuli, the dog will eventually stop attempting escape. The animal appears to give up. It does not attempt to find new ways of coping. Once this learned helplessness has occurred, exploration ceases. With the cessation of exploration, the chance for new learning and positive reinforcement vanishes. In a sense, the depression has ensured its own survival. A very similar process may occur in humans, perhaps, made even more damaging by the uncanny ability of the human to cognitively reframe such interactions into self-derogatory beliefs such as, "Obviously, nobody likes me," or "I don't even know why I bother."

The interviewer can search for evidence of interpersonal dysfunction and learned helplessness with questions such as the following:

a. Do you find yourself going out as frequently as you used to?
b. Tell me what it is like for you when you are around people at work?
c. When you talk with people what kinds of feelings do you have, like if you meet a friend on the street?
d. How do people seem to be treating you?
e. Do you find yourself easily irritated or "flying off the handle" recently?
f. Does it require much energy to be around people such as your friends?

At this point one of the more fascinating elements of interviewing presents itself. I am referring to the fact that not only are the friends and family of the patient affected by the patient's depression, but also the interviewer cannot escape the process. It benefits clinicians to periodically look within themselves at their own emotional responses. In the first place, such intuitive responses may be the tip-off that one has encountered a depression or a depressive equivalent. In the second place, both negative feelings generated in the interviewer or overly empathic feelings can seriously damage engagement. The interviewer may inadvertently distance the interviewee by tone of voice or nonverbal cue. Put differently, the interviewer needs to adjust to the needs of the patient in a continuous, adaptive creativity. To accomplish this process, interviewers must be aware of the impact of patients on themselves and vice versa.

There exist several emotions commonly felt by interviewers besides generally acknowledged reactions such as sympathy, empathy, or a desire to help. For instance, the depressed patient's slowness of movement and speech, caging, and hesitancy to answer questions can create a sense of frustration in the interviewer. Questions may have to be asked repeatedly. Answers may be vague. The interview may loom as a long and tedious process. Such feelings of frustration may be useful indicators that the clinician should be on the lookout diagnostically for depression while being wary of countertransference. In a similar fashion, the patient's depressive manner of interaction may create anger in the interviewer as well as frustration. At times interviewers may subsequently feel guilt because they suddenly catch themselves being "noncaring." This resultant guilt may provide the initial clue to a diagnosis of depression. This guilt also provides the interviewer with a vivid, experiential glimpse into the world of family members and friends who interact with a depressed patient on a daily basis. Occasionally, the first suggestion that one has encountered an atypical depression may be a growing sense of unexpected sadness within the interviewer.

The preceding interactions also emphasize the need for interviewers to adjust both their pace and their expectations. The interview with the depressed patient requires both a calm and a calming style. Indeed, any suggestions of haste or irritation may be interpreted in a highly disengaging fashion by the depressed patient. A frustrated interviewer may be perceived as, "Just like everyone else, you find me irritating." Such an interaction hardly sets an ideal platform for a therapeutic alliance.

So far I have been describing the impact of the patient on the therapist, generating feelings such as sadness, annoyance, or guilt. Flipping the coin, one finds that the therapist can unwittingly affect the patient's presentation. With regard to depression, this phenomenon occurs most frequently with dysthymic disorder and in characterologic depression. People with these disorders are often highly responsive to the immediate surroundings. A patient with dysthymic disorder or a histrionic personality can sometimes be cheered up deceptively rapidly, if the patient feels that someone is showing an interest. Therefore, an overly warm or extroverted interviewer can unknowingly shift the patient's affect.

To such an interviewer the presentation of the patient may not seem very sad or depressed. Such an initial impression might mislead the interviewer into downplaying the significance of the depressive complaints. It should also be remembered that "happy people" are often very annoying to depressed people, being perceived as incapable of understanding how miserable they feel. The interviewer best approaches the patient from the calming middle ground of gentle warmth and interested listening.

While interviewing depressed patients, the clinician will undoubtedly encounter tearful patients. The first time a patient cries in an interview, it is generally comforting to allow the patient to cry for a brief period. If the patient is on the brink of tears, statements such as, "You seem sad right now," or as MacKinnon and Michels[20] suggest, "Are you trying not to cry?" may be very helpful. Said with a soft tone, they will offer the patient a chance to ventilate, thus decreasing a sense of discomfort. Many patients feel embarrassed or vulnerable at such moments. I generally address this unstated issue with a statement such as, "It's all right to cry. We all cry at times. It's our body's way of telling us we are hurting; (after a brief pause) maybe you can tell me a little more about what is hurting you."

I generally will also ask, "Would you like a tissue?" while simultaneously offering one in my outstretched hand. Such an interaction has many metacommunications. The clinician is conveying an acceptance of crying as a normal aspect of sadness. Simultaneously, respect is given to the patient's current needs. Rather than just giving the patient a tissue, the clinician asks if one is needed. By the process of asking, the clinician conveys confidence that the patient is still in control, fully capable of making decisions. Generally, such an interaction usually results in the end of tearfulness in about a minute or two.

As the tearfulness subsides, the interviewer has an ideal chance to learn about the core pains of the patient. Tearfulness tends to decrease the use of defenses. At such a point, pertinent and startling information may emerge. If the clinician had prevented the tearfulness by cutting it off abruptly or by changing topics, then valuable information might have been lost.

Of course, at times, one might find a patient whose uncontrollable crying prevents progress. To further the interview, statements said reassuringly but firmly such as the following may be effective, "Mr. Jones this is obviously very upsetting and would be to anybody. Take a moment to collect yourself. It's important for us to talk more about what is bothering you."

But, generally speaking, interviewers tend to prematurely shut down crying perhaps because it is disturbing to feel another person's pain. Another emotion may also contribute to this premature shut down, for the patient's tearfulness can make the interviewer feel awkwardly helpless. On a deeper level, it remains important for interviewers to understand their spontaneous feelings when someone cries. In this regard part of the interviewer's basic training should be a search for answers to questions such as the following:

a. What do I feel when someone cries?
b. Do I ever perceive crying people as weak or ineffectual?
c. How often do I cry and how do I feel about myself when I do?
d. Have I ever seen my parents, family, or friends cry, and how did I feel then?

By exploring such questions, the interviewer decreases the risk that countertransference issues will adversely affect the ability to deal with a crying patient. In the last analysis, many a powerful therapeutic alliance has been forged by a clinician's calming and mature response to a patient's first tears.

A final feeling that an interviewer may experience while interviewing a depressed patient arises from both the withdrawal of the patient and the shrinking of the patient's active world. In short, as the patient introverts, the interviewer may feel ineffectual or out of touch. Such feelings are to be expected. They do not necessarily suggest that the interview is going poorly.

IV: FAMILY SYSTEM AND OTHER GROUP SYSTEMS

Sometimes depression seems to possess a life of its own, independent of the person labeled as depressed. It is within the family that this phenomenon comes most vividly to mind. To understand a depression fully, one must understand its role in the family. Family interaction may be the primary root of the depression, as in a hateful sibling rivalry. At other times the depression may have its roots in a biochemical process, yet the ramifications of this process will reverberate throughout the family. A case in point would be a spouse laid off from work secondary to a severe endogenous depression. Surely, all members of the family will feel the pains of this depressive process, almost as if the biochemical imbalance were in their own neurochemistry. Finally, the family pathology may feed a depression already caused by another system, such as the biochemical or psychological system. In this section the focus will be specifically on the impact of depression on other family members as it pertains to the initial interview.

I will introduce this topic by describing an interview that I supervised in person. The interviewer was talking with the identified patient, whom I shall refer to as Mrs. Ella Thomas. In the same room the husband and son of Mrs. Thomas were also present. Mrs. Thomas was a gray-haired woman with angry eyes that seemed resentful of all 70 of her years. She fidgeted and cried throughout the interview. At times she would suddenly change topics, whining out such statements to her husband as, "You've got to help me, Leonard! I can't go on. The pain! The pain!" She complained about the hospital and warned that, "I had better get my sleeping pills or I'll leave."

As the interview proceeded, an atmosphere of increasing tension pervaded the room. Her husband had refused to have a chair brought for himself. Consequently, he stood throughout the interview, stationed reservedly behind the interviewer. As the interview proceeded, he tightly rolled his lips upon each other, while his arms closed over his chest. Mrs. Thomas' son sat down, his body turned sideways to his mother. He occasionally tossed a glance at her when his eyes were not staring at his shoes or the floor. Later in the interview, with an angry tone plucking each word, he challenged the clinician, "Why can't she have those meds?" I felt a growing sense of discomfort inside me. The poor interviewer was nervously breaking eye contact with Mrs. Thomas, while he sheepishly performed a mental status.

I can safely say that no one in that room was comfortable. That room represented a classic reflection of the impact of depression on the family system and even on the hospital system itself. Diagnostically, Mrs. Thomas had an agitated major depression. In reality, this entire family was experiencing the depressive process. But it did not stop at the boundary of her age-spotted skin. Depression is often reflected in the actions and words of family members. Her husband and son demonstrated the frustration and anger often generated in those who love the patient. These people experience a sense of helplessness, fearing that nothing will change, despite their best efforts. Not personally experiencing the patient's anhedonia and loss of energy, they cannot understand why the patient does not help himself or herself. They also find their own daily activities continuously interrupted by the complaints and actions of the depressed person. Occasionally, secondary to such frustration, they will develop a depression of their own. In a sense, the depression will have replicated itself. As illustrated above, their anger may be expressed not only towards the patient, but also towards the interviewer. Unfortunately, as described earlier in the section on dyadic process, the negative feelings generated by Mrs. Thomas may backfire upon her, creating a hostile environment even within the hospital.

If the interviewer meets family members, their statements and nonverbal messages may be the first clue that depression is the diagnosis. At a different level, the interviewer should keep in mind that other family members may need help. The problem is not "just Ella's problem." Viewed at an even more sophisticated level, the family system may in some way need Mrs. Thomas' depression as a stabilizing force, as theorists such as Bowen or Minuchin have discussed.[23] All of these points emphasize the need for the interviewer to carefully explore the family in order to understand the depression.

Within the individual interview, family tensions may be spontaneously brought up by the patient. But at other times questioning may be needed to illuminate the issues. Questions such as the following represent some good jumping off points:

a. Who in your family seems to understand you?
b. Who in your family are you concerned about right now?
c. How do you think your family members view your depression?
d. What kinds of suggestions have your family members been making to you about how to feel better?
e. What kind of pressures has your spouse been coping with recently?

Questions such as the above will often yield information about the state of the family. They may elicit interpersonal tensions towards specific family members, where more direct questioning might have elicited denial. For instance, when answering the question about pressures on the spouse, the patient may relate feelings of guilt for being a burden, feelings of anger towards the spouse for perceived neglect, or disgust at the spouse's overattention to work or other family members, or may seem detached and uninterested in the spouse. From such a question one may also learn valuable information about situational stressors in the family system as well.

Fields of interaction other than the family can experience depression. On a direct level, reflections of depression will be seen in systems such as the job environment, church groups, and social organizations. From a different perspective, such systems may act as the major stressors triggering the depression in the first place. On the other hand they may act as important supports, buffering the patients from their depression. Society itself can be an integral system involved in depression. Careful questioning might reveal that the husband of Mrs. Thomas had been forced to retire secondary to economic lay offs. Or perhaps her family had recently relocated because of increasing taxes in their former state. Likewise the hospitalization of Mrs. Thomas will ultimately affect the Medicaid and Social Security systems.

Thus depression leaves its mark throughout all these interlocking systems. The sensitive interviewer understands these interrelationships and attempts to make a reconnaissance of each system during the initial interview. Through this diligent search the puzzle of depression may become clearer, and avenues of therapeutic intervention more apparent.

V: FRAMEWORK FOR MEANING

During an initial interview one can become so involved in the diagnosis that issues of major concern to the patient may be overlooked. In particular one should attempt to understand how patients view their problems, their life, and their beliefs. Such views represent the patient's framework for meaning as described in Chapter 4. In an initial interview, one will seldom have the time to explore this framework in any depth, but even a few minutes of discussion may provide clues for engagement or for future therapeutic discussion. Such questioning may also further convey interest in the interviewee as a person, not as a "case." Failure to have evolved a framework for meaning or a sudden breakdown in a pre-existing framework can function as triggers or perpetuators of the patient's depression, representing an existential crisis.

To investigate these areas of existential framework, several regions of information may be of value. At times demographic questions concerning religious background may act as springboards for further inquiry. Significant information may present itself following questions such as, "What role does religion play in your life?" If asked with a nonjudgmental tone, people generally respond naturally and specifically. Very quickly, the interviewer will register the role of religious doubt or ambivalence in the current crisis.

Religion is not the only axis upon which a framework for meaning is built. Other areas include family, job, community, charities, patriotism, and subcultures such as those associated with sports and rock music.

Ignorance of these factors can result in markedly disrupted engagement. Moreover, these systems can have a very powerful influence on whether the patient will comply with treatment recommendations. Consequently, it remains critical for the initial interviewer to understand these factors, as illustrated below:

> **Clin.:** What kinds of things do you like to do in your spare time?
>
> **Pt.:** When I felt better, I used to love to sing.
>
> **Clin.:** Oh . . . (with an increased interest in tone of voice) What kinds of music did you like to sing?
>
> **Pt.:** All types, but I really loved gospel music. What a beautiful way to bring God to people . . . I think if you put all of your trust in God, He will help you. Man is not the answer. Man provides artificial answers.
>
> **Clin.:** Have you been praying recently in an attempt to gain some guidance?

Pt.: Yes I have. Every day. It helps, but I wonder if maybe I ask for too much. Perhaps I am to blame.

This vignette provides a wealth of information for the clinician. In the first place, religion obviously plays a major role in this person's life. The interviewer may want to further examine the possible therapeutic supports that religion could provide, such as meetings with a minister or choral church activities. On the other hand, religion may be feeding some guilty ruminations that are part of the depressive process itself. Perhaps even more important, the clinician has some clues concerning where engagement could go wrong. In particular, the patient's statement, "Man is not the answer. Man provides artificial answers," serves as a warning to the clinician. Specifically, the patient may find treatment modalities such as psychotherapy or medication as clearly "artificial answers." Premature reference in the interview to such treatments could easily rupture engagement. The clinician will need to proceed cautiously, trying to gently find out what this particular patient wants in the way of help.

It is beyond the scope of this chapter to discuss the numerous ramifications that the search for meaning may play in depression. I refer the reader to authors such as Frankl[24] and Yalom[25] who discuss these issues in the detail they deserve. In closing, I am reminded of another example in which understanding the patient's framework for meaning helped in the initial interview of a patient with depressive complaints. I had been asked to see this patient as a psychiatric consultant in a medical ward.

Mr. Kulp (as I shall refer to him) was a 55-year-old man with alcoholism suffering from moderately severe Parkinson's disease (a progressive form of muscular rigidity). He had been admitted with suicidal ideation following a drunken spree. He had many stressors, not the least of which was a markedly battered self-image created by the stiffening of his body from Parkinson's disease. Mr. Kulp had always prided himself on being an energetic bread winner for his family. He viewed himself as a tough, former Marine. This latter role affiliation surfaced when I asked him if he liked to read. He mentioned that he loved to read, pointing to his books. When I asked if I could see them, he enthusiastically showed them to me. All of them concerned Marines and various war heroes, which led to a discussion of his former Marine days, including his boot camp experiences. At the time I did not exactly know what to make of this information. Later its usefulness became apparent.

By way of understatement, Mr. Kulp did not respond positively to my recommendations that he needed to enter a local alcohol rehabilitation center. As the discussion proceeded, I felt that he would decide against entering the program. He balked, stating that it would be too big of a time commitment and too tough. At which point I made a comment to the effect, "Well Mr. Kulp I guess you're right. It's a tough commitment, but not your first. It's sort of like boot camp was a tough commitment. But you needed boot camp. It made a good soldier of you. Maybe you and your family need this program." This statement appeared to affect Mr. Kulp. He eventually decided to enter the rehabilitation program. Perhaps he would have entered anyway, but the understanding of his framework for meaning certainly seemed to help. Suddenly the rehabilitation program was not viewed as a foreign entity; it was akin to his familiar and respected boot camp. Mr. Kulp had been given a chance to be a soldier again.

References

1. American Psychiatric Association: Diagnostic and Statistical Manual of Mental Disorders, 4th ed. Washington, DC, APA, 1994, p. 327.
2. DSM-IV, 1994, p. 349.
3. DSM-IV, 1994, pp. 332 and 338.
4. Renner, J. A.: Alcoholism. In *Inpatient Psychiatry, Diagnosis and Treatment*, edited by Lloyd I. Sederer. Baltimore, Williams & Wilkins, 1983, p. 185.
5. Klein, D., Gittelman, R., Quitkin, F., and Rifkin, A.: *Diagnosis and Drug Treatment of Psychiatric Disorders*. Baltimore, Williams & Wilkins, 1980, p. 226.
6. Bernstein, J. G.: Medical psychiatric drug interaction. In *Massachusetts General Hospital Handbook of General Hospital Psychiatry*, edited by T. Hackett and Ned Cassam. Saint Louis, C. V. Mosby, 1978, p. 502.
7. Anderson, W. H.: Depression. In *Outpatient Psychiatry: Diagnosis and Treatment*, edited by A. Lazarre. Baltimore, Williams & Wilkins, 1979, p. 259.
8. Akiskal, H., and McKinney, W.: Research in depression. In *Major Psychiatric Disorders, Overview and Selected Readings*, edited by F. Guggenheim and C. Nadelson. New York, Elsevier Science Publishing Co., 1982, p. 77.
9. Cohen, R. L.: History taking. In *Basic Handbook of Child Psychiatry*, Vol. 1, New York, Basic Books, 1979, p. 495.
10. Kolb, L., and Brodie H. K.: *Modern Clinical Psychiatry*. Philadelphia, W.B. Saunders, 1982, p. 408.
11. Renner, J. A., 1983, p. 188.
12. Klein, D., et al., 1980, p. 225.
13. Nelson, J., and Charney, D. S.: The symptoms of major depressive illness. *American Journal of Psychiatry* 138:1–13, 1981.
14. Akiskal, H. S.: Dysthymic disorder: Psychopathology of proposed chronic depressive subtypes. *American Journal of Psychiatry*. 140:11–20, 1983.
15. Jaspers K.: Symptom complexes of abnormal affective states. In *General Psychopathology*. Manchester, Manchester University Press, 1923, p. 598.
16. Minkowski, E.: Findings in a case of 'schizophrenic' depression. In *Existence*, edited by Rollo May. New York, A Touchstone Book, 1958, p. 133.
17. Beck, A. T.: *Cognitive Therapy and the Emotional Disorders*. New York, The American Library, 1976, p. 105.
18. Minkowski, E., 1958, p. 132.
19. Beck, A. T., Kovacs, M., and Weissman, A.: Hopelessness and suicidal behavior. *Journal of the American Medical Association* 234:1146–1149, 1975.
20. MacKinnon, R., and Michels, R.: *The Psychiatric Interview in Clinical Practice*. Philadelphia, W.B. Saunders, 1971.

21. Akiskal, H., and McKinney, W., 1982, p. 73.
22. Akiskal, H., and McKinney, W., 1982, p. 74.
23. Gurman, A. S., and Kniskern, D. P. (ed): *Handbook of Family Therapy*. New York, Brunner/Mazel Publisher, 1981.
24. Frankl, V. W.: *The Doctor and the Soul*. New York, Vintage Books, 1973.
25. Yalom, I.: *Existential Psychotherapy*. New York, Basic Books, 1980.

CHAPTER 6

Interviewing Techniques While Exploring Psychosis

*A*nd then a Plank in Reason, broke,
And I dropped down, and down—
and hit a World, at every plunge,
And finished knowing—then— . . .

Emily Dickinson

*O*ne wonders what the world is like when a plank in reason
splinters, as Emily Dickinson describes the slip into psychotic process. To the degree that the clinician possesses a feeling
for this world, it becomes easier to uncover subtle psychotic states.
As intuitive understanding increases it also becomes easier to understand the needs of the patient, an understanding that leads directly into a more compassionate interview.

To begin our exploration we will turn to Gérard De Nerval, a
poet of extreme talent, who had the misfortune of falling through a
plank in reason sometime during the middle of the Victorian Era.
De Nerval was a gifted Symbolist poet, who was also a world trav-
eler and a man deeply interested in philosophy, blessed with a
child-like awe of nature. In 1841 he experienced his first psychotic
break. Eventually, some 14 years later, psychotic process would
lead him on a cold winter night to an iron gate bordering an alley
near the Boulevard St-Michel. He would be found in the morning
hanging from a railing with his neck fatally embraced by an apron
string.[1]

285

On the morning after his suicide, fragments of a work entitled *Le Rêve et la Vie* were found in his pocket. It is this piece that provides us with our first glimpse into the world of psychosis.

*F*irst of all I imagined that the persons collected in the garden (of the madhouse) all had some influence on the stars, and that the one who always walked round and round in a circle regulated the course of the sun. An old man, who was brought there at certain hours of the day, and who made knots as he consulted his watch, seemed to me to be charged with the notation of the course of the hours . . .

I attributed a mystical signification to the conversations of the warders and of my companions. It seemed to me that they were the representatives for all the races of the earth, and that we had undertaken between us to re-arrange the course of the stars, and to give a wider development to the system. An error, in my opinion, had crept into the general combination of numbers, and thence came all the ills of humanity. . . .

I seemed to myself a hero living under the very eyes of the gods; everything in nature assumed new aspects, and secret voices came to me from the plants, the trees, animals, the meanest insects, to warn and to encourage me. The words of my companions had mysterious messages, the sense of which I alone understood.[2]

In some respects, it is De Nerval's last statement that provides one of the most telling clues as to the nature of psychotic process. As psychotic process becomes more intense, the patient's world becomes progressively more unique to the patient, receding further from the experience of the world as witnessed by others. In this sense, psychosis can be defined in simple terms as a breakdown of perceptual, cognitive, or rationalizing functions of the mind, to the point that the individual experiences reality very differently than other people within the same culture.

De Nerval's world became filled with a maelstrom of curious and disturbing sensations. His words sensitively depict a variety of classic symptoms of psychosis, including delusions, ideas of reference, and hallucinations. It also demonstrates the fact that some aspects of psychotic process may be exciting and even beautiful. But, and this is an important but, psychosis is almost invariably ultimately accompanied by an intensely painful collection of fears. The patient senses impending catastrophe. For instance, De Nerval states, "An error, in my opinion, had crept into the general combination of numbers, and thence came all the ills of humanity." Such paranoid perception can create a tremendous sense of urgency and responsibility in those experiencing psychotic process. Perhaps for De Nerval it was the realization that he could not correct this heinous error in the universe that led him to believe that his life should be ended, because he had failed both god and humanity.

There are many aspects of psychotic process that, in my mind, demarcate it from the innovative workings of eccentric men and women, whose thought is clearly at variance with the world view of most people but is not a psychotic process. Creative thinking may bear a resemblance to psychotic process, but it is not identical to it. We shall see that it is not so much the content of the psychotic thinking that is pathologic, but more the way in which the thinking occurs that marks the process as psychotic.

Now that we have arrived at a working definition of psychosis, an important point needs to be emphasized. The word "psychosis" is not a diagnosis. Psychosis is a syndrome that can result from any number of psychiatric disorders delineated in the DSM-IV. It is never enough to simply state that the patient appears to be psychotic, because one must proceed to determine what diagnostic entity is causing the psychotic process.

The following chapter, like the preceding chapter, is divided into two sections. In the Diagnosis of Psychotic States, we will look at seven case vignettes, which illustrate the diversity of agents that may be responsible for a psychotic presentation. Once again, the emphasis will be upon a discussion of practical points that help the initial clinician to both uncover and diagnose psychotic states. In the Understanding of Psychosis, systems analysis will be used to expand an understanding of psychosis as a uniquely human process. To begin our discussion let us meet some people who have had the misfortune of falling through a plank in reason.

SECTION I: DIAGNOSIS OF PSYCHOTIC STATES

Case Presentations

CASE 1: MR. WILLIAMS

Mr. Williams presents to the emergency room accompanied by three police officers. His behavior has not put the officers in particularly good spirits. As one officer states it, "This guy is wacko. Every once in awhile he tries to bolt as if something was after him." The officer has no idea what the "thing" is that appears so disturbing to Mr. Williams. In the interview, Mr. Williams presents as a 33-year-old male, who initially appears relatively calm despite the beads of perspiration on his forehead. He is just finishing supper from his dinner tray and is neatly wiping his mouth with a napkin. His pants are torn and soiled; obviously, they are not strangers to the harshness of street life. He appears oriented to person, place, and time. As he begins to talk he becomes more animated, displaying tangential speech with occasional glimpses of a loosening of his associations. He denies any recent drinking or drug use, but his story is vague, concerned primarily with the appearance of some creature that has been following him. Suddenly, in the middle of the interview, his eyes widen as he stares down at his feet. He cannot attend to the interview, because his attention is riveted to the floor. He begins kicking at some invisible object and angrily looks at the clinician, yelling, "Get rid of that thing!"

CASE 2: MR. WALKER

Mr. Walker is a 20-year-old male. He is thin and his clothes tend to hang on his gaunt frame. Beneath his black hair a rather handsome face sits quietly darkening with a day's worth of beard. As the interviewer enters the room, Mr. Walker acknowledges him with a slight nod of his head. His speech is soft and mildly slowed. He appears almost shy. As he speaks, there is barely a hint of facial expression, his voice painted gray by a conspicuous lack of highlights. All seems bland. Mr. Walker proceeds to describe a chaotic situation at home. He is being avidly pursued by three filthy women who enter his house at night. They attempt to force sex on him. When asked if he knows who these women are, he nods, stating that one is "that devil Miss Brown." He proceeds to describe a recent party he attended, where sex games were played. He relates that he had been tricked into going. As he entered the kitchen three men tied him to a chair and stripped him. When asked what happened, he pauses and proceeds to say, "They violated my anus." As he says these words a slight smile steals across his face. His speech is without any evidence of loosening of associations, tangential thought, thought blocking, or illogical thought. He is alert and well oriented. Both he and his family deny that he has used any street drugs. During the interview the clinician feels uncomfortable and somewhat frightened.

CASE 3: MS. HASTINGS

Ms. Hastings walks into the clinic with a disgruntled look on her face. She is 50 years old and appears a bit bedraggled. The first words out of her mouth are, "Can you help me with my husband?" Her speech is fluent, without any evidence of loose associations, illogical thought, or bizarre ideation. In actuality she is somewhat eloquent but clearly upset. When asked to elaborate, she responds with an indignant snort, "It's the divorce game, that's all!" She proceeds to relate an elaborate tale of infidelity on the part of her husband. At the present time, she says, he has hired a variety of men to harass her into a state of insanity. Her craziness will provide grounds for his sought-after divorce. The men are using "conventional spy tools," and she is beginning to feel that her own mother may be in on the plot. Her story is literally illustrated by a journal filled with drawings and time schedules she has compiled on the activities of her husband and "his goons next door." She denies hallucinations or a previous psychiatric history. She also denies most depressive symptoms except, "I'm edgy of course, wouldn't you be?"

CASE 4: MISS FAY

Miss Fay is a 23-year-old divorced woman who presents to the Assessment Center for the second time in 2 weeks. She is casually dressed in jeans and a yellow blouse that tends to overshadow her curly, dull blonde hair. She has come alone to the Center and relates, "I just had to talk to someone again. I'm a nervous wreck." Indeed, she appears somewhat of a nervous wreck, in that she wriggles uneasily about in her chair while incessantly picking at her nails. It seems difficult for her to maintain eye contact. She states to the male clinician, "You make me nervous. These are hard questions." She relates that things are terrible at home, where she lives with her mother and her two children. She never gets a moment's rest and reports significant problems falling asleep, as well as a general inability to relax. Her speech is mildly pressured and characterized by an evasive style, which clearly frustrates the interviewer. She bluntly denies any delusions or hallucinations but seems greatly concerned with an incident of sexual abuse from her distant past, which she prefers not to discuss at the moment. As the interviewer proceeds she becomes intermittently more anxious and coyly giggles at times, perhaps out of nervousness. One senses that if she could burrow beneath her chair to escape scrutiny, she would most surely do so. At the time of her first evaluation, she was diagnosed as having a relatively severe generalized anxiety disorder.

CASE 5: MR. LAWRENCE

Mr. Lawrence is a good looking man about 30 years of age. Despite his good looks he is not particularly attractive at the moment, because he is in the midst of a rage. He was found in his apartment smashing a typewriter through the bedroom window. He had trashed the apartment, madly throwing white paint over his furniture. The landlord found him screaming. Mr. Lawrence has a long-standing history of paranoid schizophrenia. He has been violent at times in the past. Tonight he refuses hospitalization, and the crisis worker has to involuntarily commit him, because he apparently seems to be in the midst of yet another acute psychotic relapse. It took two policemen to bring Mr. Lawrence into the emergency room, and on the way in he managed to creatively coin a few new obscenities.

CASE 6: KATE

The moment that one sees the look of concern on the faces of this young girl's parents, one feels that something is very wrong. Kate is 14 years old. She is slightly overweight. Her blond hair drops in a tangle down her back. Her parents relate that they feel she is very depressed and that she has become more depressed over the past 2 months. Things had reached a crisis when 5 days earlier Kate had thrown a slumber party. No one came. Since then she has been acting oddly, talking about "reality" and wandering about the house. The most bizarre incident occurred 2 nights ago, when Kate knocked at her parents bedroom door at 2:00 A.M. When they opened the door, Kate stood topless, stating in a dull monotone that she felt a need to talk. At no time had Kate been delusional or heard voices. Kate's parents had taken her to two emergency rooms in the past week. At both places her parents were told that she was hysterical. Referrals were made for outpatient therapy.

CASE 7: MISS FLAGSTONE

Miss Flagstone walks into the clinic dressed in a stylish fashion, sporting a cigarette in hand, waving it about like a baton of sorts. During the interview, her affect changes periodically, as she relates a long-standing history of "just not going anywhere in my life." At times she is tearful but is able to quickly pull herself together. She is very dissatisfied with her poor relationships with men, despite her good looks and thick black hair. Her speech rate and volume are within normal limits. Although mildly tangential at times, she does not display any loosening of associations or thought blocking. She is well oriented and denies any history of delusions. When asked about hallucinations she denies any except for one episode 2 years earlier. She continues as follows. "I've really never told anyone this story, but it has had a profound affect on me. At the time I was extremely upset. Everything was horrible in my life. Fortunately, I was not taking any drugs or else I might not have found God. I was in my kitchen doing the dishes when a sudden light filled the room. I just knew it was a message from God. He had come to bring me back to the His flock. From inside the light I heard the angel Gabriel speak. He said, 'Janet, you are with child.' I knew this was a test from God and I showed strength by accepting the mission. He talked with me, and I convinced him of my great love of God. At that point the angel told me that all was well and that I was back with God, my father. A blinding light moved in and out of the room many times. The whole thing only lasted about 15 minutes, but my life has never been the same since." This episode is the only time that she has ever heard a voice, and she denies that she has any special mission for God other than to be a good Christian.

Discussion of Case Material

As with the last chapter it is assumed, for the sake of discussion, that the preceding clinical material was obtained during an initial assessment interview. Before proceeding with this case material, it may be of value to review the DSM-IV criteria for schizophrenia, because schizophrenia may very well represent the classic example of a psychotic illness. One could say that one of the main goals in the approach to any psychotic patient remains the determination of whether or not schizophrenia is present. To this end the DSM-IV criteria are as follows:[3]

Diagnostic Criteria for Schizophrenia*

A. *Characteristic symptoms:* Two (or more) of the following, each present for a significant portion of time during a 1 month period (or less if successfully treated):
  1. Delusions
  2. Hallucinations
  3. Disorganized speech (e.g., frequent derailment or incoherence)
  4. Grossly disorganized or catatonic behavior
  5. Negative symptoms, i.e., affective flattening, alogia, or avolition

Note: Only one Criterion A symptom is required if delusions are bizarre or hallucinations consist of a voice keeping up a running commentary on the person's behavior or thoughts, or two or more voices conversing with each other.

B. *Social/occupational dysfunction:* For a significant portion of the time since the onset of the disturbance, one or more major areas of functioning such as work, interpersonal relations, or self-care are markedly below the level achieved prior to the onset (or when the onset is in childhood or adolescence, failure to achieve expected level of interpersonal, academic, or occupational achievement).
C. *Duration:* Continuous signs of the disturbance persist for at least 6 months. This 6-month period must include at least 1 month of symptoms (or less if successfully treated) that meet Criterion A (i.e., active-phase symptoms) and may include periods of prodromal or residual symptoms. During these prodromal or residual periods, the

signs of the disturbance may be manifested by only negative symptoms or two or more symptoms listed in Criterion A present in an attenuated form (e.g., odd beliefs, unusual perceptual experiences).

D. *Schizoaffective and Mood Disorder exclusion:* Schizoaffective Disorder and Mood Disorder With Psychotic Features have been ruled out because either: (1) no Major Depressive, Manic, or Mixed Episodes have occurred concurrently with the active-phase symptoms; or (2) if mood episodes have occurred during active-phase symptoms, their total duration has been brief relative to the duration of the active and residual periods.

E. *Substance/general medical condition exclusion:* The disturbance is not due to the direct physiologic effects of a substance (e.g., a drug of abuse, a medication) or a general medical condition.

F. *Relationship to a Pervasive Developmental Disorder:* If there is a history of Autistic Disorder or another Pervasive Developmental Disorder, the additional diagnosis of Schizophrenia is made only if prominent delusions or hallucinations are also present for at least a month (or less if successfully treated).

Specify Classification of longitudinal course (can be applied only after at least 1 year has elapsed since the initial onset of active-phase symptoms):

Episodic With Interepisode Residual Symptoms (episodes are defined by the re-emergence of prominent psychotic symptoms); *also specify if:* **With Prominent Negative Symptoms**

Episodic With No Interepisode Residual Symptoms

Continuous (prominent psychotic symptoms are present throughout the period of observation); *also specify if:* **With Prominent Negative Symptoms**

Single Episode In Partial Remission; *also specify if:* **With Prominent Negative Symptoms**

Single Episode in Full Remission

Other or Unspecified Pattern

---

*Reprinted with permission from the Diagnostic and Statistical Manual of Mental Disorders, 4th ed., pp. 285 and 286. Copyright 1994 American Psychiatric Association.

It should be noted that there also exists a diagnosis, schizophreniform disorder, that is applied when a patient meets criteria A, D, and E of schizophrenia but the symptoms do not last for 6 months nor necessarily result in a marked decline in functioning. In the schizophreniform disorder the symptoms (including prodromal, active, and residual phases) must last at least 1 month but less than 6 months. Many patients who have received this diagnosis provisionally will eventually receive the diagnosis of schizophrenia if their symptoms last longer than 6 months. The diagnosis of schizophreniform disorder is not used if the psychosis is caused directly by a stressor, as seen in a brief reactive psychosis.

Now that we have examined the criteria for schizophrenia, let us begin our discussion of the case material.

DISCUSSION OF MR. WILLIAMS

Mr. Williams was the wild-eyed man brought in by the police. While with the police he appeared to be responding to visual hallucinations, a process that reappeared during the interview itself. And herein lies the first clue to the diagnostic entity causing his immediate psychosis, for the presence of visual hallucinations should alert the clinician to the possibility that a general medical condition may be causing the disorder. Schizophrenia may cause visual hallucinations, but auditory hallucinations are more frequent. On the other hand, general medical causes of psychosis (e.g., endocrine disorders, infections, toxins, and seizures) frequently present with extremely vivid visual hallucinations.

Fish has suggested that the quality of the visual hallucination may tend to vary depending on whether schizophrenia or a general medical process is present,[4] but no specific characteristics clearly differentiate the visual hallucinations seen with general medical states from those seen with more classic psychoses such as schizophrenia or bipolar disorder. On the other hand, some characteristics seem to be more common in each category and may provide clues to etiology. Visual hallucinations in patients, whose psychosis is caused by a general medical condition, presenting with delirium, tend to vary from the classic psychoses by preferentially occurring at night, by being briefer in duration, and by being more frequently perceived as moving. They may also have little personal significance to the patient. For example, the patient with schizophrenia may hallucinate about a recently deceased relative, whereas the delirious patient may see snakes.[5]

With patients for whom the psychosis is caused by drugs or other general medical conditions, the hallucinations may appear more frequently and more vividly when the patient is in a darkened room or has his eyes shut. This is not the case with people with schizophrenia, who tend to see their hallucinations with eyes open or who experience little change whether the eyes are open or closed.[6, 7] In this sense it is of value to ask patients, "When you see your hallucinations, what happens if you close your eyes?" With a hospitalized patient it is of value to check with the nursing staff concerning whether the patient is hallucinating more at night.

With people suffering from schizophrenia visual hallucinations seldom occur by themselves. They usually present with auditory hallucinations or hallucinations from some other sensory modality.[8] Also of interest to the interviewer is the fact that schizophrenic hallucinations are frequently superimposed on an otherwise normal-appearing environment or may even appear with the surrounding environment absent. In hallucinogenic drug-induced psychoses the entire environment frequently seems distorted with numerous illusions and hallucinations.[9] In a similar vein the visual hallucinations of schizophrenia tend to appear suddenly without preceding visual illusions or less formed visual hallucinations. Visual hallucinations caused by a general medical condition, as seen in delirium, tend to have a prodrome of visual illusions, simple geometric figures, and alterations of color, size, shape, and movement.[9]

Patients with schizophrenia tend to see concrete things such as faces, body parts, or complete figures as opposed to geometric patterns or poorly formed images. On the other hand, once patients, whose psychosis is caused by a general medical condition, begin seeing concrete images, it has been my experience that the images frequently appear extremely real to the patients. The delirious patient may look on with terror pointing towards the hallucination, eyeing it warily or moving away from it as it appears to approach. Occasionally the patient's affective response may be pleasurable, as experienced with hallucinations of miniature people, so-called Lilliputian hallucinations, sometimes seen in the early stages of delirium tremens (DTs) and other medically related states.[10]

In Mr. William's case, the interviewer asked him if he could point more closely to the creature in question. Mr. Williams hesitantly obliged by cautiously moving his hand towards the open space in front of his feet. Abruptly he halted, "I ain't getting no closer!" It became even more apparent that the hallucination was vivid and quite real. At times these types of hallucinations can create a peculiar sensation in the interviewer, because the actions of the patient, like the movements of a mime, create the feeling that one ought to be seeing something.

Sometimes the terms "hallucination" and "illusion" are misunderstood. Mr. Williams presents with a true hallucination, because his perceptual image is arising from an open space and is not being triggered by an environmental stimulus. With illusions the image is triggered by some actual object or stimulus in the room. For instance, one patient vividly described watching the face of a man standing beside him on the bus. He saw the man's face begin to twist in a grotesque fashion and saw his eyeballs shatter and begin to bleed. This experience represents a visual illusion and also emphasizes that such illusions may be as striking and terrifying as true hallucinations. We have seen that the appearance of vivid visual hallucinations ought to arouse suspicion that an organic agent may be at work. Mr. Williams represents one of the more typical organic causes of psychosis that the initial interviewer must constantly keep in mind, abuse and withdrawal from street drugs or medications. It is important to realize that there exist two different manners in which drugs may precipitate a psychosis—by acute intoxication or by withdrawal. First, let us look at the issue of withdrawal, because Mr. Williams is suffering from an alcohol withdrawal delirium, also known as DTs.

This book is not intended to represent a thorough review of drug abuse, and the reader should study these states elsewhere in detail. However, there are some basic facts with which all assessment clinicians should be familiar. With regard to withdrawal states, alcohol and sedative/hypnotic drugs are the most likely to present with psychotic features. They are also the most likely to result in death if not recognized and treated. Withdrawal from these drugs is significantly more dangerous than withdrawal from drugs such as heroin or amphetamines. Some estimates of the mortality rate of patients in definite DTs from alcohol, who have been hospitalized, have been as high as 15%, although with good management this number should be markedly lower.[11]

As people begin to withdraw from alcohol and sedative hypnotics, they generally move from mild symptoms of withdrawal towards progressively more severe states such as DTs. As withdrawal occurs, patients frequently experience sleep disturbances, nausea, anxiety, overalertness, tremulousness, and a peculiar intensification of their sensory modalities.[12] Even if patients such as Mr. Williams deny recent drug abuse, they may willingly admit to these symptoms if asked matter of factly and without the suggestion that they have "a personal problem." In this regard, questions such as the following may be useful:

a. Have you been noticing problems with your sleep?
b. Have you been feeling edgy over the past couple of days, you know, just can't seem to relax?
c. Over the past couple of days have you been feeling sick in your stomach?
d. Do you find yourself being startled by noises or upset by people moving or talking around you?

To develop DTs, the patient must use alcohol for long periods of time. It typically does not occur under the age of 30, although it clearly can, and it usually requires consistent use of large amounts of alcohol for several years.[13] This chronic use of alcohol sets up a complex set of compensatory physiologic changes in autonomic body regulation. When the alcohol is abruptly stopped, these compensatory changes go unchecked, resulting in such abnormalities as increased pulse, increased temperature, normal or elevated blood pressure, rapid breathing, muscle twitching, and sweating. As the syndrome becomes more serious, the patient may become so tremulous that walking appears to be difficult.[14]

While interviewing the psychotic patient, the clinician should do a quick survey to see if any of these physiologic signs of withdrawal are present. With Mr. Williams, he was noted to appear sweaty. The clinician also knew that his pulse rate was elevated at 100 with a mild increase in temperature. This emphasizes an important point. In general, a patient presenting with an acute psychosis should have his vital signs taken before the clinical interview, thus alerting the clinician that an acute organic process may be at work.

Mr. Williams proceeded to become more agitated, claiming that some kind of bug was crawling on him and that some "wires are running around on the floor. They're shocking the hell out of me, man!" It is not uncommon for people with DTs to hallucinate about small animals and sometimes large objects such as trains or the proverbial pink elephant. Tactile hallucinations or illusions such as mice or lice crawling about one's skin also occur, as seen with Mr. Williams.[14]

The clinician astutely cut this interview short, proceeding rapidly with a physical examination and appropriate medical management, which raises another important point. These people need prompt medical attention. If one is not a physician, then one must quickly have such a patient seen. An appointment for "later in the day or tomorrow" is totally inappropriate.

Before leaving the topic of DTs, a few more points seem worth mentioning. Seizures ("rum fits") sometimes precede DTs, usually occurring during the first 2 days after the cessation of drinking. More than one of three patients who have withdrawal seizures will go on to develop DTs. DTs usually begin 24 to 72 hours after the cessation of drinking but can appear much later, even as long as 7 or more days later.[14] Moreover, while performing an initial assessment on a psychotic patient in the hospital a few points are worth considering.

Some patients may have a temporary drug source, such as a friend, who eventually stops bringing drugs. In these cases, DTs may not appear until much longer into the patient's hospitalization. Keep in mind that patients with a higher income may purposely lie about alcohol consumption and may consequently develop withdrawal problems only as the hospitalization proceeds. Curiously, surgery may delay the appearance of DTs as well. All these facts considered, clinicians should be alert to the possibility of drug withdrawal in any patient who develops a psychosis at any time during a hospital stay, especially if the patient's vital signs are abnormally elevated.

Thus far the material gained from the actual interview with Mr. Williams has been the focus of discussion. However, in addition, one of the most important interviews to perform when a patient is brought to the emergency room by the police is with the officers, and there is an art to this process. The first trick is training oneself to take the time to perform this interview. Both the police and the clinician are frequently harried, but nevertheless this interview can provide invaluable information. In particular one wants to establish the following: (1) What were the circumstances in which the patient was found?; (2) Is the patient a known alcohol or drug abuser?; (3) Do the officers know the patient's family, and has the family been contacted?; (4) Did the patient appear disoriented or demonstrate any signs of psychosis?; (5) Has the patient appeared drowsy or been unconscious?; and (6) Has the patient been in a fight involving a possible head blow?

This last question raises an important aspect of interviewing the police. The clinician should always consider whether an officer may have delivered a head blow either justly or unjustly. Uncovering a history of a physical confrontation can help alert the clinician to the possibility of a subdural hematoma or an intracranial bleed as the source of the psychosis, especially in older patients who have been struck. It may also help the clinician understand and perhaps decrease the patient's fear that more violence may follow.

A savvy clinician approaches these topics in a manner that puts the officers at ease and decreases any sense that the clinician is antagonistic towards the officers. It is important to remember that most officers would resort to violence only when necessary. Angry countertransference feelings directed towards the police can only get in the way of gaining valid information from them. The following type of approach may be useful:

> **Clin.:** It really looks like you had your hands full with this guy.
>
> **Police:** You can say that again, that guy's nuts. It took three of us to get him down.
>
> **Clin.:** Yeah, he's wound up, maybe he's on something. Listen, did any of your officers get hurt? We'd be glad to take a look at them and check them over.
>
> **Police:** No, don't worry about it, thanks anyway.
>
> **Clin.:** By the way when you were wrestling this guy down, did he accidentally get struck on the head?

Police: No, can't say that he did.

Clin.:   The reason I ask is that if he got a blow on the head we need to make sure he didn't get a small fracture or something like that?

Police: Hmmm . . . Well, you might want to take a look, this guy was wild, someone might have used a stick on him. He was out of control.

Clin.:   O.K., thanks a lot for all your help. We'll take a look at him. I hope the rest of your night goes better than this.

This matter-of-fact type of inquiry tends to yield accurate answers while unobtrusively reminding the officers of the dangers of a head blow.

Violently psychotic patients, frequently brought in by the police, serve as a bridge to the next topic, patients who are acutely intoxicated by a psychosis-producing agent. This list of agents is extensive and includes common agents such as speed, lysergic acid diethylamide (LSD) and other hallucinogens, marijuana, cocaine, crack, and phencyclidine (PCP). For a concise and practical discussion, the reader is referred to articles by Goldfrank and Lydiard.[15, 16]

By way of example I will briefly describe some of the more typical aspects of a patient intoxicated on PCP, a drug originally developed in the 1950s as an anesthetic-analgesic agent. These patients frequently present as markedly psychotic, although they can present without any psychotic features. In addition they can be extremely violent. In this regard any violent patient should alert the clinician to the possibility of PCP abuse. Even at low doses this drug can produce the three As of PCP use: analgesia, amnesia, and ataxia (problems with gait). The analgesia can result in self-mutilatory behaviors such as eye gouging. If use of PCP is even remotely suspected, the initial interviewer should have safety officers informed and immediately available during the interview.

On a behavioral level, the psychotic features of these patients may be quite bizarre, such as running naked in public or crawling around on all fours like an animal. They may develop paranoia, disorientation, auditory hallucinations, and visual hallucinations.

The physical examination may provide important clues, such as the various types of nystagmus (abnormal eye jerks) and hypertension reported as occurring in 57% of these patients.[17] These patients generally show miosis (smaller than normal pupils) but may also present with mydriasis (larger than normal pupils), especially if they also ingested an anticholinergic agent. Increased muscle tone and increased salivation are also common. Rather than presenting as agitated, these patients may present lethargically or in a coma if they have ingested high doses of the drug.

Returning in a more general sense to psychosis as precipitated by drugs, a few more points are worth mentioning. The rapid appearance of a full-blown psychosis in a matter of hours should make the clinician very suspicious of a drug-induced psychosis. Processes such as schizophrenia tend to develop more slowly. Some patients may not know that they have been given a drug; it may have been slipped to them or sprinkled on a joint. In this regard it is always worthwhile checking with friends who may know more about the actual circumstances surrounding the drug ingestion. One should always be on the look-out for two possibilities when faced with drug-intoxicated, psychotic patients:

1. Is the patient actually under the influence of more than one street drug?
2. Has the patient possibly ingested not a street drug but a medication that is precipitating the psychosis?

I am reminded of a young woman with a chronic history of paranoid schizophrenia. She had been doing very well in the hospital and was consequently sent home on a pass. Within a few hours of returning from her pass, she began to appear agitated and reported feeling apprehensive. In another 30 minutes she became grossly psychotic and reported that small dragons were chasing her. Indeed she was seen racing down the hall as if pursued by a bevy of such monsters. The physical examination revealed dilated and poorly responsive pupils, a dry mouth, and an elevated pulse. It was discovered that she had taken "a few extra" Cogentin (benztropine mesylate) tablets while at her apartment. Cogentin is a commonly prescribed anticholinergic agent that helps to alleviate some of the side effects of antipsychotic medications.

If taken in excess, these anticholinergic agents can quickly precipitate a delirium, as was the case with this patient. Elderly patients appear to be particularly susceptible to such anticholinergic deliriums. It is therefore important to inquire about both prescription and nonprescription medications. Keep in mind that specific medications may have a mild anticholinergic effect, but that when given together these medications may have an additive effect strong enough to precipitate a delirium.

Classes of medications that may have some anticholinergic property include some over-the-counter hypnotics and "cold medicines," certain antidepressants, some antipsychotics, certain antiparkinsonian medications, some medications for peptic ulcer disease, and even antihistamines.[18] A classic story of medication-induced delirium would begin with an elderly patient being treated with an antidepressant such as Elavil (amitriptyline hydrochloride), who becomes mildly psychotic related to the depression. The patient would then be placed on Mellaril (thioridazine hydrochloride), an antipsychotic. This medication would relieve the patient's psychosis but could also create a significant parkinsonian syndrome. To relieve this side effect the clinician might add Cogentin. By now the patient would be on three different medications with anticholinergic effect—Elavil, Mellaril, and Cogentin. Such a patient might soon be delirious and plagued by impish demons, compliments of the treating clinician. The clinician must always carefully elicit a medication history from both the patient and the patient's family.

The clinician should also keep in mind one other broad category of agents that could precipitate a drug-induced psychosis, namely, herbs and other natural agents. A naturally occurring source of anticholinergic agents is a family of plants known as the Solanaceae. Such an innocuous sounding name actually houses a variety of not so innocuous plants, including *Atropa belladonna* (commonly called deadly nightshade), jimsonweed, mandrake, and henbane. Historically, ointments and potions made from such agents may have resulted in the psychotic states that, at least partially, functioned as the source of the wild phenomena reported by the witches of the Middle Ages. In the present, it remains important to consider the ingestion of herbs and other "natural foods" while evaluating an unexplained presentation of psychosis.

Perhaps at this time it is best to return to the presentation of Mr. Williams. An interview with the police revealed that Mr. Williams had a long history of alcohol dependence, although he did not appear intoxicated presently. They also thought that he had a history of "stuffing his face with any drug he could get his hands on." Further interviewing with Mr. Williams revealed that he had a history of DTs. The physical examination and lab work revealed no other probable cause for the psychotic presentation. He was felt to be in the early stages of DTs and was begun on Valium (diazepam). In a matter of several hours he calmed down, and all psychotic symptoms vanished. His case would be summarized as follows:

Axis I: Alcohol withdrawal delirium 291.00
           Alcohol dependence (unspecified) 303.90
           Rule out Unknown Substance Abuse 305.90
Axis II: Deferred 799.9
Axis III: Rule out a variety of alcohol-related diseases such as
           hepatitis, gastritis, and pancreatitis

As we leave the discussion of Mr. Williams, several key points are worth summarizing.

1. Visual hallucinations, especially if they appear to be particularly vivid and real to the patient, are frequently seen in psychoses caused by physiologic insults to the brain, including drugs and medical disease.
2. Despite the fact that such organic psychoses may tend to have some features that distinguish them from entities such as schizophrenia, all psychoses can present in a similar fashion. Consequently, any patient presenting for the first time with psychotic features should be promptly medically evaluated.
3. One of the most frequent physiologic causes of psychotic symptoms is the use of street drugs or alcohol.
4. Withdrawal from alcohol, in heavy drinkers, may lead to an alcohol withdrawal delirium (commonly called DTs). DTs can be fatal if not treated promptly.
5. The onset of a marked psychosis in a matter of hours, in a previously normal individual, is strongly suggestive of a drug-related etiology.
6. Both over-the-counter and under-the-counter medications may cause psychotic states, especially in the elderly. Anticholinergic medications are notorious for precipitating deliria.
7. If police bring in the patient, they should be questioned thoroughly.
8. Any patient who presents violently should be thoroughly evaluated for evidence of psychotic process and the possible use of PCP.

DISCUSSION OF MR. WALKER

Mr. Walker was the young man who was being harassed by abusive women like "that devil Miss Brown." He also described brutal scenes of sexual abuse with a peculiar blandness. This blandness represents an important diagnostic clue, because Mr. Walker is suffering from schizophrenia. Criterion A-5 from the DSM-IV states that patients with schizophrenia may present with affective flattening. This type of peculiar affect can be seen in other psychotic states, but it is very common in schizophrenia.

A useful interviewing habit consists of asking oneself if the patient seems to be appropriately disturbed while describing traumatic incidents. In the case of Mr. Walker, as he related his rape, there was little display of fear, anxiety, or anger. His affect changed very little. When present to a moderate degree, this type of unresponsive affect is usually called blunted. If the patient demonstrates essentially no change in affect, it is usually referred to as a flat affect. Mr. Walker also nicely demonstrates the concept of an inappropriate affect. Rape victims do not generally smile as they describe their assaults. This peculiar combination of flattened affect and inappropriate affect is not infrequent in schizophrenia. It is one of the qualities that can create an unsettling emotional response in a clinician, as it did in this case.

An important point to remember concerning blunted affect remains the ironic and sometimes confusing fact that some antipsychotic medications frequently also cause a blunting of affect as a side effect. The wary clinician keeps this point in mind, because a patient inappropriately labeled as having schizophrenia by a previous clinician may present with a blunted or flat affect related to current medication. This blunted affect may be misinterpreted by the new clinician as further "proof" that the patient has schizophrenia, resulting in a perpetuation of the first diagnostic error.

Perhaps even more striking than Mr. Walker's blunted affect is the fact that he is clearly delusional. The appearance of delusions of any kind should always alert the clinician to the possibility of schizophrenia.

These delusions are frequently bizarre in the sense that they are patently absurd and have no possible factual basis. The patient may feel that forces are controlling his or her body or that thoughts are being inserted or withdrawn from his or her body. Other delusions tend to be concerned with magical, grandiose, or intensely religious themes. In this light, a patient may believe that God wants the patient to cut off a finger and sprinkle the blood over the earth in order to bring flowers into bloom. In paranoid schizophrenia, the patient may present with delusions of persecution or jealousy, as did Mr. Walker.

But this point raises an important diagnostic issue, for how does one separate paranoid schizophrenia from a different class of psychopathologic states collectively called the paranoid disorders? The distinction is actually somewhat easier to make than one might assume, if one keeps the following guideline in mind.

In paranoid schizophrenia, the paranoid delusions are only part of the pathologic process. Other aspects of psychotic process are generally present in addition to the disorder in the patient's belief system. In paranoid schizophrenia, as delineated by the DSM-IV, the paranoid delusions are usually accompanied by one or more of the following: some type of prominent hallucination, by evidence of a severe formal thought disorder, grossly disorganized or catatonic behavior, or "negative symptoms" such as the affective flattening seen with Mr. Walker. The thought disorder may manifest itself as incoherence or as a marked loosening of associations. Sometimes the patient presents with only one major psychotic symptom such as bizarre delusions, but in true schizophrenia this is invariably accompanied by a marked social and/or occupational dysfunction.

A comment should be made about the term "negative symptoms," which is new to the DSM-IV system. In the DSM-III-R much emphasis was placed upon those symptoms, such as hallucinations and delusions, that people with schizophrenia show that most people do not experience. These "extra" phenomena are now called "positive symptoms," indicating that they are an unwanted "excess."

We are now aware that schizophrenia also afflicts brain structures in such a way that the person loses certain normal functions. These lost functions are referred to as "negative symptoms" or "deficit symptoms," a term that I prefer. Such symptoms include affective flattening (decreased facial animation), alogia (decreased speech production and interest in speaking), and avolition (decreased drive and ability to sustain interest). Although not included as DSM-IV criteria, many clinicians view anergia (loss of energy) and anhedonia (loss of interest in pleasurable activities) as other types of deficit symptoms. As we shall see later in this chapter, these deficit symptoms are frequently devastating to both functioning and self-esteem and are in some instances more disabling than active psychotic symptoms, such as hallucinations and delusions.

With these ideas in mind, Mr. Walker's presentation becomes even more clearly typical of schizophrenia following an interview with his mother.

Clin.: What does your son do down in his room all day long?

Moth.: That is what is so peculiar. He talks with her.

Clin.: How do you mean?

Moth.: He talks with this devil woman. I'll hear voices that sound like a woman's voice coming up out of the basement. It is really weird. Late at night I can hear him arguing with her, swearing at her, and sometimes it sounds like holy hell is breaking out down there. I'm terrified, I never go down there.

Clin.: When he is with you, does it ever look like he is hearing voices?

Moth.: Oh yes, he's always mumbling to himself like he's answering someone. But the strange thing is that he's not always like this. Sometimes he seems so calm and almost normal and other times he's in a frenzy. Just last night he came screaming up out of that basement with a butcher knife in his hand. He kept screaming at me that I'd better make them stop. I couldn't take it anymore so I brought him in.

From the above it is apparent that Mr. Walker is hearing voices and clearly fulfills the criteria for schizophrenia. It also serves to stress the importance of carefully interviewing family members or other significant others. For whatever reasons, psychotic patients may withhold information critical to the diagnosis, and the family may gratefully provide the missing pieces.

Mr. Walker also illustrates the fluctuating nature of psychotic process, even in schizophrenia. The severity of the psychotic process may vary substantially. Many an interviewer has been lulled into a belief that a patient is not psychotic during the interview. In such cases it is always wise to listen carefully to the family, because the interviewer may simply be catching the patient during a period of decreased psychotic process. Moreover, patients with psychotic process may not be too eager to tell the "shrink" that they are plagued by voices. Their more rational side warns them that such talk may provide a quick ticket to the "looney bin." We may not agree with such a choice of words, but the truth of the matter remains that the patient is right.

At this point it may be useful to turn our attention to one of the exclusion criteria for schizophrenia as delineated by the DSM-IV. Exclusion D directly addresses the issue of affective symptoms. Several points are worth remembering here. In the preceding chapter we noted that a major depression may eventually manifest psychotic symptoms, representing an important diagnosis to rule out when psychosis is suspected. The particular psychotic symptoms may be either mood congruent or mood incongruent. It is important to note that in a major depression with psychotic features, the psychotic symptoms generally appear a considerable time period after the onset of the mood disorder. It is almost as if the depressive or manic process builds with a slow crescendo that culminates with the blooming of psychotic process.

Guze reports that most people suffering from schizophrenia experience affective syndromes at some time during the course of their illness.[19] Moreover, anhedonia is frequently seen in schizophrenia.[20] But in contrast to the time course of psychotic features in a major depression, the psychotic symptoms in schizophrenia tend to appear early in the process, usually predating any striking mood symptoms. While interviewing it becomes critical to spend considerable time attempting to delineate the actual history of the present illness, as discussed in Chapter 5.

Two points are worth emphasizing here. First, family members and the records of other mental health professionals can be invaluable in gaining a clear history of which came first, the psychotic symptoms or the mood symptoms. Second, it is always important when evaluating a patient who has had numerous psychotic breaks to return to the first break in an attempt to determine the role of depression in the chronology of the illness. Sometimes patients are mislabeled as having schizophrenia who in actuality have a bipolar disorder or major depression. These people might benefit from lithium or antidepressants. American psychiatrists have tended to over-diagnose schizophrenia while underdiagnosing bipolar disorder.[21] With chronic patients whose initial diagnosis may have been made 30 or 40 years ago, bipolar disorder may not have been considered as strongly, because lithium was not available.

The role of the timing of mood versus psychotic symptoms is also important in the differential between bipolar disorder (manic phase) and schizophrenia. A patient can be manic without being psychotic. The mania itself is manifested by excessive energy, unstable mood, agitation, decreased need for sleep, pressured speech and other classic manic symptoms. The mania does not become psychotic unless reality contact is disturbed, as manifested by the presence of delusions, hallucinations, or other psychotic symptoms such as grossly disorganized thought. It has been estimated that about 50 to 70% of manic patients display psychotic symptoms.[22] As with depression, psychotic symptoms in mania tend to appear significantly later than the mood symptoms. This point once again helps to ease the difficulty of distinguishing between schizophrenia and mania with psychotic process.

We can now look at a curious diagnostic dilemma. We have seen that in schizophrenia the psychotic symptoms usually predate marked affective symptoms. And in the mood disorders the psychotic symptoms generally appear later in the process, after the affective symptoms have been around for a while. But what diagnosis is appropriate when the psychotic symptoms appear at or near the same time as the affective symptoms? Here the reader's guess is about as good as the opinions of the numerous writers on the subject. The issue is controversial.

The diagnosis that helps to fill this gap is "Schizoaffective Disorder," and it is defined in the DSM-IV as follows:[23]

Diagnostic Criteria for 295.70 Schizoaffective Disorder*

A. An uninterrupted period of illness during which, at some time, there is either a Major Depressive Episode, a Manic Episode, or a Mixed Episode concurrent with symptoms that meet Criterion A for Schizophrenia.

Note: The Major Depressive Episode must include Criterion A1: depressed mood.

B. During the same period of illness, there have been delusions or hallucinations for at least 2 weeks in the absence of prominent mood symptoms.
C. Symptoms that meet criteria for a mood episode are present for a substantial portion of the total duration of the active and residual periods of the illness.
D. The disturbance is not due to the direct physiologic effects of a substance (e.g., a drug of abuse, a medication) or a general medical condition.

Specify type:
   Bipolar Type: if the disturbance includes a Manic or a Mixed Episode (or a Manic or a Mixed Episode and Major Depressive Episodes)
   Depressive Type: if the disturbance only includes Major Depressive Episodes

---

*Reprinted with permission from the Diagnostic and Statistical Manual of Mental Disorders, 4th ed., pp. 295 and 296. Copyright 1994 American Psychiatric Association.

The vagueness of this definition certainly would be at home in the campaign speech of any presidential candidate. But then at this stage of current diagnostic knowledge, this degree of vagueness may be appropriate. It serves to remind us that diagnostic categories are not necessarily real-life entities but represent our labels for observed behaviors sometimes arbitrarily forced to confirm diagnostic labels.

Clinicians vary on what they really feel that the schizoaffective disorder will prove to be. For instance, Tsuang feels that this diagnosis represents a heterogeneous category with two probable subtypes, an affective subtype and a schizophrenic subtype. According to this theory it does not really represent a genetically distinct category.[24]

The bottom line with this diagnosis is that people with schizoaffective disorders have many of the striking psychotic processes seen in schizophrenia but also have persistent and significant mood disturbances. They differ from people who have bipolar disorder or major depression in that people with schizoaffective disorder have periods when they are quite psychotic but their mood is fairly normal. This latter state is seldom seen with people suffering from a pure mood disorder, in which case psychotic process tends to "rear its head" only during a marked disturbance in mood.

On a practical level there exists some relevance to making these subtle diagnostic distinctions. If one labels the patient as demonstrating schizophrenia, this tends to bias subsequent clinicians to not think of the use of antidepressants or lithium and other mood stabilizers. The diagnosis of schizoaffective disorder serves to remind clinicians that the patient may have an affective component to the illness, suggesting medications such as those just mentioned. The diagnosis may also have some prognostic importance, because some authors feel that schizoaffective disorders have a significantly better prognosis than does schizophrenia.[25]

Concerning Mr. Walker, a diagnostic summary seems in order. No history suggestive of a personality disorder or a medical problem was found upon further interviewing. Apparently he had been displaying a downhill course for almost a year, thus fulfilling the time criteria for schizophrenia. His family reported that he appears intermittently depressed, and they were not entirely clear about the time course of the interplay between depressive symptoms and the psychotic process, but they did not feel that Mr. Walker had been consistently depressed. Once within the hospital, lab tests and other medical examinations would need to be ordered to rule out a general medical condition, such as street drugs or hyperthyroidism, as the cause for his psychosis, but his history does not particularly suggest such an entity. Consequently, the working diagnostic formulation would probably look as follows:

Axis I: Schizophrenia, paranoid type (provisional) 295.30
            Rule out schizoaffective disorder
Axis II: None V71.09
Axis III: None

Before leaving the discussion of Mr. Walker, several key points are worth summarizing:

1. A blunted or flat affect is frequently seen in schizophrenia.
2. Some antipsychotic medications can cause a blunted or flat affect. Consequently, when a patient is on an antipsychotic, it is difficult to determine whether the unusual affect is secondary to the medication or a psychopathologic process.
3. In order for a patient presenting with paranoid delusions or other nonbizarre delusions to fulfill the criteria for schizophrenia, the patient must also demonstrate one of the following: hallucinations, disorganized speech, grossly disorganized or catatonic behavior, or the negative symptoms of schizophrenia (e.g., affective flattening, alogia, or avolition).
4. Psychotic process frequently fluctuates. The interviewer should keep in mind that the patient may not be strikingly psychotic during the interview itself.
5. Collateral interviews with family members may provide invaluable diagnostic information.

Mr. Walker has provided a good example of the paranoid process that frequently appears in paranoid schizophrenia. It should be noted that the DSM-IV recognizes five major types of schizophrenia: disorganized type, catatonic type, paranoid type, undifferentiated type, and residual type. It is not infrequent for a patient to fluctuate among these types over the course of years. At present it remains unclear as to how valuable these subclassifications will be with regard to prognosis and treatment planning, but in any case, the clinician should be aware of their various presentations.

The concept of schizophrenia, residual type, is used when the patient has a history of schizophrenia but does not appear grossly psychotic in the near past or the present. These patients do not demonstrate psychotic symptoms such as hallucinations, a moderate or severe formal thought disorder, or delusions, but they do show residual signs of schizophrenia such as a blunted or inappropriate affect, a mild loosening of associations, eccentric behavior, or social withdrawal. This category emphasizes the point that one can be suffering from schizophrenia without being actively psychotic all the time. Many patients treated with antipsychotic medications eventually move into a prolonged remission and may be labeled as having schizophrenia, residual type.

At this point it is worthwhile moving to the next case history, because it adds a new twist to the diagnostic issues arising when a patient presents with paranoid symptoms.

DISCUSSION OF MS. HASTINGS

Ms. Hastings was the 50-old woman who presented with the chief complaint of, "Can you help me with my husband?" She then proceeded to describe an elaborate delusional system, which she alluded to as the "divorce game."

Unlike Mr. Walker, Ms. Hastings did not present with a blunted or odd affect. On the contrary, she seemed convincingly quite normal. Her affect was appropriately upset for someone believing that she was the object of foul play. She did not complain of any hallucinations, and subsequent interviewing revealed that she had none. There was no evidence of a formal thought disorder or the other psychotic symptoms frequently seen in schizophrenia. Furthermore, she had no evidence of any psychotic disorder before the age of 50.

The only psychopathology that she displayed was a concrete delusional system. Such a delusional system alone does not fulfill the criteria for schizophrenia unless the delusion is extremely bizarre and accompanied by a marked decline in daily functioning. Instead, Ms. Hastings brings us to a curious collection of disorders referred to as delusional disorders. In the DSM-IV these disorders include seven types: persecutory type, jealous type, erotomanic type, somatic type, grandiose type, mixed type, and unspecified type. All seven of these disorders share the following criteria of a delusional disorder:[26]

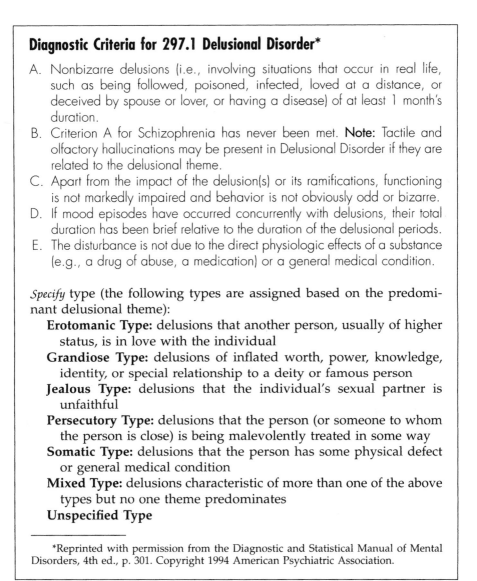

Diagnostic Criteria for 297.1 Delusional Disorder*

A. Nonbizarre delusions (i.e., involving situations that occur in real life, such as being followed, poisoned, infected, loved at a distance, or deceived by spouse or lover, or having a disease) of at least 1 month's duration.
B. Criterion A for Schizophrenia has never been met. **Note:** Tactile and olfactory hallucinations may be present in Delusional Disorder if they are related to the delusional theme.
C. Apart from the impact of the delusion(s) or its ramifications, functioning is not markedly impaired and behavior is not obviously odd or bizarre.
D. If mood episodes have occurred concurrently with delusions, their total duration has been brief relative to the duration of the delusional periods.
E. The disturbance is not due to the direct physiologic effects of a substance (e.g., a drug of abuse, a medication) or a general medical condition.

Specify type (the following types are assigned based on the predominant delusional theme):

Erotomanic Type: delusions that another person, usually of higher status, is in love with the individual

Grandiose Type: delusions of inflated worth, power, knowledge, identity, or special relationship to a deity or famous person

Jealous Type: delusions that the individual's sexual partner is unfaithful

Persecutory Type: delusions that the person (or someone to whom the person is close) is being malevolently treated in some way

Somatic Type: delusions that the person has some physical defect or general medical condition

Mixed Type: delusions characteristic of more than one of the above types but no one theme predominates

Unspecified Type

---

*Reprinted with permission from the Diagnostic and Statistical Manual of Mental Disorders, 4th ed., p. 301. Copyright 1994 American Psychiatric Association.

Ms. Hastings demonstrates many of the classic findings seen in an interview with a patient suffering from a typical delusional disorder. These patients frequently appear surprisingly normal. One would hardly suspect any psychopathology until one uncovers the topics engulfed by the delusional system, at which point, these patients often describe elaborate ramifications and subplots that would gratify the needs of any soap opera buff. Their delusions are generally unshakeable. They simply do not believe that there is anything wrong with them, as evidenced by the fact that Ms. Hastings did not seek help for herself but for the problem she was having with her husband. In the long run this striking lack of insight can make these patients frustratingly resistant to therapy.

Their delusions are frequently of a persecutory nature, but other variants exist. One such variant has been referred to as "the Othello syndrome," in which the patient becomes convinced that his or her spouse is having a sexual affair, referred to as the jealous type in DSM-IV.[27] In erotomania, sometimes referred to as Clérambault's syndrome, the patient, usually a woman, comes to believe that a man has fallen madly in love with her. She may proceed to pursue him across the country or into the bedroom. One can imagine that such patients are seldom popular with the wives of the men they so diligently pursue.

Another type of delusional disorder consists of an unshakeable belief that one has a serious medical illness, the so-called hypochondriacal paranoia or somatic type of delusional disorder. These patients differ from the person suffering from simple hypochondriasis by the fact that the belief has reached a truly delusional proportion and is essentially unshakeable. These patients may also believe that a plot has evolved to hide the truth from them.

The somatic type of delusional disorder may also present with the belief that the patient is deformed, infected, ugly, or smells badly, referred to in the literature as a monosymptomatic hypochondriacal psychosis. One of our patients was convinced that "my muscles of mastication are disordered." He had carefully produced a beautifully drawn anatomic atlas illustrating the problems with his jaw. At the interview he just happened to bring along a human skull, which he used to demonstrate in a disturbingly convincing fashion his specific anatomic defects. Sometimes these patients proceed to develop schizophrenia. If there is a preoccupation with an imagined defect in appearance, but this preoccupation is not of delusional intensity, then a diagnosis of Body Dysmorphic Disorder is made.

The term "mixed subtype" applies when no one delusional theme predominates. Unspecified Type applies when the clinician cannot determine the underlying delusional belief or is convinced that the patient's belief is fairly unique and does not fall into one of the previous categories.

Brief mention should also be made of the shared psychotic disorder. In this relatively rare condition, sometimes poetically referred to as "folie à deux," two patients share the same delusion.

One of the patients develops the delusion after the other patient has evidenced it for some time, and in this sense, the other patient is said to be induced into a delusional system. Frequently one of the patients is a dominant and powerful personality while the second patient tends to be dependent and suggestible. The second patient's delusion may even crumble if not in the presence of the dominant figure.[28]

Diagnostically, if a patient presents with a delusional disorder, it is critical to rule out a psychotic disorder due to a general medical condition. This is particularly true in patients who first develop delusional symptoms over the age of 40. There exist numerous medical illnesses that can present with delusions. Perhaps at the top of the list one should consider a brain tumor, because these tumors tend to occur in adult life. Indeed, malignant gliomas tend to arise in middle age, while metastatic tumors from other parts of the body are more common in the elderly.[29] Other frequent general medical causes include medications, endocrine disorders, infections, and temporal lobe epilepsy.

Especially with the elderly, the interviewer should also consider dementia. Roughly 20% of patients with Alzheimer's disease demonstrate paranoid symptoms at some point. Paranoid delusions tend to occur later in the process with these patients, although suspiciousness may occur early on.[30]

The issue of paranoid symptoms raises a pertinent diagnostic point. Some elderly patients present with concrete paranoid delusions frequently accompanied by auditory hallucinations and some other features common in schizophrenia, almost as if these patients were presenting with a late-onset schizophrenia.

This particular syndrome raises some problems for the DSM-IV, because these patients could technically be called schizophrenic (the DSM-III-R removed an upper age of onset limit of 45, which was present in the DSM-III for schizophrenia). But it is unclear whether these geriatric psychoses are genetically or phenomenologically the same as true schizophrenia. In the DSM-IV, if the hallucinations are not prominent, one could probably use the diagnosis delusional disorder, persecutory type. With prominent hallucinations, the diagnosis of psychotic disorder not otherwise specified could probably be used reluctantly.

I say reluctantly because such presentations are neither uncommon nor atypical as the "grab-bag" diagnosis of psychotic disorder not otherwise specified suggests. One study revealed that at least 10% of patients who were admitted with psychotic features over the age of 60 presented as described above. It is here that European psychiatry may be able to offer some clarification. In Europe this type of presentation is frequently viewed as a separate diagnosis called paraphrenia.[31, 32]

Paraphrenia typically presents in late life with well-organized paranoid delusions associated with hallucinations. In more severe illness the delusions may also become grandiose. Before these overt psychotic symptoms appear, the patient may show prodromal symptoms for months or even years. These symptoms include suspiciousness, irritability, seclusiveness, and odd behavior. Unlike patients with schizophrenia these patients, even when grossly psychotic, do not usually show problems with peculiar affect or demonstrate a formal thought disorder. They also tend to respond reasonably well to antipsychotic medications.

An unusual associated finding is the fact that about 15 to 40% of these patients have some degree of hearing loss. It has been suggested that a hearing loss may predispose the patient to misinterpret the conversation of others in such a way as to create paranoid ideation. The clinician should be on the look-out for this syndrome while interviewing the elderly. The diagnosis of paraphrenia may be included in future editions of the DSM.

For a moment let us review the diagnostic issues associated with Ms. Hastings. In this particular interview there was little time to explore for personality disorders, and the clinician would need to defer on this axis. She complained of peptic ulcer disease, chronic bronchitis, and the recent onset of a hacking cough associated with a long history of heavy smoking. With such a history of smoking the issue of lung cancer is certainly worth considering. Her diagnostic formulation would appear as follows:

Axis I: Delusional disorder (persecutory type) 297.1
Rule out Psychotic disorder due to a general medical condition 293.81
Axis II: Defer 799.90
Axis III: Peptic ulcer disease
Chronic bronchitis
Rule out lung carcinoma

On Axis III, as mentioned earlier, numerous entities should be ruled out; however, for the sake of conciseness, it is probably more practical to only list those diagnoses for which the initial interview has raised some specific suspicions, as with the cigarette smoking history suggesting lung cancer in the case of Ms. Hastings.

Let us review the major issues that surfaced with the case of Ms. Hastings.

1. The diagnosis "delusional disorder" can be classified into seven subtypes: persecutory, jealous, erotomanic, somatic, grandiose, mixed, and unspecified type. (It should be noted, that at this time, it is not yet clear whether these subcategories will prove to have any association with etiology or treatment response.)
2. Outside of the delusional content of their speech, people with delusional disorders frequently appear and behave quite normally.
3. In any patient diagnosed as having a delusional disorder one should rule out a general medical cause (e.g., a brain tumor) of the delusional symptoms.
4. Paranoid symptoms are not uncommon with people suffering from primary degenerative dementia (Alzheimer's disease).
5. Paraphrenia, although not currently recognized as a DSM-IV diagnosis, may well represent a specific syndrome in elderly patients. It is characterized by a delusional system that is associated with hallucinations.

In the next case, we shall return to the basic definition of psychosis, because a thorough understanding of this term may have significant clinical importance as we shall see.

DISCUSSION OF MS. FAY

Ms. Fay was the 23-year-old woman who had been seen 2 weeks earlier and given a diagnosis of generalized anxiety disorder. As she had appeared at her previous interview, she currently presents with an overwhelming sense of anxiety succinctly stated by Ms. Fay as, "I'm a nervous wreck." She flatly denies any overt signs of psychosis such as delusions or hallucinations. She does not demonstrate any marked evidence of a formal thought disorder such as a gross loosening of associations. She does not appear overtly psychotic, rather she seems consumed by her own anxiety.

It is this anxiety that warrants more careful exploration, because anxiety stands as one of the most frequent early signs in a developing psychosis. To further our understanding it may be useful to review what one might call the "life cycle" of psychotic process.

In the first place, there exist certain overt signs of psychotic process, which, when present, are essentially conclusive evidence that the patient is psychotic. These hard signs of psychosis include the following: hallucinations, delusions, moderate to severe loosening of associations or other marked evidence of a formal thought disorder, gross disorganization, gross disorientation, and bizarre gesturing. In a strict diagnostic sense, unless these signs are present one does not call the patient psychotic by DSM-IV standards. This conservative approach is probably good, because it eliminates the dangerous habit of loosely labeling people as psychotic. Such sloppy clinical work can lead to problems such as the inappropriate use of the diagnosis schizophrenia when the diagnosis schizotypal personality is more appropriate.

On the other hand, in a clinical sense, a patient can be quite psychotic without demonstrating these hard signs. The reason for this phenomenon can be found in the life cycle of a psychotic process. More specifically, most patients do not abruptly develop the hard signs of psychosis, as if the light switch of reason was suddenly snapped off. Instead patients generally move more slowly into the world of madness.

An excellent example of this concept can be provided by looking at one possible mode of development of a single psychotic symptom such as a delusion. The phenomenologist Lopez-Ibor has discussed this specific process in detail[33] (Fig. 6). In the following discussion we will follow his model with some minor adjustments.

In the beginning of a psychotic break the patient frequently develops what Lopez-Ibor calls a "delusional mood." During this phase the patient begins to feel that something is not quite right. There may be an intensification of perceptions such as sight and sound. In a sense, the world is almost clearer than before, because the environment appears more vivid. New details never before recognized take on new significance, for they may never have even been noticed before. There frequently exists an unsettling feeling that something ominous may be about to happen, although at other times life may seem refreshingly vibrant. The following excerpt captures this peculiar state of affairs:

*I*f I am to judge by my own experience, this "heightened state of reality" consists of a considerable number of related sensations, the net result of which is that the outer world makes a much more vivid and intense impression on me than usual. . . . The first thing I note is the peculiar appearance of the lights. . . . They are not exactly brighter, but deeper, more intense, perhaps a trifle more ruddy than usual. Certainly my sense of touch is heightened. . . . My hearing appears to be more sensitive, and I am able to take in without disturbance or distraction many different sound impressions at the same time.[34]

Eventually this process becomes more intense, developing a second phase, which can be called "delusional perception," a term clarified by the phenomenologist Kurt Schneider. With delusional perception, the perception itself may be normal in a sensory sense, but the patient's interpretation of the perception is clearly distorted. The anxiety of the patient begins to snowball, as the patient becomes convinced that something is not right and that danger is present. In this phase, not only is the environment noticed in a more intense

LIFE CYCLE OF A DELUSION

delusional mood ⟶ delusional perception ⟶ concrete delusion

___

POSSIBLE INDICATORS OF PSYCHOTIC PROCESS

A) SOFT SIGNS

↓

Suggestive of Psychosis

↓

Can be caused by a variety
of non-psychotic processes

B) HARD SIGNS

↓

Conclusive for Psychosis

___

HARD AND SOFT SIGNS OF PSYCHOSIS

SOFTS SIGNS

unusually intense affect

angry or agitated affect

glimpses of inappropriate affect

guardedness or suspiciousness

vagueness

evidence of a very mild formal
thought disorder

pre-occupation with an incident
from distant past

expectation of familiarity
from interviewer

inappropriate eye contact

long latency before responding
or thought blocking

HARD SIGNS

delusions

hallucinations

moderate or severe formal
thought disorder

gross disorientation

bizarre mannerisms and
body language

Figure 6

Life cycle of a psychotic process.

fashion, but also the details of the environment are felt to be directly related to the patient. The world becomes at once both highly personalized and terrifying. Ideas of reference occur. In a sense, patients feel that people are talking about them but do not yet know why.

*N*ot knowing that I was ill, I made no attempt to understand what was happening, but felt that there was some overwhelming significance in all this, produced either by God or Satan. . . . The walk of a stranger on the street could be a "sign" to me which I must interpret. Every face in the windows of a passing streetcar could be engraved on my mind, all of them concentrating on me and trying to pass me some sort of message.[35]

At this point the patient may already be showing marked changes in daily functioning, avoiding this person or that person, meticulously checking on people's behaviors, staying awake at night, and ruminating endlessly. In a very real sense of the word, these patients are already psychotic, because their perception of reality is markedly different than the reality of those around them. No hard signs of psychosis in a diagnostic sense have appeared yet, but they are just around the corner.

In the third phase, the phase of "delusional ideas," the slippery suspicions of the first two phases are transformed into concrete beliefs. Patients suddenly know what people are saying about them and why. The paranoid feelings become concrete delusions that are both more elaborate and entrenched. Here, indeed, the classic hard signs of psychosis flower. In a sense, as Clérambault stated, the psychosis is already old when the delusions have begun.

As mentioned earlier, psychotic process tends to fluctuate, and patients may move in and out of these various phases. For these reasons, the initial interviewer needs to pay keen attention to any evidence that the patient may be in one of the less obvious phases of psychosis. If such soft signs of covert psychosis are present, then the interviewer more carefully explores for the harder signs. These soft signs of psychosis are frequently overlooked by clinicians, as was the case with Ms. Fay during her first visit to the evaluation center. For this reason they shall be examined in more detail.

In the first place it is important to emphasize that the presence of the soft signs of psychosis does not imply that the patient is necessarily psychotic. Rather, their appearance suggests that psychotic process may be present and the clinician should thoroughly hunt for it. There exist many other nonpsychotic etiologies for the soft signs of psychosis, such as anxiety, an immature interpersonal style, or somewhat idiosyncratic interpersonal habits. For instance, a mild and infrequent loosening of associations, one of the soft signs, does not necessarily indicate that a patient is actively psychotic. Schizotypal personalities may routinely demonstrate this finding, in which case it represents an ingrained personality style, not evidence of psychosis (Fig. 6).

There exist a variety of soft signs of psychosis, including the following: (1) mild or infrequent evidence of a formal thought disorder, such as a mild loosening of associations, infrequent bits of illogical thought, idiosyncratic speech, or mild to moderate tangential speech, (2) unusually intense affect, (3) angry or agitated affect, (4) infrequent glimpses of inappropriate affect, (5) guardedness or suspiciousness, (6) vagueness, (7) preoccupation with an incident from the distant past, (8) immediate discussion of personal details as if the interviewer already knew the patient well, (9) long latency before answering questions, (10) poor eye contact in a patient who does not appear depressed, and (11) inappropriate staring. The list could certainly be made longer, but the above signs serve as a good introduction. Note that both verbal and nonverbal clues may suggest underlying psychotic process (see Fig. 6).

When a clinician notices some of the soft signs of psychosis, the clinician may want to expand the region of psychotic questioning in more detail, delicately probing for the hard signs of psychosis, such as evidence of delusions and hallucinations. The belief that psychotic patients will always spontaneously reveal their hallucinations and delusions is patently false. Frequently, one must ask for specific symptoms before they are proffered.

A few other points are worth mentioning. If the patient appears unusually affectively charged about a particular topic, it is often rewarding to gently guide the patient into a further discussion of this topic by showing interest and asking clarifying questions. With this technique one structures very little. Instead, an attempt is made to unleash further affect, because as the patient becomes more and more involved, defenses may decrease, allowing more dramatic evidence of psychotic process to emerge. Eventually, as the patient senses a friendly ear, delusional material may be shared. It is not infrequent for interviewers to simply run-over these areas of intense affect, thus robbing themselves of a natural gate into the patient's psychotic world.

In a similar vein, when a patient uses an illogical or idiosyncratic phrase, it is often wise to ask for further elaboration. It is paramount that this request for clarification sound nonjudgmental and carry a tone of true interest. As the patient proceeds to explain the ideas behind the reasoning, it is not infrequent for further and more substantial evidence of psychotic process to emerge. The psychotic patient essentially guides the interviewer into regions of questioning more likely to unearth substantial evidence of psychosis.

At this point we can return to Ms. Fay, because an excerpt of her initial interview proves to be germane. In it we shall see some of the soft signs of psychosis; in particular the interviewer will follow up on an isolated piece of illogical thought.

> **Clin.:** Tell me a little bit more about what your anxiety has been like.
>
> **Pt.:** (giggles inappropriately) That's very hard to say ... I get uptight and I just don't know what to do with myself. I suppose it all has to do with self-image and all that stuff.
>
> **Clin.:** How do you mean?
>
> **Pt.:** Sometimes when I'm alone I just get really frightened and ... I don't know ... well, I ... I don't know if I'm coming or going. I guess I'm just too anxious to be a woman. I don't know what else to say. What else do you want me to talk about?
>
> **Clin.:** When you say that you are too anxious to be a woman, what exactly are you referring to?
>
> **Pt.:** I get panicky, you know all goose flesh all over. I never know exactly when it is going to happen but it always does.
>
> **Clin.:** But how does that tie in with your being a woman?
>
> **Pt.:** It just does. Women have to do certain things and I'm unclear what exactly they are. It was all so much simpler years ago when my mother was growing up. But today what with short skirts and rock videos, it is all more confusing and there is a lot more responsibility out there, so I'm just too anxious to be a woman and I'm also too anxious to be a man, so there you have it!

The phrase "I'm just too anxious to be a woman," is a curious one. The patient did not appear cognizant of this fact and made no spontaneous attempt to explain herself. At which point the clinician wisely asked for further clarification. Her subsequent explanation was also vague, although one can surmise to what she was probably alluding. Her subsequent reply was also somewhat illogical, giving even further suspicion that a psychotic process was at hand.

As the interview progressed she appeared to become more anxious, but she never displayed or related any hard signs of psychosis. Of course, during the interview she did display a variety of soft signs, including vagueness, guardedness, a few inappropriate giggles, some small bits of illogical thought, and the hint of a preoccupation with a distant past sexual event with her brother.

She described a variety of sustained symptoms of generalized anxiety, while denying any regularly occurring panic attacks. She also described periods of fleeting paranoia and magical thinking, but said she had always had such feelings " 'cause I grew up in a bad family." She denied any persistent symptoms of depression or mania. But she did describe episodes of angry outbursts and periods of being very moody. She was evasive when questioned about previous suicide gestures.

Ms. Fay represents an excellent example of a person who leaves the interviewer with the feeling that psychotic process is lurking beneath the clinical facade but cannot be clearly identified. Because of the presence of a large number of soft psychotic symptoms, the clinician would tend to arrange for both rapid and close follow-up care.

At the end of this interview her diagnostic conceptualization was as follows:

Axis I: Generalized anxiety disorder (provisional) 300.02
            Rule out psychotic disorder not otherwise specified
Axis II: Rule out schizotypal personality
            Rule out borderline personality disorder
Axis III: Defer

The diagnosis of psychotic disorder not otherwise specified (atypical psychosis) was employed because there were no strong indicators of an affective illness nor clear-cut signs of schizophrenia or paranoid disorder, but the clinician was suspicious of some underlying psychotic process.

This suspicion proved to be well founded, because several weeks later Ms. Fay was admitted to the hospital with several striking paranoid delusions concerning her brother accompanied by many of the symptoms of mania. Apparently the clinician had caught her at a time when she was actively psychotic but had not yet developed the hard signs of psychosis. He had in essence seen her before the storm erupted, during the phase of delusional mood or delusional perception. Or she may have actually already had delusional ideas that she was not yet ready to share. Figure 7 summarizes the inter-relationships among the stages of the life cycle of a psychosis and the appearance of soft and hard signs of psychotic process. It also re-emphasizes the point that psychotic phenomena tend to fluctuate.

Figure **7**

Evolution of a psychosis.

Later interviews with Ms. Fay and with her family revealed a history of intermittent affective instability with both manic and depressed features. Her psychotic symptoms appeared early on in the process. It was unclear exactly which appeared first, affective symptoms or psychotic symptoms. Consequently, her Axis I diagnosis was changed to schizoaffective disorder rule out bipolar disorder. Further observation and history would eventually determine whether she was experiencing a true bipolar disorder or not.

Fortunately, Ms. Fay eventually stabilized upon a combined treatment of lithium and Haldol (haloperidol). Even during periods of stability, she continued to appear very manipulative. She also continued to have significant problems with anger and impulsive control. Her parents related these symptoms were lifelong in nature, lending further support to the idea that Ms. Fay might also have some severe characterologic problems such as a borderline personality disorder.

Ms. Fay serves as an example of an intriguing study in the subtle signs of psychotic process and the need for the initial interviewer to constantly seek out the soft signs of psychosis. At times such a dedicated diligence, associated with prompt subsequent treatment, may help prevent the patient from suffering the full-blown wrath of a psychotic illness.

Before leaving her case it is worth summarizing some of the major points it highlights.

1. A person may be psychotic in a clinical sense without demonstrating the hard signs of psychosis such as delusions or hallucinations.

2. The so-called soft signs of psychosis should always alert the clinician to the possibility of a smoldering psychotic process.
3. In the life cycle of a psychosis, hard signs of psychosis generally do not erupt without a prodromal phase of psychosis in which the patient's experience of reality is clearly abnormal but only the soft signs of psychosis are apparent.
4. Generally it is best to follow up on areas of intense affect because such areas may be outward manifestations of delusional material.
5. If the patient uses an illogical or idiosyncratic phrase, it is often useful to ask for clarification. In the process of clarifying, the patient may reveal further evidence of psychotic process.
6. A patient may have a severe psychotic illness on Axis I, such as schizophrenia, and still have a personality disorder on Axis II.

We can now leave the outpatient assessment clinic and return to the emergency room where Mr. Lawrence was hauled in by the police and a crisis worker. Mr. Lawrence was apparently suffering from an acute exacerbation of his chronic schizophrenia.

DISCUSSION OF MR. LAWRENCE
At first Mr. Lawrence presented in an agitated and violent manner. At one point he literally threatened to beat one of the nurses, and he subsequently tried to do so, eventually requiring restraints. There was a suspicion that somehow the nurse had been incorporated into a delusion, although the patient denied the typical delusions he had demonstrated in the past.

By the time I had arrived on the scene I was surprised to find that Mr. Lawrence was laying calmly on a cart and appeared quite cooperative. He denied any hard signs of psychosis and also denied any recent suicidal gestures, although he commented that he had been thinking of killing himself several days earlier. Eventually we were able to remove the restraints, at which point Mr. Lawrence took a peculiar turn in his clinical course.

He related that he needed to go to the bathroom. As he walked towards the toilet he appeared to stagger a bit. Once he reached his destination, he looked about as if plopped into an unfamiliar space and asked, "What am I doing in here?" When told that he had wanted to go to the bathroom, he appeared puzzled and denied ever making such a request.

As the interview proceeded Mr. Lawrence began to appear drowsy, which he attributed to being up all night as well as drinking heavily. He could only repeat three or four digits forwards, whereas he had been able to repeat seven forwards earlier. He also began clutching at some invisible objects near his feet.

If at this point Mr. Lawrence is beginning to sound similar to our first patient, Mr. Williams, who presented with DTs, it is because Mr. Lawrence is also suffering from a delirium, a delirium that would eventually threaten his life. The interview was promptly stopped at this point. An electrocardiogram (ECG) revealed some subtle abnormalities. Roughly 30 minutes later Mr. Lawrence stopped breathing. Fortunately, his life was saved through the effective use of an artificial respirator.

In retrospect, the correct diagnosis was a tricyclic overdose leading to a paradoxic rage response. This rage was followed by a delirium. His case provides a springboard into a discussion of several important points. In the first place, it is important to note that it was assumed initially that Mr. Lawrence was merely experiencing an exacerbation of his paranoid schizophrenia, because he had frequently presented with violence in the past. Therein lies one of the more dangerous clinical traps when dealing with a patient who has been labeled with a chronic psychotic process. It is both easy and natural to assume that the old etiologic agent is at work without vigorously searching for a new one.

A useful point to remember concerns the idea that psychotic processes caused by a single etiology, such as schizophrenia, frequently present in a relatively similar fashion during each episode for a given individual. The soft signs, or early warning signs, are frequently similar from episode to episode, as are the subsequent hard signs. The psychotic process tends to leave an identifying fingerprint of sorts with each patient. Consequently, in any patient in which a new episode of psychosis appears distinctly different than in previous episodes, the clinician should become suspicious that something new has been added to the picture etiologically. In the case of Mr. Lawrence, he usually presented with delusions and hallucinations. In this case neither symptom was present. This is one area in which previous hospital charts can be useful, providing a history of the patient's past episodes.

The second major point has been stated earlier but certainly warrants repeating. Any patient presenting with a delirium requires an immediate medical evaluation. This represents a clinical situation that frequently faces the crisis worker and for which the crisis worker must constantly be on the look-out. It is critical for all initial evaluators to become adept at recognizing the clinical presentation of a delirium. With knowledge and common sense it is not necessarily difficult to recognize, yet this diagnosis is frequently missed, often by physicians themselves.

We can begin our exploration of the presentation of a delirium by reviewing the DSM-IV criteria, which appear below:[36]

Diagnostic Criteria for 293.0 Delirium Due to . . . (Indicate the General Medical Condition)*

A. Disturbance of consciousness (i.e., reduced clarity of awareness of the environment) with reduced ability to focus, sustain, or shift attention.
B. A change in cognition (such as memory deficit, disorientation, language disturbance) or the development of a perceptual disturbance that is not better accounted for by a pre-existing, established, or evolving dementia.
C. The disturbance develops over a short period of time (usually hours to days) and tends to fluctuate during the course of the day.
D. There is evidence from the history, physical examination, or laboratory findings that the disturbance is caused by the direct physiologic consequences of a general medical condition.

Coding note: If delirium is superimposed on a pre-existing Dementia of the Alzheimer's Type or Vascular Dementia, indicate the delirium by coding the appropriate subtype of the dementia, e.g., 290.3 Dementia of the Alzheimer's Type, With Late Onset, With Delirium.

Coding note: Include the name of the general medical condition on Axis I, e.g., 293.0 Delirium Due to Hepatic Encephalopathy; also code the general medical condition on Axis III (see Appendix G for codes).

---

*Reprinted with permission from the Diagnostic and Statistical Manual of Mental Disorders, 4th ed., p. 129. Copyright 1994 American Psychiatric Association.

It is important to note that not all delirious patients are disoriented.[37, 38] Generally these patients develop disorientation, but at times, especially in the early stages of the process, they may be completely oriented. In this sense, deliria can present in a variety of fashions, which is part of the reason why they can be misdiagnosed.

The following guidelines provide a practical platform for clinical assessment. In the first place a delirium occurs when there exists a rather diffuse pathophysiologic dysfunction in the brain. Such a diffuse dysfunction will frequently show itself in one of two ways—a fluctuating level of consciousness or a marked problem with attending to the environment. These two processes represent the keynotes that should alert the clinician to the possibility of a delirium. Indeed, if either of these processes appears in a patient demonstrating the soft or hard signs of psychosis, then one should strongly consider a delirium work-up.

It therefore becomes critical to evaluate these two points during the initial interview of any psychotic patient. Unfortunately, it is easy to overlook their significance if the patient is agitated, as was the case with Mr. Lawrence. Let us begin with the evaluation of the level of consciousness.

People with a delirium tend to present in one of three ways: (1) hypoactive, (2) hyperactive, or (3) a mixed picture of the previous two states. In the hypoactive state, which represents the most common state, the patient may appear drowsy or may literally be hard to arouse. This type of "quiet delirium" is common in geriatric patients. Their somnolent behavior does not bother anyone, and consequently their condition may be overlooked. In the hyperactive state the patient is "wired." The patient appears unusually responsive to any stimulation from the environment and tends to appear driven. This is sometimes accompanied by marked agitation or aggression. We saw this presentation earlier with Mr. Williams, the man suffering from DTs. Finally, patients may present with a mixture. One of the hallmarks of the delirious patient is the tendency for the level of consciousness to fluctuate. This fluctuation may be so extreme as to move the patient back and forth between hypoactive and hyperactive states.

If one is actively looking for changes in the level of consciousness, they are not hard to spot. But in a busy clinical situation the trick is to be aware of their importance. A problem arises in the fact that patients tend to move in and out of delirious states relatively quickly. An alert nurse may note a brief episode of delirium that will simply not be present during clinical rounds the following morning. A frequent physician error is to assume that if the patient looks good on rounds, then, "What's the fuss?" Unfortunately such a patient may be developing permanent brain damage during the periods of delirium. Consequently, this type of patient needs a medical work-up despite a good appearance during rounds.

In association with the tendency for the delirious patient to demonstrate a fluctuating level of consciousness, this phenomenon is usually paralleled by changes in the electroencephalogram (EEG).[39] In the hypoactive state, the EEG usually demonstrates a generalized diffuse slowing of the background activity. During the hyperactive state, fast activity is often seen. At times a normal EEG may be found.

With regard to determining whether or not the patient is having trouble attending to the environment, the task becomes more difficult. The difficulty lies in the fact that subtle problems with attention and concentration may not be apparent unless tested. At times the clinician may be able to determine that concentration is reasonably good, by noting the patient's ability to converse in a natural and intelligent fashion. At other times more formal testing is required, especially if the evaluator is truly suspicious of the presence of a delirium.

Four tests come to mind, which as a battery will generally pick up any significant problems with attending to the environment. These four tests are digit spans forwards and backwards, the vigilance test, constructions, and an examination of the patient's handwriting.

In the digit span test, one asks the patient to repeat a series of digits. The clinician begins with two digits and continues in successive steps to seven digits if the patient proceeds to answer correctly. It is important to say the digits in a steady rhythm. If said like a telephone number, the patient may find them artificially easy to remember. This test can then be done by giving a series of digits and asking the patient to repeat them backwards. With the digit span one should expect an average adult to be able to repeat about seven digits forwards and four to five digits backwards.

In the vigilance test, the clinician recites a string of letters from the alphabet. The patient is asked to make a hand tap on the table every time the letter "A" is said. If the patient is experiencing problems attending to the environment, both errors of omission and commission will tend to occur. A normal adult should make few if any errors. As the series continues, some delirious patients will even forget what letter they are hunting for.

The patient may also be asked to make copies of constructions, such as a cross or a cube. Once again the delirious patient may find such a task difficult. Finally, problems with writing (dysgraphia) are common and include spelling errors, clumsily drawn letters, reduplication of strokes in letters such as "M" or "N," and problems with alignment and linguistics.[40]

These four tests represent an excellent screen for deficits in attending abilities, but one may have difficulty using them with a hostile patient. Not too many hostile patients are eager to demonstrate their artistic abilities or play word games. When these tests may be inappropriate, one can learn a great deal by carefully observing the patient. The delirious patient may demonstrate attention difficulties through an inability to follow commands, a problem remembering questions, a tendency to appear overly sensitive to noises and other outside stimuli, or simply an appearance of confusion, as was the case with Mr. Lawrence in the bathroom. The trick is in remembering to look for these processes on a routine basis when encountering a psychotic patient.

Thus far the focus has been on the two key characteristics of a delirium. It may be valuable to review a few of the more common clinical characteristics.[41, 42]

1. Hallucinations or illusions have been estimated to occur in 40 to 75% of delirious patients. Visual and auditory hallucinations are

frequent, and the presence of visual hallucinations should always arouse suspicion of a delirious or organic state.
2. Rapidly changing delusions, especially of a paranoid nature, are common. These delusions tend to be of a much more fleeting and malleable nature than the delusions seen in schizophrenia or one of the paranoid disorders.
3. Other problems with a formal thought disorder such as a loosening of associations or illogical thought may appear.
4. Short-term memory and orientation are frequently impaired.
5. Deliria tend to fluctuate. In particular, patients tend to be more disoriented and delirious at night, a process that has been referred to as "sundowning."
6. Deliria tend to emerge in a matter of hours or days, but this is not always the case. Insidious onsets can occur.
7. Although deliria are generally believed to be related to organic etiologies, it is believed that stress and psychological mechanisms can lead to a delirious presentation in some instances.
8. Affect is typically abnormal, with a high incidence of emotions such as fear and anxiety.
9. A characteristic phenomenon is the tendency for the patient to misidentify the unfamiliar as familiar. For instance, a nurse's aide may be identified as a brother or sister.

A variety of other odd behaviors have been reported during deliria, ranging from wandering aimlessly about the hospital to drinking copiously from the toilet. A particularly peculiar process has been reported in which the patient continues habitual behaviors in totally inappropriate places. For instance, in an "occupational delirium," patients perform behaviors in the hospital that are normally only done at their place of work. The term "carphology" has been coined for the behavior of picking at one's bedclothes, another abnormal behavior sometimes seen in deliria.

With regard to etiology the list is extensive. In Table 3 a practical list of common causes is presented. It is beyond the scope of this book to elaborate on the medical differential and on the appropriate laboratory and physical examination. The first and crucial step remains the uncovering of the delirium during the interview itself.

In a practical sense, interviewers must train themselves to rule out delirium any time a patient presents with a psychosis. Unless this active process of viewing delirium as a part of the differential becomes a clinical habit, one runs the risk of missing it. The patient is the one who pays for such an error, and the cost may be permanent brain damage or worse.

At this point let us summarize the DSM-IV diagnosis on Mr. Lawrence.

≡ TABLE 3	COMMON CAUSES OF DELIRIUM

Metabolic

1. Hypoxia, hypercarbia, anemia
2. Electrolyte imbalance, hyperosmolarity
3. Hyperglycemia or hypoglycemia
4. Abnormal levels of magnesium or calcium
5. End-stage liver or kidney disease
6. Vitamin B_1 deficiency (Wernicke's encephalopathy secondary to a thiamine deficiency)
7. Endocrine disorders (hyperthyroidism or hypothyroidism, hyperparathyroidism, and adrenal disorders)

Infections

1. Systemic (e.g., pneumonia, septicemia, malaria, and typhoid)
2. Intracranial (e.g., meningitis, encephalitis)

Neurologic Disorders

1. Hypertensive crisis, stroke, subarachnoid hemorrhage, vasculitis
2. Seizures
3. Trauma

Drug Withdrawal

1. Alcohol hallucinosis, rum fits, delirium tremens
2. Other withdrawal states (e.g., from barbiturates, as well as acute intoxication with street drugs)

Intoxication

1. From agents such as digoxin, levodopa, anticholinergics, and street drugs

Postoperative Sequelae

1. Especially following cardiac surgery

Axis I: Substance-Induced Delirium (overdose on antidepressant) 292.81
Paranoid schizophrenia in remission 295.35
Axis II: None V71.09
Axis III: Respiratory arrest secondary to overdose

Major points worth reviewing include the following:

1. Psychoses such as those seen with schizophrenia or bipolar disorder often present in a similar fashion from episode to episode.
2. If a patient's psychotic presentation seems different than is typical from previous episodes, then the clinician should strongly consider the possibility of a new etiologic agent.
3. The presence of a delirium always warrants an aggressive medical evaluation and can easily be missed in chronic patients.
4. The clinician should always consciously look for evidence of a

fluctuating level of consciousness or a significant problem with attending to the environment in all psychotic patients, because these two characteristics are tip-offs that a delirium may be present.

At this point we shall look at a clinical case in which the outcome was unfortunately not as good as with Mr. Lawrence.

DISCUSSION OF KATE

Kate was the 14-year-old who had been depressed and was acting oddly. Her most bizarre behavior consisted of appearing at her parents' bedroom door topless. At several emergency rooms she had been diagnosed as hysterical and in need of outpatient psychiatric care.

During the interview it was easy to see why hysterical traits had been reported. She seemed preoccupied, as if pulled into an autistic cocoon. At one point she turned, and while looking me dead in the eye she dramatically said, "Tell me Doctor, what is reality?" She denied hallucinations, delusions, and other hard signs of psychosis. Her speech was halting and was interspersed with inappropriate giggles. At times she displayed thought blocking and seemed distracted. She was completely oriented, demonstrated an alert and stable consciousness, and when pressed, displayed no marked problems with attending to the environment, although her method of handling the conversation suggested that she might prove to have some problems in this area.

Her numerous soft signs suggested that a psychotic process was present, and she was hospitalized. Her physical examination was normal, and we were suspicious of drug abuse. Approximately 1 week after her admission, she lay dying in the intensive care unit. Her diagnosis was viral encephalitis. Her admission bloodwork had revealed evidence of an infection, and a subsequent spinal tap revealed evidence of central nervous system involvement.

Diagnostically speaking, Kate did not present with a delirium. Not all general medical causes of psychosis manifest as a delirium. While looking over the spectrum of general medical etiologies of psychotic process outlined in Table 4,[43] it is important to remember that a psychosis secondary to a general medical condition like encephalitis can present in a fashion suggestive of essentially any classic psychosis, such as schizophrenia or bipolar disorder. Frequently, delirium is not a part of the picture. This point once again emphasizes the need to "think organic" when evaluating a patient presenting with the onset of psychotic symptoms.

More important, in the emergency room, and even in the private office, one of the critical triage decisions involves ruling out a life-

≡ TABLE 4	ORGANIC CAUSES OF PSYCHOSIS*

Space-Occupying Lesions of the CNS

Brain abscess (bacterial, fungal, tuberculosis, cysticercosis)
Metastatic carcinoma
Primary cerebral tumors
Subdural hematoma

Cerebral Hypoxia

Anemia
Lowered cardiac output
Pulmonary insufficiency
Toxic (e.g., carbon monoxide)

Neurologic Disorders

Alzheimer's disease
Distant effects of carcinoma
Huntington's chorea
Normal pressure hydrocephalus
Temporal lobe epilepsy
Wilson's disease

Vascular Disorders

Aneurysms
Collagen vascular disease
Hypertensive encephalopathy
Intracranial hemorrhage
Lacunar state

Infections

Brain abscess
Encephalitis and postencephalitic states
Malaria
Meningitis (bacterial, fungal, tuberculosis)
Subacute bacterial endocarditis
Syphilis
Toxoplasmosis
Typhoid

Metabolic and Endocrine Disorders

Adrenal disease (Addison's and Cushing's disease)
Calcium-related disorders
Diabetes mellitus
Electrolyte imbalance
Hepatic failure
Homocystinuria
Hypoglycemia and hyperglycemia
Pituitary insufficiency
Porphyria
Thyroid disease (thyrotoxicosis and myxedema)
Uremia

Nutritional Deficiencies

B_{12}
Niacin (pellagra)
Thiamine (Wernicke-Korsakoff syndrome)

Drugs, Medications, and Toxic Substances

Alcohol (intoxication and withdrawal)
Amphetamines
Analgesics (e.g., pentazocine [Talwin], meperidine [Demerol])
Anticholinergic agents
Antiparkinsonian agents
Barbiturates and other sedative-hypnotic agents (intoxication and withdrawal)
Bromides and other heavy metals
Carbon disulfide
Cocaine
Corticosteroids
Cycloserine (Seromycin)
Digitalis (Crystodigin)
Disulfiram (Antabuse)
Hallucinogens
Isoniazid
L-Dopa (e.g., Larodopa)
Marijuana
Propranolol
Reserpine (Serpasil and others)

*Adapted from Bassuk, E. F., and Beck, A. W. (eds.): *Emergency Psychiatry.* New York, Plenum Press, 1984.
    CNS = central nervous system.

threatening cause of psychosis. The most common life-threatening illnesses that present with an acute psychosis include the following:[44]

1. Hypoglycemia
2. Hypertensive encephalopathy
3. Poor oxygenation (perhaps related to a heart attack, pulmonary embolus, anemia, or a hemorrhage)
4. Infections such as encephalitis or meningitis
5. Drugs, including medications, street drugs, withdrawal states, industrial toxins, and actual poisons
6. Intracranial trauma (including hemorrhage, actual trauma related to head injury, and other causes of increased intracranial pressure)
7. Wernicke's encephalopathy (not generally life threatening but should be viewed as a medical emergency, because if untreated, permanent brain damage can occur)

Other serious entities to keep in mind include hepatic failure, uremia, subacute bacterial endocarditis, and a chronic subdural hematoma. Fortunately, this list does not represent a particularly extensive differential. If the clinician remembers to think of these entities, they are generally easy to rule out—but that is an important "if." In actuality, these entities are rare enough as causes of acute psychotic process that they are likely to be overlooked, unless clinicians train themselves to consistently consider them.

A brief, well-directed physical examination should uncover many of the life-threatening processes mentioned above. In fact, a patient presenting with the onset of new psychotic symptoms should seldom, if ever, leave an emergency room without a screening physical examination.

This examination can be performed quickly and is geared towards uncovering evidence of a life-threatening dysfunction. To this end, it focuses on the following five areas: (1) vital signs, (2) autonomic system dysfunction, (3) heart and lung dysfunction, (4) neurologic dysfunction and head trauma, and (5) abnormalities of the eyes.

Abnormal vital signs should be retaken. If they remain abnormal, an etiology for the dysfunction should be sought. Keep in mind that the pulse may be naturally elevated in an agitated patient, but agitation alone seldom causes pulses over 120 to 130.

Autonomic dysfunction is frequently present during a life-threatening illness. Agents such as the anticholinergic medications mentioned earlier frequently cause the patient to present with hyperthermia, blurred vision, dry skin, facial flushing, and delirium. The mnemonic "hot as a pepper, blind as a bat, dry as a bone, red as a beet, and mad as a Hatter" has been used to describe this toxic state.

A note of caution should be added, because the anticholinergic syndrome is often incomplete, or it may be hidden by other active agents such as opiates. For instance, Mr. Lawrence, who overdosed on Elavil, an antidepressant with many anticholinergic properties, presented with an increased pulse and a dry mouth, but his pupils were normal in size and reactive. His skin color was pale, not flushed, as would be expected in a classic anticholinergic syndrome.

This discussion also emphasizes the usefulness of looking at the patient's eyes. The clinician should look for abnormal size or responsiveness of the pupils as well as asymmetry. Horizontal and vertical nystagmus should be sought. The eye grounds may reveal evidence of increased intracranial pressure.

Neurologically, one scans for evidence of focal weakness and changes in reflexes. Reflexes, including the suck reflex, snout reflex, palmomental reflex, and the Babinski sign, can be quickly screened. The clinician should check for signs of neck rigidity as well as for hemotympanum of the ears or other signs of a small skull fracture.

Finally, the clinician should listen to the heart and lungs if an abnormality of the cardiovascular or respiratory system is suspected.

A screening physical examination as described earlier can quickly flush out a serious physical condition, sometimes even in the early stages. A common error in this regard is to admit an extremely agitated patient directly to a seclusion room and subsequently fail to perform a follow-up physical examination when the patient has calmed down. Once the patient has calmed, the physician should attempt a screening examination no matter how late it is at night. If Mr. Lawrence had been sent to a seclusion room to calm down and a follow-up physical examination had not been performed, he could easily have died. At times when one is strongly suspicious of the presence of a serious illness, the patient may need to be physically restrained to allow for examination.

At this point we can return to Kate in an effort to summarize her DSM-IV diagnosis. At the time of her admission, before any lab work had returned, her differential may have looked as follows:

Axis I: Psychotic disorder Not Otherwise Specified (provisional) 298.9
Rule out (1) Unknown substance-related disorder 292.9, (2) Unknown substance-induced mood disorder (depressed) 292.84, (3) Major depressive disorder (single episode with psychotic features) 296.24

Axis II: Defer 799.9

Axis III: Rule out general medical causes of psychosis

Before leaving the topic of Kate's presentation, it may be of value to summarize some key points.

1. A delirium is not the only way in which a medical illness may manifest as a psychosis. Diseases such as encephalitis frequently mimic processes such as schizophrenia.
2. The clinician should routinely consider the various life-threatening illnesses when evaluating a patient who is psychotic.
3. A screening physical examination should be performed on any patient presenting with psychotic features.
4. The absence of all the typical signs of the anticholinergic syndrome does not rule out this syndrome, because it may present with only some of the physical signs.

Let us now move on to our final case presentation, because Miss Flagstone represents an anomaly among our other cases. She is not acutely psychotic.

DISCUSSION OF MS. FLAGSTONE

The reader will recall that Ms. Flagstone was the woman in her mid-30s who presented with a dramatic flair and a long cigarette in hand. She related that several years earlier she had heard the voice of the angel Gabriel proclaim her with child. Upon further interviewing, the entire episode seemed to last roughly 15 to 30 minutes; moreover, the voice of the angel was loud and distinct. At one point the voice actually conversed with the voice of God. Apparently, near the time of this episode, Ms. Flagstone had been fired from a job and had also been feeling "slightly paranoid near my co-workers."

She also related that she undergoes periods in which she feels, "not quite myself, as if I wasn't quite real." These episodes last only for about 10 minutes and occur during times of stress. She finds these episodes very disturbing. Further interviews would reveal that no true Axis I pathology existed with regard to Ms. Flagstone, yet how does one explain the voices and the episodes of depersonalization?

The answer lies in the fact that psychotic process is not limited to Axis I. A variety of personality disorders may present with "micropsychotic episodes." These episodes tend to last from minutes to hours. At times they may extend longer, but as soon as the episodes appear to be lasting a day or longer, one should immediately begin suspecting a process on Axis I. It is much more characteristic for these events to be short-lived, as demonstrated by Ms. Flagstone, who upon further interviewing seemed to fulfill many of the criteria for a histrionic personality disorder, but this diagnosis is difficult to verify in a single hour and will require further interviewing.

Micropsychotic episodes are characteristically precipitated by stress, or they may be unleashed by drug abuse. Processes such as fleeting paranoid ideation, depersonalization, and derealization are frequently experienced. If drug abuse or stress is frequent, then both the frequency and duration of the micropsychotic episodes may increase.

Diagnostically speaking, the following personality disorders may demonstrate micropsychotic episodes: narcissistic personality, histrionic personality, paranoid personality, schizotypal personality, and the borderline personality. These phenomena are frequent companions of the last three disorders mentioned.

This case also raises the important question as to whether this episode of voices should even be viewed as psychotic. Perhaps her religious beliefs suggest that this process is a normal one. At times subcultures may assert beliefs that other cultures do not accept. For instance, in North Carolina, where I trained in medicine, it was not unusual for people to believe in "rootwork." This was a magical belief similar to the idea that one has been cursed. In this subculture, a belief in rootwork did not necessarily indicate the presence of psychosis.

To help the clinician decide whether a belief is delusional, two avenues suggest themselves. One method is to explore vigorously to what degree the reported episode is typical for the culture in mind. It is advisable to talk with friends or family. At times the clinician will discover that people holding the same belief system feel that the patient in question is "beyond this belief system." By way of example, one of my patients suffering from chronic paranoid schizophrenia and troubled by delusions of demon possession, routinely attends an Evangelical church in which her father is the minister. Despite the intensity of the Evangelical practices, such as speaking in tongues and exorcism, both the patient and her father can tell when her religiosity is becoming abnormal.

The second avenue for clarification is borne from an understanding of the life cycle of a psychotic process as discussed earlier. As had been noted, patients are frequently engulfed by psychotic process long before the hard signs of psychosis, such as delusions and hallucinations, manifest concretely. When talking with the patient, the interviewer may elicit information suggesting that soft psychotic signs were not a part of the process. If processes such as delusional mood and delusional perception are absent as was suggested by the lack of soft signs, it gives further weight to the idea that the process is cultural, not psychotic. Looked at in context of the Evangelical movement, "speaking in tongues" is a special but normal aspect of an Evangelical religious life. In contrast, if the patient were psychotic then speaking in tongues may have become a nagging preoccupation, which develops an ominous significance for the patient long after the patient leaves the church.

With regard to Ms. Flagstone, her voices and depersonalization episodes probably warrant the label of micropsychotic episodes. They are always brought on by stress, and further interviewing revealed that they tend to be preceded by mood states suggestive of the soft signs of psychosis. It should be borne in mind though that micropsychotic episodes, unlike their counterparts on Axis I, can occur fairly abruptly.

After the first interview, the differential on Ms. Flagstone looked something like the following:

> *Axis I:*   Defer–probably none 799.90
>   (Because of her tangential speech and mood shifts, an entity such as cyclothymic disorder or dysthymic disorder could be kept in mind.)
> *Axis II:* Histrionic personality disorder (provisional) 301.50
>   Rule out personality disorder not otherwise specified (mixed with histrionic, schizotypal, and borderline traits)
> *Axis III:* Rule out temporal lobe epilepsy

The Axis III diagnosis may surprise the reader, and rightfully so, because I have not yet included some pertinent information. Ms. Flagstone reports that she has become extremely interested in a variety of philosophical and religious issues. She has filled nearly 20 journals with her thoughts, none of which are psychotic. She also reports brief episodes of feeling very uncomfortable in her abdomen, a sensation that seems to move upwards into her throat area. All of these phenomena could be components of temporal lobe epilepsy, including her periods of depersonalization and her mood shifts.

Temporal lobe epilepsy is the "masquerader par excellence." It can mimic essentially any psychiatric disturbance and is particularly good at presenting as a psychotic disturbance. A query should be made for temporal lobe epilepsy in any patient presenting with psychotic symptoms.

Psychotic symptoms may emerge during the seizure itself or between seizures (the period known as the interictal phase). The seizure activity sometimes begins with a phase known as the aura, in which patients may experience a variety of odd sensations, including fear and anxiety. Patients may feel that they are experiencing a given situation for a second time (known as déjà vu), or they may have the opposite feeling that nothing is familiar (known as jamais vu). Strange and pungent odors may also be a predominant symptom. Peculiar abdominal feelings are very frequent. In some cases, these feelings are the only symptoms, and the patient is said to have "abdominal seizures."

As the seizure develops, the patient loses consciousness and usually displays various automatisms such as picking at himself or herself, wandering about, and displaying bizarre mannerisms or odd behaviors. To uncover such processes, a useful question remains, "Have you ever found yourself somewhere and you didn't know how you got there?" Two other pertinent questions are, "Have you ever had periods of losing consciousness?" and "Have your friends or family ever told you that they have seen you doing very odd things that you don't remember?"

Curiously, personality changes or psychotic-like activity may appear between seizures.[45] Ms. Flagstone reported some of the more common interictal phenomena: preoccupation with religious or moral issues, a tendency to write copiously, decreased sexual drive, intense mystical experiences, a deepening intensification of emotions, and what has been called interpersonal viscosity. This latter term refers to a tendency to want to keep talking and being near people.

It is certainly not always possible to explore all these issues during the initial interview because of time constraints. However, in later sessions, these questions should be rigorously pursued. It is an unfortunate error to label someone as having schizophrenia when the actual problem is temporal lobe epilepsy. Such a person would be robbed of the chance to benefit from a course of antiseizure medications.

At this juncture we are rapidly drawing to a close on our case discussions. It seems appropriate to summarize some of the points brought forward by the case of Ms. Flagstone.

1. Some personality disorders may present with psychotic symptoms, so-called micropsychotic episodes.
2. These micropsychotic episodes tend to extend from minutes to hours and are often triggered by stress or drugs. Paranoia, depersonalization, and derealization are common.
3. Temporal lobe epilepsy may present with psychotic symptoms, both during seizures or between seizures.
4. Consequently, questions should be asked concerning both the symptoms commonly seen during a seizure as well as the interictal personality change.

We have now concluded our survey of diagnoses that may present with psychotic symptoms. Figure 8 illustrates the rich diversity of etiologic agents that may present as a psychosis. As mentioned earlier, the word "psychosis" is not a diagnosis. The presence of psychotic symptoms forces the clinician to delineate the possible etiologic agent or diagnosis, as seen in Figure 8.

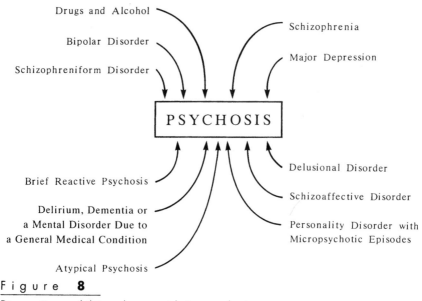

Figure **8**

Diagnostic possibilities when considering psychosis.

In order to interview effectively, we must possess a sound and flexible knowledge base concerning diagnosis. The first part of this chapter has attempted to provide just such a base. We can now turn to the equally important issue of understanding what it is like to experience a psychotic process. From such an understanding, both our interviewing skills and our abilities to empathize will undoubtedly mature. Moreover, few topics are more fascinating or puzzling.

SECTION II: UNDERSTANDING OF PSYCHOSIS

*I*n this unnerved—in this pitiable condition—I feel that the period will sooner or later arrive when I must abandon life and reason together, in some struggle with the grim phantasm, Fear.

Edgar Allan Poe
The Fall of the House of Usher

Poe aptly describes the fear and anxiety that so frequently walk hand-in-hand with the process known as psychosis. In this section we will attempt to move system by system, as we did in the previous chapter on depression, in an effort to better comprehend the intense fear associated with "going mad."

Fields of Interaction

I: PHYSIOLOGIC SYSTEM

One of the major physiologic moorings of our daily lives is the routine appearance of the phenomenon known as sleep. If one's sleep patterns are disturbed, one quickly begins to feel "not quite oneself." It appears as no surprise then that a sleep disturbance often appears early in the psychotic process.

As psychotic process begins to gain momentum, the patient often experiences severe problems falling asleep. In some instances the patient will eventually undergo a day/night reversal, in which sleep occurs during the daylight hours and the night becomes a bed of agitation. The patient may also experience other sleep disturbances, such as early morning awakening, especially if the psychosis is part of a major depression.

This difficulty with falling asleep stands as a sensitive sign of impending psychosis, frequently appearing during periods of delusional mood or delusional perception. The patient sometimes denies this sleep disturbance. Consequently, it is useful to ask family members about the patient's sleep, because they have frequently been awake themselves, coping with the growing restlessness of their relative.

Psychotic process tends to disrupt the normal control of activity levels, resulting in patient behavior ranging from agitated catatonia, in which the patient cannot stop moving, to stuporous catatonia, in which the patient shows little movement at all. It is to this peculiar state of stuporous catatonia that we shall turn our attention briefly.

At one time catatonia was generally believed to be primarily associated with schizophrenia. More recently, it has been viewed as a symptom complex that is not only seen in schizophrenia but also in affective disorders, hysterical dissociation, and in a variety of medical illnesses.[46]

Stuporous catatonia is often associated with mutism, lack of movement, negativism (as shown by a tendency to not comply with any requests), and ambitendency. This latter trait reveals itself as a hesitancy to complete behaviors, demonstrated by actions such as extending one's hand to shake and then removing it. All of these behaviors have been referred to as the "negative symptoms of catatonia." Stuporous catatonia is also associated with the so-called positive symptoms, such as the holding of bizarre postures, the senseless repetition of the clinician's words, and waxy flexibility. This latter phenomenon manifests itself as a bizarre willingness to hold one's body in any position to which it is moved.

The initial interviewer is faced with the question of how to approach a catatonic patient. It is not clear exactly what such patients are experiencing, and most likely the experience varies from one patient to another. Apparently some patients seem well aware of what is going on around them whereas others may be lost in peculiar feelings of timelessness and autism.

In the previous chapter various verbal techniques for dealing with the catatonic patient were discussed. A logical question arises as to whether one should attempt a nonverbal technique such as touching the patient. Generally speaking I believe that in an initial interview the answer is no, primarily because one simply does not know what these patients are experiencing. If delusional or actively hallucinating, the patient may perceive the clinician as attacking. Moreover, some of these patients can move almost immediately from stillness into hyperactive states.

I am reminded of one such patient who I inadvisedly touched. She was lying on the floor in an unresponsive state. We were concerned about the possibility of an overdose. When she did not respond to loud questions, I shook her shoulders. To my shock she immediately grabbed me and attempted to bite me. Apparently, drugs were not the issue.

On the other hand, in certain unusual instances the clinician may decide that it would be useful to touch the catatonic patient. If such a decision is reached, then some simple principles should be followed. In the first place someone else should be in the room, and safety officers should be aware that the patient may be unpredictable. The patient should be told in a calm and reassuring voice exactly who the clinician is and what the clinician is about to do. Patients should also be told why they are being touched and that if at any point they want to be left alone they should simply say so. The clinician should be prepared to quickly take evasive action.

I am reminded of a woman in her mid-30s, suffering from schizophrenia. During the interview she sat with her head wrenched straight back while wincing with pain. For about 10 minutes she refused to answer any questions. Her neck continued to hyperextend, as her face further contorted in pain. A second clinician stepped in at this point and said the following, "Ms. Jackson, I am one of the physicians here. I can see that you are in some kind of pain. I am concerned that you may be having a type of drug side effect (dystonic response to her neuroleptic), and I would like to see if I can help relieve your pain. In a moment you will feel me touching the back of your head. I will be trying to see if I can get your neck to move more freely. If you want me to stop, just tell me." The clinician proceeded to do just as he said, while continuously informing the patient as to his next move. In about a minute, the patient's neck straightened, allowing the interview to continue, although she proceeded to speak in a disorganized fashion. Her neck spasm was hysterical, not medication related.

Leaving the area of catatonia, one is confronted with another possible somatic concern of the patient suffering from psychotic process. Namely, these patients frequently have literal problems with determining the limits of their bodies and in a parallel sense the limits of their sense of self, their "realness" so to speak.

It has been suggested that patients experiencing psychotic process often regress to an infantile state in which the body is viewed as part self and part object.[47] At such points the person may experience intense feelings of depersonalization or derealization. This type of experience was vividly described by one patient as follows:

I look at my arms and they aren't mine. They move without my direction. Somebody else moves them. All my limbs and my thoughts are attached to strings and these strings are pulled by others. I know not who I am. I have no control. I don't live in me. The outside and I are all the same.[48]

When intense, these feelings of depersonalization may be associated with a terrifying sense of impending annihilation. Perhaps this is the almost otherworldly fear that Roderick Usher felt was his destiny in Poe's story. It is important to realize the intensity of these fears because they provide insight into the sometimes violent and drastic measures of psychotic patients.

The above quotation also leads into an extension of the concept of poor ego boundaries. One can view psychotic patients as possessing a "porous ego." The world seems to invade their skins in a distinctly unpleasant fashion. They experience a variety of sensations, which seem to enter from the outside world while becoming one with them. It is this unidirectional invasion of their integrity that is partially responsible for their fear and anxiety.[49]

Schneider included these types of invasion experiences in his list of first rank symptoms of schizophrenia. He mistakenly thought that the presence of any of these symptoms guaranteed the presence of schizophrenia. This did not prove to be the case (although they are frequent in schizophrenia), but his symptoms are an excellent inventory of common psychotic phenomena whatever the etiology, and questions concerning them should be part of any interviewer's repertoire.

Schneider described 11 symptoms, of which seven are characterized by this odd feeling of invasion by the outside world. These seven symptoms are somatic passivity experiences, thought withdrawal, thought insertion, made feelings, made impulses, made volitional acts, and delusional perception. The remaining four Schneiderian symptoms are audible thoughts, voices arguing, voices commenting upon one's actions, and thought broadcasting. These four symptoms will be described later.

With somatic passivity experiences the patient is the reluctant recipient of bodily sensations, such as suddenly feeling that his intestines are wriggling about inside his abdomen against his will. It is easy to see how such a peculiar sensation could subsequently plant the seed of delusional material, such as a paranoid fear that someone is purposely twisting the patient's insides.

Unfortunately, the patient's porous ego may also leak outwards. The result may be fears that aggressive fantasies will be heard by others in the room, or even worse, that in a magical sense, these violent ideas may automatically become reality. A common feeling is that the patient's thoughts are being broadcast, one of the four remaining Schneiderian symptoms, as poignantly described below:

*M*y difficulty is an outgo of my silent thought. It goes as it comes. I may think whatever I please, but whatever I do think goes as it comes. I suppose the constant irritation and annoyance they have kept up around me has affected the tension of nerve, so that unlike others who have the same phenomenal power, it goes as rapidly as my mind thinks. I have but to think a thought and it reaches other minds in sound without an effort on my part, and is sounded for a distance, I suppose, of 2 or 3 miles.[50]

One can quickly sense the inherent strangeness of a world encountered with a porous ego. One can more easily intuit why these patients frequently seem preoccupied or lost in thought. It requires tremendous attention to try to sort out the meanings of so odd and intrusive a world. The clinician must also bear in mind that these patients are frequently attempting to determine which of their sensations are real and which are false. To the degree that they possess a "distance" from their psychosis, they will realize that much is unreal. As the psychosis deepens, this distance is lost, and the inexplicable becomes a reality that needs no explanations.

Thus far the focus has been on the somatic sensations and physiologic ramifications of psychotic process. However, with the advent of neuroleptic medications, which have remarkably enhanced our ability to decrease psychotic process, a new set of problems has unfortunately appeared. Patients may develop significant side effects, especially with traditional antipsychotics, such as Haldol and Prolixin, much less so with newer antipsychotics, such as Risperdal and Zyprexa. Earlier the side effect was discussed in which the patient's affect becomes blunted secondary to an antipsychotic-induced Parkinson's syndrome. This blunting could be mistaken for the blunted affect so characteristic of schizophrenia.

A second side effect, akathisia, can also confuse the initial interviewer, because it can be mistaken as evidence of psychotic agitation. Akathisia represents a symptom in which patients feel that a part or all of their body needs to move. It is a deep-seated feeling of restlessness. Generally it will show itself as the physical sign of moving about in an agitated fashion, sometimes with a prance-like step. It is important to remember that akathisia is a subjective symptom and not a physical sign. In this sense the patient may not always appear agitated but may still be feeling extremely restless. By way of illustration, if in addition to akathisia the patient has also developed the stiff-like Parkinson's syndrome described above, the patient may move very little despite an intense drive to move. Needless to say this type of paradoxic situation creates an extremely discordant sensation for the patient.

It is easy to mistake akathisia for psychotic agitation; consequently the interviewer must be alert for it. In a severe form akathisia represents a new and bizarre sensation that a patient, already having problems with psychotic process, certainly could do without. Some authors have reported incidents in which they felt that akathisia either worsened a psychotic state or at times predisposed the patient to inflict self-damage.

In the following direct transcription a young professional describes his experiences with akathisia. At the time of the transcript he was no longer psychotic. When the medication had been utilized, he had been suffering from a frightening delusional system. He had also been told about akathisia and its transitory nature, but his psychotic process appears to have disrupted this information. I have never heard akathisia or its interplay with psychotic process so eloquently described:

> **Pt.:** I was very aware of a different kind of feeling from what I usually have. It felt as if it was most immediately recognizable in the morning, in that I felt that I just couldn't go through with my normal morning routine, like taking a shower and shaving and everything I do to get ready for work. It felt more like I couldn't do it because I couldn't stand to wait that long, to go through those things which were such routine motion.

> **Clin.:** Like, what are some of things that were routine?

> **Pt.:** Well, like standing under the shower. It just seemed impossible to stand under the shower for any much longer and once I got done with the shower it seemed impossible to stand there and dry myself.

> **Clin.:** Ok. What do you mean when you say it wasn't

> possible. What was it that you felt would happen if you did stay there?

Pt.: That I would break out of my skin or something like that. But, uh, that I would be so upset and unsettled that I would just be totally destroyed I think. It's just very unsettling.

Clin.: Now, did the experience change over time? In other words, were there parts of the day where you would feel worse than other parts?

Pt.: It was pretty much general all day. When I got to work, I have a sit-down job. I do remember that it was hard to stay put. It was really hard to sit. I do a lot of reading in my job and it was very hard to concentrate on the things I have to read, and as a consequence it made me feel ineffectual in my work. I just felt totally wiped out at work. I felt like I really couldn't keep working if I were to keep having this feeling.

Clin.: You mentioned the ineffectual feeling. Did you start to feel upset about being ineffectual?

Pt.: Oh, sure. Yeah, I felt that I was going to be a failure, really, if I were to keep feeling this way. I thought it would become evident right away to all the people around me that I was really screwing this up and that I really couldn't do my job anymore. And, in fact, I even got a little panicky about that.

Clin.: Describe that to me.

Pt.: Yeah, I just felt like being between a rock and a hard place because the feeling was that I had to sit there and keep doing my work because I was at work. On the other hand, my body felt like I just couldn't keep doing that anymore, and, uh, it was like you were in a crisis every second is what it was really like. Between wanting to stay there and do your job and being unable to do so.

Clin.: Did you have any fears that somehow or other that this state would not go away? You know, that this was going to continue?

Pt.: Definitely. I had the fear that the drug had set off something in my system whereby, even if I stopped the drug, that I was going to continue to have this feeling. What was definitely very much a part of the feeling was the fact that how could I go through the rest of my life feeling this way? That was very much a part of it.

Clin.: Now, what types of things did this sort of lead you to think then, that you couldn't do your work and that this state might not change?

Pt.: Uhm, I felt depressed about it, and, uh, it led me to feel scared and afraid that something was going to happen.

Clin.: Do you think that you got more frightened or nervous than you had been before? In other words, did the unpleasant sensation increase your own anxiety just because you were having it?

Pt.: Oh, yes. Definitely. I was very anxious being around other people, that they might perceive that I was in this agitated state.

Clin.: Did you have any feelings that you should try to hurt yourself or that you might hurt yourself? . . . because of the . . .

Pt.: Yes, it did seem, it did occur to me that it would be easier not to live than to live this way. That probably seems really heavy, but that did occur to me. I did, I had a resurgence of suicidal thoughts during those feelings.

Clin.: What kinds of things were you thinking at the time?

Pt.: Uh, usually blowing my head off. Really, I was thinking about that and just ending it all because it just, I think every drug I ever took, I always had the fear that it would do something, that it would never go away again.

One aspect that can help the interviewer attempt to sort out aka-thisia from psychotic agitation is the fact that akathisia represents a true bodily sensation. Patients will generally describe a need to move, an actual restlessness within the limbs. This is not generally the case when the agitation is caused by psychotic process. If the patient lacks other psychotic symptoms that could be triggering intense anxiety, then it is also more likely that akathisia is the main problem. But at times the only way to distinguish akathisia from psychotic agitation is to attempt to treat one or the other process. Fortunately with the patient described above the akathisia was greatly relieved by lowering the dose of the neuroleptic.

II: PSYCHOLOGICAL SYSTEM

Auditory hallucinations remain one of the trademarks of psychotic process. To the lay person, the presence of "voices" is practically synonymous with madness. In actuality, auditory hallucinations represent one of the true hard signs of psychosis.

But the determination of whether a patient is having hallucinations is not as easy as one might think, because the clinician must, for the most part, depend on the patient's self-report. Errors in validity appear more frequently when one must depend upon patient opinion as opposed to the elucidation of behavioral incidents. To clarify this dilemma, it may be best to start with a definition of an auditory hallucination.

For quite some time, clinicians tended to clump reports of auditory hallucinations into two categories: pseudohallucinations and true hallucinations. This distinction may well have found its most fertile roots in the writings of Karl Jaspers, who we have discussed before in Chapter 5. Jaspers seemed to believe that there was no continuum between hearing one's thoughts and hearing true hallucinations. Patients either had hallucinations, or they did not. With true hallucinations he felt that two elements were always present. First, the hallucination was substantial in the sense that it seemed real and had many of the perceptual qualities of a real perception. Second, the hallucination seemed to occupy space. With an auditory hallucination, this suggests that the voice came from a given area outside the head.

But Jaspers may not have been correct, as Fish and others have pointed out, and modern clinical experience has borne out.[51-53] There does appear to be a continuum, and I have talked with many patients with schizophrenia who describe their voices as "being in my head." In some instances, as the psychotic process progresses, these voices move out into space and truly seem more real at that point. In other cases, the voices always seem to be originating from outside the patient's head. But the bottom line remains that auditory hallucinations can be experienced in both ways. And the DSM-IV accepts both voices from inside and outside the head as representing hallucinatory phenomena.

In an even more classic sense, the concept of the apparent localizability of a hallucination is probably best viewed with regard to whether a voice is heard within the mind (which has no location) or outside the mind (where a location can be assigned). In some hallucinations, the voice is only within the mind. In many hallucinations the voice can be physically located, and this location may even be reported as being inside the patient's head as with "A radio transmitter is broadcasting from inside my head, where my neighbor implanted it." The internal terrain of the body can actually represent a geographic space and a source of hallucinatory phenomena in this regard.

It is also interesting to explore what is meant by the word "real," because patients may tell the clinician that the voices are quite real but do not sound exactly like normal voices. It is not uncommon for psychotic patients to be able to identify their hallucinations as abnormal voices. Sometimes they may even possess names for them.

If a clinician is attempting to decide whether or not a patient is faking hallucinations, these points become important. A patient who is malingering may tend to describe the voices as sounding just like normal voices, which remains possible in psychosis but not typical. The malingerer may also describe the voices as happening all of a sudden, unaware that hard psychotic symptoms usually have subtle prodromal phases such as delusional mood and delusional perception. Moreover, the voices found in processes such as schizophrenia are frequently hostile in nature and often hurl unusually obscene insults at the patient.

Because of the importance of auditory hallucinations, 3 of Schneider's 11 first-rank symptoms concern voices. One of these symptoms consists of the patient experiencing audible thoughts, in which the patient's thoughts are repeated aloud. The patient, on the other hand, may hear an undecipherable voice whose content becomes clear a few seconds after hearing it. The other two symptoms consist of arguing voices and voices commenting on the patient's activities.

The following excerpt vividly presents the eerie world created by such phenomena.

*S*eated on a steamer chair on the boardwalk of Coney Island, I heard the voice for the first time. It was as positive and persistent as any voice I had ever heard. It said slowly, "Jayson, you are worthless. You've never been useful, and you've never been any good." I shook my head unbelievingly, trying to drive out the sound of the words, and as if I had heard nothing, continued to talk with my neighbor. Suddenly, clearer, deeper, and even louder than before, the deep voice came at me again, right in my ear this time, and getting me tight and shivery inside. "Larry Jayson, I told you before you weren't any good. Why are you sitting here making believe you're as good as anyone else when you're not? Whom are you fooling? You're no good," the voice said slowly in the same deep tones. "You've never been any good or use on earth. There is the ocean. You might as well drown yourself. Just walk in and keep walking." As soon as the voice was through, I knew, by its cold command, I had to obey it.[54]

In the last analysis, there exists no better method of learning about hallucinations than the experience of asking questions about auditory hallucinations to numerous people, ranging from psychotic to normal. Only in this manner will the clinician develop a sound sense of the range of normal and abnormal responses. The following types of questions can both convey to patients that the interviewer is genuinely interested in their experiences, as well as helping the clinician learn about hallucinations themselves:

a. When you are feeling very distressed, do your thoughts ever get so intense that they sound almost like a voice? (If answered "yes," consider the following.)
b. Tell me what the voices sound like to you.
c. What do they say to you?
d. Do they sometimes taunt you or say mean things about you?
e. Are they male or female voices?
f. Do you have names for them?
g. Do they seem to be inside your head or do they come from outside your head?
h. Are they loud or soft?
i. When you first heard the voices, what did you think they were?
j. What feelings do you have as you hear the voices?
k. Do you ever hear several voices talking to each other about you?

The wording of the first question allows the topic to be broached in a fairly nonaffrontive fashion, because the interviewer is tying the phenomena directly into the patient's pain. The clinician asks if the patient's thoughts sound *like* a voice, a phrasing that offers a back-door to the reluctant patient who fears being viewed as crazy. In a typical first assessment, the interviewer may not have time to ask all of these questions, but as time permits the clinician can pick and choose, constantly learning more about the phenomenology of hearing voices.

Besides abnormalities of perception, the psychotic patient's thought process itself is often disrupted by the psychotic process. Thoughts may become speeded up and racing in nature, as is also seen in mania. It becomes difficult to concentrate as evidenced by the following patient description:

I just can't concentrate on anything. There's too much going on in my head and I can't sort it out. My thoughts wander around in circles without getting anywhere. I try to read even a paragraph in a book but it takes me ages because each bit I read starts me thinking in 10 different directions at once.[55]

This excerpt also hints at another disquieting characteristic sometimes seen. Psychotic thinking has an internally "contagious" quality to it, in the sense that it triggers a multitude of associations, sometimes close in nature and at other times distant and disjointed. This abnormality in thought process will frequently show itself with a loosening of associations in the patient's speech. This trend of creative but dystonic associations, which are not under the patient's control, is nicely captured in the following excerpt:

$\mathcal{M}$y trouble is that I've got too many thoughts. You might think about something—let's say that ashtray—and just think, oh yes, that's for putting my cigarette in, but I would think of it and then I would think of a dozen different things connected with it at the same time.[56]

At other times thought processes may become, perhaps because of the previously mentioned abnormalities, somewhat disrupted. Patients may stop in midsentence and be unable to return to their original topic. This process is known as thought blocking. It represents a strongly suggestive soft sign of psychosis. It is useful to quietly ask patients what has happened at these moments. Sometimes the patient has been derailed by an auditory hallucination. If the clinician suspects this process, the clinician can ask if this was the case.

It is important to know if a patient is actively hearing voices during the interview, because the patient may feel that the clinician is producing the messages. Generally, it is not good for rapport to be perceived as calling the patient a drunken slob or threatening to chop off the patient's fingers and other appendages. This active state of hallucinosis represents the type of situation in which violence can erupt.

It has already become apparent that the patient's thought processes are frequently affected during a psychosis, although this is not always the case. One common problem is the presence of truly illogical thought. One of the more frequent breakdowns in formal logic is the appearance of what Rosenbaum has called predicative thinking. This means that the person views things as similar or identical because they are connected by the same predicate (verb). The following example shows this process at work:

Major premise: Jesus Christ was persecuted.
Minor premise: I am persecuted.
Conclusion: Therefore, I am Jesus Christ.[57]

Other distinct problems with logic, as well as the emergence of magical thought, as seen in young children, frequently accompany psychotic process. But it is not necessarily a black or white phenomenon. Many patients will demonstrate varying degrees of normal logic.

This knowledge that the psychotic patient may be losing an ability to think logically is of immediate practical use when approaching patients who are both psychotic and agitated. It is probably a mistake to immediately assume, before talking with the patient, that the patient either can or cannot be talked down. Instead the interviewer should gently attempt to engage the patient in conversation. While doing this, the clinician can decide to what degree the patient's logic is intact. If it is reasonably intact, the interviewer may try to talk with the patient and perhaps alleviate some of the patient's anger. If, with this technique, the patient's anger begins to escalate or if the patient's logic is severely impaired, it is probably best to quickly back off from the patient and proceed with appropriate safety procedures.

To further attempt to reason with such a patient does not make much sense, because the patient is not processing the clinician's words in a normal fashion. Further interaction may push the patient towards violence. The key lies in carefully assessing the impact of one's interaction and proceeding appropriately.

A similar situation arises if the clinician discovers that the patient has incorporated the clinician into a delusional system. This brings to mind a patient with whom I observed the interview as a supervisor. She had a ragged appearance and sat in her chair spitting her words into a hostile world. As soon as I sat down she yelled out, "You're the one who called me a prostitute the other day. You're the one who has been spying on me!" I had never seen her before and even if I had, I doubt I would have spoken to her as she was suggesting.

No matter what I said in my defense she immediately grew angrier, and so I quickly shut up. Such a retreat is not only the better part of valor, but also represents a sound clinical maneuver, because this patient was not hearing a word that I was saying. It becomes easier to understand her hostile position, if the clinician realizes that she truly believed that I had belittled her publicly. Clinicians cannot quickly detach themselves from such a delusional web.

In most patients the initial interviewer has much more access to the process of blending. The question then becomes one of how does one broach topics like paranoia without offending the patient. Paranoid ideation is often easily entered by keying off the content of the patient's conversation, utilizing natural, implied, or referred gates as follows:

> **Pt.:** I don't know what to do with myself. I just, I just feel the whole thing is a mess. Probably, I don't know, probably the baby is even aware of our arguments. When we were first married, everything was so much better. But when the mill shut down a third time and he lost his job for good, well it all became history.

Clin.: It sounds like an ugly situation at home. Has the tension ever gotten so bad that he has struck you?

Pt.: Thank God no. I'd leave him, honestly I would.

Clin.: Do you think that in any way he is trying to hurt you, perhaps even trying to get your friends against you?

Pt.: Oh he's tried to hurt me in the sense of making me feel guilt, but he knows better than to mess with me or my friends.

In this fashion, the clinician has smoothly made a foray into the paranoid region. The patient's comments do not suggest paranoid ideation. There is probably no need to explore further. By now most paranoid patients would probably have nibbled at the "bait." The clinician has scouted for paranoid ideation without the patient having any idea that such an exploration of psychotic material has occurred.

This point leads to the more general issue of broaching other psychotic topics in a nonthreatening fashion. For most interviewers this type of questioning is most difficult when interviewing a patient in whom the clinician doubts the presence of psychotic process. Some authors have suggested that interviewers should never ask questions about voices and other psychotic phenomena unless they strongly suspect the presence of these phenomena. To do so, they argue, will disengage the patient.

But I have my doubts about such a blanket admonition, and in practice I generally ask all patients about psychotic process at some point in the initial interview. I believe this represents a sound practice for three reasons. (1) A patient whose psychotic process is fluctuating or whose psychotic process is part of a character disorder may look remarkably intact during any given interview. For instance, to not ask about ideas of reference or episodes of depersonalization invites the cover-up of diagnoses such as a schizotypal personality. (2) I have seldom, if ever, seen such questioning result in any lasting problems with engagement in a nonpsychotic patient. I have seen patients balk at it, but with skillful engagement techniques, the blending is quickly restored. Moreover, most patients do not seem offended at all. (3) When patients do balk at such questioning, their emotional overreactions provide an open window into their defenses and psychodynamics. This psychodynamic window is one of the best reasons to routinely ask such questions, as seen in the following:

Pt.: Let's get it straight, things have been tough all over for everybody involved and I've been damn upset.

> **Clin.:** When you are really feeling upset, have your thoughts ever gotten so intense and bothersome that they sound almost like a voice?
>
> **Pt.:** Oh great, here come the crazy questions (said angrily). Well I got news for you. I'm not crazy and I've been asked all those questions before. (The patient reaches over and squeezes her boyfriend's hand, smiling at him while subsequently tossing a little sneer to the clinician.)

This hostile display is not a typical response to this question. Indeed, it suggested to the interviewer that the patient might have some type of personality disorder, as evidenced by her sense of entitlement and manipulative actions. Such a response may suggest the expansion of diagnostic categories not considered earlier. In this case, further interviewing revealed a full-blown borderline personality disorder.

Once entering the psychotic region it is not necessary to beat it into the ground. Quickly, the clinician will achieve some idea as to whether the region is worth expanding further. If hints of psychotic process emerge, then a full expansion may be warranted. If no hints emerge, the topic may be left quickly after only a few probing questions. Part of the art lies in learning how to smoothly enter these psychotic regions.

Some questions that may be used effectively as gates into psychotic material are shown below.

a. Have you had experiences that seemed odd or frightening to you?
b. Earlier we talked about your nightmares. Have you ever had similar types of frightening images bothering you during the day?
c. You had been talking about some of your talents. Have you ever felt that you had some unusual abilities such as ESP?
d. You mentioned earlier that one of your favorite activities is watching TV. Have you even been frightened by the TV? (Depending on what the patient says, one might pursue this with a question such as follows.) Did it ever seem like the people on TV were watching you or that they literally were aware of private aspects of your life?
e. You had mentioned earlier that your sister had apparently been hearing voices. Have you ever had similar experiences?

Another excellent method of entering psychotic material is through the discussion of religious issues as shown below:

> **Pt.:** I have always been a fairly religious person. My

father was a devout Lutheran. Religion runs in our family.

Clin.: On a moment by moment basis, how much is God a part of your life?

Pt.: (long pause) He is my life and my breath, so be it.

Clin.: It sounds like He is a very important part of your life. Sometimes people who are close to God feel that He has a special mission or role for them to play. Do you feel that you may be lucky enough that God has such a role for you?

Pt.: Yes, I do. I am to bring peace to all nations. And I shall bring a calmness to all that I touch.

Clearly it would be worth exploring the psychotic region more thoroughly with this patient. But the important issue from our viewpoint is the naturalness of the gate provided by religious discussion. Even as the topic was first entered, the intensity of the patient's feelings probably suggested to the clinician that something was up.

Thus far we have focused on the complex impact of psychotic process on specific aspects of psychological functioning, such as perception and thought process. This impact is indeed both terrifying and terrible. But what of the "self"? What is the impact of chronic psychotic process and of the deficit symptoms of diseases like schizophrenia upon a person's self-image and self-respect?

In many ways I feel that this impact is the most damaging of all. As we had seen earlier, the negative symptoms of schizophrenia, such as low interest, low drive, and low energy are powerful and insidious, often lingering indefinitely, long after the voices and delusions have faded. Almost all people coping with schizophrenia initially view these symptoms not as part of the disease but as symbols of their own inadequacy as people. As the deficit symptoms make it difficult and at times impossible to work, people frequently begin a vicious process of self-belittlement. Sometimes frustrated and weary family members feed this cycle by misinterpreting these negative symptoms as laziness and psychological weakness, "The voices are gone so why doesn't he just get a job and get on with his life?"

As patients watch their siblings and friends go on to develop successful marriages, careers, and identities, they find themselves left behind in a race that seems unwinnable. It is very easy, and all too human, to decide it is not worth the risk of failure to enter such a race. The patient soon finds himself or herself intensely afraid of

further humiliation. Many patients find themselves lost in a laby-
rinth of self-doubt, and they often adopt a role as "the black sheep"
in the family. This intense demoralization, which is often at its
worst between psychotic episodes when the negative symptoms
adamantly persist, is often the prelude to suicide, as we shall discuss
in Chapter 8.

Schizophrenia rapes the soul. From the very first interview, it is
important for the clinician to remember that one of the main tasks
involved in intervention is to help the patient heal this pain and to
believe in himself or herself again. People with schizophrenia should
not be pitied. Indeed some of the most courageous and "tough"
individuals whom I have had the pleasure to meet are coping with
this traumatizing disease with dignity and resourcefulness. This
recovery process begins in the very first interview.

For the clinician it begins with the realization that we are all
"people" first. The patient's "diagnosis," albeit very important,
plays a secondary role in our understanding. This feeling grows,
with experience, as we clinicians truly realize that the person in
front of us is not a medical term but a person just like ourselves.
We, too, or our friends or family members could develop bipolar
disorder or schizophrenia. Like death, mental illness honors no
walls.

For the patient it begins with a realization that he or she is not
a disease entity but a person coping with a disease. In this sense, I
think that it is best for both the clinician and the patient to abandon
terms such as "schizophrenic." Such terms insidiously lead into
stigmatization and identification with the disease. I have never met
a schizophrenic. I have met a person coping with schizophrenia.
This distinction may be subtle, but it is telling.

I am convinced that this sense of respect and empowerment,
from a clinician, shows through in the very first encounter with the
patient. Clinicians who convey this perspective often have much
more success both in the initial interview and in all subsequent
work. Clinicians who do not convey this feeling are often sitting
alone in their offices during follow-up appointments.

This perspective is elegantly described by Patricia Deegan in an
article that I highly recommend, *Recovery: The Lived Experience of
Rehabilitation*:

*I*t is important to understand that persons with a disability do not "get
rehabilitated" in the sense that cars "get" tuned up or televisions "get repaired."
Disabled persons are not passive recipients of rehabilitation services. Rather,
they experience themselves as recovering a new sense of self and of purpose
within and beyond the limits of the disability. This distinction between
rehabilitation and recovery is important. Rehabilitation refers to the services and

technologies that are made available to disabled persons so that they might learn to adapt to their world. Recovery refers to the lived or real life experience of persons as they accept and overcome the challenge of the disability.[58]

The understanding, from this section, of the psychological damage caused by schizophrenia is at the very heart of the healing process that first begins in the initial interview. It also conveys the delicate interplays that occur between individuals dealing with chronic psychotic disorders and the people around them. Let's take a closer look at these interactions in a broader sense.

III: DYADIC SYSTEM

It is not infrequent for people with psychotic process to become socially withdrawn. In particular, when the psychosis is secondary to schizophrenia, episodes of social withdrawal are extremely frequent.[59] This social withdrawal could be related to the tendency for the patient to enter a more autistic world. In an effort to sort out the tremendous number of peculiar sensations and thoughts, the person suffering from a psychotic process may find it necessary to withdraw. Social contact becomes painfully disruptive. In other patients in whom aggressive drives may be building to a pitch, people may be avoided because of a fear of loss of control.

However, there is another aspect to this entire issue, which brings us directly to the dyadic system itself. Frequently, these patients will display behaviors that are, indeed, socially inappropriate. As we had seen in the chapter on nonverbal behavior, psychotic patients generally show some disturbance in the normal nonverbal rules for conversation. This may range from sitting or standing inappropriately close to the clinician to displaying markedly abnormal affects. Because of the tremendous need of these patients to attend to the troubled thoughts in their own minds, their ability to empathize is frequently strikingly diminished.

Clinicians should also be aware of their own feelings of confusion that may develop as they interview patients experiencing psychotic process. This confusion in the clinician may be caused by psychotic processes in the patient, such as a subtle loosening of associations. If the clinician can recognize the subjective feeling of confusion, then a more thorough pursuit of psychotic process and content may be suggested. The confusion in the clinician mirrors the confusion or disorganization of the patient.

A word of caution seems in order here. Clinicians lucky enough to be gifted with an intuitive sense of empathy can fall into a trap. The patient may be displaying subtle signs of disorganized thought, but the clinician ignores these signs because he or she understands "what the patient is thinking." Indeed the clinician might understand; however, the patient is still psychotic. When hunting for evidence of formal thought disorder, the question is not whether we understand the patient but whether a normal person would be confused or not. At the other extreme, sometimes a well-trained clinician will recognize a formal thought disorder before it would even be evident to a layperson.

All of the above disturbances in dyadic communication may lead to an uncomfortable sensation in a clinician. The sensation has been described as not being able "to feel" with the patient, in short, an inability to experience an empathic bond with the patient. This peculiar sensation has been called the "precox feeling."[60] It is felt to be particularly suggestive of schizophrenia. Used in the appropriate sense, as an intuitive guide suggesting the need to carefully explore for the criteria of schizophrenia, the precox feeling is a useful tool. It should never be used as a criterion of schizophrenia or as a justification for labeling someone as having schizophrenia.

People with psychotic process can also create feelings of frustration in the initial interviewer. This may result when the patient's lack of insight pushes the patient to reject various avenues of help such as medication or hospitalization. It can be particularly frustrating to work with a paranoid patient who clearly needs help but feels strongly "nothing is wrong with me."

In these instances, it is important to accept the naturalness of one's frustration while avoiding a demonstration of this frustration to the patient. These countertransference problems tend to surface as extensive and sometimes heated attempts to convince the patient of his or her illness. Such attempts are probably far more counterproductive than productive. It is often best to calmly discuss one's views and then acknowledge openly that the patient and oneself seem to have a difference of opinion. The patient should know that if he or she feels a desire to talk again or experiences a change of opinion, that the clinician is always available for another appointment.

Frustration may also evolve when the interviewer feels that the patient is somehow in control of the psychotic process, "flipping it on" when it is advantageous to do so. At some level this manipulation may actually occur at both the conscious and unconscious plane. I remember a man about 30 years old who would begin talking in a disorganized and delusion-littered fashion. As he felt more comfortable with me, his thinking would become more organized. If I then probed even in a subtle fashion into his personal life, he would quickly become disorganized and mumble about "the cheesedogs that were going to drop a nuclear warhead on Pittsburgh." Oddly enough I do not think he was particularly conscious of this process.

One can better conceptualize such behavior if one assumes that at some level, to the degree that the patient has both insight and motivation, the patient may be able to partially rein in psychotic process. This self-modulation must require a considerable amount of effort and concentration. Perhaps at times, and depending on the interpersonal situation, the patient might find it simply easier to just let things go as they may. At such points the psychotic process may emerge in a more pressing fashion as seen above. To the degree that we understand this process, our frustration levels may decrease.

Frustration may also arise with patients suffering from schizophrenia who are persistently negative during the interview. As Michels suggests, the interviewer may gently point out that automatically saying "No" to everything is as much a relinquishment of control as saying "Yes" to all the clinician's requests.[61] Jointly agreeing upon a topic to discuss may also open up avenues for better engagement.

Thus far the emphasis has been on the patient's effect on the clinician. With patients dealing with psychotic process, it is also important to realize that clinicians may need to monitor their own impact on the patient. In earlier chapters we have already discussed in detail some of the changes in style that may help to facilitate blending with paranoid patients, such as decreasing the use of complex empathic statements. It is also important to realize that because of disturbances in logic and reality testing, normally well-received statements by a clinician may be hostilely received. Michels points out, for instance, that with one of his patients the word "leg" had taken on a highly sexualized meaning.[62] Consequently, when the clinician would use the word, it was received as a sexual topic, probably carrying a variety of unwanted overtones.

Sometimes when people struggling with psychotic process are cooperative but frightened, it goes a long way to simply reassure them that they are in a safe environment. Especially if such patients are disorganized as well as frightened, it is useful to tell them what is happening, ask them to bring up any questions they may have, and structure the interview for them. If the patient is forced to handle an unstructured interview, filled with open-ended questions, gentle commands, and pregnant pauses, the interview itself may become traumatizing. Gentle structuring will sometimes actually result in a more organized production of speech as the psychotic defenses recede.

Along similar lines, in some instances an empathic interviewer may so decrease the anxiety level of a subtly psychotic patient that the observable psychotic process temporarily disappears or recedes significantly. Ironically, the clinician's style will have distorted the clinical picture, amply reminding us that as the interview proceeds we become a part of the dyadic system, whether we intend to or not. In a similar fashion, an involvement with the psychotic process itself awaits the friends and family members of the patient. Unfortunately, unlike clinicians, they are not generally trained to handle such bizarre interactions.

IV: FAMILY SYSTEM AND OTHER GROUP SYSTEMS

Psychosis, despite its propensity for autistic withdrawal, is a family matter. No person in the immediate vicinity of the patient will be able to remain uninvolved for long. Few processes can so ravage a family and its underlying structure. This is particularly true when the process is chronic in nature, such as with schizophrenia or a bipolar disorder. For these reasons, family members will become an important source of information as well as a targeted group for therapeutic intervention.

Most family members are sorely ill equipped with the knowledge that could help them understand and cope with the bizarre behaviors of their loved ones. One can imagine what it is like for family members to become the object of the penetrating hatred that may erupt when one is perceived as part of a patient's delusional system. In some instances family members are physically assaulted, and in rare instances they are killed by the very people they have loved most. Obviously, both family and friends must cope with powerfully ambivalent feelings, including embarrassment, guilt, fear, compassion, helplessness, bitterness, love, and the desire to abandon the patient.

I remember working with one family whose plight illustrates some of the many processes at work in the family system. The family was of Creole background. The patient was an attractive woman in her mid-30s who sat with a defiant jut to her jaw. Upon her head she wore a faded scarf that lent a sad elegance to her. She had become progressively depressed, and her mind was swarming with religious delusions. She had had to stop work and had been living with her mother and a brother, both of whom were taking care of her children. These family members had not wanted her to seek professional help, because they felt that she would get over it with God's help.

But she had recently spent several days with another brother who had angrily insisted that help be sought. Already the psychosis was beginning to dig its claws into the structural foundations of the family. It is common for family tensions to crystallize around issues such as, "What to do with Jim or Sandy."

While waiting in the emergency room, the patient, who we shall call Ms. Jenkins, stood up and began to perform a ritualistic chant. It was sad indeed to watch the mother and brother hide their embarrassment as they struggled to get her back in her seat. Later, this same mother and brother would undercut our efforts to hospitalize Ms. Jenkins. Her mother wearily looked at us saying, "I don't think there is much really wrong with her. I don't think she needs to be in a hospital. She'll pull out of it on her own. But thank you for your help." Her thanks were sincerely given.

The next day the Jenkins family was back. Ms. Jenkins had been acting bizarrely throughout the night. In the waiting room the mother sat with her arm around her daughter, her eyes red from the painful recognition that her daughter was no longer the same person she had raised.

In this regard, it appears useful to remember that at some level family members will be mourning the loss of "the person they knew." As with any mourning process, various stages such as denial, anger, mourning, depression, and acceptance will intermingle and be entered at different times. The Jenkins family highlights a common problem facing the initial interviewer, the presence of a powerful system of denial among family members. By understanding the mourning of family members, it may help decrease the angry countertransference feelings arising from their rejection of the clinician's help.

From the above discussion, it can be seen that in few cases does the initial interview with a psychotic patient end with the patient. At some early point, the family warrants an assessment as well as a chance for later counseling. Keep in mind that some family members may become seriously depressed and perhaps even suicidal. Psychosis is indeed a family affair.

The tensions of the family may at some level precipitate or aggravate the psychotic process itself. Research such as the Environmental/Personal Indicators in the Course of Schizophrenia (EPICS) Project has shown that families in which members are overly involved or antagonistic to the patient may hinder recovery even when the patient complies with medication use.[63] Family counseling seemed to significantly decrease relapse rates. This emphasizes the importance of assessing the family and beginning an alliance with them. Frequently, the initial interviewer is the first person to meet the family and consequently represents a key person in the attempts to build the much needed alliance described above.

Not only is the family affected, but also other important social networks may begin to collapse around the patient. Jobs may be lost, and friendships may become tattered. It is difficult to remain friends with a person who has developed a severe psychotic process. Frequently, both friends and family members may be dealing with feelings of guilt. A simple phrase said early during an interview may be comforting such as, "I just finished talking with your friend, who seems very disturbed. I bet you've gone through a lot recently. It was nice of you to come with him today." As with the patient, engagement issues remain critical during the opening phases of corroborative interviews.

Along these lines, it is important to remember that many parents (as well as siblings and children) of patients with schizophrenia and bipolar disorder come to us with a checkered history with mental health professionals. They have often met many fine professionals, but, more often than not, they have also, unfortunately "been put through the wringer" not only by the disease afflicting their children but also by some of the professionals supposedly helping with this disease.

It is critical in the initial corroborative meeting to win these parents over. The goal is to help them with their immense pain and also to set the stage for a joint effort to help their child as he or she recovers.

During the course of this first meeting, many parents will have some of the following unexpressed fears. Some will have all of these fears, and some will have none. However, as the interview proceeds, the clinician should take the time to try to sensitively address and dismantle these concerns. Some of these concerns are listed, directly followed by samples of clinician statements that can help to allay them:

1. This clinician doesn't really care what I have to say:
   Clinician Intervention: "One of the things I want to emphasize early on is how important your input and background information is in our helping John. There is no one in the world who knows him better than you. We are dependent on your input. I also really want to know what you think has worked and what you think doesn't work."
2. This clinician thinks that we are the problem:
   Clinician Intervention: "You know, there are some people out there who think parents somehow cause schizophrenia. Let me assure you of one thing. I don't buy that for one minute. Schizophrenia is a brain disease like epilepsy. Some of the most loving parents whom I have ever met have children who develop schizophrenia. Just in talking with you today, I am struck by how much you love John. I think he is very lucky to have you. Some parents would have abandoned him by now."
3. This guy is not going to understand how much pain we've been through:
   Clinician Intervention: "You must have gone through a lot over the years. I'm sure it just must seem like it goes on and on.

I have no miracles to offer, but I promise you that we will do our very best to help you and your son. How have you coped with all this? Have you had very much support?"

4. This "Bozo" is going to change these meds:

Clinician Intervention: "One of the most foolish things a physician can do is to change the meds before talking with parents and the patient about what is working. Your input is vital. I have no intention of changing these meds until after we talk in detail. By the way, if your son agrees, I would like to always try to talk with you and get your thoughts about any potential major med changes. What is your opinion about this particular set of medications?"

5. This guy is closed to our ideas and thinks he knows it all:

Clinician Intervention: "If you have any new ideas about helping John, please let me or the case manager know. If you find interesting articles or hear about new treatments, please let me know, and I'll find out about them, if I'm not familiar with them for some reason. I like to stay on top of new treatments."

It always pays to find out at an early stage what the family has experienced with other mental health professionals. The best way to find out is to simply ask. Your inquiry also metacommunicates that it matters to you what they think of your care. A question such as the following can help, "I'm wondering what your experience with previous psychiatrists has been like?" It is also useful to ask, "What are some of the things I can do that would help you? For instance how frequently would you like to meet with me?"

The first meeting is also a good time to refer the family to a local chapter of the National Alliance for the Mentally Ill (NAMI) if they are not already aware of it. NAMI is an ongoing support group run by family members, who have a relative with a serious mental illness. It is a superb organization and has chapters all over the United States.

Before leaving the area of the first meeting with a family member, it is worth addressing a topic that we mentioned in the last chapter. With depressed patients we had talked about the importance of understanding the patient's subculture. This is equally true with patients dealing with chronic psychotic process. Here, though, we encounter a new and somewhat disturbing twist, because patients with chronic psychotic processes such as schizophrenia frequently become a new subculture. As these patients lose their friends, spend long stays in hospitals, and wear out their welcome with relatives, they end up spending progressively more time with each other.

The society, through stigmatization, fear, and ignorance, gradually pushes people with chronic mental illnesses into a social caste of sorts. The patients frequently become outcasts from the mainstream of the society. It is important for the initial interviewer to understand these dynamics, because they may appear as a veiled hostility from the patient. And sometimes this animosity is not so veiled.

Each subculture, composed of people coping with schizophrenia and other chronic illnesses, may affect the views of the patient towards treatment itself. It is useful for the clinician to learn about these biases. For example, the local patients may develop prejudicial views on certain medications. If all of the patient's friends hate the drug Thorazine (chlorpromazine hydrochloride), it does not make a lot of sense to send the patient home on Thorazine, when a different neuroleptic may be just as effective, but not blackballed by the subculture.

V: FRAMEWORK FOR MEANING

In the arms of a psychosis the problem is not so much a world that is meaningless but rather a world that is too meaningful. As the patient copes with a suffocating mixture of bizarre and unscreened sensory experiences, the world is gradually transformed into a desert filled with burning bushes. The patient finds little rest from the intensity of the delusional world, and this intensity creates the driven quality so characteristic of psychotic process.

One of the saddest aspects of psychotic process remains the irony that it can make a patient so religiously preoccupied that religion is no longer a practical support system. Instead of providing a calm guidance, religious issues become disturbing. This type of overzealous religious ideation is frequently seen with schizophrenia.

In this regard, the clinician should not be afraid to hear about the patient's religious beliefs. These areas can provide avenues for entrance into psychotic process, as mentioned earlier, and more important, may help us to understand the patient's world view. By listening attentively and nonjudgmentally, the blending process may also be facilitated. If for some reason this type of discussion seems to be agitating the patient, then the clinician can skillfully guide the conversation to other topics.

Psychotic religious preoccupation may represent an intensified effort to replace previous areas that had provided a sense of meaning to the patient. For instance, the patient's family ties may have become critically weakened, thus depriving the patient of a powerful framework for meaning. In some unfortunate instances, patients may actually come to view themselves as burdens upon their families. In such situations, one can easily see why a grandiose religious delusion may serve as a source of much needed solace. It could represent a very real resurrection of sorts, a resurrection of the patient's self-esteem.

This process brings to light a curious aspect of the psychotic patient's search for a framework for meaning. With some patients the psychotic delusions literally become the focal points of their lives. When these delusions disappear, so can the meaning behind life.

In this regard I worked briefly with a young man suffering from schizophrenia, who believed he could broadcast his thoughts. As he phrased it, "I'm the best there is. Nobody can send their thoughts faster or further than I." As he came out of his psychosis, his delusion began to fade. One day as we talked by his bedside he turned to me saying, "I've come to realize that I can't really send my thoughts out like I told you I could. And you know what I also just realized, I realized that I'm just not a very special kind of person." At which point, he began to cry. I have since discovered that several years later he shot himself to death.

I raise these issues, because the initial interviewer will undoubtedly be working with patients in various stages of belief and disbelief of their delusions. It is useful to attempt to understand the significance of these beliefs to the patient at the time of their presentation.

Even if the patient's psychosis is being caused by primarily biologic dysfunction, the fact remains that the content of the delusions are directly related to the patient's psychological constitution, including the patient's upbringing, memories, values, and beliefs. In that sense, one may find important clues to underlying fears and issues in these seemingly illogical fantasies.

In closing, the reader will recall that we began this chapter with the writings of Gérard De Nerval, who would eventually take his own life. Who knows what the voices were saying to him or in what personal hell he found himself. What we do have are his words. As we reread them, perhaps from the understanding gained from this chapter, we will hear them with a new respect for both their brilliance and their sadness:

I seemed to myself a hero living under the very eyes of the gods; everything in nature assumed new aspects, and secret voices came to me from the plants, the trees, animals, the meanest insects, to warn and to encourage me. The words of my companions had mysterious messages, the sense of which I alone understood.

References

1. Hammacher, A. M.: *Phantoms of the Imagination.* New York, Harry N. Abrams, 1981, pp. 136–138.
2. Symons, A.: Essay on Gérard de Nerval. In *The Symbolist Movement in Literature.* New York, E. P. Dutton, 1985, pp. 14–17.

3. American Psychiatric Association: Diagnostic and Statistical Manual of Mental Disorders, 4th ed. Washington, DC, APA, 1994, pp. 285–286.
4. Fish, F.: *Clinical Psychopathology.* Bristol, Britain, Wright, 1967, pp. 19–26.
5. Roberts, J. K.: *Differential Diagnosis in Neuropsychiatry.* New York, John Wiley, 1984, p. 263.
6. Asaad, G., and Shapiro, B.: Hallucinations: Theoretical and clinical overview. *American Journal of Psychiatry* 143:1088–1097, 1986.
7. West, L. J.: A clinical and theoretical overview of hallucinatory phenomena. In *Hallucinations: Behavior, Experience, and Theory,* edited by R. K. Siegel and L. J. West. New York, John Wiley, 1975, p. 308.
8. Lehman, H. E., and Canero, R.: Schizophrenia: Clinical features. In *Comprehensive Textbook of Psychiatry IV,* 4th ed., edited by H. I. Kaplan and B. J. Sadock. Baltimore, Williams & Wilkins, 1985, p. 683.
9. West, L. J., 1975, p. 308.
10. Roberts, J. K., 1984, p. 262.
11. Sellers, E. M., and Kalant, H.: Alcohol intoxication and withdrawal. *New England Journal of Medicine* 294:757–760, 1976.
12. Sellers, E. M., 1976, p. 758.
13. Hackett, T. P.: Alcoholism: Acute and chronic. In *Massachusetts General Hospital Handbook of General Hospital Psychiatry,* edited by T. P. Hackett and N. H. Cassem. St. Louis, C. V. Mosby, 1978, p. 19.
14. Hackett, T. P., 1978, p. 20.
15. Goldfrank, L. R., Lewin, N. A., and Osborn, H.: Dusted (PCP). *Hospital Physician,* May 1982, pp. 62–67.
16. Lydiard, R. B., and Gelenberg, A. J.: Treating substance abuse, Part I. *Drug Therapy* April 1982, pp. 57–66.
17. Goldfrank, L. R., 1982, p. 65.
18. Goodman, L. S., and Gilman, A.: *The Pharmacological Basis of Therapeutics.* New York, Macmillan, 1975, pp. 514–532.
19. Guze, S. B.: Schizoaffective disorders. In *Comprehensive Textbook of Psychiatry IV,* 4th ed., edited by H. I. Kaplan and B. J. Sadock. Baltimore, Williams & Wilkins, 1985, p. 657.
20. Lehman, H. E., 1985, p. 690.
21. Haier, R. J.: The diagnosis of schizophrenia: A review of recent development. *Schizophrenia Bulletin* 6(3):417–427, 1980.
22. Guze, S. G., 1985, p. 757.
23. DSM-IV, 1994, pp. 295–296.
24. Tsuang, Ming T.: Schizoaffective disorder. *Archives of General Psychiatry* 36:633–634, 1979.
25. Guze, S. B., 1985, pp. 756–759.
26. DSM-IV, 1994, p. 301.
27. Walker, J. I., and Brodie, H. K.: Paranoid disorders. In *Comprehensive Textbook of Psychiatry,* 4th ed., edited by H. I. Kaplan and B. J. Sadock. Baltimore, Williams & Wilkins, 1985, pp. 747–755.
28. Walker, J. I., 1985, p. 75.
29. Bannister, Sir R.: *Brain's Clinical Neurology.* New York, Oxford University Press, 1978, p. 197.
30. Walker, J. I., 1985, p. 751.
31. Raskind, M.: Paranoid syndromes in the elderly. In *Treatment of Psychopathology in the Aging,* edited by C. Eisdorfer and W. E. Fann. New York, Springer Publishing Company, 1982, pp. 184–191.
32. Bridge, T. P., and Wyatt, R. J.: Paraphrenia: Paranoid states of late life: European research. *American Geriatrics Society* 28(5):193–200, 1980.
33. Lopez-Ibor, J.: Delusional perception and delusional mood: A phenomenological

and existential analysis. In *Phenomenology and Psychiatry*, edited by A. J. J. Koning and F. A. Jenner. New York, Grune and Stratton, 1982.

34. Bowers, M. B.: *Retreat from Sanity: The Structure of Emerging Psychosis*. Baltimore, Penguin Books, 1974.
35. McDonald, N.: Living with Schizophrenia. *Canadian Medical Association Journal* 82:218–221, 1960.
36. DSM-IV, 1994, p. 129.
37. Roberts, J. K.: *Differential Diagnosis in Neuropsychiatry*. New York, John Wiley, 1984, p. 158.
38. Murray, G. B.: Confusion, delirium, and dementia. In *Massachusetts General Hospital Handbook of General Psychiatry*, edited by T. P. Hackett and N. H. Cassem. St. Louis, C. V. Mosby, 1978, p. 98.
39. Roberts, J. K., 1984, p. 164.
40. Murray, G. B., 1978, p. 96.
41. Murray, G. B., 1978, pp. 93–116.
42. Roberts, J. K., 1984, pp. 161–164.
43. Barsky, A.: Acute psychoses. In *Emergency Psychiatry: Concepts, Methods, and Practices*, edited by E. F. Bassuk and A. W. Beck. New York, Plenum Press, 1984, pp. 195–218.
44. Barsky, A., 1984, pp. 195–218.
45. Bear, D., Freeman, R., Schiff, B. A., and Greenberg, M.: Interictal behavorial changes in patients with temporal lobe epilepsy. In *APA Annual Review*, vol. 14, edited by R. E. Hales and A. J. Frances. Washington, DC, APA, 1985, pp. 190–210.
46. Roberts, J. K. A., 1984, p. 239.
47. Hedges, L. E.: *Listening Perspectives in Psychotherapy*. New York, Jason Aronson, 1983, pp. 239–243.
48. Mendel, W. M.: A phenomenological theory of schizophrenia. In *Schizophrenia as a Lifestyle*, edited by A. Burton, J. J. Lopez-Ibor, and W. M. Mendel. New York, Springer Publishers, 1974, pp. 106–155.
49. Lopez-Ibor, J., 1982, pp. 135–152.
50. Landis, C., and Mettler, F. A.: *Varieties of Psychopathological Experience*. New York, Holt, Rinehart and Winston, 1964.
51. Fish, F., 1967, p. 16.
52. Asaad, G., 1986, p. 1091.
53. West, F. J., 1975, p. 307.
54. Landis, C., and Mettler, F. A., 1964.
55. McGhie, A., and Chapman, J.: Disorders of attention and perception in early schizophrenia. *British Journal of Medical Psychology* 34:103–117, 1961.
56. McGhie, A., and Chapman J., 1961, pp. 103–117.
57. Rosenbaum, P.: *The Meaning of Madness*. New York, Science House, 1970, pp. 73–99.
58. Deegan, P. E.: Recovery: The lived experience of rehabilitation. *Psychosocial Rehabilitation Journal* 11:11–19, 1988.
59. Lehman, H. E., and Cancro, R.: Schizophrenia: Clinical features. In *Comprehensive Textbook of Psychiatry IV*, edited by H. Kaplan and B. Sadock. Baltimore, Williams & Wilkins, 1985, pp. 680–713.
60. Lehman, H. E., and Cancro, R., 1985, p. 704.
61. MacKinnon, R., and Michels, R. P.: *The Psychiatric Interview in Clinical Practice*. Philadelphia, W. B. Saunders, 1971, p. 236.
62. MacKinnon, R., and Michels, R., 1971, p. 235.
63. Hogarty, G. E., Anderson, C., Reiss, D., et al.: Family education, social skills training, and maintenance chemotherapy in the aftercare treatment of schizophrenia. *Archives of General Psychiatry* 43:633–642, 1986.

CHAPTER 7

Personality Disorders: Reflections of the Social History

*T*he passionate hand is fleshy, resisting, hard, sometimes dry, always strong. The fingers are thick and rather short. . . . The passionate character is believing, powerful, active, inspired. It proceeds by a feeling for things and produced by a natural abundance. Capacity for work. Keen, enthusiastic, absorbed worker.

Anonymous
The Encyclopedia of Occult Sciences

*A*s the above quotation illustrates, for ages humans have enthusiastically attempted to classify each other. Such behavior seems to represent a trademark of the species, for better or worse. In previous centuries cheirologists attempted to determine the currents of personality in the physical characteristics of the hand. Today, such viewpoints have been appropriately relegated to the niche of the historically curious, an intellectual antique of sorts.

However, personality theory remains as intriguing today as it did for the cheirologists of the 18th century. In a sense, tremendous advances have been made in understanding both the normal and abnormal aspects of personality development. On the other hand, much remains to be learned. To be successful in the art of personality assessment, it is important to understand the limitations of current conceptualizations. It is also of value to arrive at an understanding of some of the controversies surrounding the various personality disorders, because probably more controversy is associated with this collection of disorders than with Axis I disorders. If these complicating factors are not understood by the clinician, they can seriously hinder the clinician's ability to utilize these diagnostic categories effectively in a fashion that may guide the clinician toward better methods of care.

Combined with the fact that there are 10 specific personality disorders in the DSM-IV, the above points suggest a slightly different approach than has been taken in the previous two chapters. Rather than attempt the exhaustive task of representing each diagnosis by a separate case presentation, smaller case illustrations will be liberally used to delineate diagnostic principles that may be generalizable to any personality disorder. The emphasis will remain on practical clinical points, utilizing both case histories and clinical dialogues. The task will consist of interweaving the controversies and subtleties surrounding these diagnoses into an understanding of the people beneath these labels.

To achieve this complex goal, the chapter is divided into two sections. In Section I, Clinical Principles Concerning Character Psychopathology, the necessary theoretical background is examined in detail, including basic definitions, a survey of the diagnoses, and discussions of various controversial issues regarding personality disorders. In Section II, Approach to the Interview, the effective utilization of this background in clinically problematic areas is directly addressed in a comprehensive fashion. Without further introduction, let us begin an exploration of an area of psychopathology that some would say represents the most enigmatic field of study that clinicians encounter on a daily basis.

SECTION I: CLINICAL PRINCIPLES CONCERNING CHARACTER PSYCHOPATHOLOGY

In Search of a Definition

To begin the discussion it is useful to look at an actual clinical presentation. We will refer to the patient as Mr. Fellows and begin by examining his history, which will then be complemented by a re-creation of a brief bit of dialogue from the initial interview.

Mr. Fellows was referred for outpatient psychotherapy. He had originally been seen in the emergency room with a subsequent referral for possible group therapy. After attending two group sessions, he left because "the therapist spent too much time listening to all those screwball people. And he was also an inexperienced therapist, that's for sure. I just didn't like him."

Mr. Fellows presented in a dirty plaid shirt and an unkempt army jacket. He was short in stature with a balding head from which his black hair emerged. His hair had clearly met a comb, but the meeting had not been for long. He quickly conveyed a feeling that he did not really want to be in the room. His handshake was overly firm and then suddenly weak, as if purposely avoiding prolonged contact. He wore a jaunty cap, which was a little worse for wear and had now found itself in his lap, a plaything for his fidgeting hands.

With regard to his history he had come from a tough neighborhood, and he had seldom felt at home there. "I didn't belong there, I'm a sensitive guy, and I felt things those other kids could never feel. But I beat it." He related having a very high IQ, and he indeed appeared quite knowledgeable and well read. However, he had always encountered intermittent problems in school. He had frequently been involved in arguments with teachers and tended to be a loner. He had had no problems with the law and seemed strongly opposed to violence and criminal activity. He considered taking drugs to be bad, yet he hesitantly admitted to drinking problems in the past.

He had never liked his father, who considered him to be a complete failure and had beaten him in the past. Over the years he had lost contact with most of his family, and he was generally not welcome in their homes. He viewed himself as talented, especially with regard to writing. Indeed, he had been working on a novel for years. He also boasted of his tendency to protect others from violence, and he carried a small canister of tear gas repellant with him.

Despite his abhorrence of violence, he reported a lifelong history of "finding the nearest argument." Apparently he often tended to dominate conversations, because "in all honesty I'm smarter than most of the people I meet." In short, he had developed the rather nifty habit of alienating people almost upon first contact. He was true to his style during our first session. The following dialogue occurred during the early phases of the body of the interview:

Pt.: That last therapist was a real loser. And I really don't see much sense in group therapy anyway. In fact if I really look at this realistically, I don't really need any help at this time.

Clin.: With that idea in mind what were some of your reasons for coming in for an evaluation today? Apparently you had been referred for outpatient psychotherapy.

Pt.:   In the first place I don't really like psychotherapists. I don't think you guys really know what you're doing anyway. I mean I had seen a therapist off and on for 6 or 7 years. He was O.K. but he charged more than he was worth. What you need to do for me today is to write a note saying that for medical reasons I need to live in a new halfway house. The one I'm at is situated in too dangerous a neighborhood. And that's all I need or want from you.

Mr. Fellows was clearly not meant for public relations work. At least he quickly got to his point. In the next session, when he was reminded that further evaluation was needed before I would consider his request, he became actively hostile and commented, "You don't give a damn do you, Doctor! For all you care, I could be mugged tomorrow, and it would be no sweat off your back. I hope someday you're being murdered and when you call the police, they say further inquiry will be necessary before we respond to your call!"

With regard to diagnosis, Mr. Fellows was eventually given the primary diagnosis of a narcissistic personality disorder. He also displayed antisocial, borderline, and paranoid traits. Indeed a rule-out secondary diagnosis was Personality Disorder Not Otherwise Specified (mixed: antisocial, borderline, and paranoid traits). On Axis I he continued to demonstrate alcohol abuse intermittently, although he had not been drinking for several months.

Subsequent therapy revealed that throughout his life Mr. Fellows had suffered from an intense feeling of vulnerability. The question, "Am I really worth loving?" was a rather constant companion, a shadow, from which he could not step away, no matter how hard he tried to inflate his self-esteem. He developed a series of defenses to protect himself from his pain, including a sense of entitlement, a tendency to put others down, fantasies and preoccupations with grandiosity, and a coolness in interpersonal contacts. This coolness could serve to protect him from the danger of imminent rejection, a rejection that had first surfaced in the form of abuse from his father.

We are now beginning to perceive the subtle workings of a disordered personality structure. In these conditions, the individual develops a series of defenses that can temporarily and in certain circumstances protect them from significant pain. Unfortunately these same defenses become rigid and small in number. The patient is left with a defensive structure that is inflexible and frequently ineffective in decreasing pain in the long term. Mr. Fellow's cool indifference and his tendency to put others down may indeed protect him from the potential pain of losing a loving figure, but it will ironically prevent him from ever developing such a relationship in the first place. Mr. Fellows does not know how to function otherwise, and therein lies the tragedy of the situation. The intensity of the loneliness and self-loathing can be enormous.

This point is important for the clinician, because it serves to reframe the obnoxious and irritating behaviors of people displaying various personality disorders in the light of a response to their pain and anxiety. Such a realization can help to decrease angry countertransference feelings, while serving to increase a sense of compassion. For instance, the same Mr. Fellows, who was so patently rude and demanding in these initial sessions, would later cry during the termination phase of his psychotherapy.

The story of Mr. Fellows also highlights another, sometimes easily missed point. The key to understanding adult psychopathology lies in an understanding of childhood and adolescent development. An adult psychiatrist cannot work in an intellectual vacuum, as if adult patients spontaneously appeared at 18 years of age. Many critical therapeutic interactions parallel parent-child behaviors and feelings. Indeed, these patients can quickly arouse parental responses in the clinician even during the initial interview. If unaware of these responses, initial interviewers can inadvertently disrupt blending.

With these ideas in mind let us look at the definition of a character disorder as viewed in the DSM-IV:

A personality disorder is an enduring pattern of inner experience and behavior that deviates markedly from the expectations of the individual's culture, is pervasive and inflexible, has an onset in adolescence or early adulthood, is stable over time, and leads to distress or impairment.[1]

The actual diagnostic criteria[2] are as follows:

General Diagnostic Criteria for a Personality Disorder*

A. An enduring pattern of inner experience and behavior that deviates markedly from the expectations of the individual's culture. This pattern is manifested in two (or more) of the following areas:
1. Cognition (i.e., ways of perceiving and interpreting self, other people, and events)
2. Affectivity (i.e., the range, intensity, lability, and appropriateness of emotional response)
3. Interpersonal functioning
4. Impulse control
B. The enduring pattern is inflexible and pervasive across a broad range of personal and social situations.

Box continued on following page

C. The enduring pattern leads to clinically significant distress or impairment in social, occupational, or other important areas of functioning.
D. The pattern is stable and of long duration, and its onset can be traced back at least to adolescence or early adulthood.
E. The enduring pattern is not better accounted for as a manifestation or consequence of another mental disorder.
F. The enduring pattern is not due to the direct physiologic effects of a substance (e.g., a drug of abuse, a medication) or a general medical condition (e.g., head trauma).

---

*Reprinted with permission from the Diagnostic and Statistical Manual of Mental Disorders, 4th ed., p. 633. Copyright 1994 American Psychiatric Association.

Several key points are beginning to emerge. In the first place, a personality disorder (or character disorder as it is sometimes described) is a historical diagnosis. The critical criteria for making the diagnosis lie in the patient's history, not in the patient's behavior in the interview itself. The patient's immediate behavior in the interview often provides important clues to underlying psychopathology, but the criteria for establishing the diagnosis lie in historical evidence. In a sense, a personality disorder leaves historical tracks.

The nature of these tracks varies significantly, but one of two elements will be present. Either the patient's rigid defenses result in behaviors, which are disturbing to other people, or in feelings, which are unsettling to the patient. By way of illustration, a person with an antisocial personality may steal the life savings of an employer who trusted the patient implicitly. The patient may have no regrets about such actions, but clearly the patient's behavior will have had a disastrous effect on the employer. Such behaviors are called ego-syntonic, because they do not disturb the patient. At the other extreme, a person with an avoidant personality may shun almost all social contact, while living in a self-imposed interpersonal tomb. This behavior may not really harm anyone else per se but results in significant personal distress. These types of behaviors are referred to as ego-dystonic, because they directly create subjective pain in the patient.

Some patients show a combination of ego-dystonic and ego-syntonic symptoms. However, in patients who display primarily ego-syntonic behaviors, an important point surfaces. These patients frequently are not strongly invested in receiving help, because their behaviors are not disturbing to them. Family members, lawyers, or administrators may have pushed such patients into therapy; consequently, these patients may be unusually difficult to engage in therapy. For the interviewer, functioning as a consultant, the presence of primarily ego-syntonic behaviors may suggest the recommendation that an experienced staff member be assigned to the case as opposed to a trainee.

But whether ego-syntonic or ego-dystonic, the behavioral manifestations of a personality disorder tend to result in specific types of interpersonal patterns, including parental relations, sibling relations, dating relations, employment patterns, and friendship patterns. In this fashion, the historical tracks of a disordered personality are usually found in the soft ground known as the social history.

The social history is not merely a sterile recording of "what job was held when" but represents an extremely sensitive mirror in which the reflections of a personality disorder may first appear to the alert clinician. Stated even more boldly, a totally normal social history is not compatible with a personality disorder. Somewhere along the line the pathologic personality traits will disrupt interpersonal relationships. Later in this chapter various methods of effectively gathering the social history in this light will be described.

In uncovering personality disturbances the clinician must actively search for consistent patterns of behavior, demonstrated from adolescence onward, without major disruption of these patterns. In this regard, Mr. Fellows serves as a suitable illustration. His defensive patterns appeared early in his life. His social history was littered with weak relationships, a poor job history, an unending string of arguments, and a maladaptive grandiosity. These behaviors were consistent over time and were undeniably crystallized by late adolescence.

A natural next question focuses on the etiology of such unchanging patterns of behavior. Theoreticians could spend—and have spent—a large amount of time discussing the numerous conflicting theories regarding etiology. However, a recapitulation of their work would not be time well spent in a text of this type. Instead a simplified and unifying approach will be described, which can help guide the interviewer toward a more sophisticated understanding of the person seeking the clinician's help.

The shaping of a personality structure can be viewed as a matrix of sorts, consisting of three interdependent factors: (1) physiologic factors, (2) psychological factors, and (3) environmental/interpersonal factors. Together, these fluctuating influences will eventually determine the anxieties and need states that will result in the development of specific unconscious defense mechanisms and conscious coping strategies of the organism.

In the physiologic realm, Thomas and Chess have emphasized the point that small infants display characteristic temperaments, which can persist into later stages of life.[3] These variables include intensity of reaction, activity level, attention span, threshold of response to stimulation, mood, and distractibility. Both genetics and intrauterine factors could influence the development of such traits. One can easily see how such factors could play a significant part in the determination of personality structure.

For example, if a child was born with a propensity to be easily distracted, the child may have significant problems with learning and also with obeying rules. The child might literally have problems attending to a parent's commands. Here we see the matrix effect, because this physiologic component will both affect and be affected by the other two realms mentioned earlier. The child's seemingly intentional disobedience and poor school performance may disturb the child's parents. Frustration and anger may result, even in high-functioning parents, who may tend to show displeasure and subtle rejection of the child. Perhaps a sibling will become "the apple of Daddy's eye."

Considerably more problems will arise if the child has been born into a family already steeped in psychopathology. An alcoholic parent may beat the child, probably only resulting in a child who is further unable to concentrate and learn secondary to fear and agitation. The cycles begin to feed and regenerate each other. Marital disharmony may intensify as arguments ensue regarding the management of the bad behavior of the child. On the other hand, a child with a relatively normal attention span may be born into such a chaotic household. Soon the child may become chronically anxious, and in this sense environmental influences may actually trigger physiologic changes.

In any case, the child will begin to develop psychological defenses in order to function at a reasonable level of anxiety. The theoretical child, described earlier, could easily become more reclusive and timid; or the child may develop a conception of himself or herself as being inferior and unwanted. The result may be the development of distancing tactics that protect the child from rejection or the development of grandiose thinking. These tactics function to buffer the child from feelings of worthlessness. Perhaps these were the types of factors that jointly combined to create Mr. Fellows, the theoretical child in the flesh.

No easy explanations exist. It is relatively meaningless to bicker over which element of the matrix was most instrumental, because with each individual this mixture will vary. Moreover, in most cases, the resultant personality is a reasonably healthy one. This chapter concerns itself with those instances in which an inflexible set of defenses emerge.

In the DSM-IV, an attempt is made to characterize behavior, not to explain it. In this modest fashion the DSM-IV may help provide more reliability in the labeling process, thus allowing research to eventually provide more clues as to etiology and hopefully improved treatment techniques. In this vein, the criteria for determining personality diagnoses in the DSM-IV are not etiologic in nature. The DSM-IV acknowledges the fact that any of the factors listed above may play a part in the development of character psychopathology.

To serve as an illustration, let us look at the criteria used in the diagnosis of a narcissistic personality disorder, the diagnosis used with Mr. Fellows.

NARCISSISTIC PERSONALITY DISORDER[4]

Diagnostic Criteria for 301.81 Narcissistic Personality Disorder*

A pervasive pattern of grandiosity (in fantasy or behavior), need for admiration, and lack of empathy, beginning by early adulthood and present in a variety of contexts, as indicated by five (or more) of the following:

1. Has a grandiose sense of self-importance (e.g., exaggerates achievements and talents, expects to be recognized as superior without commensurate achievements)
2. Is preoccupied with fantasies of unlimited success, power, brilliance, beauty, or ideal love
3. Believes that he or she is "special" and unique and can only be understood by, or should associate with, other special or high-status people (or institutions)
4. Requires excessive admiration
5. Has a sense of entitlement, that is, unreasonable expectations of especially favorable treatment or automatic compliance with his or her expectations
6. Is interpersonally exploitative, that is, takes advantage of others to achieve his or her own ends
7. Lacks empathy: is unwilling to recognize or identify with the feelings and needs of others
8. Is often envious of others or believes that others are envious of him or her
9. Shows arrogant, haughty behaviors or attitudes

---

*Reprinted with permission from the Diagnostic and Statistical Manual of Mental Disorders, 4th ed., p. 661. Copyright 1994 American Psychiatric Association.

These criteria are fairly representative of the criteria used in the DSM-IV for the delineation of personality disorders. The criteria range from those traits of a more subjective nature, such as fantasies of unlimited success, which the clinician would depend on patient self-report to determine, to more objective criteria such as arrogant, haughty behaviors or attitudes, which are more behavioral in nature and could be reported by friends or family. Of special interest is what is not here. Specifically, the DSM-IV purposely avoids criteria that would be tied to a specific etiologic theory.

For example, one does not find criteria such as "the patient has not adaptively integrated his grandiose imago with his idealizing imago." This particular criterion would represent one of several psychoanalytic models, in this instance the work of Heinz Kohut. It can be seen that the inclusion of such criteria could lead to many problems, including clinician bias away from diagnoses because of a disagreement on theoretical grounds, clinician ignorance of the meaning of specific terminology, and the need for clinicians to "read into" the facts in order to recognize a diagnostic criteria. All of these factors could lead to disturbingly poor inter-rater reliability, a flaw that essentially prohibits productive research. In this attempt to produce more reliable criteria, the DSM-IV represents an important advance.

As with most advances, there are some accompanying limitations, and the DSM-IV system is no exception. As clinicians, it is important to remember that these diagnostic labels do not necessarily shed significant illumination on the person behind the label. This is the penalty that one pays for not basing the diagnoses on dynamic formulations. It also emphasizes the fact that these diagnostic labels serve a valuable function only when the clinician understands their development and limitations. They do provide a foundation for predicting treatment selection and a powerful method of learning from the writings of previous clinicians who are using the same criteria; however, they do not explain the person sitting in front of us. The DSM-IV has never purported that diagnoses should be used as explanations. Instead they serve as useful maps, suggesting possible avenues of exploration, as the clinician attempts to understand the reasons that this particular patient has developed these particular behaviors.

In order to use these diagnoses intelligently, another ramification of their development deserves attention. Some of these diagnoses, such as the antisocial personality, are based on extensive empirical research and historical validity. Other categories, such as the narcissistic personality, have less empirical research behind them. Indeed, some authors feel that this lack of empiricism may result in the inclusion of diagnoses that will not survive the "test of time"; in short, they may lack validity.[5] For instance, the DSM-III-R diagnosis of "passive-aggressive personality" was dropped from the DSM-IV for such reasons, yet may be added to future editions if research data validate it. Diagnoses under consideration, such as passive-aggressive personality, are described in Appendix B of the DSM-IV.

But let us see how all this controversy can affect the clinician directly. The narcissistic personality serves as a good example. A significant problem consists of the fact that in attempting to read about a specific diagnosis, various authors may be describing strikingly different types of people, while applying the same diagnosis. For example, the criteria for the narcissistic personality tend to follow the conceptualizations of Theodore Millon. The emphasis is on a person who tends to exude a sense of overconfidence and superiority. As long as the patient's abilities parallel the existing expectations, these people may be reasonably happy and certainly may function at a high level of achievement. The personality structure is supposed to develop from a parenting pattern of overattention and favoritism. This is the classic "spoiled child," who can be so frustratingly pompous and demanding as an adult.

In contrast to this relatively well-functioning individual, albeit a rigidly structured personality, the DSM-IV criteria could also be met by a person with a remarkably different history and psychological structure. Kohut and colleagues have elegantly described this type of personality. These people also appear grandiose and demanding, but these defenses are the result of poor self-esteem. The world is seen as hostile and threatening, a place teeming with rejection and competition. Their poorly evolved sense of self results in marked periods of depressed mood, even in relatively benign environments. Anger and resentment are daily personality accessories. Mr. Fellows is an excellent example of such a person. These people are strikingly more disturbed than many of the narcissists described by Millon, and yet both types of people could conceivably fulfill the criteria of the DSM-IV for a narcissistic personality. This overlap suggests a diagnostic category whose criteria are too broad to ensure appropriate discrimination.

We have reached a point in which our search for a definition has begun to wind down. An attempt has been made to demonstrate that to intelligently utilize the diagnoses subsumed under the category of personality disorders, one must understand the development and limitations of the system. The case of Mr. Fellows has served to illustrate some of the complexities inherent in the system. In retrospect one could say that just as a species must evolve, each individual personality must also undergo a gradual evolution. This development can be affected by the elegant interplay of various factors, including physiology, environment, and psychology. When such evolution is disrupted, maladaptive behavior patterns emerge, which have been described as personality disorders. To understand the pain of these patients, the clinician must move beyond the label into a study of the patient's personal development. In this idiosyncratic history, the interviewer will find the constellation of factors that have spawned the aberrant behavior, essentially trapping the individual in a prison defined by the unyielding walls of his or her own personality structure. At this point it may be valuable to take a closer look at these puzzling disorders as they actually present to the clinician.

Survey of DSM-IV Personality Disorders

One cannot begin a discussion of these disorders without touching upon the unifying concept of Axis II itself. In DSM-I and DSM-II, a multiaxial approach was not taken. This unidimensional scheme of conceptualization ran the risk of leading unwary clinicians into simplistic formulations. One of the great advances of the DSM-III was the introduction of a diagnostic formulation that essentially forced clinicians to view the patient as an integrated whole, not just as a "case study." On these five axes the clinician was to explore not only evidence of hard-core psychiatric illnesses such as schizophrenia but would also consider the patient's personality structure, the physiologic factors, the immediate stressors, and the abilities of the patient to function adaptively.

Axis II was created in an effort to emphasize the importance of assessing the patient's character structure in all instances. In certain individuals, it was felt that disorders of personality could be primarily responsible for psychiatric dysfunction, without an accompanying Axis I diagnosis. Even in the presence of Axis I psychopathology, such as a bipolar disorder or an anxiety disorder, it was felt that the underlying character structure could significantly affect the manner in which the Axis I disorder would manifest itself. For instance, the development of a bipolar disorder, at age 25 in a person with an underlying borderline personality, may present a strikingly more complicated picture than a bipolar disorder in an otherwise high-functioning individual. Questions also began to arise as to whether certain personality disorders might predispose individuals to develop specific Axis I diagnoses.

The DSM-III also advocated an extremely flexible system of nomenclature, which has been further developed in the DSM-III-R and DSM-IV. If the patient fulfilled the criteria for more than one personality disorder, then each disorder should be listed separately. A separate category was created for those individuals who did not fulfill the criteria for any specific disorder but who demonstrated a personality disorder that seemed to be created from bits and pieces of different disorders. These patients are to be listed as having a personality disorder not otherwise specified (mixed personality disorder) with the specific traits listed. It should be noted that this diagnosis is only for patients who do not fulfill the criteria of any of the already described personality disorders. A common mistake would be exemplified by taking a patient who fulfills the criteria for both an antisocial personality and a histrionic personality and labeling him or her as a mixed personality. Instead, such a patient should have both diagnoses listed separately, as mentioned above.

The DSM-IV demonstrates ultimate flexibility by also allowing the clinician to essentially use diagnostic labels not even delineated in the DSM-IV itself. For example a clinician may find a utility in the diagnosis of an inadequate personality, which is not listed in the DSM-IV. The clinician could utilize this diagnosis by writing personality disorder not otherwise specified (inadequate personality). Theoretically, one could even coin new personality disorders under this heading. In this regard several potentially new personality disorders, such as the "depressive personality disorder" and passive-aggressive personality disorder (which may still prove to be valid), have been included in Appendix B of the DSM-IV.

Further flexibility appears, in the DSM-III and subsequent editions, with the listing of maladaptive personality traits on Axis II. This allows a clinician to target a specific trait, such as narcissistic entitlement, for therapeutic intervention, even though the person does not display a full-blown narcissistic personality disorder.

In a similar attempt to provide a more realistic picture of the patient, the DSM-IV also suggests the listing of defense mechanisms (e.g., denial, isolation, and repression) on Axis II. All in all, it can be seen that the development of Axis II, despite some of its problematic issues, represents many important innovations in clinical emphasis, which many would say were long overdue.

With the above ideas in mind, we can begin our survey of the diagnostic entities themselves. It is crucial that the clinician become thoroughly familiar with the actual criteria, because the diagnoses are made by a careful expansion of these diagnostic regions. On the other hand, the criteria are somewhat sterile sounding in nature. One of the first steps in gaining a proficiency is the development of a general sense of what the core characteristics of each disorder actually look like. The clinician must gain a sense of these disorders not as checklists but as living individuals. In the following survey an effort will be made to provide some flesh to the individual disorders, while pointing out some of the distinguishing characteristics between similar disorders. The reader should supplement the following descriptions by a parallel reading of the actual DSM-IV criteria.

To aid in the familiarization process, I have placed the 10 specific personality disorders recognized by the DSM-IV into three broad groups. These groups contain disorders that have some similar core characteristics with regard to how the patient experiences life. If during the course of the initial interview, the clinician recognizes these more pervasive world views, then an immediate cluster of diagnostic regions for more extensive expansion suggests themselves. Each clinician can determine his or her own ways of organizing the personality disorders. The following system merely represents a method that I have found practical. In any sense, the three broad categorizations are as follows: (1) anxiety prone disorders, (2) poorly empathic disorders, and (3) psychotic prone disorders (referring to a more frequent tendency to develop micropsychotic episodes as described in the previous chapter). It should be noted that the DSM-IV uses a very similar set of clusters (i.e., odd-eccentric (Cluster A), dramatic-emotional (Cluster B), and anxious-fearful (Cluster C).

ANXIETY PRONE DISORDERS

This cluster includes the following three disorders: obsessive-compulsive personality, dependent personality, and the avoidant personality. All three of these disorders share the common thread of an existence riddled with tension and anxiety. They differ in how this anxiety manifests itself and with which methods it is controlled. This is not to say that other personality disorders do not cause anxiety, because they can. Instead it merely suggests that anxiety is often a keynote feature of these three disorders. These patients are also susceptible to intermittent bouts of depression, which may occur when their needs are not met or their defenses are not adequate.

Obsessive-Compulsive Personality Disorder

A person who has an obsessive-compulsive personality sees life from the inside of a pressure cooker. It is a pressure cooker constructed from the patient's own set of perfectionistic goals and demands. In short, these patients are hard on themselves. Driven by an internal sense that any failure is an ultimate failure, they help to form the army of workaholics, who both love and resent their work. In a sad sense, these people frequently function under a covert belief system that they must prove themselves worthy of being loved. Thus there is no time for fun, and they often appear too serious for their own good, while presenting a somewhat cool and distant exterior. Deep inside there seems to be a fear that they are about to lose control. Consequently, life becomes a series of contests that are won through discipline and endless lists and work schedules. Patients with an obsessive-compulsive personality truly show their colors when they produce an innately paradoxical "schedule for play." Even free time is a commodity to be well spent. Moreover, major decisions rapidly become major hurdles, because the patient becomes terrified of the chance of making a wrong decision. Life is viewed as a long corridor of one-way doors, few of which lead to "success." It is a costly lifestyle, filled with stress. It is a way of life in which tears may not be shown but are felt nevertheless.

Dependent Personality Disorder

As with the previous disorder, a person with a dependent personality views the world as a place filled with disaster; however, the resultant anxiety is handled in a different fashion. The compulsive person throttles the anxiety by fiercely attempting to control all possible situations. The passive-aggressive individual mutes the anxiety by saying, "I never expected much from this lousy show anyway." In contrast, the dependent personality runs from the anxiety, straight into the arms of some unsuspecting surrogate parent. Life is spent hunting for this savior. White knights are not the inhabitants of fairy tales; they are the invited dinner guest. These patients are exquisitely sensitive to rejection, but they are willing to risk humiliation if the reward is eventual safety. Consequently they are often warm and giving, bordering precariously on the cusp of obsequiousness. They are more than willing to bend to the needs of others; indeed, they thrive on receiving the chance to prove their irreplaceable devotion. Because they view themselves as weak and ineffectual, they do not want to make decisions. Moreover, their intensely low sense of self-esteem traps them into a fear that they could not make it on their own. This type of person is unable to leave the spouse-abuser, and his or her unfortunate answer to insecurity is the safety of slavery.

Avoidant Personality Disorder

Affection and love are two conditions that people with an avoidant personality hope for desperately. Unfortunately these goals remain mere dreams, because these patients suffer from such low self-esteem that they dare not risk making an attempt at friendship. If ever there were people who followed the credo "Any club that would accept me, I wouldn't want to belong to," it is this group of patients. Like dependent personalities, they feel inadequate, but their low self-esteem seems laced with a more brutal self-ridicule. These people literally do not generally trust themselves and essentially become socially phobic. Unlike the person with a dependent personality, they frequently appear aloof and cool, so as to protect themselves from the rejection they feel is a future certainty. They also tend to alienate other people with self-denigrating comments such as, "You probably don't want me along, but can I come to the movies too?" Such testing comments beg for a statement of acceptance from their targets, who may quickly tire of providing reassurance. Their timid demeanor may provoke ridicule from bullies and those predisposed to cruelty. Moreover they do not search for the "white knight" of the person with a dependent personality, because they would not even dare to address such a figure if found. It is a lonely existence. These are the patients who live in cities for years without making an effort to secure a friendship unless they feel absolutely certain that rejection will not occur. Every night is lost in the white flickering of television characters, who have no method of inflicting pain and who will reliably show up for the next date.

POORLY EMPATHIC DISORDERS

People with these personality disorders share a peculiar inability to empathize in the same sense, or with the same regularity, as most people. Their personal history may be littered with a trail of people who have felt betrayed and manipulated. On the other hand, the lack of empathy may be a reflection of a true lack of interest in human contact, as seen with the schizoid personality. In any case, during the initial interview, one may catch glimmers of a world in which the feelings of other people are of little worth to the patient. The manner in which this self-centered approach manifests may vary strikingly among the following four disorders comprising this group: the schizoid personality, the antisocial personality, the histrionic personality, and the narcissistic personality.

Schizoid Personality Disorder

The person presenting with a schizoid personality structure represents the classic picture of the quiet loner. If one were to picture an animal analogue, some type of mollusk comes to mind—one that is slow moving, has limited ability to reach out, yet is more than capable of living a shell-like existence, content to function as an isolated unit. There is a blandness to the world of these patients, both in their internal and external worlds. They tend to form few relationships and prefer the role of a wallflower. Emotions run neither high nor deep. Tenderness tends to be neither felt nor sought. They exhibit a relatively bland indifference to what others may think of them. Their lack of affective color may suggest the cool stamp of one looking down from the pedestal of superiority. This is seldom the case. In actuality, their "colorless" quality represents a muted palette. These people tend to lack both the need and the social skills to actively engage other people.

On the surface, they may sound somewhat like people with avoidant personalities. But the avoidant personality is a hotbed of anxious emotions stirred by a perpetual duel with predicted humiliation. A person with an avoidant personality actively flees people, whereas a person with a schizoid personality effortlessly glides through people with a minimum of contact. There is no fear of rejection, because there is no desire for acceptance.

Some mention should be made of another diagnosis with which the schizoid disorder is sometimes confused, but which, in reality, shares little resemblance, except with regard to the spelling of their names. A person with a schizotypal personality, like a person with a schizoid personality, may also have few friends and appear somewhat aloof and distant. But these patients are generally but not always rejection sensitive, much more like a person with an avoidant personality. Moreover, their world is seldom bland. On the contrary, it is extremely active, rich with bizarre and idiosyncratic emotions and conceptualizations, a bit like a dream on feet. Furthermore, the diagnosis of the schizotypal personality seems to be somehow related to schizophrenia and may later develop this Axis I diagnosis. To the contrary there appears to be no striking relation between the person with a schizoid personality and one with schizophrenia. Indeed the person with a schizoid personality is not generally prone to the micropsychotic episodes seen with certain other personality disorders.

Antisocial Personality Disorder

A person with an antisocial personality is a chameleon. At times he or she may appear somewhat withdrawn like the schizoid, but more frequently the person appears actively involved with others. With certain people this individual may appear belligerent and nasty. On a different night or with a different person, the individual may present as the epitome of charm. The reason for the deftness in style lies primarily in the fact that these patients are participating in a continual game in which other individuals exist as pieces to be manipulated and utilized as deemed fit. As a result, people with antisocial personalities are frequently at odds with the law and are noted for lying, cheating, drug fencing, job hopping, and paternity suits. Sex is a one-night affair, and the word "responsibility" is not listed in their dictionary. At their worst, these patients may be cruel, sadistic, and violent. It has been suggested that they seldom feel anxiety and certainly infrequently feel the anxiety born from guilt. Indeed, they live a life in which a superego seems to have never set foot in their psyche. In a surprising sense, these people frequently see their problems as arising from flaws in other people, as opposed to their own inadequacies.

Obnoxious as these patients may sound, Vaillant makes the humanizing point, that, in reality, they probably do or at least did feel pain.[6] Indeed, their amoral behaviors and world view probably are at least in part a reflection of defenses developed to deflect relatively intense pain. For instance, the apparent callousness of their relationships may in some cases represent a defense, protecting the patient from a fear of being engulfed by intense dependency needs. Ironically, people with an antisocial personality may very well be as entrapped as their victims, their distancing defenses taking them so far from human emotion that they may appear as monsters. But in the last analysis, they are all too human.

Histrionic Personality Disorder

There are probably few people who are as pleasant as a person on a "good day," who has a histrionic personality disorder and few as miserable as an unhappy one on "a bad day." On this adult see-saw, these patients attempt to live life as a child, hoping to find a perch on Daddy's knee. The world is seen through the eyes of an Impressionist painter, popping an occasional hallucinogen. They do not look at details and seldom remember them. The past is a blur of impressionistic images. Whereas the person dealing with an obsessive-compulsive personality collects the world in neat categories and cages, the histrionic patient gleefully unlocks all the doors. These patients feel little responsibility and demonstrate an unnerving sense of devil-may-care. With a forced eviction lying only days ahead, the histrionic patient may be focusing attention on courting a date met on last Friday night's dance floor. Somehow or another a new apartment is supposed to materialize.

There is no doubt that life is exciting for them, because they view themselves as if their life were part of a movie. They tend to demand center stage, and if lucky enough to be good-looking or talented, they may well end up center stage. Their life is a long string of over-reactions, tantrums, and lost loves. Beneath the dramatics is a painfully fragile self-esteem that is easily crushed. Behind the glamour, intense feelings of inferiority and neediness hide. They are powerfully dependent upon the applause of others for their own sense of self-worth. Keenly sensitive to rejection, they are constantly searching for reassurance and praise. People are manipulated to achieve these needs, and a person with a histrionic personality can little afford to empathize with the needs of those who may lie in his or her way. Suicidal gestures are not uncommon, but these gestures may be followed several days later by a bright smile, if "Mr. or Mrs. Right" has entered the picture. This ability to change moods rapidly, depending on environmental circumstances, is a hallmark feature. Like a child throwing a tantrum, one needs only to distract a person with a histrionic personality in order to make things better. Somehow, there is tragedy in all this glamour. Adults were not made to live as children.

Narcissistic Personality Disorder

As mentioned earlier, this category seems to house two rather distinctive types, which, for want of a better title, can be referred to as the stable and unstable variants. In the stable variant, the patient's narcissism appears to be well rooted. These patients actually view themselves as superior and frequently enjoy their own company. In contrast to this picture, with the unstable variant, the narcissism appears more as a defensive front, a type of pseudonarcissism. With these patients the grandiosity is more of a charade, hiding an intensely frightened ego.

Let us look at people with a stable narcissistic personality first. To these patients, other people exist as objects, whose reason to be is to comfort the patient. Other people are objects made to serve the "self" of the patient. This tendency, seen in both stable and unstable narcissistic personality disorders, has been referred to as conceptualizing the world through "self-objects." A person with this type of narcissism finds it difficult to view others as having needs. The world revolves around one god, and the god is "I." Like a small child, the narcissist's views of others may rapidly change from idealizing to denigrating. Mother is great if she buys the toy airplane and is a hated object if she denies the purchase. People with a stable narcissism are often the product of a spoiled upbringing, in which sharing was not common. Consequently, they never develop the ability to think of other's needs. It simply does not cross their minds. Naturally, few people locked into a narcissistic perspective are born with nearly the talents and skills they feel they have. Daddy's little girl may merely be another average kid to the rest of the world. To deflect this painful realization, these patients may preoccupy themselves with grandiose fantasies. It has been said that people who are neurotic build castles in the air, whereas people who are psychotic live in them. People with a narcissistic personality structure try to rent them. In many respects people with a stable narcissistic personality structure, especially if talented, may be reasonably happy, although they may be difficult to get along with. Problems arise if, for whatever reason, adulation and subservience do not come their way. In such instances they may pout, stomp about, or become depressed.

In contrast, a person with an unstable narcissistic personality tends to live in a much more hostile world. The sense of ego is actually poorly developed, and life is a constant threat. There lurks an incipient feeling of annihilation and a piercing feeling that the individual is truly worthless. This is defended against by the production of a grandiose style, not unlike that seen in the person with a histrionic personality. But the stakes are high, and these patients are easily wounded. Their defense may consist of a vicious rage, and they can turn on a friend in moments. Few people are trusted, and bitterness becomes a way of life. They are constantly fleeing humiliation, while gloating over the embarrassment of others. If dinner is not on the table on time, then one may find it angrily thrown on the floor. Tantrums and rages become second nature. They expect to be at the head of the line, and when this does not happen, a scene is to be expected. They are almost impossible to please and are prone to severe depressive episodes, because their needs are not met. Their personality structure is quite primitive, and they are prone to micropsychotic episodes. People with unstable narcissism are often not successful in life, because their behavior prevents advancement, while their mood swings make consistent work difficult. In other instances, they may demonstrate reasonably good impulse control in public or on the job, demonstrating their more primitive qualities in specific relationships such as with their therapist. Unlike the stable narcissist, the unstable narcissist is frequently sad and angry. Every day is a battlefield. They pretend to be Napoleon, but deep in their hearts they know they are a sham. Worse yet, they fear that others recognize the sham as well.

PSYCHOTIC PRONE PERSONALITY DISORDERS
This collection of disorders includes the borderline personality, the schizotypal personality, and the paranoid personality. If one looks at the patient's sense of self in these disorders, as indicated by their ego structure and spontaneous coping defenses, one finds that these people appear to be seriously delayed developmentally. Their defensive structure is reminiscent of the defenses used by tiny children, including magical thinking, preoccupation with internal fantasy worlds, and tendencies to act impulsively or out of rage. When pressured, they may experience micropsychotic episodes, as these defenses sweep them into a false reality. For this reason they are clustered as "psychotic prone." They could just as easily be referred to as the primitive personality disorders referring to the developmental immaturity of their ego structure. In this regard the histrionic personality and the unstable narcissistic personality, of the last section, at times may also function as primitive personalities. Let us begin our survey of these disorders with a special attention to the intense pain that coats their reality with a distinctive sense of impending chaos.

Borderline Personality Disorder
The person coping with a borderline personality structure experiences life as if there were no sense of inner self. If one could feel inanimate, like a piece of clothing hanging forlornly in a closet, then one can begin to appreciate the hollowness that haunts these people. Like the clothing, they feel empty unless filled by the presence of others. Like the clothing, they depend on others to give meaning to life. Consequently, they intensely dislike being alone, because it can

lead to sensations of impending annihilation and destruction. As a friend leaves the apartment, they may literally feel empty, as if a part of themselves were now absent. Their need for others is so great that they cannot understand how anyone who really cares about them could leave them alone. Thus their dependency quickly becomes a hostile one, as they resent the pain that others inflict upon them. When they feel slighted, they can rapidly escalate into rages, throwing glasses, breaking furniture, and screaming profanities. In this sense they are unpredictable, because they are so exquisitely sensitive to being hurt, that friends and lovers quickly tire of apologizing and eventually grow angry themselves. A high level of interpersonal stress is the standard price required to befriend these patients.

Without the presence of others, these patients frequently view life as colorless and boring. Consequently, coupled with their intense feelings of weakness and self-loathing, they may ceaselessly seek stimulation using drugs, sex, and eating to satisfy their feelings of emptiness. Their impulsive behaviors unfortunately may bring them into contact with superficial people, who promptly proceed to abuse them, thus fulfilling their worst fears. Fear of abandonment becomes a nagging companion, stoked by the fact that their unpredictable behavior and manipulative attitude frequently result in actual rejection.

Suicidal thought arises almost with a predictability. It may be coupled with a peculiar tendency to enjoy self-mutilation. These patients are notorious for delicately cutting at their wrists, burning themselves with cigarette butts and matches, and overdosing. When cutting themselves, they frequently report no pain. The self-mutilation seems to serve as a release for intense feelings of rage. Such bizarre gestures are often preceded by an argument or broken date. These periods of analgesia, while cutting themselves, probably represent fleeting periods of psychotic depersonalization. Other common micropsychotic processes include derealization and paranoia. In the last analysis these patients face a harsh world over which they feel they have little control. The picture is further darkened by the sense that they themselves are also out of control. They represent the stuff of which soap operas are made. They are "the glass people," delicate to touch, easily broken, and dangerous when shattered.

Schizotypal Personality Disorder

Like the person with a borderline personality, the individual with a schizotypal personality seems to lack a core. This person also is stalked by a rather unsettling sensation that he or she is somehow empty. This blandness becomes an invitation to an inpouring of vivid fantasy and psychotic-like process. The world becomes peopled with clairvoyant messages, ghost-like presences, magical hunches, and secretive glances. Like a child withdrawn into a world peopled with pretend playmates, the person with a schizotypal personality silently retreats from life. Unlike a person with a schizoid personality described earlier, a person struggling with a schizotypal personality disorder is frequently sensitive to rejection. This person wants contact but does not know how to make it. There is a desperate quality here, in which the eccentric professor finds more solace in his books than with others of his species. One of my adolescent patients would spend endless days running with stray dogs in the woods near his house. Apparently they were kinder companions than the children at his school. Moreover, he was "the king" of his dogs, whereas he was merely "the dog boy" at his school. Thus these fantasy wanderings may provide a firmer sense of self-esteem to these patients. Because of their withdrawal into their private worlds, these patients may develop idiosyncratic ways of thinking and using words, tending to become metaphoric and vague. Unfortunately, these traits result in further problems with socialization. When stressed, the person with a schizotypal personality may decompensate into micropsychotic episodes, including delusions and hallucinations. In a sense, this individual lives life from "the inside of the bottle," peering at others as if watching a different species, worried that someone may poke a finger or two into his or her private world.

Paranoid Personality Disorder

The world of the person with a paranoid personality is blanketed by a thick covering of restless worrying. Probably more than any other disorder discussed so far, these patients see the world as a hostile environment. These patients have never evolved the ability to trust other people. As a consequence they are suspicious and guarded by nature. They scour their interactions with others for the subtlest hints of deception, often ignoring the bigger picture as they fixate on a slip of the tongue or an errant look. Their paranoid ideation, except during micropsychotic episodes, is not delusional in quality, but nevertheless, they seem driven by it. It is as if they feed on their own concerns. One is left with the feeling that without their fears, they would feel awkward and without purpose.

Their defensive guardedness has generally arisen to protect them from a deep-rooted sense of inferiority. Moreover, they fear that their weaknesses will leave them vulnerable to attack. In response they become haughty, finding it extremely difficult to admit mistakes. All new faces represent potential enemies, not potential friends. Everything needs to be checked out. By way of illustration, during an initial interview one of my patients suddenly produced a notebook in which he began vigorously scribbling down our dialogue. He related that, "I'm just keeping a record so that people on the outside know what's going on in here." It is a lonely existence. It is also one in which delusional thinking can erupt, because the paranoid patient's isolation prevents him or her from receiving corrective opinions from others. These brief delusional micropsychotic breaks are often accompanied by tremendous feelings of rage and indignation. These patients are also predisposed to more severe disorders on Axis I, such as a paranoid disorder. In the final analysis they are exquisitely unhappy. In a true sense they lead tortured lives, because everywhere that they look they see men with black hoods. Ironically, it is the hands of their own projections that weave the hoods.

We have now completed our survey of the various personality disorders. The above descriptions are meant to convey a general feeling for the manner in which these disorders may present. An attempt has also been made to convey, in a phenomenological sense, some of the ways in which these patients experience life. Only with this type of compassionate feeling for the patient can the clinician become skilled at detecting the possibility of a personality disturbance during the initial interview. It remains important to realize that the above descriptions are, in actuality, caricatures of a sort, useful as they may be. In reality patients present with nuances and variations that a short description cannot hope to convey. Only by listening carefully to many patients while attempting to actively empathize can the clinician gain a clearer understanding of the individuality of the person seated across from him or her.

Having completed our survey, it may be useful to examine some of the problems associated with the diagnostic system in actual practice.

Common Problems Associated with Determining an Axis II Diagnosis

A variety of problematic issues arise when attempting to utilize the concepts described thus far. These problems cluster into two main areas: (1) problems with diagnostic reliability and validity, and (2) problems created by the interviewers themselves.

Looking at the first area, one difficulty that strikes the eye is the fact that many of the personality disorders seem to share characteristics with each other. All the disorders that we have collected under the heading of psychotic prone personalities also tend to experience anxiety on a frequent basis. In this sense they share this quality with the disorders described as the anxiety-prone disorders. On a more specific level, a significant degree of people with a borderline personality will also fit the criteria of a histrionic personality. The more overlap found in a diagnostic system, the more likely that the system will have trouble distinguishing between entities. At some level this is a problem of sorts for the DSM-IV, which manifests as a propensity for patients to carry multiple diagnoses on this axis. It is hoped that in the future this overlap will be decreased, but some overlap is a natural outcome of the complexity of personality structure. One would expect to see considerable overlap in this area because, in actuality, these diagnostic categories are merely labels into which reality is sometimes uncomfortably forced to fit.

This criticism leads to a related problem. Some of the criteria used in the diagnostic descriptions tend to be vague or depend on subjective interpretation by the interviewer. For example, in the diagnosis of a person with a histrionic personality we find the following types of items listed:

1. Is suggestible; that is, easily influenced by others
2. Shows self-dramatization, theatricality, and exaggerated expression of emotion
3. Interactions with others are often characterized by inappropriate sexually seductive or provocative behavior.[7]

Although these characteristics appear simple enough, one wonders how flirtatious one has to be in order to fulfill criterion 3. And what exactly does an exaggerated expression of emotions look like in order to be viewed as pathologic? Obviously each clinician is left to decide these issues somewhat idiosyncratically. One of the real dangers arises when clinicians are unaware of their own personality traits both pathologic and not pathologic. In these instances the clinician may accept clearly pathologic behavior in the patient as not bad enough to fulfill a specific criterion. For example, a clinician may possess a hefty dose of dramatic and reactive behavior. This clinician may subsequently view the patient's dramatic behavior as "quite all right, I might do the same thing myself if feeling pressured." Such blind spots can significantly affect the inter-rater reliability of the Axis II diagnoses.

This discussion leads into the second category of diagnostic problems, those problems related not so much to weaknesses in the diagnostic system but to the clinician's misconceptions. The first common problem to be avoided is the tendency to make personality diagnoses too rapidly, without actually determining whether the patient truly fulfills the criteria or not. This problem manifests itself frequently, when clinicians diagnose in an impressionistic fashion, saying things such as, "That patient is clearly a borderline, she was so manipulative during that interview." The behavior of the patient in the interview and the clinician's intuitive feeling for the patient's pathology are extremely useful tools. But they are tools whose usefulness rests in guiding the clinician towards diagnostic regions that merit further detailed exploration, perhaps even in future interviews if time does not allow appropriate immediate exploration. The major point remains the fact that personality disorders are historical diagnoses, and the patient's behavior in the interview provides suggestive, not conclusive, evidence.

This point is far from academic in nature. It is extremely important clinically. So far we have emphasized the overlap among various Axis II diagnoses. In actuality, superficial overlap may exist between diagnoses on Axis I and Axis II when one considers the immediate behavior of the patient in the interview itself. A patient may present in a dramatic fashion with a seductive blouse and brightly colored pants. The patient may talk with a mild pressure to her speech, demonstrating a knack for telling a colorful tale. The same patient may act coyly and may be caught by the clinician in several trivial lies.

An inexperienced clinician may immediately label this patient as having a histrionic personality, but this diagnosis is being made on the recent and immediate behavior of the patient. In actuality, the patient may be in the early stages of a first break manic episode. A careful interview might have uncovered that this extroverted behavior is quite atypical for this patient historically. In addition, the patient may have a long history of depressive episodes as well as a positive family history for bipolar disorders. With regard to treatment, this patient may benefit significantly with a trial of lithium. Unfortunately the impressionistic diagnostician may not "get the point" until the patient turns the corner into a blatant manic crisis. A dramatic patient presentation could also be seen with other Axis I diagnoses, including an atypical bipolar disorder, a cyclothymic disorder, and amphetamine abuse or some other drug-related disorder. An even more ominous problem would exist if this abnormal behavior was secondary to an organic agent such as a brain tumor.

The impressionistic diagnostician can also run into problems around the issues of countertransference and labeling theory. Stated simply, the various diagnoses on Axis II often carry a connotation to them, frequently pejorative in nature. If a clinician takes a rapid dislike to an abusive patient, then the patient may rapidly become "just another god damned sociopath." One would like to think that one is "above that process," but few if any clinicians are. In this sense it is important for clinicians to explore what these diagnoses mean to them on a personal and emotional level. It also serves as a reminder that these diagnoses should not be made casually, because they can greatly affect the future course of therapy for the patient. I have certainly seen patients refused by a clinic because "he's a borderline and we don't treat borderlines."

It also serves to warn us not to fall into the trap of using these diagnoses as stereotypes. In a positive sense they can provide valuable information that allows the clinician to learn from the writings of others and to eventually lead to a better understanding of the patient. However, they do not delineate the specific characteristics or prognosis of any patient. It may be true that people with an antisocial personality tend to do poorly in therapy, but it does not necessarily mean that the patient sitting in front of the clinician will do poorly. Within each of these personality disorders there exists a wide range of characteristics and responses.

The above cautionary points are important in guiding the clinician toward a wise use of these diagnostic entities. But if these cautionary points are taken to their extreme interpretation, they become damaging in themselves. In this sense clinicians can become essentially phobic toward the idea of making a personality diagnosis in a single hour. One might hear the clinician state, "I never make a personality diagnosis in an hour; it takes much longer to know a person and make sure they present in the same way over several sessions." Ironically this misinterpretation of the concept of a personality disorder hinges on the same error in thinking seen with the impressionistic interviewer. Specifically, the clinician is stating that the diagnosis is being made primarily upon how the patient presents. But we have just seen that a hypomanic patient could present for months in a style totally consistent with a histrionic personality.

The pertinent point remains that personality disorders are not made primarily upon the basis of the patient's presentation. They are historical diagnoses. The issue is not whether the patient presents for seven sessions with histrionic behaviors but whether the patient has displayed histrionic behavior consistently for years dating back to adolescence.

In this light the limiting factors in making the diagnosis in the initial session are two-fold: (1) Does the clinician have enough time to explore the past history of the patient appropriately? and (2) Is the patient providing reasonably valid information? If the above two criteria are met, then one can safely make a personality diagnosis in an hour. The truth of the matter appears to be that some diagnoses are more easily made in an hour and some may be difficult to make in an hour. Those that are easier tend to have behaviorally oriented criteria that do not depend much upon the subjective opinions of the clinician. For instance, the antisocial personality, the borderline personality, and the schizotypal personality depend heavily upon fairly concrete criteria. As a case in point, either the patient has or has not been suspended from school. Either the patient has demonstrated self-mutilating behaviors outside of periods of Axis I pathology or no such behaviors have occurred. These behaviorally oriented diagnoses can fairly frequently be made in a single hour, as long as the patient is telling the truth.

On the other hand, those disorders in which the criteria are highly subjective may be quite difficult to make in an hour, for the clinician must cover a wide variety of historical circumstances in order to determine whether or not the patient typically demonstrates the behaviors in question. This category of disorders, which are difficult to diagnose in an hour, includes entities such as the histrionic personality and the narcissistic personality.

In actual practice a talented clinician who actively pursues clues to personality dysfunction and who persistently hunts for diagnostic criteria will usually have a good idea as to whether a personality disorder is present or not. With the more behavioral diagnoses, this may result in an actual diagnosis or perhaps a provisional diagnosis or at least a set of rule-out diagnoses. In the more elusive diagnoses the clinician should at least have a feeling for possible rule-out diagnoses and, at times, even the elusive diagnoses may be made in an initial assessment. Interviews with family members and other sources are particularly valuable in clarifying personality diagnoses when the picture is not clear.

The interviewer who appears overly cautious risks a variety of consequences. In the first place the attitude itself tends to make these interviewers sloppy in approaching these diagnoses because, "if you can't make the diagnosis, then why try?" In a sense they become self-fulfilling prophets. Because they do not practice delineating the skills needed to make these diagnoses efficiently, they indeed cannot make them efficiently in one or two interviews. But even more important is the fact that it may be a disservice to the patient to not spot these diagnoses until it is too late.

This is particularly true in the case of the consultant or the intake interviewer, who may be asked to suggest treatment approaches or may actually triage the patient. If the patient is determined to either fulfill or nearly fulfill the criteria of a borderline personality, the head of an outpatient psychotherapy clinic would be ill-advised to refer this patient to one of the inexperienced clinicians or worse yet to a clinician demonstrating serious psychopathology. In short, it is of value to recognize these diagnoses early. As another example, a psychotherapist may significantly change such parameters as the frequency of sessions, depending on the presence or absence of a primitive personality disorder. It might be detrimental to accept for therapy such a patient if the clinician intended to move from the area in the next 6 months.

We have ended our discussion of the numerous factors that can affect the clinician's ability to utilize Axis II diagnoses effectively. It is hoped that the survey of the disorders also provided a beginning sense of the enormous pain that sometimes envelops these patients and the people who care about them. In the next section we shall get down to the actual art of interviewing these patients, who represent a complicated challenge even for the experienced clinician.

SECTION II: APPROACH TO THE INTERVIEW

*S*ometimes she [Emily Dickinson] would only talk to acquaintances from behind a closed door. She fled from approaching visitors and refused to appear when friends or guests came to see her. She surprised one visitor, who was permitted to see her, by allowing him to choose between a glass of wine or a rose from the garden. Whenever possible, she avoided conversation, preferring to communicate with people in writing.

A. M. Hammacher
Phantoms of the Imagination[8]

Validity Techniques: Keys to Eliciting Sensitive Material

When one speaks of the approach to the interview, one is in some sense speaking of the clinician's approach to life as well. More precisely, a clinician who is prone to passing moral judgments will probably have great difficulty in both interviewing and subsequently working with people who have developed the character structures that we label as pathologic. A gentle compassion is needed in order to convey the unconditional positive regard of Carl Rogers discussed in Chapter 1.

This point is important because many of the traits that the clinician must explore in order to detect the presence of character pathology are traits that may arouse considerable guilt in the patient. If the clinician conveys a judgmental attitude, this guilt will generally be intensified, frequently to the point that the patient will feel uncomfortable, undergoing not a therapeutic exchange but a public humiliation. A clinician's parental glance may punish as effectively as a scarlet letter.

Besides unsettling the patient, such behaviors by the clinician serve to sabotage the interview itself, because the more that the patient's self-system is activated, the more likely it is that information will be distorted or withheld. Indeed the skill of a clinician to uncover character pathology seems to greatly parallel the ability to ask questions regarding sensitive material in an unassuming and natural fashion. The sensitive material may range from inner feelings of despair, which are not necessarily viewed in a negative light by society but that are viewed as intimate feelings by the patient, to activities such as drunkenness, promiscuity, and criminal activity, which are clearly frowned upon by the society. It is not that the clinician condones such activities, but rather that the clinician views them as aspects of the human condition and as reflections of human pain. The clinician listens in an effort to understand the patient, not in an effort to chastise the behaviors chosen by the patient.

In this regard a variety of techniques exist that can help the clinician to approach sensitive material without conveying that the clinician is "digging for bad material." Some of these techniques are also specifically geared to decrease the likelihood of deception, thus increasing the likelihood of a valid database. When utilized effectively, these techniques can result in the elicitation of sensitive material that one might think would never be revealed in an initial assessment. And indeed it would not be revealed had not the patient been provided a safe environment for sharing.

SHAME ATTENUATION AND RELATED TECHNIQUES

Let us look at one technique, "shame attenuation," which operates upon a clever premise. The problem with many sensitive questions lies in the fact that if the patient answers positively he or she is in essence admitting a failure. The natural result is a feeling of shame, which can clearly act as a deterrent to open expression on the part of the patient. For example if the clinician asks, "Do you have a drinking problem?", many patients will answer negatively, unless they have already reached a degree of insight that has led them to acknowledge their alcohol abuse. But in the following example we will see a different approach:

> **Pt.:**   I guess some of my best times are with my friends. I really would rather be with my male friends than with my wife and some of her losers. Talk about boring, they invented the word.

> **Clin.:**   Are these the same guys who are your drinking buddies?

> **Pt.:**   Yep. They're the ones.

> **Clin.:**   Well where do you guys like to go for a brew?

> **Pt.:**   All over the place (patient chuckles). We'll tie one on anyplace anytime.

Clin.: Well it sounds like you enjoy your drinking and your friends. You know, some people have problems holding their liquor, and others are pretty good at it. How about you, are you pretty good at holding your liquor?

Pt.: Oh, I don't have any problems holding my liquor. I'm not the best mind you, but I can hold my own.

Clin.: Can you hold down a pint or a fifth in a single night?

Pt.: Sure, a pint, no problem.

Clin.: How often in a given week do you put down a pint or more, in all seriousness.

Pt.: In all seriousness . . . I'd say 2 or 3 nights a week. Well, make that 2 nights. It's usually only on weekend nights that I really go after it.

In this example the clinician has phrased the question in such a way that if the patient answers affirmatively, then he or she is actually stroking the ego as opposed to admitting a flaw. In fact to admit that "I have problems holding my liquor," represents the answer more likely to produce shame: In this example the shame has been attenuated (indeed, it was almost reversed; in the first edition of this book, this technique was called "shame reversal"), hence the name "shame attenuation." This exchange is both more comfortable for the patient while also much more likely to yield valid data than a standard question such as, "Are you an alcoholic?" Of course one must also make sure that the patient is not purely bragging. This can usually be accomplished by subsequently delineating the actual drinking history via specific questions aimed at eliciting behavioral incidents, as this interviewer was just beginning to do.

This technique is so valuable that we ought to see it in a different context. In this instance the clinician is suspicious that the patient has had problems with angry exchanges on the job and has probably been fired several times. However, the patient appears somewhat cagey around this topic. Consequently the clinician utilizes the technique of shame reversal to create a safer environment for the patient.

Clin.: What have your jobs been like?

Pt.: Oh, nothing special, I've always gotten along O.K.

Clin.: Ever have any problems on the job?

Pt.: Nah, none worth mentioning.

Clin.: How about with bosses, have you had any bosses who really seemed like they needed to be "big shots," you know, the kind that just like to get on somebody's case?

Pt.: Now that I've been asked, more than I care to think about.

Clin.: What do you do, do you tend to take the abuse or are you the kind of guy who likes to let the boss know where you stand?

Pt.: Oh, I let them know where I stand alright, nobody is going to just push me around.

Clin.: Well, what might you do if the boss seemed out of line?

Pt.: I'd tell him to get off my back, that's what I'd do.

Clin.: How do they usually react?

Pt.: Most of them back off.

Clin.: Any of them ever get mad and fire you?

Pt.: A couple have, but I didn't want to work for them anyway.

Clin.: How many times have you been fired, would you say five times, ten times?

Pt.: Hmm . . . maybe around five times, somewhere around there.

The actual phrase that represents the shame attenuation was, "What do you do, do you tend to take the abuse or are you the kind of guy who likes to let the boss know where you stand?" Once again the technique takes away the judgmental shame associated with a positive answer. Imagine the difference in response that might have followed a line of questioning that began with, "Are you unreliable at work or have you ever been fired?"

Patients who have abused their children infrequently during episodes of anger may find it very difficult to share this material, even though they feel they need help. Shame attenuation can ease their anxieties and lead gracefully into abuse issues with questions such as:

a. It can be pretty difficult to control a temper sometimes. Have you ever done anything that you really regretted when you flew off the handle, such as striking your wife or your child?
b. Sometimes parents can really be pushed to their limit, and they're

so upset they just feel like hitting their kid if they just cry one more time. Have you ever felt like that yourself?

An important point to remember with regard to the technique of shame attenuation is that the clinician must be careful not to side with the patient or condone the described behavior. Such overidentification gives a false impression to the patient and also conveys an inaccurate moral judgment. Instead, the clinician attempts to suspend judgment, while voicing the question in such a manner that the patient may respond from the perspective of how the patient sees it. Thus, although the sociopath frequently sees other people as the trouble makers, the clinician neither agrees nor disagrees with this stance. Moreover the phrasing of the question allows the person with sociopathic structure to express the world as it is seen through the patient's own eyes.

In their outstanding text, *The Clinical Interview Using DSM-IV*,[9] Ekkehard and Sieglinde Othmer demonstrate a technique that they call "induction to bragging," which takes shame attenuation one step further. As with shame attenuation, they believe that it is quite effective with people displaying a sociopathic character structure. In its simplest form, the clinician attaches a positive adjective to a behavior with a negative association, as with the following question, "Were you a good fighter?" In this simple form it is no different than shame attenuation. But when the clinician actually passes on a complement to the patient, in a statement preceding the question, then "induction to bragging" represents a new and distinct validity technique.

In this use of induction to bragging, the clinician begins with a complimentary statement, which makes it easier for the patient to "almost brag" about a behavior that is somewhat less than exemplary. Othmer and Othmer give an example such as, "You seem to be sly like a fox ...," a description that a person, shall we say, prone to deceit might find a bit more to his or her liking than, "You're a deceitful son of a bitch, aren't you?", not that a clinician would say the latter, although many of us have thought it. After making the above compliment, the clinician can then proceed to inquire about deceitful behavior in a more productive fashion, fueled by the patient's desire to live up to the compliment.

Let's see how induction to bragging can help a patient share self-incriminating information:

Clin.:   What other types of things did you and your buddies do back in high school?

Pt.:   Oh, we hung out together. I'm not saying we were a

gang or something, but we were somebody you don't mess around with.

Clin.:   Well, you are obviously very big and clearly work out regularly, I bet you don't take any shit from anybody? (induction to bragging) How many fights have you actually been in?

Pt.:   Oh, a lot. I could really hold my own.

Clin.:   Did you ever use a knife on anybody?

Pt.:   Don't need to. I got these (patient holds fists up and smiles). I used a tire chain on some guy once.

Unlike Othmer and Othmer, I like to limit the use of the term "induction to bragging" to those situations in which the clinician literally compliments the patient in a prefatory statement, so as to clearly distinguish it from shame attenuation. Another clarifying distinction between the two techniques can be seen when shame attenuation, like induction to bragging, is used as a preparatory statement. When used in this fashion, shame attenuation never conveys praise as with induction to bragging. Instead, with shame attenuation the clinician conveys that he or she understands the difficult conditions, as rationalized by the patient, that may have led to the problematic behavior as with, "It sounds as if the depression was really making you irritable at work (shame attenuation). How frequently did you get into an argument with your boss?"

Sometimes, despite our best efforts to convey unconditional positive regard, it is obvious that an overly conscientious patient is suddenly feeling an inordinate amount of shame about a "bad" behavior, that he or she has just revealed. Although the behavior may seem fairly insignificant to the interviewer, the interviewer should never forget that the accompanying shame in the patient may be far from insignificant. Such painful moments, experienced in the initial interview, may drive the patient away from the entire process of therapy if not addressed. At such times Othmer and Othmer sometimes employ another validity technique, which they call "exaggeration."[10]

Exaggeration is a technique for immediately decreasing a patient's inordinate shame, so as to increase the likelihood that he or she will continue to share sensitive material, while simultaneously securing engagement. In this sense the technique of exaggeration is probably best viewed, not so much as a validity technique, but as an engagement technique for increasing blending.

Exaggeration works by helping the patient understand that when his or her "shameful activity" is put into perspective with other types of human "wrongdoings," the patient's activity is not of great magnitude, highlighting the fact that you, as an interviewer, are far from aghast at the patient's revelation. Effective "exaggeration" requires a well-timed sense of humor by the clinician. When done well, as demonstrated below, it can release a marked amount of interpersonal tension that otherwise could have resulted in disengagement.

In this vignette, the patient is a conservatively dressed woman with her hair tied into a meticulous bun. She is a successful department store manager with a portable "time-clock" for a superego. She strives for perfection and expects it of herself. She has unfortunately developed a nagging generalized anxiety disorder, for which she has reluctantly sought treatment, despite the admonitions of her superego that "strong people do not go to therapists." In her social history she shares what for her is a major sin of the past, stealing a candy bar from a drugstore, when she was 10 years old. And even worse she got away with it. Up to this point the interviewer has established a nice rapport with her, but senses the surprising intensity of her shame:

Clin.: In the past, have you ever had any problems with the law or arrests?

Pt.: I was never arrested (pauses, eyes briefly turn to the floor). But I did steal something once. I know it was a wrong thing to do.

Clin.: Oh, what did you steal?

Pt.: I stole a candy bar when I was about 10. I feel badly about it. I know it wasn't right to do (patient appears clearly uncomfortable with herself and hastens to add): I haven't stolen anything since.

Clin.: So let me get this straight. At 10 years old you entered a store, pulled out a knife, stole $200 worth of clothing, pocketed $500 of jewelry, and, as you left, kicked the store owner's half-blind cat (clinician smiles).

Pt.: (Absolutely aghast) Oh my gosh no! (She suddenly catches on to the humor and smiles for the first time in 20 minutes.) Of course not (sheepishly smiling). I guess it wasn't that bad after all.

Clin.: Not bad (said with a feigned sternness). Why, you stole a Milky Way bar, didn't you! One of the big ones too, I bet. My gosh, I have a mind to call the cops right now, but the statute of limitations has probably expired.

Pt.: (Laughing and smiling) Okay, okay, I get the point. I take things too seriously sometimes (continues to chuckle).

Clin.: (With a normal tone of voice) You know, Jane, let me go out on a limb here. I bet you tend to get down on yourself pretty hard.

Pt.: Well, I guess you could say that (smiling).

Clin.: Maybe that is something we can take a look at in the therapy. It may be one of the reasons that you are so anxious. Does that sound like a good idea to you?

Pt.: Yes. I think that would be a very good thing to do. Although I'm a little bit afraid to do it.

In most cases, "exaggeration" is utilized by employing much shorter phrases. When it is done well, as with this delightful bit of interviewing, it can effectively transform some difficult moments.

SYMPTOM AMPLIFICATION

This technique is based on the fact that patients sometimes downplay the frequency or amount with which they have disturbing behaviors, such as the amount that they drink or the frequency with which they gamble. This distorting mechanism is bypassed with the technique of symptom amplification, without upsetting the patient by challenging his or her minimization. In fact, the clinician allows the patient to naturalistically use minimization as a defense. This task is accomplished by setting the upper limits of the quantity in question at such a high level that, when the patient downplays the amount, the clinician is still aware there is a significant problem. For a question to be viewed as symptom amplification, the clinician must suggest an actual number.

For instance, the clinician can, as was demonstrated in an earlier excerpt, ask about drinking behavior as follows, "How much liquor can you hold in a single night, a pint, a fifth?" When the patient responds, "Oh no, not a fifth, I don't know, maybe a pint," the clinician is still alerted that there is a problem despite the patient's minimizations.

Here are some other examples of symptom amplification:

a. How many physical fights have you had in your whole life, 20, 30, 40?

b. How many times have you tripped on acid in your whole life, 25, 50 times?

c. How many times have you actually struck your wife, 10, 20 times?

There is one important caveat to the use of symptom amplification. Be sure that you do not set the upper limit at such a high number that it seems absurd or creates the appearance that you don't know what you are talking about. Perhaps the funniest example of this error that I've had the fortune or misfortune to encounter was when a trainee asked a street-wizened junkie the following question, "When you've used peyote buttons, how many have you used at a time, 100, 200?" Besides providing an extremely hearty chuckle for the junkie, who immediately began imagining the single most nauseated human being in recorded history, it also provided the clinician with a mildly uncomfortable moment when the patient queried, after containing his glee, "You don't know much about peyote, do you Doc?"

DENIAL OF THE SPECIFIC

In denial of the specific, the clinician avoids asking generic questions. Instead, a series of quite specific questions about a list of activities are asked, which essentially force the patient to deny specific acts, while jogging the patient's memory. For example, instead of asking, "Have you ever used any street drugs?" the clinician asks a series of questions concerning specific drugs. It is generally more difficult to shade the truth in response to a specific question as opposed to a generality. In the following example, after asking a generic question, which yields very little information, the clinician will use a series of denials of the specific:

Clin.:   Have you used many street drugs in the past?

Pt.:   Oh . . . Not much, really.

Clin.:   How about coke (denial of the specific)?

Pt.:   No no, not really, it's too expensive.

Clin.:   How about if someone gives it to you?

Pt.:   (Patient smiles) Hey, I'm no fool. Sure, I'll run in the snow if it's falling.

Clin.:   Would you say 5, 10 times a week? (Note the symptom amplification.)

Pt.:   Nah, maybe three, four times a month.

Clin.: How about when you were younger, has there ever been a time when you used more coke?

Pt.: Oh sure, when I was in the first couple of years of college, I was probably snorting a couple of lines a day.

Clin.: Have you ever used speed (denial of the specific)?

Pt.: Now that's a drug that I can take or leave.

Clin.: What's it like for you?

Pt.: I just don't like it that much. I don't like coming down off it, crashing is no fun.

Clin.: Even though you don't like it very much, how many times have you used it in the last month?

Pt.: The last month, let's see, hmm, maybe two or three times.

Clin.: Was there ever a time in the past where you speeded for days at a time?

Pt.: Sure, when I was in college I might speed for 2, 3 weeks at a time. Hey, I was a Hunter S. Thompson. I was on the road to Vegas (patient chuckles), sort of wish I was there now.

Clin.: Have you ever used some type of downer like Quaaludes or valium (denial of the specific)?

Pt.: Well . . . some . . . not a lot. When I was speeding I'd sometimes use some ludes if I needed to come down. But nothing in years.

Clin.: How about marijuana, have you ever used marijuana (denial of the specific)?

Pt.: Yea, now that's something I've used a little more of.

The clinician's persistence is paying off. It is not infrequent for patients initially to deny or downplay the use of a drug. But if asked specifically about past use, a patient may then admit to heavier usage. Thus it is often a good idea with a drug history to probe both for the recent past and the distant past.

GENTLE ASSUMPTION

Pomeroy, Flax, and Wheeler[11] describe a technique, gentle assumption, which is powerful in its simplicity. It can be used any time the clinician feels that there is sensitive material that the patient may be hesitant to share. Such material may range from sexually related material to suicidal ideation, where it is particularly effective as we shall see in the next chapter.

In this technique the clinician assumes that the suspected behavior is occurring and frames a question based on this assumption. The technique was developed as a tool for doing research on sexual activity, where it was noted that questions such as, "How frequently do you find yourself masturbating?" were much more likely to yield valid answers than, "Do you masturbate?" If the clinician is concerned that the patient may be "put off" by the assumption, it can be softened by adding the phrase "if at all" as with, "How often do you find yourself masturbating, if at all?" If engagement has gone well, patients are seldom bothered by gentle assumption. Let's look at some examples:

a. What other ways have you thought of killing yourself?
b. What other street drugs do you like to use?
c. How frequently are your wife and yourself arguing?

With adults, gentle assumption can help open the door into the difficult area of sexual abuse with a question such as, "What type of sexual encounter have you ever had that you regret and perhaps was even forced upon you?"

On the other hand, gentle assumption should be avoided in any patient who is trying to please the interviewer or is prone to be easily led. Such patients may feel pressured by the use of gentle assumption to admit to behaviors that were not actually performed. In particular, I feel that gentle assumption is counterindicated with children, when questioning about abuse, because I feel that it can lead to false memories.

NORMALIZATION

In this technique the clinician phrases the question so that the patient realizes that he or she is not the only person who has ever experienced the behaviors or problems under scrutiny. This technique can be very useful in eliciting the sexual history as with, "It is not unusual for men at some point in their lives to have experienced problems with maintaining an erection. Have you had this type of experience?" But the technique is not limited to the sexual arena as evidenced below, starting with a question we had previously seen in Chapter 6 on psychosis:

a. People sometimes tell me that when they are extremely anxious, their thoughts sound almost like voices to them. Has this happened to you at all?

b. Sometimes when people get really angry they say things they later regret. Has that ever happened to you?
c. Sometimes when people are really worried about their weight, they will do things to make sure they don't gain weight like force themselves to vomit after a meal. Have you ever tried that?

Some students tend to confuse normalization with shame attenuation. Such confusion makes sense because they are both based on the same principle of unconditional positive regard and rationalization, but structurally they are easily distinguished by the base for the rationalization. In shame attenuation, the rationalization is always cued to the *patient's perceptions of the difficulties* that necessitate their need to do the problematic behavior, such as with, "Considering the marked financial disasters you've encountered over the past year, have you felt a need to be less than truthful on your income tax this year?" Contrast this with the following use of normalization where the question is *always* related to what *other people sometimes do,* "Sometimes people tell me that they feel comfortable withholding information on their income tax, have you sometimes felt that way or even filed a somewhat false report?"

A family practitioner described a useful variant of normalization in which the person referred to as the normalizing point of reference is the interviewer himself or herself. He uses this technique with patients suffering from severe diseases, such as AIDS or cancer, in which he feels the patient needs some help in moving past some denial, which has outlived its usefulness. An example would be, "Mike, I know that if I had learned that I had AIDS it would scare me a lot, I'm wondering if you are having some of those types of feelings?" This technique is simply called, "self-normalization."

FURTHER TECHNIQUES FOR ELICITING THE SEXUAL HISTORY

Taking a good sexual history can be uncomfortable for both the beginning clinician and the patient. Some of the techniques described earlier can be of value, but it takes practice with these techniques before one feels progressively at ease. In this regard the familiarization process can be speeded up by the use of role-playing or practicing the questioning while in front of a mirror. These drills help the clinician to focus on his or her paralanguage and body language, both of which play a pivotal role in helping the patient to relax during the sexual history. The clinician's nonverbal behavior should be identical to his or her nonverbal behavior during the rest of the interview. Sexual questions asked with a calm matter of factness usually result in matter-of-fact responses.

Some forms of leading questions can put patients on the spot as well. For instance, the question, "Do you have orgasms about

80% of the time?" may suggest to the patient that a response of less frequency is unusual or abnormal. This unwanted effect can be minimized simply by asking, "How frequently do you reach orgasm during sex?" But some clinicians feel that this totally open-ended approach can also generate anxiety, because it leaves the patient alone with his or her projections of what he or she thinks the clinician is expecting. This can be alleviated by asking a question that provides a range without any indication of what is wanted, but communicating, via the range, that any number is fine. By combining this approach with the use of normalization, the question takes on a nonthreatening tone as with, "Women vary a great deal on how frequently, if ever, they have an orgasm. What percentage of the time do you think you have an orgasm—5%, 20%, 80%, or almost never?"

Concerning sexuality, some patients will feel guilt about activities for which there is not necessarily a reason to feel guilt, such as homosexuality. Once again the clinician attempts to raise the topic in such a way that the patient does not feel awkward. For example, one useful method of approaching homosexuality is via the developmental history, utilizing normalization, as follows, "As adolescents mature they frequently experiment with different lifestyles and sexual preferences. When you were an adolescent, did you ever experiment with homosexual contact, perhaps to see what it was like?" One can continue the questioning into adulthood simply by asking, "In the long run some people prefer a homosexual or bisexual orientation to a heterosexual one, or vice versa. Do you have any preference at this point in your life?"

Moving to a different topic, the question of childhood sexual abuse can be difficult to discuss at times. Naturally, the topic will be spontaneously raised in some instances; however, sometimes there is nothing to suggest its presence. In these cases, a good way to screen for a history of sexual abuse often presents itself while the clinician is taking the family history for other psychiatric disorders. Suppose it has been uncovered that a parent has had alcoholism, then the following question, using a natural gate, can be quite effective, "With your Dad's problems with drinking, it is not uncommon for people to tell me that there was also a history of violence in the family or sexual abuse. Was that true in your family?" By now you will have recognized the timely use of normalization again, which further decreases the risk of disengagement with this approach.

Thus far we have reviewed various validity techniques that are useful in uncovering a diversity of phenomena, ranging from normal sexuality to pathologic drinking behavior. Perhaps, at this point, an interview excerpt can help to bring these techniques to life for us.

INTERVIEW EXCERPT ILLUSTRATING VALIDITY TECHNIQUES

In this example the patient was a lanky male approximately 27 years of age. He had come to the evaluation center on his own initiative because, "I just think things are going poorly at Trellway House (fictional name for a local drug rehabilitation center)." Although the patient complained of feeling depressed, he gave the impression that all of his problems were the result of the weaknesses of others. He was dressed in jeans and a faded plaid shirt. Apparently he was in the process of growing in a goatee that was tugged at intermittently. We will pick up the conversation well into the body of the interview, at a point at which the clinician decided to expand the antisocial personality region. Besides looking for the techniques just discussed, keep your eye out for a validity technique that we described in Chapter 1—that is, the behavioral incident.

Clin.: Tell me a little more about what is bothering you the most back at Trellway House.

Pt.: To begin with man you got to understand that I been living at Trellway for a couple of years now. And it used to be that we were really trying to get off the drugs and if you didn't pull your own way, hell, they'd let you have it, really have it. But not now, now they let them get away with too much, hell, I've seen guys regularly toking up on the back porch.

Clin.: It sounds like you don't really like some of the new people who moved in. Have you tried to talk to any of them about the changes that are happening?

Pt.: Hell, I talk to them man and they don't listen. These guys don't give a damn.

Clin.: Do some of them try to hassle you (shame attenuation)?

Pt.: Yeah sure, but that's all part of the game.

Clin.: Have any of them tried to push you around (behavioral incident)?

Pt.: Yeah, a couple of them but I set them straight.

Clin.: How do you mean (behavioral incident)?

Pt.: I kicked their asses.

Clin.: Well, you look like you're in pretty good shape, I imagine you can take care of yourself pretty well (induction to bragging). What about in the past, what types of fights have you been in (gentle assumption)?

Pt.: Oh, I been in a few now and then. People know not to mess with me. I grew up in a tough neighborhood and you had to know how to fight to survive.

Clin.: When you were fairly young, let's say between the ages of say 15 and 25, how many fights do you think you were in, 20, 30 (symptom amplification)?

Pt.: I'm bad but not that bad . . . oh, let's see, maybe about 15, who knows, it could have been as high as 20.

Clin.: Did you ever get hurt?

Pt.: Nah, not really, but I did a number on a few of those guys.

Clin.: Did you ever put anyone in the hospital (behavioral incident)?

Pt.: Yeah, there was one dude that I cut up pretty good, but he really deserved it, trust me.

Clin.: Earlier you told me that you drank a fair amount in the past but have completely stopped now, which you deserve a lot of credit for. Back when you were drinking, did you sometimes feel on edge almost like you needed a good fight, so you went looking for one, perhaps the alcohol making it a little more difficult to control your anger (shame attenuation)?

Pt.: Sometimes, yeah sometimes . . . especially if I was pretty strung out I would be just plain nasty, and I started my fair share of fights. But usually I was just protecting myself or the guy really had it coming to him.

Clin.: It certainly sounds like you know how to handle yourself in a fight (induction to bragging). Did you use to run in a gang or how did you learn how to defend yourself so well?

Pt.: Like I said, where I grew up you had to learn how to fight, and I did hang out with a gang for a couple of years.

Clin.: Oh, what were they called?

Pt.: The Blades. And we were a tough group, but not crazy, no way crazy, not like . . . like some gangs.

Clin.: If people hassled your gang or caused you problems (shame attenuation), how frequently did you do things to get back at them, like slashing their tires or smashing their windows (gentle assumption)?

Pt.: Yeah, we did that kind of shit. It looks pretty stupid now.

Clin.: Did you ever get suspended from school because you were out with the gang and the gang got you into trouble (shame attenuation)?

Pt.: Oh yeah, I was suspended maybe three, four times.

Clin.: What for (behavioral incident)?

Pt.: Fighting, cutting classes, the usual stuff.

Clin.: How do you look back at this stuff now?

Pt.: Well, I think a lot of it was pretty stupid, but it's what I needed to do. There were a lot of stupid people in that school and the principal came on way too strong.

Clin.: How did all the hassles at school affect your grades (shame attenuation)?

Pt.: I did all right, grades weren't a big hassle.

Clin.: What types of grades did you get (behavioral incident)?

Pt.: Mostly Bs and Cs. You see, I did some growing up back then and I eventually left the gang. I even did pretty good in history.

Clin.: Oh, what kinds of grades did you get there (behavioral incident)?

Pt.: Mostly Bs and I even pulled a couple of As.

Clin.: Sounds like you did real well there. What did you like about history?

Pt.: Uh, I liked learning about the past and I got into things like the Korean War and the Civil War. It's interesting, and the way I figure it you got to learn from the past, even from your own past, like my father he never learned from his mistakes, and that's why he is and always will be a jerk. But I learn from my mistakes.

Clin.: You mean sort of like how you turned your drug habit around?

Pt.: Exactly. I don't mess with nothing now, and I don't intend to in the future.

Clin.: You really did do well in history, did you ever have some difficulty with some courses?

Pt.: Sure, didn't everybody?

Clin.: What courses did you ever fail (gentle assumption)?

Pt.: I flunked algebra and I also flunked social studies, but that teacher was a farce. I'd like to catch up with her now.

Clin.: Did you ever have to repeat a year (behavioral incident)?

Pt.: No, but I had to go to summer school twice (chuckles). What a joke, I skipped out on that more than I skipped out during the regular school year.

Clin.: Jim, you mentioned earlier that your father had given you a rough time and that he would beat you if he felt you were pulling a fast one. Did you find that in order to protect yourself, you had to lie to him, keep him in the dark if you know what I mean (shame attenuation)?

Pt.: Yeah he was easy to fool. I could lie to him all over the place. I once told him that I was staying at school during remedial period for help in math, but that they had begun remedial periods an hour earlier than they used to. The old man bit on that one.

Clin.: What about now, do you feel like if you have to you are pretty clever at deceit or are you a lousy liar (shame attenuation)?

Pt.: (Chuckles) I can lie if I have to.

Clin.: In what kinds of situations would you lie if you had to?

Pt.: Well I'll tell you one thing, I ain't telling the old lady if I'm having an affair (patient chuckles). I ain't that dumb.

Clin.: You had been telling me about your childhood and it sounds like both of your parents were unpredictable and tough to be around at times. Did you ever run away to get away from it all (shame attenuation)?

Pt.: Yeah.

Clin.: How many times—5, 10, 15 times (symptom amplification)?

Pt.: I don't know, maybe around five or six times. But I always came back in a day or two. I don't know why, but I did.

Clin.: To get back at them, did you ever do things like set fires (behavioral incident)?

Pt.: No.

Clin.: Did you ever try to get revenge by sort of punishing them, perhaps by hurting one of their pets (behavioral incident)?

Pt.: No, but I did like to tease cats for awhile, a couple of us were doing that.

Clin.: What would you do (behavioral incident)?

Pt.: We'd stick a cat in a can and then kick it or sometimes we sprinkled the cat's tail with lighter fluid and then lit it.

Clin.: How do you view those behaviors now when you look back?

Pt.: That was weird and I don't think I'd do any of that now. I've learned that there's no use hurting things in this life man, and I'm really pretty much of a pacifist. I'm not out to push anybody around.

Clin.: Now if a boss was pushing you around or taking advantage of you (shame attenuation), how often would you get back by not showing up or slacking off some (gentle assumption)?

Pt.: Oh, I do that. If a guy is dumping on me at work, I just don't show up for a couple of days. See how he likes that. I'm nobody's stooge.

In this excerpt the clinician is eliciting a powerful history, filled with evidence of antisocial behavior, and yet the patient appears to feel comfortable. Part of this comfort may be related to this patient's tendency to not feel guilt, but a considerable part seems to be related to the clinician's skill at handling sensitive material. It certainly warrants taking a closer look in an effort to see the smooth intermingling of the various techniques utilized by the clinician.

In the first place the clinician is not taken in by the patient's superficial appearance of "being a good guy just minding my own business." In this light, people presenting with an antisocial personality frequently see themselves as the victims of circumstance, highlighted by a tendency to point their finger at a variety of nearby villains. This type of rationalization opens the gate for the use of shame attenuation, which allows a patient to utilize his or her rationalizations. In this interview the patient presents himself as a rehabilitated drug addict who is incensed that the rehabilitation program is not as strong as it ought to be. He may actually have many of these feelings, but there is more to the picture than he spontaneously presents, such as the fact that he has been in fights with several of his fellow residents. The deftness with which this clinician manages to uncover the underlying material results in many ways from his ability to take advantage of the patient's trait described above, namely of seeing others as the cause of his problems.

For example the clinician chooses to enter the potentially loaded topic of fighting, via the conduit of shame attenuation, by asking, "Do some of them try to hassle you?" referring to the patient's fellow residents who are supposedly abusing the system. In this fashion the topic of fighting has been brought up in a manner in which the patient will openly discuss his participation in fights, because no accusation has been made that he is starting them. And this is probably exactly the fashion in which this patient views most of his fights.

Once the patient is talking freely about fights, the clinician takes the opportunity to focus the interview towards a historical perspective by asking, "When you were fairly young let's say between the ages of say 15 and 25, how many fights do you think you were in, 20, 30?" It is important to focus the patient on specific periods of his life as opposed to just asking generally about the past. With a more specific focusing the clinician will gather much more data efficiently. Moreover, this question also illustrates the effective use of symptom amplification.

The clinician needs to discover whether the patient is indeed someone who is involved in fights primarily because of a violent neighborhood or whether the patient is frequently the instigator. This is not done by prematurely asking questions such as, "Do you pick a lot of fights?" Instead the clinician has waited until fighting itself has become a topic that has been discussed in detail and with ease. At this point the clinician moves towards uncovering the patient's role in these fights. If the patient denies any provocative role, the clinician does not know whether to believe the patient or not. On the other hand, if the patient openly admits to self-incriminating behavior, then the validity of the information is probably reasonably high. Towards this end the clinician's phrasing has associated the tendency to pick fights with the use of alcohol, thus providing the patient with something else to blame, in this case the bottle, for his own tendency to lose control. This is another example of shame attenuation.

Shame attenuation is used again when entering the issue of grades. The clinician asks, "How did all the hassles at school affect your grades?" as opposed to asking something such as, "Did you have any problems with grades at school?" Once again the clinician has allowed the patient to blame the hassles at school as the culprits as opposed to poor study habits. At this point we see the implementation of an important principle in effectively expanding a personality disorder region.

The clinician has been gently but persistently focusing the interview into the content region of antisocial behavior. But when the patient brings up a bright spot in his academic career, the clinician flexibly takes time to talk about this bright spot and to stroke the patient for his accomplishment with the question, "Sounds like you did real well there. What did you like about history?" This ability to skillfully pepper the expansion of the content region with facilitatory excursions and empathic interludes is pivotal to the development of the powerful blending needed to pursue sensitive material.

After allowing the patient to describe his interests in history and providing some positive feedback, the clinician returns to the topic of poor grades. This transition is made upon the tail of some positive reinforcement with, "You really did do well in history, did you ever have some difficulty with some courses?" The clinician eventually asks specifically about any failing grades. This quiet persistence frequently pays off with material that would otherwise be hidden or downplayed. Indeed this patient had previously stated that, "I did all right, grades weren't a big hassle." If the clinician had accepted this self-evaluation by the patient, then the truth that this patient had failed several courses and been required to attend summer school twice would never have surfaced. This is a reminder of the need to hunt for behavioral incidents when the emphasis is upon validity.

Eventually the interviewer utilizes a referred gate to bring the discussion back to the patient's childhood in an effort to search for evidence of early sociopathic traits. The referred gate was as follows, "Jim, you mentioned earlier that your father had given you a rough time and that he would beat you if he felt you were pulling a fast one. Did you find that in order to protect yourself, you had to lie to him, keep him in the dark if you know what I mean?" With this transition, the clinician has also managed to inquire about deceit in a fashion that is not antagonistic, once again offering a possible rationalization for the activity to the patient through the use of shame attenuation.

With his follow-up query, the clinician effectively utilizes the technique of shame attenuation yet again, "What about now, do you feel like if you have to you are pretty clever at deceit or are you a lousy liar?" With these techniques the clinician has actually reached a point in which the patient is openly admitting negative traits without any significant lowering of the blending process. This situation is providing a more valid database for the clinician, while also making the interview far less threatening for the patient. It is more likely that this patient would return to this interviewer than to one who probed for sociopathic material in a rigid and checklist fashion, as if interrogating the patient.

In the last question asked by the clinician, the interviewer illustrates the use of two validity techniques in tandem, an often powerful technique. The phrase, "Now if a boss was pushing you around or taking advantage of you" is a clear-cut shame attenuation. This proffering of a shame-reducing rationalization sets the stage for the effective use of gentle assumption, "How often would you get back by not showing up or slacking off some?" The two techniques re-enforce each other, helping to create an effective wedge into the patient's history of antisocial behaviors.

This example also illustrates a major point. Although this represents a rather lengthy excerpt, the actual time involved in the interview is probably no more than around 10 minutes. In this relatively short span the clinician is already close to having enough information to make not just a tentative diagnosis of sociopathy but an actual diagnosis of an antisocial personality disorder. This diagnosis could probably be solidified in another 5 minutes. In this regard a personality disorder is being uncovered in roughly 10 to 15 minutes of interviewing time, emphasizing that lengthy interviews or multiple interviews are not always needed in order to make these diagnoses.

We have completed a review of some of the techniques that may be useful in delineating a specific personality disorder as well as gathering sensitive material in general. What remains is to examine the methods through which the clinician first gathers hints as to which personality disorders may be present in the patient. We will also examine the reasoning that helps the clinician to choose the specific disorders to expand in detail, for the clinician can only hope to fully expand a few personality disorders or perhaps only one in a given hour.

Passively Scouting for Clues to Personality Dysfunction

The first step in making an Axis II diagnosis in the initial interview consists of limiting the field of diagnostic possibilities. No clinician could gracefully and sensitively explore the criteria of all 10 personality disorders in 60 minutes. The resulting interview would be hurried, stilted, and inviting of a "no show" at the next appointment. Instead, the clinician must figure out one or two (maybe three) diagnoses that are more probable. The second step consists of subsequently exploring these diagnoses in a thorough and sensitive fashion.

Throughout the interview the clinician has the opportunity to reflect upon both the patient's words and actions. In this sense, without actively searching for clues to personality dysfunction, the astute clinician frequently picks up on a variety of hints as to which disorders may be worth pursuing in more detail. In this regard the clinician can focus on the patient's behaviors and style of interaction (clinical signs) or on the patient's related complaints and history (clinical symptoms). Both areas are rich with implication, providing pertinent clinical hints, pointing the direction toward which Axis II diagnoses are most likely, for any interviewer who cares to read them.

SIGNAL BEHAVIORS

Since personality disorders represent long-standing patterns of behavior, it is not unusual for patients to reveal some of their pathologic behaviors during the interview itself. This does not always occur, but it frequently occurs. I am consistently amazed with the frequency of times that these signal behaviors occur in the first 5 to 10 minutes of the interview during the scouting period. This early appearance of characteristic defensive behaviors may result from the patient's anxiety stimulated by meeting a clinician. This self-system anxiety probably triggers many of the most ingrained defenses of the patient.

Earlier we discussed the mnemonic PACE as representing the mental activities of the clinician during the scouting period. If the reader will recall, the "A" stands for an assessment of the patient's mental status and behaviors. An important part of this assessment process is the clinician's careful openness to the presence of signal behaviors. Signal behaviors may also appear during any subsequent phase of the interview as well.

The signal behaviors represent signs suggestive of specific personality disorders that may warrant further investigation. They do not indicate that the patient necessarily has these disorders, because these behaviors may be present in personality disorders other than the ones listed or in people without character pathology at all. But what the signal behaviors do suggest is the increased likelihood that a particular disorder may be present.

Each clinician could probably develop a long list of signal behaviors gleaned from experience. In this chapter I am sharing some of those that have been most useful for me. Many others exist, and I am not attempting an exhaustive study here. The following observations are derived from clinical experience and do not represent research-validated data. Nevertheless, I think that they provide a useful jumping-off point for clinicians who are attempting to master the fine art of delineating character pathology.

One of the more peculiar signal behaviors is the presence of comments made by the patient during the interview about the interview itself or the interviewer. Most patients do not make such process comments, because they are inhibited by the newness of the situation and do not want to do something that is wrong. I remember a young man who was being interviewed by a student in front of a group of fellow students. The patient had a dramatic intensity and related several times that he was an extremely sensitive individual. It has been said that if one has a good trait, one never needs to tell others about it. Such was the case with this "sensitive" patient, for in the middle of the interview he turned to the obviously struggling interviewer saying, "You sure seem to be having a lot more trouble with this interview than me." If the clinician was not feeling awkward enough already, then this statement certainly pulled out a few more beads of sweat.

This practice of commenting on the process of the interview, frequently in a somewhat caustic fashion, is often a dead giveaway that the clinician is speaking with a person exhibiting one of the following three disorders: an antisocial personality, a histrionic personality, or a borderline personality.

A somewhat related signal behavior arises when the patient makes some type of unwarranted complaint during the interview itself. These complaints may be coupled with demands of a subtle nature and sometimes of a not so subtle nature. For example, a patient may walk in the door for the first appointment announcing that he or she does not intend to sit in the waiting room so long the next time. Or the patient may begin, "You really should get better parking arrangements for your patients, although I'm sure you've already looked into this matter before (topped off with a pleasant smile)." Such behaviors are often the window dressings of a person with a disorder such as the following ones: a borderline personality, a narcissistic personality, a paranoid personality, or an antisocial personality.

At the other extreme one may encounter the patient who seems a little too pleased with the clinician. These are the patients who drop gentle sexual innuendoes during the interview. This may consist of overly frank discussions of sexual adventures or may be more blunt, such as overt offers for a date or the request of a telephone number. In other instances the patient may turn on the charm with phrases such as, "Well, I've always seemed to be fairly attractive to the opposite sex, as I'm sure you have found to be true for yourself." These types of comments represent signal behaviors for disorders such as the following: an antisocial personality, a histrionic personality, and a narcissistic personality. If the innuendoes become more lewd or intrusive, one should become even more alert to the possible presence of an antisocial personality structure.

This type of behavior is similar to the patient who presents with a dramatic bravado. The patient may be boldly dressed in bright colors or a sinewy scarf. Breasts may be nearly bursting from tight sweaters or legs may be sensually wrapped about each other. The patient is frequently quite enthralled with the very act of talking about the history of the present illness while animatedly gesturing. Frequently the patient may rapidly become tearful and even more rapidly shut off the tears when the clinician asks a new line of questioning. These types of behaviors should serve as an indication that one may be in the presence of a person with a histrionic personality or a borderline personality.

Another type of signal behavior consists of the patient who appears child-like and helpless. These patients may speak with a quiet meekness, accompanied by an earnest attempt to please the interviewer with statements such as, "Is this what you wanted to hear?" As one would suspect such behaviors are often the trademarks of a dependent personality structure. Such helplessness is sometimes also seen episodically in people with histrionic personalities and with borderline personalities.

As a final example of a signal behavior, we can look at those patients who become openly manipulative during the interview itself. They may attempt to make the clinician grant them a request or make a condemnation of another clinician. For instance the patient may say, "My current therapist is very bossy. Don't you think that is strange for a therapist?" The patient then waits anxiously for the clinician to make a disparaging comment that will undoubtedly be fired as a verbal salvo at the therapist in question. Other types of manipulations may consist of various methods of controlling the interview or bargaining with the clinician, "Look it's getting late, if we must talk let's do it quickly and I need a cigarette first." Once again we've hit the province of the more primitive disorders, such as the borderline personality, the histrionic personality, and the narcissistic personality. Such "sighing compliance" may also mark a person presenting with passive-aggressive traits. (See Fig. 9 for a summary of signal behaviors.)

To wrap up this discussion of signal behaviors, an actual clinical example may serve to consolidate some of the ideas. The following activities occurred primarily in the minutes directly preceding the interview and in the first few minutes of the interview itself. The interview was taped for supervision purposes. The patient, who we had discussed earlier in the chapter on nonverbal behavior, had come to the Diagnostic and Evaluation Center because "I'm having problems coping." For the sake of convenience the patient will be

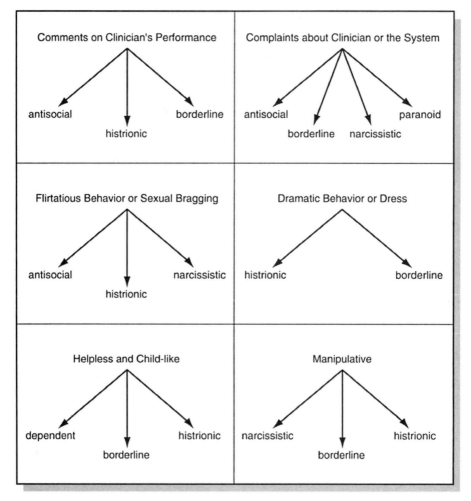

Figure **9**

Signal behaviors suggesting fan-like diagnostic possibilities.

called Ms. Dole. Ms. Dole was dressed somewhat shabbily with worn-out corduroy trousers and a faded blouse. Her dull brown hair seemed to "come with the outfit" in the sense that it too had seen better days, as it hung in long folds. Her lengthy hair accented her lanky body.

Both she and the clinician began placing their respective microphones. Ms. Dole fumbled repeatedly with her microphone, until her awkward machinations attracted the eye of the interviewer. Immediately before the clinician looked at Ms. Dole a most curious process unfolded. Ms. Dole had actually managed to get the microphone on, but she promptly pulled it off. As the clinician asked if she could manage, Ms. Dole looked up with pleading eyes and nodded her head from side to side, never saying a word. She looked like a 3-year-old asking her mother for help. And help was quickly on the way, because the clinician proceeded to attach the microphone for her.

When the interviewer began the actual interview, Ms. Dole quietly handed her some notes, mumbling that these would help the interviewer to understand. "I wrote them a few days ago," she meekly related. At which point the interviewer watched as Ms. Dole fumbled with the papers, taking about a minute to find the passage she wanted read.

Ms. Dole was managing to rapidly gain control of the interview by utilizing a mixture of helpless ineffectuality and manipulative staging. Her helplessness may have represented a signal behavior suggestive of the presence of a borderline personality or a dependent personality. Her manipulative gestures would also be consistent with a histrionic personality or a borderline personality. Subsequent detailed interviewing resulted in a diagnosis of a mixed personality disorder with histrionic and dependent traits. Thus the first 3 minutes of interaction provided powerful clues as to which diagnostic regions needed further exploration. Sometimes an interviewer's eyes are more useful than his or her questions.

SIGNAL SYMPTOMS

As the interview proceeds, the patient frequently relates symptoms or pieces of behavior that may function to guide the clinician toward consideration of specific personality disorders. Once again, as with signal behaviors, the clinician is not actively eliciting these symptoms. Instead, the patient is spontaneously providing them; the clinician needs to only passively recognize their importance.

Some signal symptoms are classic for certain disorders. This does not mean that these symptoms are seen only in these disorders but rather that they are frequently characteristic of these disorders. For instance, the presence of a history of self-mutilation or of frequent suicide gestures should always alert the clinician to the possibility of a borderline personality disorder. People with borderline personalities are notorious for behaviors such as wrist slashing, burning themselves with cigarettes, headbanging, and frequent overdoses.

Another classic signal symptom is the reporting by the patient of an extreme need for perfectionism. This is frequently accompanied by a nagging sensation that the patient has never done enough. It is the mark of a superego run amok and should strongly suggest the presence of an obsessive-compulsive personality or at least some compulsive traits.

A third relatively classic signal symptom is the reporting of a history of run-ins with the law. Repeated arrests, burglary, or frequent fights all strongly suggest the need to expand the antisocial personality region. Other areas to explore include fencing drugs, prostitution, and arrests for disorderly conduct or drunken driving. When asked about arrests, patients frequently conveniently fail to mention the last two types of incidents. It is often best to specifically inquire about disorderly conduct and drunken driving as well as speeding.

Other signal symptoms suggest not just one disorder but a variety of disorders. In a sense these signal symptoms suggest a fan-like differential diagnosis. The presence of frequent feelings of anger, sometimes accompanied by actual physical violence, alerts the clinician to the likely presence of either an antisocial personality or a borderline personality. Other less likely components of the fan include the paranoid personality, the narcissistic personality, and the histrionic personality.

A different signal symptom consists of an extreme feeling of low self-esteem. Such intense feelings of worthlessness and inadequacy are frequently seen in people with a dependent personality, avoidant personality, schizotypal personality, or borderline personality. Figure 10 illustrates some of the various signal symptoms and the possible diagnoses they suggest.

It should be kept in mind that the characteristics that were used earlier to group the various personality disorders may also serve as signal symptoms. Thus the reporting by the patient of powerful and persistent feelings of anxiety should alert the clinician to the possible presence of the obsessive-compulsive personality, the dependent personality, and the avoidant personality. In a similar fashion the antisocial personality, the histrionic personality, the schizoid personality, and the narcissistic personality are all suggested by a tendency for the patient to demonstrate a poor ability to empathize effectively. Finally, the presence of frequent micropsychotic breaks should alert the clinician to the potential presence of the primitive personality

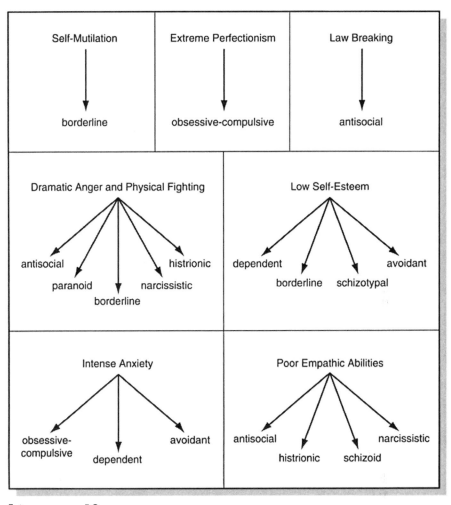

F i g u r e   **10**

Signal symptoms suggesting diagnostic possibilities.

disorders including the borderline personality, the schizotypal personality, and the paranoid personality.

It takes some time for clinicians to begin to routinely recognize the significance of signal behaviors and signal symptoms; however, with experience, the ability to utilize these invaluable clues becomes almost second nature. It should be readily apparent that many patients will in the course of 30 minutes practically point the way for the clinician as to the most likely paths to provide concrete evidence of personality psychopathology. However, the clinician does not have to rely solely on spontaneous clues by the patient;

rather, the interviewer can actively try to draw out evidence of personality dysfunction.

Active Scouting and the Finalized Delineation of Specific Personality Disorders

There is one other method of accomplishing the first step in personality assessment, that is, to limit the field. This technique consists of asking so-called probe questions[12] concerning a specific disorder. If the patient answers negatively to the probe questions, the clinician does not further expand that specific disorder. On the other hand, positive answers suggest that further questioning may uncover a specific disorder. The craft of delicately and thoroughly substantiating a personality diagnosis requires both skill and a sense of timing. The talented interviewer doggedly pursues the evidence needed to make the diagnosis but does so in a manner that fosters both a more powerful blending and an increased understanding of the patient not as a label but as an individual.

First let us examine a list of probe questions for personality disorders, several of which were developed by Jeremy Roberts.[12]

1. Obsessive-Compulsive Personality
   a. Do you tend to drive yourself pretty hard, frequently feeling like you need to do just a little more? (yes)
   b. Do you think that most people would view you as witty and light-hearted? (no)
   c. Do you tend towards being perfectionistic? (yes)
   d. Do you tend to keep lists or sometimes feel a need to keep checking things, like is the door locked? (yes)
2. Passive-Aggressive Personality (currently in DSM-IV Appendix)
   a. Do you frequently feel like your friends or employers tend to take you a little too much for granted? (yes)
   b. Sometimes have bosses tended to nag you, you know, ask you to do something a couple of times? (yes)
   c. If your boss asks you to do something that is stupid or that you disagree with, do you sometimes try to make a point by doing it slowly or without your full effort? (yes)
   d. When others are overly optimistic, do you tend to be the one who shows them the problems with their plans? (yes)
3. Dependent Personality
   a. Is it sort of hard for you to argue with your spouse, because you're worried that he or she will really get mad at you and start to dislike you? (yes)
   b. When you wake up in the morning, do you tend to plan your day around the activities of your husband or wife? (yes)
   c. Do you enjoy making most decisions in your house or would

you prefer that others make most important decisions? (prefers others to make the decisions)

   d. When you were younger, did you often dream of finding someone who would take care of you and guide you? (yes)
4. Avoidant Personality
   a. Throughout most of your life, have you found yourself being worried that people won't like you? (yes)
   b. Do you often find yourself sort of feeling inadequate and not up to new challenges or tasks? (yes)
   c. Do you tend to be very careful about selecting friends, perhaps only having one or two close friends in your whole life? (yes)
   d. Have you often felt hurt by others, so that you are pretty wary of opening yourself to other people? (yes)
5. Schizoid Personality
   a. Do you tend to really enjoy being around people, or do you much prefer being alone? (much prefers being alone)
   b. Do you care a lot about what people think about you as a person? (tends not to care)
   c. Are you a real emotional person? (no, feels strongly that he or she is not emotional)
   d. During the course of your life have you had only about one or two friends? (yes)
6. Antisocial Personality
   a. If you felt like the situation really warranted it, do you think that you would find it pretty easy to lie? (yes)
   b. Have you ever been arrested or pulled over by the police? (yes)
   c. Over the years have you found yourself able to take care of yourself in physical fights? (yes)
   d. Do you sometimes find yourself resenting people who give you orders? (yes)
7. Histrionic Personality
   a. Do people of the opposite sex frequently find you attractive? (answered with an unabashed "yes")
   b. Do you frequently find yourself being the center of attention, even if you don't want to? (yes)
   c. Do you view yourself as being a powerfully emotional person? (yes)
   d. Do you think that you'd make a reasonably good actor or actress? (yes)
8. Narcissistic Personality
   a. Do you find that when you really get down to it, most people aren't quite up to your standards? (yes)

    b. If people give you a hard time, do you tend to put them in their place quickly? (yes)

    c. If someone criticizes you, do you find yourself getting angry pretty quickly? (yes)

    d. Do you think that compared with other people you are a very special person? (answered with a self-assured "yes")

9. Borderline Personality

    a. Do you frequently feel let down by people? (yes)

    b. If a friend or a family member hurts you, do you sometimes feel like hurting yourself, perhaps by cutting at yourself or burning yourself? (yes)

    c. Do you find that other people cause you to feel angry a couple of times per week? (yes)

    d. Do you think that your friends would view you as sort of moody? (yes)

10. Schizotypal Personality

    a. Do you tend to stay by yourself, even though you would like to be with others? (yes)

    b. Do you sometimes feel like other people are watching you or have some sort of special interest in you? (yes)

    c. Have you ever felt like you had some special powers like ESP or some sort of magical influence over others? (yes)

    d. Do you feel that people often want to reject you or that they find you odd? (yes)

11. Paranoid Personality

    a. Do you find that people often have a tendency to be disloyal or dishonest? (yes)

    b. Is it fairly easy for you to get jealous, especially if someone is making eyes at your spouse? (yes)

    c. Do you tend to keep things to yourself just to make sure the wrong people don't get the right information? (yes)

    d. Do you feel that other people take advantage of you? (yes)

Responses in the indicated direction to one or two of these questions suggest that it would be worth the clinician's time to pursue the personality disorder in more detail. Some of these questions may overlap, and positive answers may be consistent with several different diagnoses. For example, if the patient responds positively to the probe question for the paranoid personality concerning jealousy, several other disorders may also be worth considering. Jealousy is commonly seen in people with narcissistic personalities, histrionic personalities, and borderline personalities. But an effort has been made in compiling these questions to list those questions that tend to be more specific for each of the diagnoses for which the question serves as a probe. If the patient responds positively to several or all of the probe questions, then it is significantly more likely that the specific probe diagnosis will eventually prove to be valid.

These probe questions are never used in a checklist fashion but are quietly woven into the fabric of the natural flow of the interview. The clinician will probably only have time to utilize a few of the specific probes for each diagnosis. Fortunately, in this sense, probe questions can often serve to quickly eliminate certain diagnoses. If one asks the following probe for schizoid qualities, "Do you really enjoy being around people or do you much prefer being alone?" and the patient responds, "Oh I love being around people, I'm a party animal" one can safely assume that a person with a schizoid personality is not in the room, unless it happens to be the interviewer. All levity aside, the point of the matter is that certain answers are inconsistent with certain diagnoses and no further probing would be required.

In point of fact, the clinician will probably not ask most of these questions, because the passive clues given by the patient as described earlier will automatically eliminate many diagnoses, while pointing the way toward those with more potential. Those areas with more potential can then be actively scouted by using several of the probe questions; and, if the diagnosis appears more likely, the clinician will proceed with a more thorough exploration in order to substantiate it.

One may wonder whether there are regions of the interview where it is best to utilize probe questions and to explore for personality dysfunction. The answer to this question is that the interviewer can utilize these techniques essentially anywhere in the body of the interview, but there is one area, the social history, in which personality pathology virtually leaps out at the interviewer, if it has not already done so in the history of the present illness.

As mentioned before, the social history represents the region of the interview in which patients inadvertently discuss the impact of their personalities on the people and jobs behind them. Many signal symptoms will be given here, and probe questions can be utilized effectively to determine which personality disorders warrant a more thorough exploration. Since the social history frequently is not taken in detail until a later part of the body of the interview, the blending has usually had time to develop strongly, thus allowing the clinician to more effectively explore the sensitive types of material frequently associated with personality disorders.

In the following example we will watch a clinician as he delineates which areas of personality dysfunction warrant more careful exploration. The dialogue occurs during the social history. Some of the clinical thinking that might be guiding such an interview is presented in brackets.

Clin.:   After you left college what happened?

Pt.:   Let's see, uh, I think the first job I took was with the electric company, but that job didn't really pan out to be what I was promised.

Clin.:   In what sort of ways?

Pt.:   Oh, the job was really boring and the pay wasn't so hot either. So I left after about 3 months and eventually got a job in sales. I liked that much better. I stayed there for, let me see, maybe a year, and then I had a whole string of jobs.

Clin.:   In the 5 years following that time how many jobs do you think you had, a couple, 20, 30? (symptom amplification)

Pt.:   Oh, pretty many, maybe close to 20 jobs. (The large number of jobs, in a relatively short period of time, certainly suggests that something is up here. An erratic job history is a signal symptom frequently suggesting the presence of an underlying antisocial personality, as well as a personality with a tendency for erratic relationships and impulsivity. Consequently the clinician asks several probes concerning sociopathy.)

Clin.:   Did anything ever happen on some of these jobs, like having a problem with the law or an arrest, that made you have to leave, because sometimes that's why people leave jobs quickly?

Pt.:   Oh no, not with me boy. I don't like the police. They terrify me. I've never been arrested or even pulled over for running a light.

Clin.:   Doesn't sound like you have a very extensive criminal record. (clinician smiles and patient laughs)

Pt.:   No, it sure doesn't. I don't break the laws. In that regard I'm a pretty straight arrow.

Clin.:   What about things like using drugs or selling drugs?

Pt.:   Nope, I wouldn't touch them, never even tried them. I just don't think it's right to use illegal drugs, that may sound sort of corny but it's true. (This patient shows little evidence of sociopathy, in fact he seems to have a fairly strong sense of what is right or wrong. Thus there must be something else going on. The clinician will now switch the focus more toward social interaction and friendships.)

Clin.: What kinds of things do you like to do for fun?

Pt.: Now that's a good question, because I don't have a lot of fun. I'm really pretty much of a loner. Sometimes I think that I just wasn't made to get along well with people, so I keep to myself pretty much. (Here various options are opening up. A person with a schizoid personality classically describes himself or herself as being a "loner," but such a person frequently holds jobs down well. Moreover, the openness and talkativeness of this patient earlier in the interview are uncharacteristic of the schizoid personality disorder. On the other hand, some of the disorders that are rejection sensitive lead to the avoidance of people as a means of protection. The clinician decides to figure out if the patient shuns people because he does not really want the company of people [as with a schizoid personality] or because he fears the company of people [as with an avoidant personality].)

Clin.: If you had some better skills at being around people, do you think you would like to do that?

Pt.: Oh yes, I have always wanted to be popular and sometimes I really do enjoy people. I love to laugh, but somehow I always end up getting hurt. (The schizoid personality disorder has been essentially eliminated, because such patients seldom if ever strive for social interaction in the fashion that this patient is describing. The feelings of inferiority and inadequacy expressed by this patient also make it unlikely that we are dealing with an entity like a narcissistic personality disorder.)

Clin.: Do you frequently feel let down or hurt by people?

Pt.: Very frequently. And to be quite frank it angers me, and that's why I've basically decided to keep my distance, but that's no fun either. And I resent that. Why should I be the one that suffers, what do they want from me anyway? (Plenty of important data are coming to light now. The patient truly sounds rejection sensitive. Entities come to mind such as the schizotypal personality, the dependent personality, the avoidant personality, the histrionic personality, and the borderline personality. That is quite a string of possibilities, but they can be decreased relatively rapidly. First, in an earlier part of the interview, when the region of psychotic material was being reviewed, the patient denied any psychotic material even of a subtle nature. Consequently the schizotypal personality is not worth pursuing. A careful sensitivity to the material already uncovered reveals another interesting point. People with dependent personalities and with avoidant personalities tend to stay in jobs for a long time, because they fear new situations and they tend to dislike the process of job interviewing or meeting new co-workers. To sort out this situation better, the clinician refers back to the job history, to see if the erratic history may be related to interpersonal problems with bosses or with co-workers. If frequent angry interactions are uncovered, then one could essentially rule out more timid entities such as the dependent personality and the avoidant personality.)

Clin.: Earlier you mentioned that you changed jobs frequently. Did you find that some of the people you were around were difficult people to work with (utilization of shame reversal)?

Pt.: As a matter of fact I did, some of them were very difficult.

Clin.: What types of arguments would you get into?

Pt.: The usual kind, you know, a boss who can't let you do your own work and who asks you to do things one way one time and another the next. I hate that. I never know what they want. Now don't get me wrong, I sometimes had something to do with it too, but not usually, at least I don't think so.

Clin.: Did some of the bosses get angry and ask you to leave?

Pt.: Yeah, I've been fired a couple of times if that's what you mean. And I think it's been 50-50.

Clin.: How do you mean?

Pt.: Fifty percent of the time my fault and 50% of the time their fault. (The demonstration of open anger, the firings, and the tendency to see a lot of other people at fault all essentially eliminate the dependent personality and the avoidant personality as suggested before. This pattern is also certainly not the job history of a person with a compulsive personality.)

Clin.: When you get angry, what do you do?

Pt.: Sometimes I really get furious. I go home and I let off steam.

Clin.: How do you mean?

Pt.: I don't know, break things, throw things . . . people just treat me like shit sometimes and it's not fair. It's not fair. That's why I get depressed all the time (angry tone of voice).

At this point the differential is becoming a good deal more manageable. We are left with the histrionic personality and the borderline personality. The patient's history is thus far consistent with both, but the histrionic personality seems less likely for several reasons. In the first place, not too many people with histrionic personalities view themselves as socially inept, and despite repeated painful experiences they seldom become more reclusive. The better bet is probably the borderline personality.

The anger-control problems are certainly consistent with borderline process. We are also starting to see, with her last statement, the possibility of the marked moodiness so often seen in people with borderline process. At this point the clinician has successfully limited the field. Time is probably best spent exploring the borderline criteria thoroughly and further checking of histrionic criteria. There is, of course, the possibility that the patient has a mixed personality disorder with borderline and histrionic traits. One could also add from the disorders in the appendix of the DSM-IV that this patient has some fairly striking passive-aggressive traits.

This example illustrates how quickly the clinician can begin to develop a differential along Axis II by utilizing passive techniques, such as recognizing signal behaviors and signal symptoms in conjunction with the more active technique of asking probe questions. What remains is for the clinician to skillfully expand the most likely diagnosis in a graceful and noninvasive manner.

To perform this second step in Axis II diagnosis, the clinician must become intimately familiar with the specific criteria for each diagnosis in the DSM-IV. Such familiarity comes both from conscientious study and, more powerfully, from experience. The process is greatly enhanced as the clinician develops a more sophisticated feel for the manner in which these diagnoses present and what it is like to be this particular patient with this particular style of "being in the world" in a more phenomenological sense. Once again the skillful blending of empathy, intuition, and analytic reasoning remains critical to the art of crafting a successful interview.

In order to delineate the principles behind performing a sensitive and thorough expansion of a personality disorder, we will focus on a single example to serve as an illustration. The enigmatic diagnosis of the borderline personality disorder will be examined in more detail. In some respects this diagnosis remains somewhat controversial. But despite its controversy, it stands as one of the diagnoses that, in certain instances, may more readily be made in a single interview, because many of its criteria are behavioral in nature. Those criteria, which are of a more subjective nature, tend to be unique enough that they are fairly easy to spot.

There is another reason to focus on this particular diagnosis. New and exciting advances have been made in helping people with borderline structure, such as Dialectical Behavioral Therapy (DBT).[13] This cognitive/behavioral strategy, which utilizes both individual and group therapy, was developed by Marsha Linehan and has shown great promise. However, you can't use it, unless you spot the diagnosis first. Fortunately, this diagnosis can frequently be made early on, even in the first session, if one knows what to look for.

Before continuing with an examination of the phenomenology of the disorder, it is of value to look at some of the thoughts regarding its etiology, because here is where much of the controversy resides. In my opinion, the radically unstable nature of the moods and perceptions of these people may truly be multiply determined. Some people who have this behavioral presentation may have developed it more from one etiology in one case and more from another etiology in a different case. Thus, some people displaying borderline structure may represent people with subaffective disorders, whose chaotic emotionality may be intimately related to biologic malfunction, much like some major depressions or dysthymic disorders. In this regard, it is not unusual to find patients who fulfill the criteria for dysthymic disorder as well as a borderline personality. Others may represent people with subthreshold seizure activity, which is missed by the equipment currently available to the electroencephalographer. Another percentage of these patients may prove to be people suffering from an unresolved attention deficit disorder as it appears in adulthood. The impulsiveness, moodiness, and inability to achieve stable relationships as seen with the borderline personality is highly reminiscent of the child with an attention deficit disorder with hyperactivity.

There may also be a subgroup of these patients whose problems stem mainly from more purely psychological and environmental difficulties. Frequently these patients have been significantly abused, often including physical and sexual abuse, at an early age. Some of these patients are best regarded as having significant developmental delays in their cognitive abilities, much as Piaget would describe cognitive deficits. This view has been championed by Gerald Adler in his book *Borderline Psychopathology and Its Treatment*.[14] For instance, these patients may not have fully developed such basic cognitive skills as being able "to see the gray" in situations as opposed to always seeing black or white, possessing an ability to consider past experiences when evaluating current experiences, or being able to develop a strong sense of object constancy (even with regard to themselves). A more thorough examination of these cognitive deficits will lead us into a richer understanding of the phenomenology of these patients, because the cognitive disturbances may actually be at the root of the rages and mood instability so commonly seen with borderline structure.

Taking just one of these deficits, the inability to see gray, the world of the person with a borderline personality becomes at once more comprehensible and intriguing. If the patient with a borderline personality must always clump experiences into extremes, then the simplest of frustrations or rejections may be interpreted quite naturally as a vicious attack. By way of example, if the clinician must cancel an appointment because of an unexpected meeting, then the borderline personality is limited, by his or her inability to see gray, into hearing from the clinician only one of two things, either "I care about you" or "I don't care about you." In this instance the words of the clinician are more on the unpleasant side than the pleasant, so they are immediately transformed into the latter cognitive interpretation, and it is no wonder that the patient subsequently slams the phone down yelling, "You really are a son of a bitch aren't you?" Such a response is no different from the small child who berates his mother for not buying the toy airplane with an, "I hate you. I hate you!" The child sees the denial as a true rejection, a black act.

Meanwhile, at the other end of the phone, the clinician sits dumbfounded, wondering what went wrong. In actuality, the "irrationally" angry response of the patient is not as irrational as it may seem at first glance. It would be irrational for a person with a normal ability to see gray to respond in such a fashion, because the normal response would be to view this cancellation as disappointing but understandable. On the other hand, if a person simply did not have the cognitive ability to see gray, then the angry response is reasonably appropriate, because this patient literally "heard" the therapist state, rather boldly, that the therapist did not care about the patient. In essence, the psychological deficit is more with the patient's ability to interpret the environment than in the patient's actual display of anger. From this viewpoint, the patient's unsettling rages may be understood from a more compassionate stance, realizing the tremendously punishing interpersonal environment that these patients must encounter on a daily basis.

This tendency for seeing only the black or the white may tip off interviewers that they are in the presence of a person with borderline psychopathology. The clinician may even see the patient rapidly change opinions about the interviewer as the interview unfolds. Such developmentally delayed manners of cognitively interpreting the world can also be seen in people with other primitive personality disorders, including the paranoid personality, the schizotypal personality, and the more regressed forms of the narcissistic personality. In mild degrees it can be seen in all of us and can lead to a variety of neurotic tensions.

To illustrate the tendency for a person with a borderline personality to display black or white perception in the course of the interview itself, I am reminded of a young woman, whom I interviewed directly after another clinician. The patient quickly began, "You know, the person I was just talking with didn't seem to know what she was doing. I didn't like her. I'm not going to have to talk with her again, am I?" As our interview proceeded, the patient seemed to warm to me relatively quickly, eventually stating that she would not mind working with me. She eventually attempted to demand placement on a specific inpatient unit, which we felt was inappropriate for her. When I told her that she would not be able to go to that particular unit, she angrily pouted. Later her boyfriend came up to me privately saying, "My girlfriend is very displeased with you, and frankly so am I." More classic borderline behavior could not be found. I jumped from Prince Charming to Idi Amin in a single bound. This type of rapid idealization-devaluation is a classic signal behavior suggestive of borderline psychopathology or some other primitive personality.

This patient also displayed a trait, commonly seen with borderline pathology, loosely known as "splitting," in which the patient attempts to pit one person against another. This was demonstrated when she told me her complaints about the previous interviewer. It was also demonstrated by her ability to eventually pit her boyfriend against me.

When considering a different cognitive delay seen in patients with a borderline personality, one can also imagine the havoc that the lack of an ability to view objects as stable could have on an individual. In this regard, having a borderline personality is a little like being a toddler who rolls a ball under a couch and believes that the ball has literally vanished into nonexistence. A good cry will

soon follow as the child finds that its favorite playtoy has disap-
peared. People with borderline personality development may have
problems believing in the constancy of those who love them. Consequently, these patients may frequently feel abandoned. Even more
curious is the disturbing quality of the person with a borderline
personality to feel almost empty inside, as if his or her own sense
of self were mercurial. They may become very dependent upon the
presence of others for a sense of security, frequently going to frantic
efforts to avoid being alone, a condition in which they feel that they
risk the same annihilation that the errant rubber ball encountered.
For people with a normal cognitive development, this type of world
view is very difficult to empathize with, but it occurs nevertheless.
I have never seen it quite so elegantly described as by D. H. Lawrence in his novel *Women in Love.*

*A*nd yet her soul was tortured, exposed. Even walking up the path of the
church, confident as she was that in every respect she stood beyond all vulgar
judgment, knowing perfectly that her appearance was complete and perfect,
according to the first standards, yet she suffered a torture, under her confidence
and her pride, feeling herself exposed to wounds and to mockery and to
despite. She always felt vulnerable, vulnerable, there was always a secret chink
in her armour. She did not know herself what it was. It was a lack of robust self,
she had no natural sufficiency, there was a terrible void, a lack, a deficiency of
being within her.

And she wanted someone to close up this deficiency, to close it up for ever.
She craved for Rupert Birkin. When he was there, she felt complete, she was
sufficient, whole. For the rest of time she was established on the sand, built over
a chasm, and, in spite of all her vanity and securities, any common maid-servant
of positive, robust temper could fling her down this bottomless pit of insufficiency,
by the slightest movement of jeering or contempt. And all the while the pensive,
tortured woman piled up her own defences of aesthetic knowledge, and culture,
and world-visions, and disinterestedness. Yet she could never stop up the terrible
gap of insufficiency.[15]

This particular character may or may not completely fit the designa-
tion of a borderline personality, but this description of the hollowness experienced by the person with a borderline personality
could not be more convincing.

Returning to an actual patient, I remember a woman who described feeling intensely angry at her partner any time that her
partner would roll over to fall asleep. Suddenly the patient was left
by herself and experienced a disquieting sense of panic, like a lost
child, who suddenly realizes that a parent is not nearby in a department store. At these moments she would feel acutely abandoned by
her partner and deeply resented her partner's need for sleep.

   With these ideas in mind let us watch a clinician expanding the diagnostic region of a borderline personality. The patient was a casually dressed woman with dark brown hair that was somewhat unkempt. She spoke with a curious blandness, as if commenting on a character viewed from afar as opposed to her own life. She tended to have poor eye contact, which seemed purposeful, as if she would look at you if she felt moved to do so. Earlier aspects of the interview had demonstrated that the patient had experienced, besides her current episode, only a single bout of major depression in her life. She also denied a history of manic episodes. The immediate reason for her presentation involved her transfer from another hospital. Apparently she had been doing reasonably well, but when she went down to the patient store, she bought a bottle of aspirin and promptly ingested all 24 tablets. She conveniently waited awhile before presenting to her physician's secretary at a time when he was out. She proceeded to casually inform the secretary that she had just overdosed. We will join the conversation roughly midway in the body of the interview:

   Clin.:   Mrs. Jacobs, tell me a little more about what led up to your overdose?

   Pt.:   In the first place, I told him I was going to do it. I really did, but I guess nobody wanted to believe me. Now Dr. Johnson claims I said that I was all done hurting myself, maybe I did, but I sure don't remember telling him that. In fact, I told him I was feeling impulsive like I might overdose, maybe he was just thinking differently, I don't know. But my husband thinks he blew it, and he's real mad that Dr. Johnson let me go down to that store. And it was so easy, I just cut off my patient wrist band and they sold me a bottle of aspirin (patient smiles).

   Clin.:   You seem to have some mixed feelings for Dr. Johnson.

   Pt.:   Do I? . . . Well I suppose I do. I really like him but I think he's dumping me by sending me here. He says he'll take me back, I don't know. You see, I liked my psychologist before Dr. Johnson and I never would have believed I could work with anyone but him, but I got along well eventually with Dr. Johnson too. I guess he'll take me back, but he's mad at me even though I told him.

   Clin.:   With both Dr. Johnson and your previous therapist you seem to have formed strong relationships. Has that been typical of yourself, say back in junior high and high school?

Pt.:   Oh yeah (said in a somewhat disinterested fashion). I always seem to have this thing for an older man who will sort of guide me, help me with my development. That's happened a lot with me, maybe I have a thing for father figures, I don't know. But I had several teachers who I was very close to and there was a minister of our church group who helped a lot too. I'd rather spend my time with these kinds of men.

Clin.: Did you ever find that some of these friends would later let you down and you learned to dislike them?

Pt.:   Oh yes, people use me for a doormat. Reverend Jenkins was a good example. I viewed him as very special, like almost a saint or something, but I wasn't special to him. He saw hundreds of other people in his congregation, I mean there I was sharing my deepest feelings and he'd soon be listening to another person's problems, just like I was one of them.

Clin.: Back around that time, during your school years, what were your friendships like?

Pt.:   They weren't so hot. My mother always told me I was the most gifted kid, but look how I turned out. I wasn't that popular, and people are all basically bastards, trust me.

Clin.: Did you form any friendships in your life that have lasted for over 4 or 5 years?

Pt.:   Not really . . . let me . . . no . . . not real friends.

Clin.: What usually happens to your friendships?

Pt.:   We end up having an argument or something like that, and I tell them off or they tell me off. For some reason people always seem to take advantage of me and it makes me angry.

Clin.: When you get angry, do you tend to keep your anger bottled up inside or do you tend to let it out, maybe by yelling at the person or throwing something?

Pt.:   I keep a lot of it in, but when I let go I can get pretty mean, I mean I have thrown things. I threw a plate at my husband when we were on a pass about 2 weeks ago.

Clin.: I know you've been feeling pretty depressed recently, how about just when you're feeling your normal self, how many times do you think you've broken things when some one angered you?

Pt.: Oh I've done that, probably more times than I could count easily. I remember throwing down my husband's camera, that set him off.

Clin.: Sounds like it would. What's the biggest thing you've ever broken?

Pt.: My husband's nose (patient smiles and both the patient and clinician chuckle).

Clin.: Pretty big nose huh?

Pt.: Yeah and it got bigger.

Clin.: Well, what about when you're feeling very angry, say back in your school days again, did you ever pound your fists into a wall?

Pt.: Oh yeah, I put my fist in the wall once, my mother almost screamed, but then she needed shaking up a bit.

Clin.: Some patients tell me that when they get really angry, they might even pound their heads against the wall, just to get the anger out. Have you ever felt that way?

Pt.: I think I've done that, yeah I think I've done that.

Clin.: What do you remember?

Pt.: A long time ago I used to do that, not a lot though, sort of sounds silly, hurt too. You know, I've done this too. (Mrs. Jacobs rolls up her sleeve and reveals some small scars on her wrist, her affect also hardens a bit, with a very mildly angry undertone.)

Clin.: Looks like you've cut at yourself at times. Is that what these marks are?

Pt.: Yeah, that's what they are all right.

Clin.: Did it hurt when you cut at yourself?

Pt.: Not really, I just sort of like to watch it bleed.

Clin.: What makes you stop?

Pt.: I've never figured that one out, somehow it just feels better, I feel like it's all over.

Clin.: Like what's all over?

Pt.: The anger, the pain, I don't know, all I know is I'm probably going to do it again, 'cause I like it. And you're not going to stop me.

Clin.: Are you worried that I'm going to try to stop you?

Pt.: No I'm not, 'cause I know you can't.

Clin.: I think you're right about the fact that I can't ultimately stop you, only you would be able to do that and right now you don't want to. So let's not focus on that right now, we'll come back to it a little later on. With all these tough times you've had, and you've had some tough ones, do you feel that your moods change pretty rapidly?

Pt.: Yeah that's something I don't like. And if you could help me with that, I'd appreciate it.

Clin.: Do your moods ever change rapidly in a single day, you know, you might wake up in one mood and somebody says something and boom you're in a bad mood and 3 hours later you're O.K. again.

Pt.: Oh yeah, I'm moody, just like that.

Clin.: Do you think your parents or friends in high school viewed you as moody?

Pt.: Sure, I've always been a moody person and people just have to learn to live with my moods. I don't try to be irritable, but sometimes I can't help it.

Clin.: What about when you're alone, what is your mood like for you when you are all by yourself, say back in your apartment?

Pt.: Sometimes I like it and sometimes I don't.

Clin.: When you don't like it, what does it feel like?

Pt.: I just don't like it, I get depressed.

Clin.: Say a friend of yours just left for the evening. As the door shuts and you suddenly find yourself alone, does your mood ever change as that door shuts?

Pt.:   Yes it does, sometimes I feel really bad, like a piece of me has been torn away, and sometimes I get angry, sometimes that's when I cut myself. I really am a moody person, and I don't know what to do about it. I guess that's why Dr. Johnson hates me now. (Mrs. Jacobs becomes quietly sadder.)

Clin.:   When you feel depressed like that, do you ever start to feel almost empty inside, like a piece of you is missing?

Pt.:   Sort of, I don't know if I would phrase it that way.

Clin.:   What does it feel like to you, that's what I'm most interested in understanding.

Pt.:   Dead. I feel dead.

Clin.:   With the deadness, do you frequently feel bored?

Pt.:   No, not really. But it's as if a part of me were not in the room, it's very hard to explain, but it is very unpleasant. My husband just simply can't understand it. He can be such a mean person, but then I guess I've let him down. I let all the people down at the hospital.

Clin.:   How do you mean?

Pt.:   I think my friends back at the hospital were disappointed that I tried to hurt myself. Maybe they're worried I might lose control. Will I be on a locked ward?

Clin.:   Yes, the ward will be locked. I guess that can be sort of scary, are you worried about it?

Pt.:   Yeah, but I guess they better lock me up.

Although this illustration is somewhat lengthy, it probably only required around 10 minutes of interviewing time. In this relatively short period of time, the clinician has uncovered a variety of characteristics seen in the borderline personality, including mood instability, chronic feelings of emptiness, tendencies for idealization alternating with devaluation (as seen with her minister), inappropriate outbursts of anger, tendencies for self-damaging acts, and a general dislike of being alone. In fact, the clinician has probably already gathered close to enough data to fulfill the criteria for a borderline personality disorder by DSM-IV standards, all in a matter of 10 minutes. In addition, the blending seemed reasonably high as indicated by shared periods of levity and a report by the patient, when the interview actually ended, that she liked this clinician.

What is of particular note is the fashion in which the clinician gently and persistently pursued the criteria needed for the diagnosis. The clinician tended to carefully search for historical data by utilizing focusing statements such as, "back in your high school years do you think you felt . . ." or "Do you think that your parents or school friends would have viewed you as. . . ." In the process of unraveling the complexities surrounding a specific personality disorder, once the interviewer has uncovered a particular trait, it is critical to search for evidence that the trait is long-standing in nature. Thus, if a patient brings up many angry periods as an adolescent, then the clinician will need to eventually guide the conversation to a point in which an exploration can be made of angry feelings during the subsequent periods of the patient's life or vice versa.

This clinician was also careful not to assume that behavior occurring during an actual episode of major depression was related to the presence of character pathology, as shown by the following excerpt:

Clin.: When you get angry, do you tend to keep your anger bottled up inside or do you tend to let it out, maybe by yelling at the person or throwing something?

Pt.: I keep a lot of it in, but when I let go I can get pretty mean, I mean I have thrown things, I threw a plate at my husband when we were on a pass about 2 weeks ago.

Clin.: I know you've been feeling pretty depressed recently, how about just when you're feeling your normal self, how many times do you think you've broken things when someone angered you?

In this fashion the clinician is trying to uncover episodes of impulsive anger that are not related to Axis I psychopathology. Sure enough, Mrs. Jacobs proceeds to describe a long-standing pattern of angry and hostile feelings. If the interviewer does not frequently make it explicit to the patient which areas of time are being discussed, then patients almost invariably begin to merge time periods. Once this inadvertent blurring occurs, the clinician is destined to gather a history that may be considerably distorted.

I have seen clinicians interview patients who acted impulsively, with angry outbursts and suicidal threats or gestures, during episodes of hypomania or mania. Sometimes these patients were subsequently inappropriately labeled as having borderline personality disorders. Certainly the behavior of these patients was consistent with a borderline personality during the manic periods, but it was the underlying mania that was causing the impulsive behavior. Careful interviewing of the patient or corroborative sources would have shown that these impulsive behaviors were not present outside of periods of acute Axis I psychopathology.

Another secret to structuring the interview effectively is remaining flexible, demonstrating an ability to side-track when the patient has a need to side-track. For instance, this clinician spent some well-used time when he joked with the patient about her husband's nose. This brief interlude helped the patient to feel more at ease, while also conveying to her the clinician's own sense of humor. This clinician was truly listening with the patient, not just attempting to complete a checklist.

Even when Mrs. Jacobs begins to turn on the so-called borderline charm with the interviewer, the interviewer does not over-react. For example, when she challenges the interviewer concerning the issue of wrist cutting with, "I don't know, all I know is I'm probably going to do it again, 'cause I like it. And you're not going to stop me," the interviewer does not reflexively counterattack, immediately telling the patient of the need not to undertake such activity. Such a display of clinician fear would be "just what the chef ordered" for a person with a borderline personality. Soon the patient would begin to push the clinician in a tug of war and nerves. Instead, this clinician calmly acknowledged the dilemma, agreed with Mrs. Jacobs' impression, and gracefully proceeded with the pertinent exploration of diagnostic information. At a later point in the interview the issue of self-cutting would be more thoroughly explored.

Besides demonstrating a method of unobtrusively expanding a specific diagnostic region, this excerpt serves to remind us of the intensely unsettling world of people with the personality structure we refer to as a borderline personality. Mrs. Jacobs' world is one of ceaselessly circular contradictions. Her husband is at one moment the good guy who will protect her from the carelessness of Dr. Johnson; at another moment, he has been transformed by her tendency to see only black or white into "such a mean person." Her minister is transmuted from a saint into a demon merely because he does not devote all of his attention to her.

She is truly frightened of the world, because she battles back an insistent feeling of "deadness," which threatens to swallow her and those around her for all she knows. Consequently she resorts to the age-old axiom of the best defense is an offense. She attacks. Even during this first encounter with a new clinician, she quickly challenges him to a duel of sorts over the issue of who will rule her wrists. Wisely he declined the verbal glove that so unexpectedly slapped his face. Even at a subtle level, she antagonizes because of her unpredictability. By way of illustration, at the end of the excerpt she suggests a fear of being placed on a locked ward. The clinician attempts to calm this fear with an empathic inquiry. No sooner does the clinician extend his concern than Mrs. Jacobs coolly responds, "Yeah, but I guess they better lock me up." This type of inconsistent interaction is what clinicians frequently report as being "jerked around" by borderline patients. Just as the clinician tries to be nice, the patient conveys a cool nonchalance.

The compassionate interviewer tries to see beneath this type of anger, realizing that the patient is coping with an ominous sense of impending doom and cannot find anything to hold on to to prevent a lethal plummet. In this sense Mrs. Jacobs represents a child trapped in an adult's body, and no one wants to play her game. The art is for the clinician to understand both the child and the adult, helping the patient to recognize that they do not need to be enemies.

Perhaps this is a good time to close this chapter. An attempt has been made to examine many of the core principles and intrigues surrounding the issues of character psychopathology. Hopefully the reader has come away with a variety of new perspectives and specific techniques that can be of immediate practical use. In the last analysis, the ability to readily recognize the presence of these disorders is probably one of the most difficult tasks facing the initial interviewer. The ability not only to recognize them but also to see the person beneath them is an even greater challenge. Without the latter skill, the former pales considerably in significance.

References

1. American Psychiatric Association: *Diagnostic and Statistical Manual of Mental Disorders*, 4th ed. Washington, DC, APA, 1994, p. 629.
2. DSM-IV, 1994, p. 633.
3. Siever, L. J., Insel, T. R., and Uhde, T. W.: Biogenetic factors in personalities. In *Personality Disorders*, edited by J. P. Frosch. Washington, DC, APA, 1983, pp. 42–65.
4. DSM-IV, 1994, p. 661.
5. Gunderson, J. G.: DSM-III diagnosis of personality disorders. In *Personality Disorders*, edited by J. P. Frosch. Washington, DC, APA, 1983, pp. 20–39.
6. Vaillant, G.: Sociopathy as a human process. In *Major Psychiatric Disorders*, edited by F. Guggenheim and C. Nadelson. New York, Elsevier Biomedical, 1982, pp. 179–188.
7. DSM-IV, 1994, pp. 657–658.
8. Hammacher A. M.: *Phantoms of the Imagination*. New York, Harry N. Abrams, 1981, p. 17.
9. Othmer, E., and Othmer, S. C.: *The Clinical Interview Using DSM-IV*. Vol. 1: *Fundamentals*. Washington, DC, American Psychiatric Press, 1994, p. 77.
10. Othmer, E., and Othmer, S. C., 1994, p. 76.
11. Pomeroy, W. B., Flax, C. C., and Wheeler, C. C.: *Taking a Sex History*. New York, The Free Press, 1982.
12. Roberts, J. K. A.: *Differential Diagnosis in Neuropsychiatry*. New York, John Wiley, 1984, p. 26.

13. Linehan, M.: *Cognitive-Behavioral Treatment of Borderline Personality Disorder*. New York, Guilford Press, 1993.
14. Adler, G.: *Borderline Psychopathology and Its Treatment*. New York, Jason Aronson, 1985.
15. Lawrence, D. H.: *Women In Love*. Franklin Center, PA, The Franklin Library, 1979, p. 12.

PART

3

Advanced Techniques of Interviewing

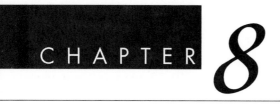

CHAPTER 8

Exploring Suicidal and Homicidal Ideation

$\mathcal{D}$ying
Is an art, like everything else.
I do it exceptionally well.

I do it so it feels like hell.
I do it so it feels real.
I guess you could say I've a call.

Sylvia Plath
Lady Lazarus

$\mathcal{T}$hese words written by Sylvia Plath invoke the coolness of death. They appear even more unsettling when one realizes that their author would eventually go on to kill herself, her words acting not so much as art but as prophecy. Her death added one more digit to the frightening statistic of more than 25,000 suicides per year in the United States, with the rate of 12.5 deaths per 100,000 and an average of one completed suicide every 20 minutes.[1] Moreover, these values probably represent conservative estimates, because they exclude dubious accidents, such as one-driver automobile fatalities, which may actually represent masked suicides. In any case, with suicide representing the ninth leading cause of death in adults in the United States, and, after accidents and homicides, the most common cause of death in 15 to 24 year olds,[2] the determination of suicidality represents a daily task for most mental health professionals.

It is a task that requires a gentle sensitivity and a tenacious

443

persistence. All of the interviewing skills previously discussed are put to their most rigorous test. If ever there were a moment of critical importance in interviewing, it is the moment when one listens for the harbingers of death. This arena is not a place for haphazard approaches or reliance solely on intuitive skills. Instead, interviewers possess two major tools that can assist their intuition in the determination of lethality. First, there exists a wealth of knowledge concerning statistical indicators of suicide potential that may help the clinician to predict increased suicide potential. Second, one can utilize interviewing techniques that may enhance the clinician's ability to elicit suicidal ideation itself.

In this chapter, we will examine the first tool by reviewing the numerous risk factors that may lead to increased lethality. A review will be generated by the use of two mock case histories, which illustrate many of the facets of suicide assessment. We will approach the second tool by looking, in depth, at a four-step strategy of sensitively probing for suicidal ideation, known as the Chronological Assessment of Suicide Events (CASE) Approach, a strategy that provides a very powerful database from which to try to determine immediate suicide potential. I doubt that one can overemphasize the importance of technique in the craft of eliciting suicidal ideation. In my opinion it is important for an interviewer to both develop and practice a flexible and consistent style of questioning, and the CASE Approach is one such system.

A consistent approach provides the interviewer with a chance to become familiar with responses to specific questions from both suicidal and nonsuicidal patients. Such a familiarity with responses offers the experiential framework from which the most subtle of nuances indicating lethality can be picked up. The same interviewing principles are also useful in delineating homicidal and violent ideation, which is an increasingly pressing problem for mental health professionals to uncover. Consequently, approaches for eliciting violent ideation and assessing homicidal risk are also explored at the end of the chapter. At this junction, it seems expedient to begin a review of risk factors by meeting our first patient.

SECTION 1: SUICIDAL RISK FACTORS

CASE 1: MR. JAMISON

Mr. Jamison is a 21-year-old male who comes to the emergency room at 1:00 A.M. accompanied by a male friend. Mr. Jamison's shaggy hair hangs to his large shoulders, which cap a body obviously shaped by the rigors of a weight-lifting room. Mr. Jamison reports feeling "odd" for months and has frequent ideas of reference. He also displays a loosening of associations sporadically. He relates, "It all comes down to the way the clouds kiss the moon." Other than this sentence, he demonstrates no illogical thoughts, tangential thought, or thought blocking, and he denies hallucinations. His speech has a gentle quality to it, with a peculiarly long latency before responses, as if he is preoccupied with a disturbing decision. His affect is guarded with periods of unusual intensity.

He denies feeling depressed and reports few neurovegetative symptoms of depression. He claims to have felt "upset" since he witnessed the brutal slaying of a friend by a motorcycle gang member. As he warms to the interviewer, he admits to recent abuse of alcohol, speed, lysergic acid diethylamide (LSD), and marijuana. When asked about whether he wants to kill himself, he replies testily, "I've no intention of killing myself (pause), that's what I'm fighting for." He refuses to elaborate. At the end of the interview, he refuses admission.

At this point, the clinician is faced with a formidable disposition problem. Does the suicide risk of this patient warrant hospitalization, or can he be treated as an outpatient? A second consideration is the fact that even if admission is warranted, the patient is refusing such treatment. Inadequate grounds for commitment are present. Can the interviewer discover adequate grounds if necessary? With these issues in mind, we can begin an examination of risk factors.

In the first place, Mr. Jamison's sex and age are consistent with an increased suicide risk. With regard to sex, men more frequently successfully commit suicide at a 3:1 ratio compared with women. On the other hand, women attempt suicide three times more frequently than do men.[3] Perhaps this increased "suicide efficiency" in men relates to the choice of the means of suicide. Men more frequently choose violent methods (e.g., guns), which provide a more certain means of death.

With regard to age, in general, suicide risk is greater for both sexes with increasing age. In women, the suicide rate increases until mid-life, after which it tends to reach a plateau. In men, the suicide rate increases precipitously with older age, the highest rate being in white men 70 years of age and older. In men, more than in women, the curve is complicated by a bimodal tendency, with a second peak occurring in late adolescence,[4] a point of special significance with regard to Mr. Jamison.

Unfortunately, in recent years there has been a disturbing rise in the frequency of suicide attempts among adolescents, with suicide representing the third highest cause of death among teenagers.[5] Between 1952 and 1992, the rate of suicide tripled in the 15- to 24-

year-old age group.[6] It has been estimated that a staggering one half million adolescents and young adults perform suicide gestures or attempts each year.[7] Moreover, a clinician should always keep in mind that, even though young children are much less likely to commit suicide, they still do. This fact is driven home by the knowledge that 255 children, from 5 to 14 years of age, actually killed themselves in 1986.[8]

However, there is more to worry about with Mr. Jamison than the implications of his sex and age, because the interviewer left the encounter feeling that Mr. Jamison might be psychotic. The presence of psychosis, with or without depression, should nag an initial interviewer when evaluating suicide potential. Psychosis should be considered a potentially major suicide risk factor, because rational thought often acts as the final obstacle to self-destruction. In particular, three disturbing processes, which could possibly push a patient towards violence to self or others, should be carefully evaluated when the clinician is suspicious of the presence of psychosis: (1) command hallucinations, (2) feelings of alien control, and (3) religious preoccupation.

Command hallucinations represent auditory commands to perform a specific act. Such commands may be egging on the patient to harm himself or herself or others. Their presence, in some cases, should strongly influence the evaluator to hospitalize the individual immediately. Often knowledge of these hallucinations is not volunteered by the patient. Consequently, the clinician must actively inquire about their existence.

During the inquiry, several phenomenological considerations merit the attention of the clinician. Command hallucinations are not black or white phenomena in the sense that the patient either has them or does not. In actuality, command hallucinations can vary in numerous fashions. Some of the defining characteristics include the emotional impact on the patient, loudness, frequency, duration, content, degree of hostility, and the degree to which the patient feels driven to follow them.

With these variables in mind, command hallucinations can vary from relatively innocuous phenomena with little frequency and impact on the patient to dangerous phenomena in which the voices incessantly hammer at the patient in an effort to provoke violence. Some people who suffer from chronic schizophrenia have adapted to their voices and pay them little heed. This type of command hallucination is probably of minimal concern. At the other end of the continuum, command hallucinations can become acutely harassing, loud, and insistent. In such cases, the clinician should always ask to what degree the patient feels in control. Patients may sometimes feel unable to resist even soft yet persistent voices. These types of acutely dystonic command hallucinations generally indicate the need for acute hospitalization. In order to determine the dangerousness of the command hallucination, the clinician must take the time to explore the numerous pertinent variables.

Over the years various papers have purported that there is little or no statistical correlation between command hallucinations and suicide.[9–13] However, if one looks at these papers, it becomes evident that none of the research carefully categorized the hallucinatory phenomena along the critical variables listed earlier. Indeed, the research is generally based on hospital charts, which are notorious for poor reporting of the nuances of patient phenomenology. No one knows whether these voices were at one end or the other end of the continuum of dangerousness. Consequently, the statistical analyses are essentially meaningless.

There was, however, an article in 1990 that utilized direct interviews of patients who had recently experienced command hallucinations.[14] Although this study by Junginger was not prospective in nature, the results are worth noting. Of the 20 patients who experienced dangerous command hallucinations, eight acted on them. These results are certainly more consistent with the observations of experienced clinicians, and they represent a first step toward a more valid and rigorous study of the phenomena of command hallucinations.

Nevertheless, to date I have not seen a prospective study that carefully operationalized the phenomenological data in such a way that the data are appropriate for statistical analysis in a valid sense. Until such a paper exists, it remains necessary for clinicians to carefully consider the fact that some patients definitely do act violently after command hallucinations. The question is what type of patient and which phenomenological experiences result in such actions.

At present, the only method available to help make this decision remains the detailed exploration of the variables discussed earlier. It is hoped that future research, well grounded in phenomenology, will provide better guidelines. However, even if better statistics become available, it is crucial to remember that the suicide of a given patient is not just a statistical phenomenon. More specifically, a patient may kill himself or herself whether the statistics suggest that he or she is at risk or not at risk. Apparently, patients are not always aware of the statistical rules that they are meant to follow.

In a similar sense, alien control, as evidenced by the feeling that one is being controlled by an outside agent, may represent a second dangerous psychotic process if this "other agent" becomes suicidally or homicidally oriented. It is not uncommon for a patient to battle off such potentially lethal urges on a minute-by-minute basis.

A third significant concern arises when the patient exhibits a specific type of excessive religious preoccupation. This type of rumination centers on ideas that God wants the patient to perform certain acts in order to prove the patient's love for God. These acts may include suicide, homicide, or self-mutilation. Such concerns may be associated with command hallucinations as described earlier. This time, however, the commands originate from an individual as ultimately persuasive as God. Patients may believe that their faith is being tested and may perhaps compare themselves with Abraham, who was commanded by God to sacrifice his own son, Isaac. This "Abraham syndrome" can prove fatal. At other times, patients may feel that Satan is pushing them toward violence.

In a related fashion, the patient may be preoccupied with specific verses from the Bible that suggest violent action. Such a biblical injunction may be interpreted from Matthew 5:29, in which lustful wanderings of the eye are handled in a rather absolute fashion, "If your right eye causes you to sin, pluck it out . . ."[15] Obviously, psychotic process can provide ample reasons for acting on such phrases. Bizarre methods of self-mutilation, such as autocastration and the removal of the tongue, may result when verses such as this one are twisted by psychotic thought.[16] If religious preoccupation is found, it may be very useful to ask simple questions, such as, "Are there parts of the Bible that seem particularly important to you?"

Before leaving the topic of psychotic process and its relation to suicide, an important and easily overlooked consideration should be mentioned. Patients with schizophrenia more frequently attempt suicide, not in relation to active psychotic processes but in relation to devastating demoralization and depression, resulting from years of pain, frustration, and low self-esteem caused by the disease process itself.[17-19] As mentioned in Chapter 6 on psychosis, schizophrenia rapes the soul of the patient, robbing an individual of the chance to pursue the dreams that motivate all of us. The core pains of losing a sense of internal control and subsequently a loss of meaning in life can prove unbearable, even for the most courageous of people. As people suffering from schizophrenia perceive themselves to be hopelessly damaged, their reasons for living are gradually extinguished. It has been postulated that patients with the following characteristics may be most at risk: young age, chronic relapses, good educational background, high performance expectations, painful awareness of the illness, fears of further mental deterioration, suicidal ideation or threats, and hopelessness.[20]

Mr. Jamison illustrates yet another important factor in the determination of lethality. He is a heavy drug abuser. The presence of chronic alcohol abuse or other drug abuse should be viewed as another risk factor, because these agents may decrease impulse control or precipitate the psychotic process. However, alcohol is not only a problem with regard to poor impulse control; it also appears to cause long-term problems with suicidal ideation. It has been shown that people with chronic depression directly caused by alcohol abuse are at a significantly higher risk of making a serious suicide attempt.[21]

The acutely intoxicated patient presents a particular problem, because the intoxication predisposes the patient toward a suicide attempt in two ways. First, impulse control may be significantly lowered. Second, because of cognitive impairment, the patient may inadvertently commit suicide in a variety of fashions, such as forgetting that a large number of pills were taken earlier in an evening and subsequently proceeding to ingest "just a few more." Such miscalculations can result in a fatal overdose. Because of these factors, even chronic emergency room abusers who present with serious suicidal ideation while acutely intoxicated should be observed until they sober up. Frequently, as the alcohol wears off, the suicidal ideation disappears and may not even be remembered.

These points also highlight the fact that significant organic impairment of the sensorium can also increase risk. Thus, fluctuating levels of consciousness or impaired concentration warrant careful attention during the mental status examination. At this juncture, Mr. Jamison presents a disturbing clinical dilemma. Too many gaps exist in the knowledge base to enable the clinician to make a sound decision. To clarify the issue, an interview with Mr. Jamison's friend unearthed the following material.

Mr. Jamison had not been himself since the murder of his friend who was, indeed, shot. Recently Mr. Jamison had seemed more distant than usual and was using a "load of uppers." He had been discharged about 3 weeks ago from a psychiatric hospital. Unfortunately, Mr. Jamison was at odds with his family; he was currently living by himself in a dingy apartment and was subsisting on food stamps. The friend knew of no previous suicide attempts.

But there was another piece of information from Mr. Jamison's friend that proved troubling in nature. It surfaced as follows:

Clin.: Any other things about Jim that might be of importance?

Friend: I don't think so—except, well it's probably not that important.

Clin.: What were you going to say?

Friend: Well, you know, he's just more wound all the time. Sometimes he looks positively wired.

Clin.:   What's he do that makes you say that?

Friend: Oh, he paces and he looks sort of, I don't know, frightened. It's really sort of weird. I guess it's just that he's so damn intense about everything. I keep telling him to chill out, but he doesn't.

The element of concern in this new information is the presence of intense anxiety in Mr. Jamison. Recent research has suggested that increased anxiety, especially if acute and intense, may play a role in impulsive suicide attempts. On inpatient units, there is evidence that patients with high levels of anxiety and agitation are more likely to kill themselves. This knowledge provides some support to the value of time-limited use of antianxiety agents at effective doses, when such patients "hit the unit." Keep in mind that almost 5 to 6% of suicides in the United States occur in inpatient units.[22] Mr. Jamison's anxiety could be related to a variety of factors, including psychotic anxiety, concurrent panic attacks, or his use of speed. No matter what the cause, there is reason for concern.

When asked whether he had seen Mr. Jamison with any type of potential weapon, his friend remarked, "I hadn't really thought about it, but he does carry a hunting knife he got after he left the hospital. But he's had hunting knives before." Mr. Jamison lost his girlfriend about a month after the murder. When asked if he could stay with Mr. Jamison until he had an outpatient appointment, the friend quietly replied "No way, I just can't do it. Maybe his mom or something could do it."

In the first place, the above data illustrate the important principle of interviewing appropriate friends or family members, because they may provide invaluable information. In an emergency room situation, it is often critical to talk with significant others before making a decision regarding a patient's safety. Don't forget that if there are serious concerns about safety, these concerns outweigh confidentiality. It is sometimes necessary to contact relatives against a person's will. These contacts should be made after consulting with a supervisor or colleague, and the reason for the decision to break confidentiality should be clearly stated in the chart as should also be the role of the consultation.

In general, corroborative sources should be asked if they have witnessed anything that suggests possible suicide intent on the part of the patient. After a general inquiry, specific questions such as the following may be useful:

a. Has he made any comments about being "better off dead?"
b. Has he joked about killing himself?

c. Have there been any statements about "things being better soon?"
d. Does he have any potential weapons in the house, such as guns or knives?
e. Has he ever tried to hurt himself before, even in small ways such as taking a few pills too many?
f. Has he appeared depressed or tearful?
g. Is he spending more time alone than usual?

In this type of questioning, other than determining lethality, one is also searching for information that would fulfill involuntary commitment criteria. Specifically, using New Hampshire criteria (criteria differ from one state to another), one checks to see if the patient has participated in behavior that is a clear danger to himself or to others. The criteria are also met if the patient has expressed a desire to harm himself or others while taking some steps (e.g., purchasing a weapon) to fulfill this desire. In the case of Mr. Jamison, his friend knew of no such behavior, except for the purchase of the hunting knife, although it was unclear as to whether the knife was bought for innocuous or dangerous purposes. It is noteworthy that with adolescents the most common method of suicide is the use of a gun, distantly followed by hanging.[23] Any household with an adolescent at risk should get rid of any guns. This may be one of the single best measures for preventing the suicide of an adolescent or adult.

The corroborative interview also provides a chance to determine stressors and social supports. With regard to stress, the clinician should search for situations such as unemployment, family disruption, rejection by a significant other, abrupt changes in career responsibilities, or a recent catastrophic stress (e.g., witnessing a murder in Mr. Jamison's case). Concerning support systems, a lack of friends, family, or societal supports, such as church organizations, has often been reported as a risk factor. In particular, one should be looking for evidence of recent losses, such as Mr. Jamison's estrangement from his girlfriend and his family.

In their practical primer on the assessment and treatment of suicidal patients, Fremouw, de Perczel, and Ellis point out that one of the more striking statistical correlations with suicide remains the increased risk associated with the absence of a spouse. The highest risk is with people who are separated, followed, in descending level of risk, by people who are divorced, widowed, or single. People who have never been married are twice as likely to commit suicide as people currently happily married. Divorced and widowed people have even higher rates.[24]

Immediately available supports are particularly important when postponing a final treatment decision until a more thorough evaluation can be done the next day. Such a situation may arise when the clinician is ambivalent about the seriousness of the lethality while simultaneously being confronted with a "stacked-up" emergency room. If a friend or family member can stay with the patient constantly until the scheduled appointment, then such a plan may be feasible.

In such cases it is critical that the family members thoroughly understand that the patient should not be left alone. Moreover, I generally find it useful also to have a discussion with the patient and the family together, talking openly about suicidal concerns and the design of the safety plan. Such a procedure helps to teach the patient and family that it is both safe and appropriate to discuss suicidal ideation frankly. To the contrary, the ideation may prove more deadly when it is not discussed.

With regard to the items discussed earlier, including long-term supports, immediate supports, and recent stressors, Mr. Jamison gives cause for increasing concern. The risk is further heightened by the relatively recent discharge of Mr. Jamison from a psychiatric hospital (which could provide "no information at this time because the medical records are closed"). In particular, the first month following the patient's discharge represents a particularly high-risk period.[25] Mr. Jamison has no known suicide history. With regard to previous attempts, corroborative informants often provide information that is withheld by the patient. Previous attempts are clearly associated with increased risk, as evidenced by a study in which more than 46% of successful suicide victims had previously attempted suicide.[26]

With regard to Mr. Jamison's clinical disposition, the interviewer investigated one more pertinent system of support—the mental health system itself. The charge nurse, when queried, related that the outpatient department was flooded with people requiring appointments and was backlogged for several weeks. She thought that it was highly unlikely that Mr. Jamison could be seen the next day. Thus, because of a lack of immediate social support and a relative lack of professional support, the clinician felt very uneasy about outpatient triage. At this point, however, despite many statistical risk factors, it is unclear how lethal a risk Mr. Jamison presents. It must be remembered that he denied suicidal intent, albeit in a somewhat quizzical fashion. Furthermore, at present, there are insufficient grounds to commit Mr. Jamison.

At this point the interviewer made a wise, but often underused, decision to interview the patient again. This time the clinician would make an even more concerted effort to bring psychotic ideation to the surface, while listening persistently for adequate grounds to commit Mr. Jamison, if indeed he appeared more imminently suicidal. The following dialogue evolved after about 10 minutes:

Pt.: I don't think there's anything that could have been done. Peace is what is needed. Peaceful mankind . . . but it all seems so weird and I try to stop them.

Clin.: To stop who?

Pt.: Bad people . . . bad people who push me and make me do things, make me watch things.

Clin.: Have you ever felt like someone or something was really trying to take you over?

Pt.: Oh . . . they take me over, or try to, but I don't let them.

Clin.: Who are you talking about?

Pt.: Something inside me, something about my heart, scratching at my heart, my muscle.

Clin.: It sounds very frightening.

Pt.: Very frightening, but I won't do it.

Clin.: What do they want you to do?

Pt.: To cut it out, to cut the scratching out of my heart, to bring peace to mankind, to wipe off the pain. But I won't do it unless I see the sign. The clouds will kiss the moon, you'll see.

Clin.: What do they want you to use to cut yourself?

Pt.: My knife.

Clin.: Have they ever made you hold the knife in your hands?

Pt.: Oh yes . . . one night, I think it was last night, they put it in my hand. I told them I didn't want to, but they made me hold it with the point pressing on my chest, just waiting.

Clin.: And what did they want you to do?

Pt.: To thrust it deep inside my heart, to let my scratching out, to let my God in, to thrust steel truth into God.

The interviewer has succeeded. He has been granted access to the patient's inner world, which proves to be grossly psychotic, as was initially suspected. By probing along the lines of alien control, the interviewer has skillfully uncovered both suicidal ideation and action. In the earlier interview, Mr. Jamison had denied suicidal ideation probably because he felt that an alien force wanted him to die, not his own will. In his mind this was murder, not suicide. Clearly, Mr. Jamison warrants hospitalization, and adequate grounds for commitment are now available if necessary. It should be noted that the interviewer had gently guided Mr. Jamison towards a concrete description of his suicidal actions in the hope that grounds for commitment would emerge. Many times a patient will not grant such information unless he or she is sensitively guided towards it.

Perhaps a review of some basic principles illustrated by Mr. Jamison may be of value here:

1. A relatively small but significant number of people who attempt suicide are actively psychotic.
2. Any evidence of psychosis warrants a thorough evaluation of lethality.
3. Three particularly dangerous areas of psychotic process are command hallucinations, feelings of alien control, and hyper-religiosity. These areas should be actively probed by the interviewer if they are not elicited spontaneously.
4. Recent evidence suggests that many suicides in schizophrenia occur in response to depressive episodes while the patient is relatively nonpsychotic.
5. Demographic material such as age, sex, and marital status may indicate risk factors for suicide.
6. Recent losses and poor social support systems also represent risk factors for suicide.
7. Alcohol, drugs, or any physiologic insult to the central nervous system may increase the likelihood of suicide or homicide.
8. When evaluating systems of immediate outpatient support, one should carefully consider whether the mental health system itself is prepared to offer adequate support.
9. Interviews with corroborative informants may yield valuable information.

At this point, it may be best to move on to our second patient, who presents some new areas of concern when considering lethality.

CASE 2: MRS. KELLY

Mrs. Kelly, a 50-year-old married mother of three, has arrived for an outpatient initial assessment, accompanied by her eldest daughter. Mrs. Kelly appears frail, walking as if each step presented a personal challenge. There remains a glint in her eye, but it is a weary one. Her hands are grossly deformed by the ravages of rheumatoid arthritis. She reports feeling very depressed, and her speech is punctuated by heavy sighs. She complains of many neurovegetative symptoms of depression. They have persisted for more than 6 months, "although I've not felt normal since the arthritis began over 7 years ago." She continues tearfully, "I'm not the same woman my husband married." She manages to smile as she wryly adds, "You know, if my memory serves me right, I used to move a little faster."

When asked about suicide, she admits to having thought of it occasionally but denies any intention of pursuing it. She has no organized plan. She relates an increasing sense of hopelessness, adding, "I think I'm starting to lose my fight. I think my husband would be better off with me dead, at least he says so." She is without evidence of psychosis and does remarkably well when tested for cognitive dysfunction.

Her daughter relates that her mother used to be a real fighter. At one time she was "the belle of the ball." With the onset of the arthritis, she had been forced into a strikingly more sedate lifestyle. Her illness has greatly affected her husband, who always wants to be active socially. They bicker constantly. Her daughter has seen no evidence of suicidal behavior in her mother but is frightened of what her mother will do when she becomes bedridden.

Mrs. Kelly's case certainly raises different concerns than those encountered with Mr. Jamison. In the first place, she appears to be significantly depressed. As expected, depression represents one of the suicide risk factors. It is important to keep in mind the possibility of atypical depression. Indeed, various somatoform disorders, such as the psychogenic pain syndrome, may be accompanied by depression. With such an atypical presentation, an interviewer can be lulled into a feeling of false security concerning suicide potential.

The presence of a severe psychiatric disorder, such as a major depression, is probably the single strongest statistical correlate with suicide risk. Sometimes clinicians ask, "What is one of your best tips for predicting suicide potential?" and one of the wisest of responses seems to be simply, "Do a good diagnostic assessment." Reviews of completed suicides have shown that as high as 95% of all suicides, including both adolescents and adults, occur in people suffering with a psychiatric disturbance.[27] Major depression leads the pack. It is followed by alcoholism, schizophrenia, and people coping with a severe borderline personality disorder.[28]

There is also increasing evidence that people who experience frequent panic attacks are at a higher risk. If the panic attacks occur in conjunction with a severe depression, then a "red flag" should go up. In a study of almost 1000 patients with a mood disorder, Fawcett found that depressed patients who experienced panic attacks demonstrated three times the suicide rate of other patients, accounting for nearly two thirds of the suicides in the first year of the study.[29, 30] Other research has supported the idea that patients with panic attacks alone have an increase in suicidal ideation. Whether this translates into a definitely higher rate of suicide attempts is unclear.[31]

With regard to physical illness, Mrs. Kelly highlights the fact that severe illnesses are often associated with increased suicide risk. The clinician should pay particular attention to illnesses that result in markedly decreased mobility, disfigurement, and chronic pain. Mrs. Kelly's rheumatoid arthritis unfortunately creates all three of these burdens. The interviewer should also note the impact of illnesses in which the patient perceives a horrifying demise. Illnesses such as Huntington's chorea, multiple sclerosis, severe diabetes, and severe chronic obstructive pulmonary disease may present more suffering than many of us can bear to accept and that some individuals would choose to accept. The interaction of medical illnesses with the patient's underlying personality structure also warrants attention. In some instances, people locked into damaging structures such as narcissistic, histrionic, or borderline personalities may have an inordinate amount of difficulty dealing with disease processes that people lucky enough to have more mature coping skills can handle better.

Leonard has described three personality types who may be predisposed to suicide when stressed.[32] The first type is a controlling personality; these patients tend to constantly manipulate their environment. They are often hard-driven and feel a need to be "on top of things." They frequently pilot their way into roles of power and authority. When such people are suddenly struck by the loss of control caused by a crippling illness, they may attempt to escape through death. Mrs. Kelly certainly may possess some of these dynamics, because she had always been an "on the go" person. Her daughter's fear of what will happen when her mother becomes bedridden represents a well-founded concern.

A second personality type is exemplified by a dependent-dissatisfied approach to life, a common element of people suffering with borderline personality disorders and people with "passive-aggressive" structures. Such people often leave a long line of exasperated caretakers in their wake. When the last source of aid finally closes the door, these people are suddenly left without any means of emotional support. Suicide may loom as the only viable option. Finally, a third predisposing characterologic type involves people who have evolved a truly symbiotic relationship with a significant other. These people are at high risk if their sustaining support dies or abandons them.

All of these examples emphasize one of the most important hallmarks of suicide. Suicide is an interpersonal phenomenon. As such, an evaluation of suicide potential not only involves consideration of the identified patient, but it also requires an evaluation of the interpersonal systems surrounding that patient. At times, this evaluation proceeds through the use of corroborative interviews. At other times, the interviewer must depend on information provided solely by the patient. In either case, a careful consideration of interpersonal factors is warranted.

In a simplistic but practical approach, the interviewer should attempt to determine whether the patient is returning to a supportive or hostile environment. If the patient's family or friends provide a caring milieu, this fact bodes well for the patient. Even in this situation, a paradoxic problem can arise if the patient begins to feel guilty "about being a burden to everyone." Phrases such as Mrs. Kelly's, "I think my husband will be better off with me dead," should perk the ears of the interviewer. In this vein of reasoning, after suicide has been broached as a topic, questions such as the following can be revealing:

a. If you would kill yourself, how do you think that would affect your family?
b. What do you think your spouse would feel if you killed yourself?
c. What are your thoughts about your responsibilities for your family and children if you kill yourself?[33]

Such questioning may lead directly to evidence of an interpersonal maelstrom or into an exploration of the framework for meaning that will keep the patient alive, such as the need to care for a child. On the darker side, as the evaluation proceeds, the interviewer seeks for clues that suggest that a supposed support system in reality may wish at some level that the patient were dead. A death wish may be unconscious or conscious, innocuous or sinister. The clinician's recognition of such death wishes is not a moral judgment passed upon a potential support system but rather an objective attempt to see the potentially lethal ramifications arising from such situations. A premature dismissal of such factors may represent a dangerous naiveté on the part of the interviewer. Certainly, in the case of Mrs. Kelly, one wonders to what degree the marital alliance has been severely strained. At some level, does Mr. Kelly "want out?"

An unconscious death wish may show itself by a lax attitude of the family towards appropriate precautions against suicide. The clinician may discover that the safety suggestions of previous mental health professionals, such as removing a firearm, have not been followed by the family. On another level, there may be resistance to hospitalizing a seriously lethal patient. Considering the perspective of psychological defense mechanisms, family members may see a falsely rosy picture because of denial or repression.

At a more disturbing level, clinicians will undoubtedly encounter, at some point in their practice, a death wish laced with true malice. Perhaps it will be a spouse who has long been denied a divorce or a battered significant other unable to retaliate. These family members, rightly or wrongly, may consciously wish the patient dead. It is not known how many times people have waited a few hours before calling for help when they have happened upon a "sleeping" family member surrounded by empty pill bottles.

In this regard, I remember one patient whom I hospitalized from the emergency room whose spouse literally yelled at her, "take the damn pills, in fact I'll stuff them down your throat, and trust me I won't call a soul." The uncovering of such vicious interaction should serve as a warning to the clinician. It may influence the clinician to hospitalize a patient who might otherwise have been perfectly safely discharged to a more supportive environment.

Another aspect of the hostile environment may be the fact that the patient might be equally angry with family members. With revenge in mind, patients may kill themselves, hoping "to show them they'll be sorry when I'm gone." Questions such as, "What have you pictured your funeral being like?" may provide revealing insights into the patient's motive for suicide. It is not at all unusual to receive answers such as, "They will all be really hurt, realizing at last what they've done to me." In a similar vein, some authors have viewed suicide as the result of a murderous impulse turned inward, a symbolic murder with an ironic satisfaction.[34]

Reasoning of the types described earlier emphasizes the importance of determining whether the patient is developing powerful interpersonal excuses for suicide. The more rational the suicide appears to the patient, the more concerned the interviewer should become. It becomes particularly ominous when the excuse has a humanistic flavor to it, as with "It's the only way I can really help my family." Such thinking may be the first note in a death toll.

Leaving the interpersonal realm and returning to Mrs. Kelly, several indicators suggest a lowered suicide risk. In the first place, she denies immediate hopelessness. Aaron Beck's work with the cognitive aspects of suicide has suggested that the presence of hopelessness may be an ominous sign. In fact, hopelessness may be an even better indicator of lethality than the severity of depressive mood.[35] Viewed from a logical perspective, suicide usually represents a last option that is taken when no other alternatives are apparent to the patient. Moreover, a sense of helplessness is often coupled to this state of despair. Patients generally kill themselves for one major reason, to escape what appears to them to be an inescapable pain.

Further questioning also revealed that Mrs. Kelly was not only raised a Catholic but also that she strongly practiced her faith and believed that suicide was a mortal sin punishable by eternal damnation. At this intensity, religion is probably acting as a major framework for meaning that precludes the suicide option. Other patients may have different frameworks for meaning, such as caring for their children or fulfilling other important societal roles. In any case, the clinician should seek out evidence of such powerful deterrents.

A peculiar and unsettling twist can enter the picture with regard to children. Some patients may decide that their children would be even worse off after the patient's suicide. For instance, the patient's spouse may have alcoholism with an active history of abusing the children both physically and sexually. In these cases, the patient may be contemplating taking the lives of the children before killing himself or herself. Although this happens rarely, one only needs to read the newspaper in order to learn about such tragedies. If suspected, validity techniques, such as normalization, may be useful when moving unobtrusively into this extremely sensitive area.

> **Pt.:** I am a total failure, a miserable mother, and I now realize that my only option is death . . . I intend to take that option.
>
> **Clin.:** You know, sometimes when people feel really angry at themselves, they also find themselves turning the anger outwards onto others (normalization). Have you felt like hurting anyone else?
>
> **Pt.:** (pause) Yes I have. I don't think I'd do it, but maybe it would be better anyway.
>
> **Clin.:** What are you referring to?
>
> **Pt.:** I've thought of killing my husband.
>
> **Clin.:** Anyone else? Such as your children?

At other times the following type of approach may be useful:

> **Pt.:** My husband will never change. He likes to hurt us. We have no future, and I now realize that suicide is my only option.
>
> **Clin.:** You mentioned "we." What do you think is going to happen to your children after you kill yourself?

> **Pt.:** (long pause) I don't really know.
>
> **Clin.:** Sometimes parents consider taking the lives of their children (normalization), has that thought ever crossed your mind?
>
> **Pt.:** Yes, it has . . . it's a terrible thought but it has.
>
> **Clin.:** What have you thought of doing?

Another positive note in Mrs. Kelly's presentation is the lack of a recent, abrupt change in clinical condition in either direction. The sudden onset of severe sleeplessness, agitation, or marked dysphoria may indicate that the patient is rapidly approaching a pain level that he or she cannot tolerate. On the other hand, one hears of the often quoted clinical observation that an unexpected improvement in clinical condition may be masking a sinister outcome. The patient's peace may be secondary to the patient's decision to commit suicide. Suddenly, the patient senses a perceivable end to the suffering. The most upsetting decision of the patient's life is over.

Another problem concerning "improvement" surfaces from the fact that sometimes depressed patients appear more likely to attempt suicide when they begin to improve. Suicide is less common while they are in the troughs of their depression. This curious finding is probably related to the fact that as they initially improve, they regain initiative and energy, even though their dysphoric mood may remain severely intense. The clinician should keep this fact in mind when encountering a patient who has recently started taking an antidepressant.

Finally, further interviewing revealed that Mrs. Kelly has no immediate models for suicide. Neither friends nor family members have ever attempted suicide. If one discovers a legacy of suicide in a family tree, this should arouse concern on the part of the interviewer.

At this point a summary of issues illustrated by Mrs. Kelly may clarify some principles.

1. The presence of disease may increase suicide risk, especially if it leads to immobility, disfigurement, or severe pain.
2. The interviewer should search for evidence of feelings of hopelessness or helplessness.
3. A hostile interpersonal environment may substantially increase the risk of suicide.
4. A strong framework for meaning, such as a deeply held religious conviction, may decrease risk. It should be sought for by the clinician.

5. Sudden changes in clinical condition, either positive or negative, may indicate an increased risk.
6. Rational excuses for committing suicide may indicate increased intention.
7. The presence of a positive family history of suicide should be actively looked into by the clinician.
8. Suicide assessment should always include a search for major psychiatric disorders, such as major depression, alcohol dependence, schizophrenia, bipolar disorder, obsessive-compulsive disorder, and panic disorder.

Chronic Versus Immediate Risk of Suicide: The Triad of Lethality

Perhaps the most important indicator that Mrs. Kelly is not imminently suicidal is the fact that she denies current suicidal intent and has no organized plan to harm herself. This point illustrates the usefulness of making a distinction between chronic suicide potential and immediate suicide potential. If a patient presents with a variety of risk factors present over a significant period of time, then the patient may well represent a chronic risk for suicide. Such is the case with Mrs. Kelly, who presents with the following risk factors: presence of a major psychiatric disorder (depression), increasing age, debilitating illness, increasing sense of hopelessness, a strained marital alliance that may actually represent a hostile environment, and the slow evolution of a rational excuse for suicide.

However, the presence of numerous risk factors does not necessarily indicate an immediate risk of suicide. More important, the absence of most risk factors does not necessarily indicate the lack of a serious risk if certain critical factors are present. By way of example, concerning the first point, Mrs. Kelly most likely could be safely triaged to an outpatient therapist despite her substantial list of risk factors (although she would probably benefit from hospitalization). Thus, the pressing question facing the clinician is to determine what factors would have suggested that she was in immediate danger of suicide.

In my opinion, the three most useful indicators, which form a lethal triad, include: (1) the presenting history of a serious suicide attempt, (2) the presence of acutely disturbing psychotic processes suggestive of lethality, and (3) an indication from the interview that the patient seriously intends self-harm. The presence of any one of these factors should warn the clinician that suicide may be imminent. With respect to triage, the clinician should strongly consider hospitalization for the patient, even if opposed by the patient.

In my opinion, the last element of the triad, which is primarily dependent upon the clinician's interviewing skills, represents the single most important indication of suicide potential. This inter-

462 Advanced Techniques of Interviewing

viewing process is so important that we will devote the entire next section of this chapter to reviewing its subtleties.

In the meantime, as we look back at the first element of the triad of lethality, the presence of a presenting serious attempt, certain points may help to determine the significance of the attempt. First, the clinician should ascertain the potential dangerousness of the method used. For example, taking a few extra aspirin is a great deal less disconcerting than shooting oneself or ingesting lye. Moreover, the threat of an overdosage by a physician, who understands the use of medications, is more worrisome than the same threat in a nonmedical person.

Second, the clinician should determine whether the patient appeared to really want to die or not. Looked at differently, did the patient leave much room for rescue? The interviewer should search for factors such as the following: Did the patient choose a "death spot" where the patient could easily be discovered? Did the patient choose a spot where help was nearby? Did the patient leave any hints of suicidal intention that could have brought help, such as an easily accessible suicide note? Did the patient contact someone after the suicide attempt?[36] The absence of the previous findings may indicate that the patient was frighteningly serious.

At this point I would like to refocus on the general issue of chronic versus immediate suicide potential. By way of illustration, Mr. Jamison and Mrs. Kelly appear to represent two ends of this continuum. Mrs. Kelly lacks all the elements of the triad of lethality. Specifically, she has no recent history of a serious suicide attempt; she has no evidence of psychosis; and she gives no feeling from the interview of current suicidal ideation. Thus, despite the fact that she has numerous risk factors, she is probably not in immediate danger. On the other hand, Mr. Jamison possessed all three elements of the triad and thus was worrisome indeed. These two cases highlight the point that there is no mechanical formula that one can use for determining suicidal potential. Instead, clinicians utilize a craft in which they carefully weigh various risk factors, historical elements, and pieces of information gleaned from the interview. Perhaps a summary of these factors and their interplay would be helpful at this time.

Statistical and Clinical Risk Factors: Summary and Use

Through the examination of the two case studies, the risk factors most often cited in the literature have been surveyed. When pressured by time constraints, clinical demands, and the other standard pressures of being a mental health professional, it is sometimes difficult to remember all these issues. To facilitate their recall, the following two acronyms can provide some reassuring structure in the most chaotic of situations. The first acronym, the SAD PERSONS Scale, was developed by Patterson, Dohn, Bird, and Patterson.[37] It serves as a useful checklist of pertinent risk factors. The second acronym, NO HOPE, developed by the author, adds further depth to the evaluation of suicide potential:

Sad Persons Scale	No Hope Scale
• Sex	– No framework for meaning
• Age	– Overt change in clinical con-
• Depression	dition
• Previous attempt	– Hostile interpersonal environ-
• Ethanol abuse	ment
• Rational thinking loss	– Out of hospital recently
• Social supports lacking	– Predisposing personality fac-
• Organized plan	tors
• No spouse	– Excuses for dying are present
• Sickness	and strongly believed

Needless to say, the acronym NO HOPE itself emphasizes the need to inquire about feelings of hopelessness.

If clinicians routinely explore the ramifications of these factors before making a triage decision, they can be assured that they are utilizing a sound knowledge base. Moreover, the presence of a large number of these factors should increase clinicians' suspicions of suicide potential. And, as mentioned earlier, the presence of any one of the factors within the triad of lethality should strongly lean clinicians towards hospitalization, even if few of the other risk factors are present. In the final analysis, despite an extensive knowledge of risk factors, it is the clinician's impression of imminent suicidal intent, garnered from the interview, that remains the cornerstone of intervention. It is to this process that we now turn our attention.

SECTION 2: ELICITATION OF SUICIDAL IDEATION

General Considerations: Resistance, Countertransference, Myths, and Tips

There exists little doubt that as mental health professionals we will all be interviewing a patient at some point in our careers who has decided to commit suicide. As we talk, the patient will have already accepted an invitation to die. The question becomes whether the patient will decide to share this decision with us.

At such a moment, the interviewer, as a measuring instrument, should be set at the highest pitch of sensitivity. The clinician essentially should try to elicit even the smallest of suicidal intentions, because such ideations may suggest important implications for disposition and treatment. In the following pages, an attempt is made to offer various principles that may significantly increase the likelihood that suicidal ideation will be shared. As usual, each interviewer must ultimately develop an individually tailored style, but these suggestions may serve as useful stimulants for thought. They are discussed within a framework built of two stages.

These two stages consist of (1) sensitively setting the platform for the suicide inquiry, and (2) eliciting the actual suicidal ideation itself. With regard to the second stage, a specific interviewing strategy known as the CASE Approach is presented in detail. As has been the practice throughout this book, an attempt is made to delineate specific techniques and concrete strategies that can maximize the clinician's skills. Thus, the query for suicidal ideation presents not as a single question but as a meticulously developed process that is gently guided by the interviewer.

Before looking at these two stages in detail, it is worth discussing some practical general considerations, because suicide is a difficult topic to discuss. It raises many factors pertaining to complex issues such as metacommunication, resistance, validity, and reliability.

In the first place, I have made it a habit always to ask about lethality at some point, using specific words such as "kill yourself," "commit suicide," or "take your life." I do not think lethality inquiries are any time to risk misunderstandings. The patient needs to know exactly what the clinician is talking about. Such calm frankness on the part of the interviewer provides a powerful metacommunication to the patient. This metacommunication states, "It is okay to discuss thoughts of suicide with me." In an immediate sense, this implied reassurance may relax the patient, increasing the patient's sense of safety. In a long-term sense, it may be the single action that brings a potentially suicidal patient to help. Several months later, if the patient becomes seriously suicidal, the patient may remember that there was one place where the patient's "horrible secret" could be shared. Such knowledge could literally save a life.

A trainee related a relevant vignette concerning the specific words chosen during the suicide inquiry. The interviewer had asked an adolescent girl, "Have you had any thoughts of wanting to hurt yourself?" The girl assuredly answered no. Because of a large number of suicide risk factors, the clinician readdressed the issue later, asking, "Have you had any thoughts of wanting to kill yourself?" To the clinician's surprise, the girl matter of factly responded, "Oh yes, I've thought about it a lot. I've stored up a lot of pills, and I may really try it some day." The clinician asked the girl why she had denied suicide earlier, and she replied, "You didn't ask me about suicide. You asked if I wanted to hurt myself, and I hate pain. Even the method I have chosen for suicide is not going to be painful."

Several other points come to mind concerning lethality questioning. They can be summarized as follows:

1. The least hesitancy in a patient's response may suggest that the patient has had such thoughts, even if he or she proceeds to deny them.
2. Answers such as "No, not really," often indicate that there has been concrete suicidal ideation. The interviewer can often break the resistance with a concerned tone of voice and a question such as, "What kind of thoughts have you had?"
3. The interviewer should look carefully for any body language clues that the patient is being deceptive or feels anxious.
4. To increase clinician awareness of such clues, there is probably no excuse for notetaking during the elicitation of suicidal ideation.
5. The clinician should avoid nonverbal evidence of any uncomfortableness with the topic of suicide, such as might be shown by increased displacement activities or looking away from the patient.

This is also an opportune time to look at a common myth concerning the search for suicidal ideation. Simply stated, the myth reads: "I might give patients the idea to kill themselves, if I talk about it."

In the first place, to my knowledge, there is not a single case example of such a process unfolding. In the second place, the idea of suicide is no secret. A patient would have to be unusually backward to have never heard of suicide before encountering the clinician. And thirdly, and probably most important, suicide is extremely hard to do. It will take a lot more than a single interviewer's discussion of the topic to lead someone to make the decision.

To the contrary, as discussed earlier, the clinician's frank discussion allows the patient to share a heavy burden, made much heavier by the isolation imposed by silence. Moreover, the demonstration that suicidal ideation can be openly discussed conveys that help may be only a spoken word away. Suddenly, suicidal ideation is no longer a sin to be hidden, but rather a problem to be solved.

It should be added that sometimes, later in the interview, it may be worthwhile to repeat the inquiry. Sometimes resistance varies with time. If the interviewer is not satisfied with the first inquiry, a second one may yield some surprises.

The topic of why patients are hesitant to talk about suicidal ideation raises some interesting points. Several specific reasons for patient resistance come to mind:

a. The patient feels that suicide is a sign of weakness and feels shame.
b. The patient feels that suicide is immoral or a sin.
c. The patient feels that discussion of suicide is a taboo subject.
d. The patient is worried that the interviewer will perceive the patient as crazy.
e. The patient fears that the patient will be "locked up" if suicidal ideation is discussed.
f. The patient truly wants to die and does not want anybody to know.

This is quite a formidable list. It re-emphasizes the importance of effective engagement and appropriate setting of the stage, which we will address shortly. It also brings up issues of how to approach navigating some of these potential resistances.

To begin with, the clinician may attempt to dissipate a patient's fears that he or she will be perceived as bizarre or unusual. An old friend of ours, the validity technique of normalization, can often serve as a gentle lead-in: "Frequently, when people are feeling very upset, they have thoughts of killing themselves. Have you had any thoughts of wanting to kill yourself?" When said matter-of-factly and sensitively, such an inquiry can be significantly reassuring to patients, indicating that they are not being viewed as odd or deviant by the interviewer.

The clinician must also be concerned that his or her own anxiety over suicidal issues is not conveyed to the patient. Such anxiety may be misinterpreted as a forewarning of moral disapproval. If, indeed, the patient picks up evidence of moral condemnation through tone of voice or body language, the patient may shut up like a frightened child before an unforgiving parent. With this problem in mind, it becomes important for the interviewer to be keenly aware of countertransference issues. An awareness of such issues may surface by asking questions of oneself such as:

a. What are my beliefs about suicide?
b. Do I feel that suicide is sinful or unnatural?
c. Do I feel that people who commit suicide are weak?
d. Do I ever picture myself as capable of taking my own life?

e. Have I known anyone in my family or friends who killed themselves? How does this fact affect the way that I approach the
  issue in my interviews?

The answers to such questions may help the interviewer to notice
stylistic elements that may increase patient resistance.

It also seems pertinent to raise a countertransference issue that
many interviewers do not like to admit, but one that I think is
present in most of us. Namely, if we uncover serious suicidal ideation, we are potentially creating a mess for ourselves. For instance,
if suicidal plans emerge, we may need to greatly prolong our assessment when we are already strapped for time. Family members may
need to be involved. We may have to deal with an irate patient or
equally irate family member if we need to proceed with involuntary
commitment. And, finally, we may have to spend a day in court if
commitment occurs. The bottom line is, if we do our job well, we
may have to pay a not-so-insignificant price. These realistic concerns
can definitely emerge as countertransference in the guise of processes such as not even inquiring about suicide, waiting until the
end of the interview to ask about it, poorly setting the stage, hur-
rying the assessment, and asking questions in a manner that decreases the sensitivity of the questions themselves.

With regard to the last concern, it is important to avoid type A
validity errors, as described in Chapter 1, such as asking questions
with a negative, as follows:

  Pt.:   Sometimes things are simply too much. My husband
        can't stop yelling, the dog is barking, kids screaming,
        too much, just too much.

  Clin.:   You've not thought of hurting yourself, have you?

  Pt.:   Why no, I haven't thought of that really.

Such a leading question, which is actually a statement of inquiry
containing a "negative," may suggest to the patient that the interviewer does not morally approve of suicide and may be judgmental
if told of suicidal ideation. In reality, it may merely represent the
hassled interviewer's unconscious prayer that nothing serious comes
up. Unfortunately, to the interviewee, it clearly indicates that this
interviewer wants "no" for an answer. As a general rule, interviewees try to please interviewers. Validity clearly becomes an issue here.
I watched such an interaction in which the patient denied suicidal
ideation to an initial interviewer. A second interviewer reap-
proached the same patient at the end of the first clinician's interview.
This time the second interviewer avoided the question begun with

a negative. He subsequently discovered that the patient had overdosed on aspirin about 5 days earlier. Technique counts.

Concerning the issue of resistance, a second general principle comes to mind that can be simply stated: Do not accept the first "no." I am consistently amazed at how many people flatly deny suicidal ideation when first asked despite the presence of such ideation. The clinician should seldom, if ever, leave the topic after a single denial. As noted earlier, all sorts of resistance issues may be at work.

With these general considerations tucked in the back of our minds, let's begin to look at the first stage in the actual interview process, a step that, if not done well, could spell disaster.

Stage 1: Setting the Platform for the Suicide Inquiry

With regard to setting the platform, the interviewer attempts to create an atmosphere in which the patient is most likely to share suicidal ideation. If one reflects upon it, the most effective atmosphere is probably a rather unusual state. In this state, the patient should feel maximally safe with the interviewer while being intensively involved, psychologically, with the painful emotion that is pushing the patient towards suicide. I have found that intense emotional involvement usually tends to lower conscious defenses, thus increasing the likelihood that suicidal ideation will be shared.

Patients will often spontaneously enter these areas of intense involvement, but at other times, the interviewer must skillfully lead them there. In our previous example of Mr. Jamison, the utility of leading the patient towards intense affective involvement was elegantly illustrated.

In the first interview Mr. Jamison essentially denied suicidal ideation, refusing to elaborate on the subject. Perhaps the stage for sharing had not been adequately set. In contrast, in the second interview, the clinician quietly entered the actively psychotic world of the patient, sensitively leading him into a discussion of his psychotic concerns. As Mr. Jamison entered this world of emotional pain his affective involvement became more intense, leading to an increased desire to relieve his pain by sharing his burdens with a compassionate listener. Obviously, to be effective this process is predicated on the fact that the interviewer has previously decreased the patient's initial paranoia. Consequently, at this delicate point where secrets are shared, the interviewer will be perceived as an ally worthy of such trust.

With regard to psychosis, such well-timed focusing upon affectively charged content may lead the patient into a mildly dissociated state, in which conscious and unconscious defenses may be diminished, with direct questions often yielding direct answers. Processes mentioned earlier, such as command hallucinations, alien control, and hyper-religiosity, may be described more openly by the patient at these times. In essence, the interviewer has created a gate with which to enter the realm of suicidal ideation.

At this junction, it may be beneficial to look at the various gates that can provide more effective access to suicidal ideation. There appear to be three primary gates that lead people toward sharing their thoughts of suicide. These gates are: (1) psychotic process, (2) depression and hopelessness, and (3) a sense of crisis, anger, or confusion. Generally speaking, it pays the interviewer to refrain from asking about suicidal ideation until the patient is obviously emotionally involved in one of these three areas. The clinician does not pop the question to the patient; the clinician leads up to it.

If the interviewer suspects that the patient has been depressed, then the interviewer may wait to inquire about suicide until the patient gives evidence of being involved in depressive affect. In some cases, the interviewer may need to gently lead the patient into these areas, because the patient may be using denial or other mechanisms to avoid such painful affect. This principle of guiding the patient towards emotional involvement also applies to the third gate, in which the patient contemplates suicide secondary to some specific emotional turmoil. Sensitively setting the stage in such a manner as described above also provides the interviewer with the time needed to have established a sound degree of blending with the patient, thus further enhancing the likelihood of eliciting suicidal intent. Generally, this evolving process reaches a peak somewhere in the middle of the interview.

On the other hand, not infrequently the interviewee will hint at suicidal ideation earlier. Such hints suggest that the stage may already be set and that the patient is ready to share. If spontaneous gates appear, they should generally be pursued by the interviewer, as follows:

> **Pt.:** My life is very different for me now. Over the past several years it seems to have gone empty.
>
> **Clin.:** How do you mean?
>
> **Pt.:** After the divorce, I was on automatic pilot, but eventually it all sunk in, it all seemed horribly empty, not worth continuing, much as it seems now. But I have managed and have had some brighter days.
>
> **Clin.:** When you say, it seemed not worth continuing, had you thought of ending your life?

Pt.:   Yes . . . and I still do.

Clin.:   What kinds of things have you thought of doing?

Pt.:   I thought of taking pills and I did that once . . .

If the clinician does not pick up on such nuances by referring to them directly, the conversation can quickly move to new topics. If this movement occurs, the clinician may have missed the most opportune spot for inquiry. By bringing up such thoughts, the meta-communication of the patient seems to be a simple one, "Ask me about suicide." When given such an open gate, it seems unwise to walk by it. By not following up, the interviewer may discover that later on, due to an unexpected problem with engagement, the interviewee will no longer feel comfortable about sharing. The suicidal ideation will remain unspoken, a most deadly situation.

Before leaving the process of setting the stage, two other technical points should be mentioned. First, if one gate fails, then the interviewer can try a different gate. For instance, the evaluation may hit a denial of suicidal intent when flowing with depressive ideation in a man with a psychotic depression. If approached by the gate of psychosis, this same man may admit to suicidal ideation.

Some interviewers may initially approach suicidality with a mildly ambiguous question, which essentially invites the interviewee to discuss suicidal ideation without spelling it out. If the patient does not follow this type of lead, the clinician proceeds to ask directly as described earlier. This technique may be of value in patients who appear exceptionally anxious about being interviewed, thus providing a back door through which the patient may feel more comfortable about entering a discussion of suicide, as follows:

Pt.:   Nothing seems to matter much anymore and everything seems wrong.

Clin.:   How do you mean?

Pt.:   I can't sleep, I can't eat, and every minute seems worse than the one before. I'm not kidding when I say I feel miserable.

Clin.:   Have you ever thought of a way of ending your pain?

Pt.:   Yes, yes I have . . . I thought of blowing my brains out (nervous laughter) but that's a little messy.

Clin.:   Sounds scary.

Pt.:   Yes it is.

Clin.:   Do you have a gun in the house?

Pt.:   Yes I do . . . beside my bed.

At this point in our discussion, it is time to look at the actual exploration of the patient's suicidal ideation, the exploration of which is both a delicate and complex art.

Stage 2: Eliciting Suicidal Ideation Using the CASE Approach

BACKGROUND AND LIMITATIONS

When one reviews the enormous literature on suicide assessment, one is first struck by the magnitude of the number of studies, scales, papers, and books. The second striking finding is the relative lack of writing about the practical aspects of "how to do the interview." The vast majority of the writings focus on such topics as statistical indicators, risk factors, what data need to be gathered, and the clinical judgment process itself, which are all very important subjects. However, one critically important subject is often given short shrift.

Few selections focus primarily on the interview process itself; in other words, how did the clinician gather the information in the interview in the first place? More specifically, was the necessary material gathered and was it gathered in a way that maximized both engagement and validity? During a suicide assessment, one can ask for all the "right data," but if it is invalid data, one might as well not be asking. In the last analysis, the cornerstone of all suicide assessments is the degree with which the clinician's interview style leads to the highest level of truthfulness from the patient: to what degree does this person, contemplating death by his or her own hands, let us into his or her secret world? The stakes are high.

The rest of this chapter attempts to fill this void in the literature. From my experience in managing a busy psychiatric emergency room, many of the errors concerning lethality assessment did not come primarily from poor clinical judgment. They often came from good clinical judgment made from poor clinical information. The two biggest errors in the suicide assessment database tended to be errors of omission, involving critical data, and errors in which the interviewer's style of questioning or engagement resulted in the patient providing misleading information.

The reason why we all make these mistakes, and I make them too, is quite easy to see. Complicated suicide assessments have a way of occurring at complicated times. They often happen right in the middle of an extremely hectic clinic day or in the chaotic environment of a packed emergency room. In these days of managed care, time pressures, and waiting lists, clinicians often find themselves in unenviable positions in which there does not seem to be enough time to do anything well. However, as we all know, a suicide assessment must always be done well.

In addition, suicide and violence assessments, which constitute another topic of this chapter, are, if we are honest, frightening. A mistake can result in an unnecessary death and a terrible tragedy. It can also result in a lawsuit which is much less important but also very disturbing in its own right. Thus in many suicide assessment scenarios, we find a harried clinician, performing an extremely pressurized task, in an unforgiving atmosphere. No wonder mistakes are made. Under such difficult clinical conditions it is very easy to see and understand why we may make mistakes, such as unintentionally forgetting to ask for important data. The truth is—we always will make such mistakes, because we are only human. However, the question is, "Are there techniques and strategies that can greatly diminish the likelihood of such mistakes?" I think that there are.

I believe that the trick lies in developing a flexible but consistent approach to exploring suicidal ideation and in practicing this approach until it becomes second nature, much like a martial artist practices a series of attack and defense movements, called katas, over and over again until they become so natural that they become "instinctive." At this point the movements have become gateways to intuition and, more important, they will be there when the martial artist most needs them: when the martial artist is tired, distressed, feeling beaten or, possibly, even fighting for his or her life. That is exactly what we want as clinicians—a set of graceful and reliable interviewing techniques that will reliably be there when we most need them, no matter how tired we are or how hectic the crisis situation.

It was with this specific intention that the CASE Approach was designed. Borrowing upon the principles of facilics and the structuring techniques that we have already discussed, a simple, easily remembered strategy of questioning was developed. The CASE Approach is not a method of gathering information about the risk factors; most of that information will have been gathered in other regions of the interview. Instead, it presents a method of gathering information about the presence and extent of suicidal ideation itself. Just how close is this person to deciding to kill himself or herself? Using the CASE Approach, the enormous number of points that a clinician needs to explore can become more easily remembered; indeed, memorization becomes minimal, because the key points make logical sense to ask.

It is also very important to remember that the CASE Approach is not a method for making a clinical decision, but rather it is a method for gathering the information from which an effective clinical decision can be made. It is the first step in a suicide assessment—the data gathering. The second step, involving what to "make" of that data and the clinical decision-making itself, constituted the topics of the first part of this chapter. The CASE Approach is presented as an easily learned framework for gathering the critical database about suicidal ideation itself.

As we have seen from our understanding of facilic analysis, one of the best ways for a clinician to avoid errors of omission is to simplify the database. With regard to suicide assessment, this simplification takes place by organizing the sprawling set of questions, which are pertinent when exploring suicidal ideation, into much smaller and more manageable regions, each of which has a well-defined body of information to gather. These separate regions are significantly easier to remember and explore. For example, we have seen earlier how the massive and somewhat chaotic-appearing database expected in an initial diagnostic assessment using the DSM-IV becomes more manageable by exploring it region by region in a sensitive and methodical fashion.

These facilic principles, when applied to the area of suicidal ideation and actions, point towards four discrete regions that are worthy of exploration. Each region represents one step in a manageable process. Each region is based on an exploration of suicidal ideation and actions within a specific time frame, hence the term "chronological" in the name of the approach. Generally speaking, each region is explored thoroughly before moving to the next. The clinician consciously chooses not to move with pivot points into unrelated material, unless there is a very good reason to do so. When the stage has been set appropriately to explore suicidal ideation, the clinician explores the following four regions in this order: (1) the presenting ideation or suicidal event, (2) the recent ideation and events (over the preceding 6 to 8 weeks), (3) past suicidal ideation and events, and (4) immediate ideation and plans for the future. Please refer to Figure 11.

This pathway seems to flow quite smoothly for most patients. Naturally one can, and should, flexibly alter it depending on the needs of any specific patient. Once the topic of suicide has been raised it makes sense, to most patients, to talk about their presenting attempt first, if one is present. It follows naturally to discuss recent ideation and subsequently past ideation. We have found that these joint explorations of the past generally improve engagement and trust, as the patient sees that it is "O.K." to talk about suicidal ideation. At this point, when the trust is maximized, it makes sense to explore current suicidal plans and intentions, because this is the single most important area of a suicide assessment. Here is the

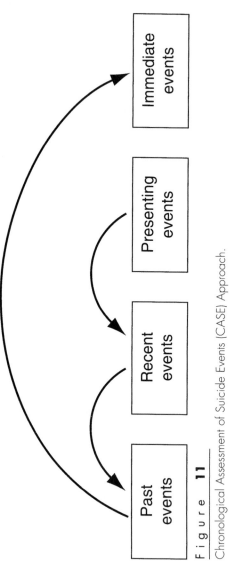

F i g u r e **11**

Chronological Assessment of Suicide Events (CASE) Approach.

region where the most subtle nuances of facial expression or hesi-tancy of speech may indicate that suicide is imminent.

This chronological approach is very simple. That is exactly why it works. It is easy to remember. In fact, it is actually hard to forget. Most clinicians tell me that once they have studied it, it naturally pops into their minds as soon as they begin an exploration of suicidal ideation. All that remains is to examine what information is important to explore in each time frame, always attempting to simplify the task by organizing the material into logical miniregions and strategies. We will now examine each chronological region in detail, in the same order we would explore them in an actual interview.

Step 1: Exploration of Presenting Suicidal Events

If a patient presents with a suicide attempt or gesture, it becomes critical to understand the severity of the event, because a serious suicide attempt represents one of the criteria of our Triad of Lethality and may well indicate the need for prompt hospitalization. But what information are we seeking? What would tell us that this was a dangerous event and that hospitalization might be necessary? The answer seems to lie in asking a series of questions that give the clinician an idea of how close the patient came to killing himself or herself and how does the patient feel about the fact that he or she did not die. The following information can help provide answers to these two pressing questions:

1. How did the patient try to kill himself? (e.g., What method was used?)
2. How serious was the action taken with this method? (e.g., If the patient overdosed, what pills and how many were taken? If the patient cut himself, where did he cut and did the cut require stitches?)
3. To what degree did the patient intend to die? (e.g., Did the patient tell anyone about the attempt afterwards? Did the patient hint to anyone beforehand? Did the patient do the attempt in an isolated area or in a place where he or she was likely to be found? Did the patient write a will or suicide note, check on insurance, or say good-bye to significant others in the days preceding the event?)
4. How does the patient feel about the fact that he or she did not successfully kill himself or herself? (A very good question here is to simply ask, "What are some of your thoughts about the fact that you are still alive now?")
5. How well planned was this attempt as opposed to an impul-sive act?

6. Did alcohol or drugs play a role in the attempt?
7. Were interpersonal factors a major role in the attempt, including feelings of failure, "people would be better off without me," and anger toward people (a suicide attempt undertaken to make others feel guilt)?
8. Was there a specific stressor or set of stressors that prompted the attempt?
9. At the time of the attempt, how hopeless did the patient feel?
10. Why did the attempt fail? (e.g., How was the patient found, and how did the patient end up getting help?)

As one can see, answers to these questions can provide a powerful window into the internal world of the patient at the time of the attempt. Such a window provides the best information available with regard to how serious the patient was during this attempt. All the statistical risk factors in the world will not tell us if a specific patient intended death. Excluding patients who may accidentally kill themselves during manipulative gestures, people kill themselves because they have decided to do so. It is not only an act of the heart, but it is also a cognitive decision of the mind. The above information gives us direct access into the shadowy recesses of this decision-making process.

Obviously, it is important to uncover the information described above, but at first glance this appears to be an intimidating list of things to remember. To some degree it is, if one tries to memorize it. We need a strategy. Fortunately, we already have one. In the first chapter of this book, we discussed the power of a validity technique, designed by Pascal, called the "Behavioral Incident." If you recall, the clinician uses this technique every time that he or she does one of two things: asks for a specific piece of data (e.g., "Did you put the gun up to your head?") or asks the patient to continue a description of what happened sequentially (e.g., "Tell me what you did next"). Using the behavioral incident technique, there is a way to gather almost all of the above data without even having to think about the separate bits for the most part. Simply ask the patient to "walk you through" the suicide incident itself, from front to back. In essence ask the patient to create a "verbal videotape" step by step. If the patient does this, then almost all of the material described above will surface naturally.

Let us see this strategy at work with a 52-year-old successful businessman, who we will call Mr. Leland. Last night he was seen in the emergency room by a member of the crisis team, following an overdose. He refused hospitalization but agreed to see a therapist the next day for possible inclusion in a crisis support group. Much of his pain arises from the unexpected loss of his wife of 30 years, who died of a ruptured aneurysm about 3 months ago.

Mr. Leland is a man who was greatly subdued by his pain. He speaks surprisingly quietly, and with a weary hesitation that one would not necessarily expect from a high-powered executive. He is nicely groomed, and as one would expect from an executive, he is all too well tooled in the fine art of putting up a pleasant front during difficult times. His short black hair, like his voice, is quietly receding. Occasionally he manages a genuine but weary smile, the look of a strong man resigned to his own weakening. Let us pick up the conversation as the clinician begins an exploration of the presenting suicide event:

Clin.: It's my understanding from the crisis worker, Elizabeth, that . . .

Pt.: By the way, a very nice person.

Clin.: Yes, she is. And very good too. In any case Elizabeth told me you had overdosed last night. Tell me a little bit about what happened.

Pt.: Well, not much to say. I just felt like I couldn't take it any more, and I took a bunch of pills.

Clin.: Why don't you sort of walk me through what happened last night, so I get a better feel for what happened. For instance when did you start to think about killing yourself yesterday?

Pt.: That's hard to say, I've been thinking about it a lot . . . (pause). I find weekends really hard. I miss her so much. I do better during the work week when I'm busy. The weekends seem endless. Anyway, after dinner I just sort of felt overwhelmed. I was listening to a song we loved, and I just couldn't stop crying.

Clin.: It sounds very very painful, well beyond words (patient nods his head in agreement). What happened next?

Pt.: Well I just took the pills.

Clin.: Now where did you keep the pills?

Pt.: In the medicine cabinet.

Clin.: Had you stockpiled any pills, you know, with the intention of maybe killing yourself?

Pt.: Yea, I'm ashamed to say so, but I had.

Clin.: What makes you say you are ashamed to say so?

Pt.: It just seems weak, an easy way out, it's not me.

Clin.: It doesn't sound weak to me, with all the pain you are feeling, it's pretty common to have thoughts of killing oneself. You know I see this less as a sign of weakness and more as a sign of how much you loved your wife.

Pt.: (tilts his head and squints his eyes) Hmm. Yea, I guess that's possible.

Clin.: But back to the overdose itself, how many bottles had you stored up?

Pt.: Fifteen, twenty.

Clin.: So you'd been thinking about this awhile?

Pt.: Oh yea.

Clin.: Had you made out your will or done other things like written suicide notes?

Pt.: As a matter of fact, I had written a note for my son, Bernie. My will, it was already in order.

Clin.: Now when you took the pills what pills did you take?

Pt.: Some Tylenol, some Benadryl, and some type of sleeping med, I forget what it was.

Clin.: How many pills did you take?

Pt.: Not a lot.

Clin.: Roughly how many, 30, 40?

Pt.: No not that much, maybe 15, 20 max.

Clin.: What stopped you?

Pt.: I'm not really sure . . . (pause). I think part of it was my son, I tore the letter up when I was done. I don't think it's fair to him, to have to deal with another death, not after what he's been through. I think I'm just going to have to deal with this (hand goes up to his brow and he begins to sob) but I'm not sure I can.

Clin.: Well I'm glad you came in. Obviously you're in a lot of pain, and you're obviously a very strong man. Maybe we can help you to deal with this better.

Pt.: I hope so . . . . God, I hope so.

Clin.: I know you've been in a tremendous amount of pain recently. Sometimes that makes people feel hopeless. Were you feeling hopeless last night?

Pt.: Pretty hopeless, but I feel a little better today, I think I need to go on, killing myself isn't the answer.

Clin.: What makes you say that?

Pt.: I stopped didn't I?

Clin.: Yes, I guess you did. I'm struck by your strength and your love for your son too. You know, when you say you stopped, what did you do after you stopped?

Pt.: Well I called my best friend, Peter. I told him what was going on. He wasn't surprised. He told me he'd been worried about me and thought we needed to go to the E.R. I was so damn exhausted I just did what he said and off we went.

Clin.: How do you feel about the fact you're still alive?

Pt.: (long pause) I don't know (pause). I guess it's O.K. I need some help of some sort, if I'm going to go on. I can't go on like this indefinitely.

Clin.: I think we can get you some help. That's why we're here. You've done a really good job of telling me about some very difficult material to talk about. One other thing I wanted to touch on. A lot of people who try to kill themselves, sort of get up the courage to kill themselves by drinking. I was wondering if you were drinking at all last night.

Pt.: Not really, maybe a couple of vodkas on the rocks, but that's it. I didn't need much alcohol to give me the courage to do it. When I reached for the pills, I wanted to die, I saw no reason to go on, until I started thinking about Bernie again.

So far the clinician has done a nice job of exploring the presenting ideation, always attending to the engagement process, while consciously sticking to the task of creating a verbal videotape of the attempt. Powerful information has been shared. And, frankly, it's a bit of a "dicey call" at present. Mr. Leland seems to have decided against suicide, but the intensity of his pain, the thought-out nature of the plan, and the hopelessness of last night (a hopelessness which could return quickly) are all disturbing. Clearly, more information is needed. Just how extensive have Mr. Leland's thoughts of suicide been recently? How close has he been to actually killing himself? Let's find out.

Step 2: Exploration of Recent Suicidal Events

In this region, the clinician will delineate the types of suicidal thoughts and actions that the patient has had during the previous 6 to 8 weeks. This glimpse of the patient's world can provide important insights into the degree of suicidal planning and intent that the patient has experienced. The more concrete and thorough the planning and the more frequent and intense the ideation, the more concerned the clinician should be about acute suicide risk. This region also provides a wonderful window into the patient's weighing of the advantages and disadvantages of suicide, including the patient's thoughts concerning what death will bring, all of which can provide insight into the patient's immediate dangerousness.

Vague forays such as, "How much have you been thinking about suicide?" and "Have you thought about any other ways?"—if left alone—are invitations for miscommunication and under-reporting of suicidal ideation. With the CASE Approach, this region is explored by concretely determining exactly what types of plans for suicide the patient has had and how far the patient has acted on these plans. Such concrete behavioral information can provide a more direct measure of lethality. The best way to approach this process unfolds in three steps: (1) Find out what plans have been contemplated, (2) determine how far the patient took actions on these plans, and (3) determine how much of the patient's time is spent on these plans and accompanying ruminations about suicide.

This database looks somewhat formidable in scope, although it is obviously of great potential value. Keep in mind that we are trying to gather the most valid and comprehensive database that will allow us to make our best educated guess about the patient's lethality, because it is always a guess. However, we want to make this guess from the best view of "where the patient is at" that we can possibly garner. Fortunately, as was the case with our exploration of the region of the presenting event, we already have the tools necessary to do the task engagingly and with a minimum of time. Once again the behavioral incident will be of great use, but this time it will be combined with some of the other validity techniques that we discussed in Chapter 7 on uncovering personality dysfunction. Specifically, gentle assumption, symptom amplification, and denial of the specific will all be utilized.

The task is rather straightforward. We will delineate the list of methods and the extent of action taken upon them by weaving these validity techniques into easily remembered strategies. I will talk about two different approaches, but the reader should feel free to design new approaches in a flexible fashion as the needs arise. There is no cookbook approach that is correct, but these principles can make the exploration of recent ideation and actions surprisingly easy and natural.

The first approach is straightforward. After the clinician has finished exploring the region of the presenting event, gentle assumption is used to delineate the next method that was considered by the patient, such as the use of a gun. The clinician then proceeds to use a series of behavioral incidents to sculpt out how far the patient acted on this method. If the patient responds with positive answers to each question, the series may look something like this: "Do you have a gun in the house?", "Have you ever gotten the gun out with the intention of thinking about using it to kill yourself?", "Have you ever loaded the gun?", "Have you put the gun up to your body or head?", "How long did you hold the gun there?", "Did you take the safety off?", "What stopped you from pulling the trigger?"

Once the clinician has a good idea of how close the patient came to killing himself or herself with this method, the clinician once again uses gentle assumption to get the third method. This method is then explored, using behavioral incidents in exactly the same manner. Gentle assumptions are then used with follow-up behavioral incidents until the patient denies other methods.

But the clinician doesn't stop here. Once the use of a gentle assumption yields a negative answer, the clinician uses a series of denials of the specific. We have seen earlier how surprisingly powerful this technique can be, even when a patient has denied sensitive material earlier in the interview. The interviewer doesn't drive this technique into the ground with a long series of methods, but simply asks about any methods that are common to the patient's culture and that have not been discussed yet. Thus, if the patient has talked about overdosing, guns, and driving the car off the road, the clinician may ask the following short list of denials of the specific: "Have you thought about cutting or stabbing yourself?", "Have you thought about hanging yourself?", "Have you thought about jumping off a bridge or other high place?", "Have you thought about carbon monoxide?" I never cease to be amazed at how often such questions uncover more ideation, and in a few cases I have actually had recent attempts uncovered, despite further suicidal ideation being denied earlier. As before, if a new method is uncovered the clinician uses a series of behavioral incidents to find out to what extent the patient took action.

This approach for generating the methods and actions taken towards suicide is shown in Figure 12. After completing these explorations, the clinician then hones in on the frequency, duration,

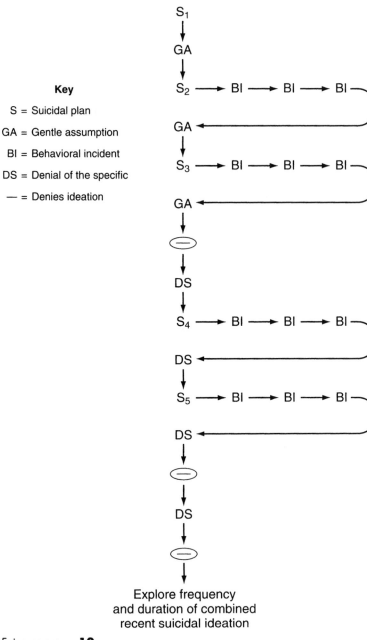

Key

S = Suicidal plan

GA = Gentle assumption

BI = Behavioral incident

DS = Denial of the specific

— = Denies ideation

Explore frequency
and duration of combined
recent suicidal ideation

F i g u r e   **12**

Exploration of recent suicidal ideation.

and intensity of the suicidal ideation with a question such as: "Over the past 6 to 8 weeks, how much time daily do you think about killing yourself, roughly?"

This approach is logical and simple to remember. It also flows imperceptibly for the patient, frequently increasing engagement as the patient is pleasantly surprised at how easy it is to talk to the clinician about material that had frequently been shouldered as a topic of shame for the patient. Let us return to Mr. Leland and see if this approach sheds more light into his suicide potential:

Clin.: You've talked about your son Bernie several times. He must mean a lot to you.

Pt.: He's a good kid. Well, he's not really a kid any more.

Clin.: How old is he?

Pt.: Twenty-three and he's gone through a lot. He's right in the middle of law school, and he's struggling a bit. Then he lost his mom. I don't think he could handle his old man killing himself right now. Maybe later. I just hope I can hold on for him.

Clin.: As I hear you talk it's clear you've been in intense pain ever since your wife died. How long have you been thinking about killing yourself?

Pt.: That's sort of hard to say. But I thought about killing myself the day she died. But I didn't really start thinking about it seriously until about 2 months ago.

Clin.: What other ways, besides pills, have you been thinking about (gentle assumption)?

Pt.: (pause) Well for awhile there I was thinking about shooting myself.

Clin.: Do you have a gun (behavioral incident)?

Pt.: Not now. I got rid of it. Too dangerous.

Clin.: How do you mean, too dangerous?

Pt.: I thought I was going to kill myself with it.

Clin.: Did you ever get it out with the intention of killing yourself (behavioral incident)?

Pt.: Yes I did.

Clin.: Did you ever load it with thoughts of killing yourself (behavioral incident)?

Pt.: Yes I did.

Clin.: What did you do after you loaded it (behavioral incident)?

Pt.: Well I only did that once. I kept the gun in the bedroom in the night stand. Bought it for burglars. My wife was always worried about burglars (pauses, looks away for a moment). Any way, about a month ago, I got the thing out. It was a Friday night, some friends had invited me over, my friends have been great. But I just didn't want to go. I got really bad. And I just went to the bed and loaded the thing.

Clin.: What did you do then (behavioral incident)?

Pt.: I put it inside my mouth. But I didn't pull the trigger.

Clin.: Had you taken off the safety?

Pt.: Yea.

Clin.: Wow, close.

Pt.: Real close.

Clin.: What stopped you (behavioral incident)?

Pt.: I don't have the foggiest idea (sighs). I just didn't do it. I gave the gun for keeping to a friend the next day. If I wouldn't have done that, I really think I would have been dead last night. I'd have used it.

Clin.: That was another example of you stopping yourself. What do you make of that?

Pt.: You know, there must be a part of me that doesn't want to do this, Lord knows why. But I've never been a quitter. I had a neighbor who killed himself once. And I remember thinking it was wrong. Deep in my gut I still feel that. I think that's why I'm here today. I don't want to kill myself. But the thoughts just keep coming.

Clin.: What other ways have you been thinking about killing yourself (gentle assumption)?

Pt.: Oh I don't think there are any other ways. That's enough isn't it (smiles)?

Clin.: Yes, that's enough (both laugh). What about cutting yourself or stabbing yourself (denial of the specific)?

Pt.: That is not appealing, never even crossed my mind.

Clin.: How about driving your car off the road (denial of the specific)?

Pt.: Thought about it briefly, but it's not a sure thing.

Clin.: How frequently did you think about it (behavioral incident)?

Pt.: Oh, not often, couple times, just fleetingly.

Clin.: Did you ever get in the car with the intention of killing yourself (behavioral incident)?

Pt.: No, can't say that I have.

Clin.: How about hanging yourself (denial of the specific)?

Pt.: Absolutely no way. Never crossed my mind. That's repellent to me.

Clin.: How about carbon monoxide (denial of the specific)?

Pt.: You know, I did think of that. Back when I was thinking of shooting myself, I also thought about that.

Clin.: Did you go to the car and check it out with thoughts of doing that (behavioral incident)?

Pt.: Sort of.

Clin.: What do you mean, what did you do (behavioral incident)?

Pt.: I went out to the garage and sort of looked things over. I wanted to see if there were doors I'd need to seal up and cracks in the walls. I even looked at my hose, but couldn't figure out how you are supposed to attach the damn thing to your exhaust.

Clin.: What did you do next (behavioral incident)?

Pt.: Nothing (smiles sort of sheepishly). I thought it would be too much damn trouble (shakes his head from side to side and smiles again in embarrassment).

Clin.: Over the past couple of months how much time have you been spending thinking about all these ways, say on a daily basis (behavioral incident)?

Pt.: That's hard to say.

Clin.: Couple of hours a day: 4, 6 hours, most of the day (symptom amplification)?

Pt.: Here's the strange thing. It's actually gotten better. Back when I was thinking about the gun, I was sometimes thinking about it most of the day. But it's been much less, not even daily and then boom, I just felt like crap last night. It was sort of strange. But I really don't want to kill myself now. If I'd wanted to, I could have done it last night after they let me go home, but I don't really want to. I'm really not a weak person. Really.

Clin.: I can see that. And I think we have a lot to offer you.

Pt.: Good. I've heard very good things about this place.

This has proved to be a powerful segment of interviewing, done nicely. Much has come to light. In the first place there are some promising signs here. Mr. Leland clearly seems to be denying current intent, and it comes across in a believable way. He also had a weapon removed from his house, which shows a real instinct for self-protection. He seems to have a strong superego, and this is helping him to feel that it is important to avoid suicide. The framework for meaning, concerning his son, sounds powerful. Ironically, it is given even more validity by his comment that maybe he would commit suicide later but not now, because his son really couldn't handle it now. This suggests that he has really given a lot of thought to his son's needs and seems committed "to living."

Also, notice that his affect has improved as the suicide assessment has progressed. There is some genuine humor there, and he is building a bond with the interviewer. This could prove to be an important point in helping him to remain as an outpatient, perhaps in a crisis support group.

On the other hand, the clinician has deftly uncovered a significant background of suicidal ideation and some significant action, which some clinicians might have missed. Mr. Leland's suicide risk is to be taken quite seriously. I believe that he could very well have killed himself if he had not disposed of the gun. Moreover, if Mr. Leland were to demonstrate any "gaminess" about his safety in the rest of the interview or look more ambivalent, the clinician now has enough background information so that he would probably lean towards hospitalization, even commitment. Note that the careful and persistent use of gentle assumptions and behavioral incidents has led to some very strong grounds for an involuntary commitment, which "would stick" if needed. A judge is much more likely to be impressed with the "gun in the mouth" than the relatively small overdose.

The excerpt also demonstrates a beneficial but rather peculiar "side effect" of using behavioral incidents to find out how far a person has taken actions towards self-harm. Not infrequently, while patients are describing their actions, they spontaneously discuss some of the advantages and disadvantages about killing themselves. This listing often provides important clues with regard to which "way they are leaning." For instance, in the above excerpt, while discussing why he stopped himself and did not proceed to use the gun, Mr. Leland raised the issue of a friend who had killed himself and we uncovered his bias that suicide is morally weak, which represents an important deterrent from his perspective.

Sometimes, at such moments, it is an ideal time for the interviewer to lead the dialogue into a deeper exploration as to what the patient hopes to achieve by his or her own death. In his wonderfully insightful and very practical book, *Suicide Risk: The Formulation of Clinical Judgment*, John T. Maltsberger points out the diversity of fashions in which patients can view their own death by suicide:

1. Suicide is a gateway leading into a dreamless sleep (nothingness).
2. It will effect reunion with someone or something that has been lost.
3. It will be a way of escaping from a persecutory enemy, interior or exterior.
4. It will destroy an enemy who seems to have taken up a place in the patient's body or some other part of himself.
5. It will provide a passage into another, better world.
6. One can get revenge on someone else by abandoning him or by destroying his favorite possession (the patient's body), and one can then watch him suffer from beyond the grave.[38]

The clinician can ask questions that explore regions such as the above, and the answers can provide insight into the drives motivating the individual patient towards death, perhaps gaining further insight into the imminent risk of a suicide attempt. These beliefs can serve as surprisingly powerful, and sometimes odd, motivators for suicide, especially in people who see no other ways of resolving their current pain or who find existence, as we know it, to be a bleak proposition. This was highlighted in the mass suicide of 39 people in a rich suburb of San Diego. The idea that suicide could provide a method of passage to a better world was the driving force behind the members of the Heaven's Gate cult. The cult members believed that their death would carry them to a better world aboard an alien spacecraft, which just happened to be tagging a ride inside the tail of the Hale-Bopp Comet.

I had mentioned there are other ways to approach the task of exploring the region of recent suicidal events. In the second most popular way that I have seen (and this is a way that I'm very comfortable with as well), the clinician first generates the entire list of suicide methods, contemplated by the patient, and then goes back to explore each one in detail.

In this approach, after the clinician has finished exploring the presenting method, gentle assumption is used to find out the second method, if indeed one has been considered. In the first approach, the clinician would have proceeded to use behavioral incidents to delineate the extent of action taken on this new method, but this is not the case in this approach. As soon as the second method is uncovered, the clinician asks another gentle assumption such as, "What other ways have you thought of killing yourself?" This use of gentle assumptions is continued until the patient answers that there are no other ways. The clinician does not stop there. The interviewer proceeds to use denial of the specific repeatedly until the list is done. It might be useful to look at Figure 13 now, because it shows this approach in detail, making it easy to see how it differs from the first approach that we discussed.

At this point the clinician then returns to each method in turn and uses a string of behavioral incidents to find out how far the patient has gone in taking actions towards self-harm. For instance, the clinician might say, using an internal referred gate, "Earlier you mentioned that you had thought of shooting yourself. Is there a gun in the house or one available to you?" A series of clarifying behavioral incidents would follow, concerning the actions taken with the gun. When the interviewer has completed his or her determination of the extent of action taken by the patient on this second suicide method, the interviewer will proceed to use the exact same tactic with the third method, and so forth.

Just as with the first strategy, after all methods are explored with behavioral incidents, the clinician checks on the frequency, duration, and intensity of the recent ideation with a question such as, "Looking at all these methods combined, over the past 6 to 8 weeks, how much of any given day are you spending on thoughts of suicide?"

Both methods are easy to remember. In the first strategy, as each method is uncovered, the clinician uses behavioral incidents to follow the extent of action taken. In the second method, a list of all the methods is uncovered first before any of them are explored in detail with behavioral incidents. You can try both methods and decide which one you prefer, or you can develop entirely new

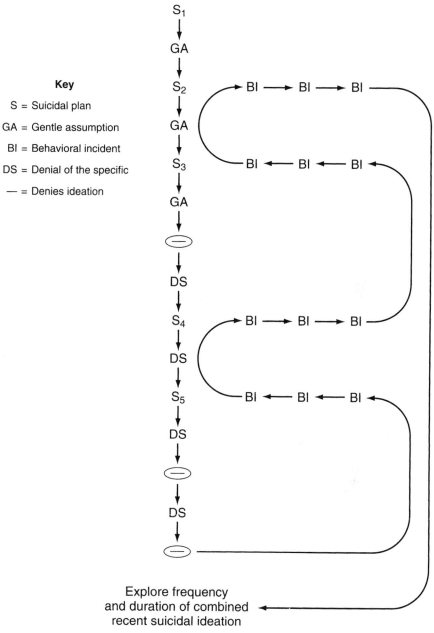

Key

S = Suicidal plan

GA = Gentle assumption

BI = Behavioral incident

DS = Denial of the specific

— = Denies ideation

Explore frequency
and duration of combined
recent suicidal ideation

F i g u r e   **13**

Alternative exploration of recent suicidal ideation.

methods. There is no right method. However, the art is to consciously develop strategies as opposed to relying solely on intuition or habit.

After the clinician has explored the patient's recent ideation, there is still more investigative work to be done, because a history of serious suicide attempts in the past could change the triage decision. One wonders what the history of Mr. Leland will hold.

Step 3: Exploration of Past Suicidal Events

In a curious sense, this is the one area where clinicians sometimes, during the initial interview, spend too much time. Patients with extensive histories of suicidal attempts and gestures, as seen with some people suffering from a borderline structure, may have enormous past histories of suicidal material. One could spend an hour just reviewing this material. It would be an hour poorly spent.

Under the time constraints of busy practices and managed care, initial assessments must usually be completed in an hour. Time is at a premium, thus the question becomes, "What past suicidal history is important to gather?" I believe the answer is: "Gather only that information that could potentially change one's decision on the safety of the patient." Using this filter, the following key points require inquiry:

1. What is the most serious past suicide attempt? (Is the current ideation focused on the same method? Practice can be deadly in this arena. Does the patient view the current stressors and options in the same light as during the most dangerous past attempt?)
2. What is the approximate number of past gestures and attempts? (Large numbers here can alert the clinician to issues of manipulation, making one less concerned, or may alert the clinician that the patient has truly exhausted all hope, making him or her more concerned. In either case, it is important to know.)
3. When was the most recent attempt?

That's about it. I don't think it is important, in the first interview, to explore this region in much more detail. The above questions will ferret out the information that could alter the actual decision about the patient's safety. For instance, if one were to discover that Mr. Leland had actually taken a very serious overdose about a year ago, requiring him to be hospitalized in an intensive care unit, this would make one more concerned about his current safety. Of even more concern would be the fact that he had not mentioned this earlier, and had, indeed, been implying that suicide was quite foreign to him. Similarly, if Mr. Leland admitted to a string of attempts or gestures in the past, one would have to question the reliability of his current assurances of safety.

Let us see what our clinician found out:

Clin.: I'm glad you've heard good things about us. A little bit later I'd like to discuss some of the options we have for helping you. To help me get a little bit better idea of how we can help, I'd like to hear a little bit more about your past, especially any past suicidal ideation. Have you ever tried to kill yourself in the past, even way back when you were a child or teenager?

Pt.: No.

Clin.: How about any vague suicidal thoughts or feelings?

Pt.: Oh way back in college I had some toying with the idea.

Clin.: What were the circumstances?

Pt.: Oh I had broken up with a girlfriend, but I got over it. Sort of felt like the end of the world then.

Clin.: What ways, if any, did you think of?

Pt.: Oh God, no way. This was just a couple of fleeting thoughts. I've never seriously thought about suicide at all until now.

Done. Not much there, which is a great sign. The clinician pushed on "any vague suicidal thoughts or feelings" just to ensure Mr. Leland was not downplaying something significant. Once the clinician has finished exploring past suicidal events, it is time to explore the single most powerful time frame—the present.

Step 4: Exploration of Immediate Suicidal Events

This region focuses on "Where is this patient, right now, concerning suicidal intent?" In a practical sense, the clinician focuses on the suicidal ideation that the patient is having during the interview and the patient's prediction of future thoughts of suicide, after he or she leaves the office or emergency room and returns home.

It cannot be emphasized enough that if there are continuing concerns about the safety of the patient or the validity of the patient's self-report, corroborative sources are critical. It is important to evaluate the support structure and, if necessary, design specific interventions and plans for the use of these supports.

In this region of the CASE Approach, this is frequently done by asking questions such as, "What would you do later tonight or tomorrow if you began to have suicidal thoughts again?" From the patient's answer one often gets a feeling of how serious the patient is about ensuring his or her own safety, as well as providing a chance to brainstorm and finalize plans for just such an occurrence.

Obviously, one also asks the patient point blank whether or not he or she is feeling suicidal at present with questions such as, "Right now, are you having any thoughts about wanting to kill yourself?"

This leads into questions about "safety contracting." The single most important thing to remember about safety contracting is that it provides no guarantee of safety whatsoever. I once had a patient overdose 2 hours after making a safety contract in my office.

Can a safety contract act as a relative deterrent? I don't believe there is any proof one way or the other. My personal bias is that safety contracts can sometimes function as deterrents. The more powerful the bond is with the clinician and the more concrete the contract (e.g., written down), probably the more powerful will be the deterrent. It is hard to kill oneself. Anything that makes it even harder can function as a deterrent. In this regard, I believe that a sense of commitment and trust with a therapist can make the patient hesitant to break his or her word.

In terms of litigation, the documentation of a safety contract in the initial assessment provides some mild forensic support in a lawsuit, by demonstrating that one asked about safety in some detail, making it harder to prove negligence on the clinician's part. This protection is probably enhanced by carefully wording your record of the use of the contract, using observations that would be valuable in defending why you believed that the safety contract was a good one. For instance, "The patient was able to make a sound safety contract with me, showing good eye contact, a genuine affect, and a natural and unhesitant tone of voice."

If one is meeting the patient for the first time, for instance in an emergency room, is a safety contract of use? As an effective deterrent, a safety contract is probably much less useful than in the context of a well-established psychotherapeutic relationship. However, if the patient has bonded quickly, as Mr. Leland did with the crisis worker, Elizabeth, or as he is apparently doing with the current clinician, it may have a mild deterrent effect.

Deterrence, however, is not the main reason to use a safety contract in the initial meeting. The main reason to use a safety contract is to utilize the process of negotiating the contract as an exquisitely sensitive assessment tool. At the time of presenting the safety contract, scour the patient's face, body, and tone of voice for any of the signs of deceit or ambivalence. Here is the proverbial "moment of truth." I believe that this moment of the interview is, potentially, the most powerful window into the patient's true suicidal intent. Look carefully.

Using the "safety contract" as an assessment tool, I have completely changed my mind about letting a person go because of hesitancy on his or her part to contract. If one notices nonverbal clues of ambivalence, one can simply ask, "It looks like this is sort of hard for you to agree to, what's going on in your mind?" The answer can be benign or pose a cause for concern.

It is also important to realize that there are certain people with whom it is best to avoid the whole issue of a safety contract. By way of illustration, some patients with borderline or passive-aggressive characteristics may become embroiled in manipulation around safety contracting issues, tossing out lines like, "I don't know what to tell you, I guess I'm safe, but on the other hand, I can't make any guarantees, do you know anybody who can?" This type of comment is usually made around 2:00 A.M. in an emergency room teeming with restless people who are waiting to be assessed. The question of whether or not to use a safety contract with a person suffering from a severe character disorder is best addressed by directly talking with the patient's ongoing treatment team or therapist.

A final note regarding the safety contract is worth mentioning. Once again, it is important to explore the patient's current level of hopelessness and whether or not the patient is making productive plans for the future or is amenable to brainstorming on concrete plans for dealing with current problems and stresses. It is important to see if the patient is interested in follow-up mental health care.

Let's take a look at an exploration of this last region of the CASE Approach with Mr. Leland:

Clin.: We've talked a lot about your thoughts on suicide today and I'm wondering what thoughts you're having right now. Are you feeling like killing yourself now?

Pt.: No. No, like I said I don't think it's the answer now. When I stopped myself last night, I really stopped myself. It's not an option now. I need to be around for Bernie. But I'll tell you, I've got to feel better somehow. I can't go on indefinitely like this.

Clin.: I know that last night you were feeling pretty hopeless, are you still feeling hopeless?

Pt.: No, not really. I actually feel better after talking about all this stuff. Don't get me wrong, I'm not feeling real hopeful either, but I think I might be able to get some help.

Clin.: That's why we're here. Do you feel as we get this help lined up that you can assure me that you'll call our crisis team, 24 hours a day, if you get any more thoughts of suicide?

Pt.: Yes. I'm not going to kill myself.

Clin.: Can you shake on that? It's really important, 24 hours a day.

Pt.: (patient smiles genuinely) Yea I can shake on that. (They shake hands.)

Clin.: Good. Let's talk a bit about some of our options.

Pt.: Now Elizabeth had told me that this support group meets at night, is that true?

Clin.: Yes, that's true. We also have a group in the afternoon.

Pt.: That's great. I can't afford to miss work. I'd be incredibly embarrassed. That makes a big difference.

Clin.: I don't know if you are aware of this, but I'm one of the therapists in our evening group, so we will be working together.

Pt.: Oh good. I feel comfortable with you. And I don't want to have to tell my whole story again.

The suicide assessment is done. Earlier in the interview, the clinician had tracked down all the important statistical risk factors, which were also weighed into the decision-making equation as the CASE strategy helped to cull more and more pertinent data. Mr. Leland, as it turns out, was not a heavy drinker. He was actually concerned about his recent increase and was willing to cut back. There was no psychotic process. He had developed a fairly severe major depression and was referred for a medication assessment, which actually pleased him. He also had a large cluster of concerned friends, several of whom Mr. Leland agreed to have involved in safety planning and providing support. His son, Bernie, eagerly agreed to visit with his Dad for a week to provide some extra support, an idea that seemed to please both Mr. Leland and Bernie. Note also Mr. Leland's spontaneous relief at hearing that the crisis group met in the evening, allowing him to attend without missing work. This was a reassuring moment, because it underscores that Mr. Leland is still concerned about how others perceive him in his future role at work, a concern that would not generally be present in someone who has decided to die.

In this chapter, the overall strategy presented consists of using the CASE Approach to sensitively and deeply enter the patient's world of suicidal preoccupation. This information is used to complement a careful review of the risk factors described earlier. Using these combined approaches, the clinician can begin to gain a deeper understanding of the potential suicide risk of the patient.

During this assessment process, something else has also been accomplished—something very important, because the interviewer has helped the patient to share painful information, which, in many instances, the patient has shouldered alone for too long. At a different level, perhaps the thoughtfulness and thoroughness of the questioning, as illustrated with the CASE Approach, have conveyed that a fellow human cares. To the patient, such caring may represent the first realization of hope. Such was the case with Mr. Leland.

NOTES ON HOMICIDAL IDEATION

Background

We live in a violent culture. Violence permeates our movies, television screens, computer games, and, most disturbingly, our newscasts and newspapers, which is hard evidence that the violence is all too real. It is sobering to realize that in the 10- to 34-year-old age group, homicide outranks suicide as the leading cause of death. In 1994 in the United States, 173 children between the ages of 1 and 4 were murdered.[39] As mental health clinicians, we encounter issues of violence daily and often try to help the victims of violence to regain a sense of safety and integrity.

This segment focuses on spotting the individual who is about to commit violence. One of the first issues of interest is the finding that violence can be inflicted by very different types of people in many different types of settings. Reid Meloy describes two of these distinctive categories—affective violence and predatory violence.[40] In the first category, affective violence, we find individuals who, because of intense anger and emotion, impulsively act out violently, often in response to interpersonal stress and frequently under the influence of alcohol and drugs. This is also frequently the arena of marital violence, child and elder abuse, and violence undertaken at the job or in the streets. This type of violence probably arises from a very "different head-set" than Meloy's second categorization. With predatory violence, the killer or perpetrator has often thought out the violence beforehand, frequently derives pleasure from the violent act itself, and feels little if any remorse. Here is the domain of many rapists, sadistic perpetrators of children, and individuals with sociopathic personality structures.

Although there are undoubtedly significant biologic underpinnings to the above styles of violence, I think it is useful to include a third category of violent behavior—"biologically induced violence." This term specifically describes those individuals whose violence is directly caused by brain pathophysiology or structural pathology. The first subcategory, pathophysiology, includes individuals who are suffering from biochemical abnormalities such as schizophrenia, mania, or acute ingestion of drugs such as lysergic acid diethylamide (LSD) or phencyclidine (PCP). The second subcategory, structural damage, includes people suffering from diseases such as brain tumors, partial complex seizures, intracranial infections, brain trauma, multiple sclerosis, and Alzheimer's disease. Violent behavior sometimes erupts from combinations of these categories as well.

By reminding ourselves of these three "domains of violence," we can sometimes increase our suspicion of when to search for violent ideation, ensuring that we are searching frequently enough. With regard to this latter point, clinicians, owing to various factors including schools of training, countertransference, and lack of familiarity, can sometimes have "blindspots." For instance, exploring for evidence of the sexual sadism often seen in predators can be unnerving and is sometimes, consequently, avoided by a clinician. It should be noted that there are times when such avoidance, if consciously chosen, is not only appropriate but wise. For instance, if a female interviewer unexpectedly uncovers a sexual sadist whose victims are female, the details of this patient's violent history may in some cases be better taken by a male clinician and vice versa for a male interviewer if men are the patient's victims. Another example of a blind spot can occur for clinicians who do not frequently work with people with psychotic processes. In such a situation it can be easy to miss the subtle indications of active psychosis, and consequently the clinician may not undertake the type of questioning that such psychotic process suggests.

Now that we have delineated what we are looking for, the question arises—are there methods for increasing our ability to look for violent ideation? I believe that there are. Fortunately we have already developed the foundation, because, as Tardiff emphasizes in his excellent pocket guide, *Assessment and Management of Violent Patients*,[41] a sound homicide assessment has much in common with a sound suicide assessment. The techniques that we found so valuable in the CASE Approach are directly applicable to an assessment of violence, which is why this segment is much shorter than the section on suicide assessment. Our main tool has already been described.

Before proceeding, though, it should be mentioned that there is a great deal of debate about a clinician's abilities to predict violence, including immediate, short-term, and long-term. It is beyond the scope of this chapter, but the interested reader will find plenty of interest in the works of Lidz and associates and other studies.[42–46]

As was the case with suicide, we will begin with a review of statistical risk factors and then proceed to look directly at techniques for eliciting violent ideation.

Risk Factors for Violence

Past Violence. The single most robust statistical indicator of violence is a history of previous violence.[47, 48] If you want to be a "betting man," here is the place to put your money. As Tardiff notes, a general tendency for marked problems with impulse control may also be part of the picture. In this regard it is also important to ask about destruction of property, criminal record, reckless driving, reckless spending, sexual acting-out, and suicide attempts.[49]

Sex, Age, and Environment. Young men have the highest rate of violent behavior. In fact, after the age of 35, homicide is no longer in the top 10 causes of death in either sex.[50] Growing up in impoverished areas, where violence is sometimes more frequent and peer pressures for violent behavior may be strong, carries a higher risk of violent behavior. It is also noteworthy that growing up in a family in which one was abused or where one watched other family members being abused may also be associated with an increased risk of violence.[51, 52]

Presence of Psychiatric Disorders. The most significant diagnosis here is the presence of alcoholism and street drug abuse. Other common correlates with violence are antisocial personality disorder; borderline personality disorder; and psychiatric disorders secondary to a general medical condition, including conditions such as mental retardation and dementia and disorders where psychotic or manic process may emerge. It should be kept in mind that most people with psychotic process, most of the time, are very safe. It is a damaging and unfortunate myth among the lay public that people with schizophrenia, by definition, are dangerous. On the other hand, during the exacerbation of specific types of psychotic process, such as paranoid delusions and command hallucinations, such patients are definitely at a higher risk of violence. We will talk more about the clinical implications, for the initial interview, of this fact shortly.

Violence is also seen with intermittent explosive disorder. However, this is a relatively rare disorder, and some clinicians inappropriately use it. It can only be applied when there is no other psychiatric disorder present that could explain the violence. Thus it is not an appropriate diagnosis in domestic violence if alcoholism or antisocial personality disorder is present.

Triad of Lethality

As was the case with suicide assessment, a clinician's final clinical judgment is not made solely from statistical risk factors. These risk factors are carefully weighed in addition to information about the patient's immediate presentation. In my opinion, three aspects of this immediate presentation can alert the clinician to the potential for violence, either during the interview itself or upon leaving the emergency room or clinic.

This triad of lethality is as follows: (1) the patient is presenting subsequent to a recent serious act of violence (often brought in by police), (2) the presence of the types of psychotic process that may precipitate violence, and (3) indication from the interview itself that the patient intends to perform violence. The reader probably recognizes that this homicidal triad looks very similar to the triad of lethality for suicide.

With regard to the first element, a history of presenting recent violence, generally the clinician should feel more concerned the more severe was the violent act and the degree with which the patient remains hostile and angry. But here we begin to see the role that an understanding of some of the differences that Meloy points out between violent individuals of an affective style versus a predatory style may play in helping the clinician to predict violence. For instance, if the patient has a history of an affective style of violence, then the continuing presence of a simmering anger during the interview should alert the clinician that hospitalization may be necessary for the purposes of a "cool down." On the other hand, an unwary clinician can be lulled into a sense of safety by the apparent calmness of demeanor of a predator, even right after or before performing an act of violence. Never forget that, in the presence of a predator, it is important to "look through" the person's presenting affect, because it is almost always a mask.

Another important aspect of history concerns the issue of whether the intended victim has been an object of the patient's violence before. If so, this fact should be disconcerting, because the risk of violence may increase in such a "powder keg" environment. Keep in mind that most homicides occur between people well known to each other.

A powder keg environment may also develop when the potentially homicidal patient is placed around other people who have poor impulse control. In short, anger may beget anger, and violence may breed violence. Furthermore, the presence of alcohol abuse or drug abuse, in either the patient or the companions, may increase the risk of violence as well. It is important for the interviewer to actively hunt for evidence of such powder keg environments. As with suicide, corroborative interviews may be revealing in this regard.

Concerning the second element, psychosis, the same three processes as seen with suicide assessment are of concern. Once again, if psychotic process is spotted, the interviewer should actively pursue evidence of: (1) command hallucinations, (2) alien control, and (3) hyper-religiosity. With regard to the latter, the clinician should pay particular attention to "missions from God to rid the earth of some evil." Such an intense preoccupation with right and wrong may be signaling underlying homicidal ideation. The search for specifics may be rewarding, as follows:

Pt.: The world is filled with scum. Derelicts and bums. I hate them all. God wants them gone.

Clin.: How do you mean?

Pt.: God has his ways.

Clin.: Has he given you any ideas of how to get rid of them?

Pt.: Yes he has. He wants me to slit their eyes out. And I might do just that.

Clin.: Have you thought of anyone in particular that you might hurt?

Pt.: Sam . . . what a scum life. I've thought of him.

Clin.: What have you thought of doing to him?

In talking about psychosis, another important avenue to pursue is the presence of paranoia. In particular, the interviewer should search for evidence that the patient so believes in the delusional material that methods of acting upon it have been pursued, as the following illustrates:

Pt.: The neighbors know everything, I can't keep their eyes out of my brain.

Clin.: What are they planning on doing to you?

Pt.:	They're going to cut off my feet but I'm not going to let them.
Clin.:	What have you thought about doing to protect yourself?
Pt.:	I'm going to scissor them.
Clin.:	How do you mean?
Pt.:	I'll stick a pair of scissors in their spines.
Clin.:	Have you armed yourself with scissors or some other weapon at home?
Pt.:	Yes I have. Last night I patrolled my house with a pair of scissors and a butcher knife.

This degree of acting, on the premise that the delusion is a real threat, should strongly suggest hospitalization. Any neighbor of this man may be in serious danger for merely accidentally crossing his path. But the point is, it is not enough to find out if a paranoid delusion is present. The clinician needs to find out what the patient intends to do about it.

With regard to the third element of the triad, the patient's self-report of violent intention and history, we will devote the entire next section to the interview process itself, as we did with suicide assessment.

Elicitation of Violent Ideation

GENERAL CONSIDERATIONS

Ironically, the first thing to remember about the information elicited from the patient, with regard to violent intent, is not to rely upon it. Family members and friends may be far superior sources of information. The police, previous and current therapists, and crisis clinicians may also hold critical pieces of information. One should not forget the immense value of previous records, looking for arrests, violent episodes, commitments, and a history of restraining orders.

The issue of records raises another important point. As Applebaum and Roth point out,[53] one of the major reasons why receiving hospitals reverse involuntary commitments at the door is because important information elicited from the patient, family, or police is not adequately recorded by the interviewer or the information is not passed on to the receiving center. It is often best not only to include these written documents but also to call the receiving institution and speak directly about your concerns with the clinician who will be assessing the patient.

With regard to the strategy for eliciting violent ideation, the flexible use of the same strategies as used with the CASE Approach can be very revealing. First, as with suicide assessment, the clinician carefully "sets the stage." Second, the clinician proceeds to explore presenting, recent, past, and immediate violent events (both ideation and behaviors) in that order.

Once again, the major goal consists of determining whether a concrete violent plan has been reached and whether any actions have been taken on it. The interviewer also looks for information suggesting that the patient is about to impulsively act out violent ideation. A point to keep in mind is that if the interviewer suspects that the patient truly intends to harm a specific person, the clinician has the legal responsibility to warn that potential victim, as mandated by the Tarasoff decision.

SETTING THE STAGE

One aspect to consider, when setting the stage for asking about violent ideation and intent, remains the wide variety of gates available. Homicide has more than the three gates that are useful when dealing with suicidal ideation. Some of these homicidal gates include: (1) psychosis, (2) interpersonal conflict, (3) need for money and other practical concerns, (4) revenge, (5) jealousy, (6) political concerns, (7) organized crime, and (8) violence for pleasure and pathologic sexual desires. Naturally, any of these gates could be used to form a window with which to explore dangerousness.

In domestic violence, one way of setting the stage is to get the patient to describe in detail his or her worst argument with the significant other. Once the patient has depicted the intensity of the anger ask, "When you and your wife are arguing like that, has she ever sort of lost her control and hit you or attacked you?" After the patient responds to this inquiry, one is much more likely to get a valid response to the follow-up, "How about you, during arguments like that. How frequently have you struck your wife or grabbed her, if at all?" By first asking about the other person's potential violence, it helps the patient, whom you actually suspect of violence, to feel equally heard and hence safer with you. This sense of safety can directly lead to more valid self-reporting. Notice also the clinician's use of the validity technique of gentle assumption with the phrase, " . . . how frequently have you struck your wife or grabbed her, if at all?" as opposed to a phrase such as, " . . . have you ever struck your wife or grabbed her?" Of course, domestic violence is sometimes a two-way affair, and this approach can also uncover this process.

Once the patient has been engaged, and the stage is set by exploring regions such as the above, then the formal exploration of violent ideation and behaviors can begin. Even if there is little suspicion of violence, as Tardiff suggests, it should be routinely screened for with nice bridging questions such as, "Have you ever lost your temper?"[54]

CHRONOLOGICAL ASSESSMENT OF VIOLENT IDEATION

Presenting Event. If the patient is brought in following a violent episode, the same principles that are used in exploring a presenting suicide attempt are utilized. The clinician should guide the patient into a creation of a "verbal videotape" through the use of a series of behavioral incidents. It is important to understand the patient's motivation for the violence and how pre-planned, as opposed to impulsive, it may have been. It is very useful to explore the patient's feelings about the act of violence with simple and direct questions such as, "How do you feel about having hit your wife?" and "How do you feel about your wife now?" It is also important to find out what happened after the violence and how the patient ended up in front of you.

The severity of the violence should be carefully delineated using behavioral incidents to avoid the minimization so often seen by abusive or violent individuals. In this light, opinion questions such as, "Did you hurt her badly?" are replaced with, "Did you leave any bruises?", "Did she need to go to an emergency room?", "Did she receive any stitches?" (ask how many), "Did she break any bones?", "Were x-rays taken?" All of these questions can help cut through minimization and denial. In this regard the validity technique of symptom amplification may also be useful, such as with, "How many times did you actually strike Mary, 5, 10, 20 times?"

After exploring this region thoroughly, the clinician smoothly moves into the arena of recent violent activity.

Exploration of Recent Violent Events. This is an extremely important region in the violence assessment, and it covers the past 6 to 8 weeks. As stated earlier, a history of violence is a powerful predictor of future violence. A history of recent violent behavior may be an even more compelling predictor. This is especially true if the object of the intended violence has recently been assaulted by the patient, as is often the case in domestic violence, both spouse battering and child or older adult abuse.

The same consistent and persistent strategy used during the exploration of recent suicidal plans is used here. Only this time, the emphasis is on generating a list of people with whom the patient is having violent ideation or fantasies and then proceeding to find out how much actual planning and action has been taken toward harming each of these people. This exploration will uncover the methods of violence, the timing of the proposed assault, the place of the assault, and whether or not accomplices are to be involved.

As with suicide, once the concrete methods and circumstances are elicited, the clinician makes an effort to determine the frequency and intensity of the patient's violent thoughts. Questions such as the following may be of use: "How many times in the past 5 or 6 weeks, have you been thinking about hurting Debbie, daily, couple times a day?" and "How close do you think you have come to actually hitting her?"

As we have started to see, when the clinician applies the CASE Approach to the assessment of recent violence, a heavy reliance is made upon the same validity techniques that were used in suicide assessment, including the behavioral incident, gentle assumption, symptom amplification, and denial of the specific. Such interviewing can be quite difficult because of the emotional charge attached to it, especially if the clinician is in the presence of a sexual predator. It is not an arena for the squeamish. Clinicians need to practice these techniques. Role-playing and group discussion of these approaches can be very useful.

It is critical that the clinician explore these regions with a matter-of-fact tone of voice and quiet confidence. When asked in a calm, straightforward manner, such questions often get surprisingly straightforward answers, particularly with a patient who has some guilt over his or her behaviors. Let's watch a demonstration of these techniques in a patient who presented to the clinic secondary to depression. He has a pleasant affect and is dressed casually in shorts and a tee shirt. His age is 27, although he looks younger. A relatively recent stressor has been a break-up with his girlfriend, which was initiated entirely by her. The patient attributes much of his pain to this break-up. To the clinician's surprise, the patient relates some stalking behavior.

As the interview proceeds, keep your eye on the clinician's clever maneuvering as he attempts to make sure that enough information has been related about the intended victim, in order that she could be alerted by the police if Tarasoff's decision needs to be invoked:

Clin.: Timothy, when you say you've been following Judy around, what exactly do you mean (behavioral incident)?

Pt.:   I . . . I . . . I sort of keep track of her, you know, where she's been, stuff like that.

Clin.:   Is that easy to do, I mean does she live near you now (behavioral incident)?

Pt.:   Yea, she's still in the city. It ain't that hard.

Clin.:   Do you follow her to work (behavioral incident)?

Pt.:   Sometimes, but more like when she comes home.

Clin.:   Now where does she work and how far is it from there to her home? I want to understand what it is really like for you, when you are following her (behavioral incident).

Pt.:   She's working at Clement's Pharmacy. She takes the subway home. It don't take her long. [Got it! If the patient's ex-girlfriend needs to be warned, there is now adequate information to find out who she is, in the necessity of a Tarasoff's warning. In this case, there is no indication that such a warning is needed yet. Later, after the violence assessment is done, the clinician will ask for the girlfriend's last name. But to do so now may "spook" the patient into withholding information, creating a potentially dangerous situation.]

Clin.:   Now when you say that you follow her at home, what exactly do you mean (behavioral incident)?

Pt.:   I wait to see if she's coming or going, see if she's with anyone.

Clin.:   Do you ever look in her windows or use binoculars to look through the windows (behavioral incident)?

Pt.:   Thought of it, but I've never done it.

Clin.:   How many nights during the past month have you done this, 10, 20 (symptom amplification)?

Pt.:   I don't think that often. Maybe six, seven times.

Clin.:   Are you thinking about hurting her when you follow her (behavioral incident)?

Pt.: No, I'd never hurt her.

Clin.: What are some of the reasons you think you follow her?

Pt.: I don't really know, I guess I miss her.

Clin.: Sounds like you really do (pause). You know, what you're doing is called stalking. It's actually illegal. Do you feel like you need to stop?

Pt.: Sort of. I guess so.

Clin.: Maybe we could help you to stop (pause). Would you like that?

Pt.: Yea.

Clin.: We'll take a look at that later. You know, earlier, you had told me that you had a sexual relationship with . . .

Pt.: Well, we didn't really have sex, I mean, we kissed a lot, but she wouldn't have sex with me.

Clin.: O.K., even so, sometimes after a break-up, people still have sexual thoughts about the other person (normalization), has that been true for you?

Pt.: Yea.

Clin.: What type of sexual fantasies do you have about her (gentle assumption)?

Pt.: I just sort of think about having sex with her, you know, that kind of stuff.

Clin.: Do you masturbate to these fantasies sometimes (behavioral incident)?

Pt.: Oh yea, I like to masturbate.

Clin.: When you masturbate to her, do you ever have fantasies of forcing sex on her (behavioral incident)?

Pt.: Sort of.

Clin.: What do you picture doing (behavioral incident)?

Pt.: I . . . I . . . I just sort of make her have sex with me.

Clin.: In your fantasies, do you ever use a weapon to do that?

Pt.: (looks uncomfortable) Sometimes I picture having a knife with me.

Clin.: I know this is very difficult material to talk about, Timothy, but you're doing a great job of explaining. I ask these questions so that I know what you are really feeling and if there is something you want help with, then I can help better. Getting back to the knife, do you ever picture cutting her with it (behavioral incident)?

Pt.: I have. Not often though, I mean that. I'd never do it. I don't think it's right.

Clin.: I can see the idea of doing it upsets you. Maybe you'd like to get rid of some of these thoughts. When you have the fantasies about her, where do you cut her? (Behavioral incident—this is an attempt to more clearly delineate the degree of lethality of the fantasy material.)

Pt.: Oh man I don't want to talk about this. I really don't picture it very often. I would never do it. (The clinician decides to "back off" a bit so as not to lose the engagement with the patient.)

Clin.: When you follow her, do you ever carry a knife or any other weapons (behavioral incident)?

Pt.: Hell no. I'm not going to do anything to her. I'm just sort of mad at her, that's all. I've never hurt anybody in my life.

Clin.: Good. That's good to hear. Well, Timothy, how about other women? What have your relationships been like over the years?

Pt.: Well there haven't been many. I get mad about that too.

Clin.: What kind of fantasies about forcing sex have you had about other women, if any (gentle assumption)?

Pt.: Not a lot. But I have them, every once in awhile.

Clin.: Timothy, have you ever followed another woman, even for a short distance, ever (behavioral incident)?

Pt.: Never.

Clin.: Have you ever raped anybody, you know, forced sex on them (behavioral incident)?

Pt.: No. (pause) Sometimes I worry about that though.

Clin.: How do you mean (behavioral incident)?

Pt.: Oh, you know, having these thoughts I've been talking about. I know they're not right.

Clin.: Are you O.K. talking about this stuff? I know it's hard to do.

Pt.: (sighs) Yea, I almost feel better. I've never told anybody this stuff.

Clin.: I'm glad you can talk about it. Maybe we can get you some help to stop the thoughts. You mentioned that you know this is bad. I'm wondering what other kinds of sexual thoughts you may have had that you feel sort of bad about having (gentle assumption)? Now might be a good time to talk about them.

Pt.: Nothing, really.

Clin.: Do you buy girlie magazines (behavioral incident)?

Pt.: Oh yea. I masturbate to the pictures.

Clin.: Sometimes those magazines have pictures that excite some people and turn off other people (variant of normalization). Do your magazines ever have pictures of children in them (behavioral incident)?

Pt.: Some of them.

Clin.: Do you look at them (behavioral incident)?

Pt.: Sort of, but they don't turn me on.

Clin.: Have you ever masturbated to them (behavioral incident)?

Pt.: (sheepish affect) A couple of times, but I really didn't get off on it that much.

The interview continues. This clinician is uncovering very important material, and there appears to be growing evidence that we may be in the presence of a predator or "predator in the making." Timothy's anger towards women is disturbing and certainly fits the profile of someone capable of rape. Obviously, pedophilia will need to be explored in much greater detail. The probability that Timothy has committed some type of sexual aggression is high, although he is currently denying it. The clinician is doing a good job of engaging Timothy, while gaining entrance to his very private and dark world.

I have provided a fairly extensive illustration here, because I find that training on uncovering violence, especially sexual violence, is frequently underemphasized in training programs across disciplines. This is somewhat surprising, because such interviewing must be done frequently in most private practices, managed care settings, and community mental health centers. Obviously, it is a daily exercise in emergency rooms and inpatient units. Any person with a history of violence of any kind should be screened for sexual violence, and there exists a disturbingly high frequency of incest and pedophilia in general, often in people who have no other history of violence.

While exploring the region of recent violence in a person who is currently committing domestic violence, keep in mind the power of symptom amplification for obtaining a more accurate picture of the frequency of the violence, which is usually minimized without this technique. For example, as mentioned earlier, a question such as, "How many times do you think you've hit her?" can become much more effective by adding, "... 10 times, 20 times, maybe more?" This technique is also useful in disrupting minimization, while eliciting the frequency of acts of violence in the more distant past, which is our next topic of discussion.

Elicitation of Past Violent Events. As with the use of the CASE Approach with suicidal ideation, because of time constraints the clinician must be careful not to overdo this section in the initial assessment. On the other hand, this section warrants some explorations that are not necessarily used in suicide assessment because of the high correlation of future violence with a history of past violence. It is also during the review of past violence that the astute clinician may find some of the best evidence that he or she is in the presence of a predator, as opposed to a patient whose violence is triggered by affective charge or brain pathophysiology/structural damage.

Key elements for review include: (1) What is the worst act of violence?; (2) Approximately how many acts of violence have occurred?; (3) When was the most recent act of violence?; (4) Has violence been done to anyone in the past against whom there is current violent ideation or fantasy?; (5) Has a weapon been used in the past and, if so, is it being considered for use presently?; and (6) Is there an arrest and jail history related to violence?

Some questions about past acts of violence may help uncover predatory violence. Specifically, one is interested in seeing if the patient has much of a superego, which may show itself by the degree of guilt and shame the patient feels about past violence. In this regard, Meloy suggests exploring the patient's thoughts and feelings before, during, and after previous violent acts.[55] This gives a potential window into superego constraints and also whether or not violent thoughts "trouble" versus "arouse" the individual, the latter finding being more disturbing.

Two other useful questions along these lines are: "Is there anything you have done that has made you feel guilty?" and "If the price were right, is there anything you would not do?"[56] The presence of sociopathy and predatory process sometimes blossom with such questioning.

After exploring this region thoroughly, it is time for the clinician to bridge into an exploration of immediate violent ideation and intent.

Elicitation of Immediate Violent or Homicidal Ideation. As with suicidal ideation, the clinician asks about immediate violent ideation with a calm and nonjudgmental tone of voice. Once again this is no time to mince words, and, if an intended victim has been mentioned, the clinician should ask directly about his or her safety with questions such as, "Timothy, right now, are you planning on hurting or killing Judy?" Other useful questions include, "How well do you feel in control of your desires to attack Judy?", "After you leave here, do you think your thoughts about hurting Judy will return?", and "If you get any violent thoughts, what are you going to do about them?" Another important issue is whether or not the patient is intending to seek out the person with whom he or she is currently angry. One can feel slightly more comfortable if the patient says, and means it, "No, I need to stay away from her. I realize that." In contrast, comments such as, "I gotta at least talk to her. She's got to understand. I know she will," are far from reassuring.

Generally speaking, safety contracts are, in my opinion, significantly less effective in this arena compared with their use as a suicide deterrent. They may serve a purpose, as a means of assessment, with certain patients who you feel are truly upset by their violence. Nevertheless, in many patients with affectively triggered violence, once they are in an angry exchange with the object of violence, all bets are off again, no matter what was genuinely intended in a safety contract.

With predators and people with antisocial structure, in most instances I believe the very act of safety contracting can often make one look naive and almost silly. Respect for the clinician can drop, as the predator silently thinks, "What a stooge." It is often much better to address the lack of trust with comments like, "Jim, I think both you and I know that from your history, I'd be very foolish to trust you—and I don't. That doesn't mean I don't want to help you, but it just means you've got to earn my trust, and vice versa. I would like to hear from you, as best you can, how dangerous you think you are right now." This type of candor may catch the predator off guard and sometimes engages him or her in the sense that you are at least seen as a more worthy opponent.

In contrast to the suicide assessment, another thing that is different, during the exploration of immediate violent ideation, is the simple fact that the patient may assault you, not only while exploring this region but also at any time in the interview. The role of the patient's immediate mental status, in predicting such an assault or the likelihood of imminent violence if released, is very important. Always be careful. Most assaults upon clinicians can be avoided, and the key is to think about safety at all times and to quit the interview if safety becomes an issue.

Although clinicians have not shown outstanding accuracy at predicting short-term (weeks to months) violence, there is evidence that immediate violence can often be predicted. Solid predictors pretty well follow common sense and include items such as irritability, boisterousness, physical threats, verbal threats, attacks on material objects, and confusion.[57]

This last point emphasizes the need during an initial interview, especially in emergency rooms, always to wonder whether or not the person in front of you may become violent because of a biologically induced violence. Keep alert for evidence of alcohol intoxication or street drug abuse, including alcohol on the breath, unsteady gait, slurred speech, dyscoordination, nystagmus, pupillary signs, and confusion. Such things as tremors, incontinence, abnormal eye movements, poor hygiene, cushingoid facies, and exophthalmos could all indicate an organic cause for violence.[58] Naturally all violent patients in an emergency room require physical examination, testing of vital signs, and laboratory tests as medically indicated.

If the above strategies have been skillfully employed, a rich database will have been achieved and the clinician will have essentially ended the assessment of violent ideation across all four chronological regions. Using this information plus the statistical risk factors gained from other regions of the interview and corroborative sources, the clinician can make his or her best clinical prediction of imminent violence. In the last analysis, the major limiting factor for the interviewer, as with suicidal ideation, remains the interviewer's own skill, tenacity, and sensitivity.

References

1. Roy, A.: Psychiatric emergencies, suicide. In *The Comprehensive Textbook of Psychiatry*, 6th ed., edited by H. I. Kaplan and B. J. Sadock. Baltimore, Williams & Wilkins, 1995, pp. 1739–1752.
2. National Institute of Mental Health: Suicide Fact Sheet (based upon completed suicides in 1993), NIMH Web Site, June 1996 update.
3. Patterson, W. M., Dohn, H. H., Bird, J., and Patterson, G.: Evaluation of suicidal patients: The SAD PERSONS scale. *Psychosomatics* 24:343–349, 1983.
4. Conwell, Y., and Duberstein, P.R.: Suicide among older people: A problem for primary care. *Primary Psychiatry* 3:41–44, 1996.
5. National Institute of Mental Health, Website, June 1996.
6. Hirschfeld, R.M.A.: Algorithms for the evaluation and treatment of suicidal patients. *Primary Psychiatry* 3: 26–29. 1996.
7. Husain, S.A.: Current perspectives on the role of psychosocial factors in adolescent suicide. *Psychiatric Annals* 20:122–127, 1990.
8. Pfeffer, C.: Clinical perspectives on treatment of suicidal behavior among children and adolescents. *Psychiatric Annals* 20:143–150, 1990.
9. Roy, A.: Depression, attempted suicide, and suicide in patients with chronic schizophrenia. *Psychiatric Clinics of North America* 9:193–206, 1986.
10. Wilkinson, G., and Bacon, N. A.: A clinical and epidemiological survey of parasuicide and suicide in Edinburgh schizophrenics. *Psychological Medicine* 14:899–912, 1984
11. Breier, A., and Astrachan, B. M.: Characterization of schizophrenic patients who commit suicide. *American Journal of Psychiatry* 141:206–209, 1984.
12. Drake, R. E., Gates, C., Cotton, P. G., and Whitaker, A.: Suicide among schizophrenics: Who is at risk? *Journal of Nervous and Mental Disease* 172:613–617, 1984.
13. Hellerstein, D., Frosch, W., and Koenigsberg, H. W.: The clinical significance of command hallucinations. *American Journal of Psychiatry* 144 (2):219–221, 1987.
14. Junginger, J.: Predicting compliance with command hallucinations. *American Journal of Psychiatry* 147 (2):245–247, 1990.
15. *The Holy Bible, Revised Standard Version*. New York, Thomas Nelson, 1971.
16. Lion, J.R., and Conn, L.M.: Self-mutilation: Pathology and treatment. *Psychiatric Annals* 12:782–787, 1982.
17. Roy, A., 1986, pp. 193–206.
18. Drake, R. E., et al., 1984. pp. 613–617.
19. Amador, X.F., Friedman, J.H., Kasapis, C., et al.: Suicidal behavior in schizophrenia and its relationship to awareness of illness. *American Journal of Psychiatry* 153:1185–1188, 1996.
20. Drake, R. E., et al., 1984, p. 617.
21. Elliott, A.J., Pages, K.P., Russo, J., et al.: A profile of medically serious suicide attempts. *Journal of Clinical Psychiatry* 57:567–571, 1996.
22. Busch, K.A., Clark, D.C., Fawcett, J., and Kravitz, H.M.: Clinical features of inpatient suicide. *Psychiatric Annals* 23:256–262, 1993.
23. Clark, D.C.: Suicidal behavior in childhood and adolescence: Recent studies and clinical implications. *Psychiatric Annals* 23:271–283, 1993.
24. Fremouw, W.J., de Perczel, M., and Ellis, T.E.: *Suicide Risk: Assessment and Response Guidelines*. New York, Pergamon Press, 1990.

25. Roy, A: Risk factors for suicide in psychiatric patients. *Archives of General Psychiatry* 39:1089–1095, 1982.
26. Roy, A., 1982, p. 1092.
27. Callahan, J.: Blueprint for an adolescent suicidal crisis. *Psychiatric Annals* 23:263–270, 1993.
28. Fawcett, J., Clark, D.C., and Busch, K.A.: Assessing and treating the patient at risk for suicide. *Psychiatric Annals* 23:245–255, 1993.
29. Fawcett, J., Scheftner, W.A., Fogg, L., et al.: Time-related predictors of suicide in major affective disorder. *American Journal of Psychiatry* 147:1189–1194, 1990.
30. Fawcett, J., et al., 1993, pp. 247–249.
31. Cox, B.J., Direnfield, D.M., Swinson, R.P., and Norton, G.R.: Suicidal ideation and suicide attempts in panic disorder and social phobia. *American Journal of Psychiatry* 151:882–887, 1994.
32. Fawcett, J.: Saving the suicidal patient — The state of the art. In *Mood Disorders: The World's Major Public Health Problem*, edited by F. Ayd. Baltimore, Ayd Medical Communication, 1978.
33. Fremouw, W.J., et al., 1990, p. 44.
34. Everstine, D.S., and Everstine, L.: *People in Crisis: Strategic Therapeutic Interventions*. New York, Brunner/Mazel, 1983.
35. Beck, A.: Hopelessness and suicidal behavior. *Journal of the American Medical Association* 234:1146–1149, 1975.
36. Weisman, A.D., and Worden, J.M.: Risk-rescue rating in suicide assessment. *Archives of General Psychiatry* 26:553–560, 1972.
37. Patterson, W.M. et al., 1983, pp. 343–349.
38. Maltsberger, J.T.: *Suicide Risk: The Formulation of Clinical Judgment*. New York, New York University Press, 1986.
39. National Center for Injury Prevention and Control: Ten Leading Causes of Death by Age Group (based on 1994 data), NCIPC Web Site, 1997 Search.
40. Meloy, J.R.: The prediction of violence in outpatient psychotherapy. *American Journal of Psychotherapy* XLI: 38–45, 1987.
41. Tardiff, K.: *Assessment and Management of Violent Patients*. Washington, DC, American Psychiatric Press, 1996, pp. 127–135.
42. Lidz, C.W., Mulvey, E.P., and Gardner, W.: The accuracy of predictions of violence to others. *Journal of the American Medical Association* 269:1007–1011, 1993.
43. Lidz, C.W., Mulvey, E.P., Apperson, L.J., Evanczuk, K., and Shea, S.C.: Sources of disagreement among clinicians' assessments of dangerousness in a psychiatric emergency room. *International Journal of Law and Psychiatry* 15:237–250, 1992.
44. Gardner, G., Lidz, C.W., Mulvey, E.P., and Shaw, E.C.: Clinical versus actuarial predictions of violence in patients with mental illness. *Journal of Consulting and Clinical Psychology* 64:602–609, 1996.
45. Mossman, D.: Assessing predictions of violence: Being accurate about accuracy. *Journal of Consulting and Clinical Psychology* 62:783–792, 1994.
46. Appelbaum, P.S., and Roth, L.H.: Assessing the NCSC guidelines for involuntary civil commitment from the clinician's point of view. *Hospital and Community Psychiatry* 39:406–410, 1988.
47. Blomhoff, S., Seim, S., and Friis, S.: Can prediction of violence among psychiatric inpatients be improved? *Hospital and Community Psychiatry* 41:771–775, 1990.
48. McNeil, D.E., Binder, R.L., and Greenfield, T.K.: Predictors of violence in civilly committed acute psychiatric patients. *American Journal of Psychiatry* 145:965–970, 1988.
49. Tardiff, K., 1996, p. 130.
50. National Center for Injury Prevention and Control, 1997, Web Site.

51. Tardiff, K., 1996, p. 131.
52. Blomhoff, S., et al., 1990, pp. 771–775.
53. Appelbaum, P.S., and Roth, L.H., 1988, p. 408.
54. Tardiff, K., 1996, p. 129.
55. Meloy, J.R., 1987, p. 41.
56. Hare, R.D.: The Hare PCL-R, Interview and Information Schedule. North Tona-wanda, NY, Multi-Health Systems, 1990, 1991, p. 10
57. Linaker, O. M., and Busch-Iverson, H.: Predictors of imminent violence in psychiatric patients. *Acta Psychiatrica Scandinavica* 92:250–254, 1995.
58. Reid, W.H.: Clinical evaluation of the violent patient. *Psychiatric Clinics of North America: The Violent Patient* 11:527–537, 1988.

CHAPTER 9

The Mental Status and Vantage Points: Bridges to Psychotherapy

*M*an designs for himself a garden with a hundred kinds of trees, a thousand kinds of flowers, a hundred kinds of fruit and vegetables. Suppose, then, that the gardener of this garden knew no other distinction than between edible and inedible, nine-tenths of this garden would be useless to him. He would pull up the most enchanting flowers and hew down the noblest trees and even regard them with a loathing and envious eye.

Herman Hesse
Steppenwolf

*D*uring the initial years of training and, indeed, during the remaining course of the clinician's career, the clinician cultivates a garden of sorts. In this garden, the clinician attempts to develop a variety of perspectives or vantage points from which to gain an increased understanding of the patient. There exists no rational reason for the clinician to become fixated upon one viewpoint. Such a narrowing of perspective is suggestive of the gardener, described by Hesse above, who does not comprehend the beauty inherent in each flower, heedlessly discarding that which may be of most value.

Instead, like the gardener, who realizes that a rose delights the eye but a lowly tomato more suitably satisfies the stomach, the maturing clinician begins to understand the advantages of differing viewpoints and schools of thought. Moreover, the maturing clinician avoids overinvestment in personal beliefs, always allotting ample time for a good laugh at himself or herself, because taking oneself too seriously is perhaps one of the most common and treacherous traps awaiting the budding clinician.

Consequently, it seems appropriate as the close of this book approaches to examine at least a few of the many vantage points available to clinicians. By vantage point I am referring to the idea that during any specific moment of the interview, the clinician can consciously concentrate upon different aspects of the ongoing interview process. These viewpoints can be classified broadly into two clusters—attentional vantage points and conceptual vantage points.

For instance, four common attentional vantage points consist of the following: (1) the clinician attempts to listen *with the patient*, seeing the world through the patient's eyes, (2) the clinician attempts to look *at the patient*, as if the patient were an organism to be studied, (3) the clinician attempts to look *at himself or herself*, in order to understand the manner in which the clinician may appear to the patient, and (4) the clinician attempts to look *within himself or herself*, in order to gain an understanding of the patient from the clinician's own emotional responses. These four attentional vantage points may be viewed as forming two axes upon which the clinician may rapidly and flexibly move during the course of the interview (Fig. 14). Each vantage point can provide information that the others may easily miss or may literally prevent from being accessible to the clinician.

Beside these four attentional vantage points, numerous conceptual vantage points can be utilized. Indeed, the number of conceptual vantage points is at least as large as the number of differing theories of counseling and psychotherapy, hardly a small dinner party. In this chapter, three of these conceptual vantage points will be explored, including the perspective concerned with attempting to evaluate the patient's suitability for dynamic psychotherapy, the perspective concerned with deciphering the underlying personality structure of the patient using Kernberg's structural interviewing, and the clinician's ongoing use of intuition and spontaneity. Earlier, in Chapter 2 we examined in detail a fourth conceptual vantage point, facilics, which represents an attempt by the clinician to focus attention on the structuring of the interview as it actively unfolds.

Each of these conceptual vantage points represents a rich new vista from which the clinician may gain fresh insights. The more of these perspectives in which the clinician feels at home, the more flexible the clinician's style and the more fascinating the art of interviewing become. The clinician becomes constantly surprised by

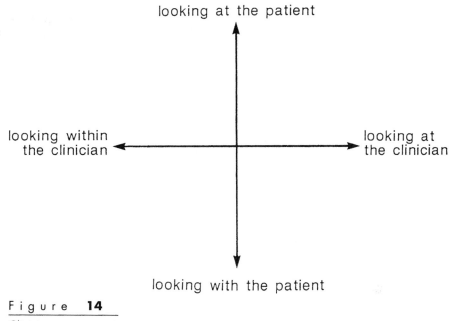

looking at the patient

looking within
the clinician

looking at
the clinician

looking with the patient

Figure **14**

Clinician vantage points.

new pathways to follow suggested by the developing characteristics of the immediate interview.

Some clinicians seem to move effortlessly among these various vantage points with little or no conscious awareness that such movements are being made. Such a natural gift for utilizing varying perspectives is not typical. The more natural course consists of slowly learning about the advantages of each perspective, first in a didactic sense and subsequently through experience. As clinicians consciously employ differing vantage points, these clinical perspectives gradually become increasingly more natural, eventually becoming integrated aspects of the interviewer's style. As more experience is gained, frequently the shifts become spontaneous and more intuitive, leading to the sense of surprise, mentioned above, as the clinician happens upon an insight that was not viewable from a previous perspective. As this stage of integration occurs, clinicians frequently report experiencing more vivid feelings while interviewing, and, indeed, the practice of interviewing is never the same again. Clinical challenges, such as encountering resistance, evoke more excitement than they do fear. In this regard, talented interviewers enjoy their work, as evidenced by the spontaneity of their mannerisms and wit.

The question becomes one of discovering a practical method of incorporating the ability to change vantage points into the development of the clinician. Towards this end we will briefly wander into a somewhat enigmatic realm, the world of the "philosopher" G.I. Gurdjieff.[1]

Gurdjieff was born in the 1870s in the Caucasus region of what is now Russia. He would eventually find his way to Europe, where he established the Institute for the Harmonious Development of Man in Fontainebleau, France. Controversy and fanatic fervor were destined to follow Gurdjieff throughout his career more dependably than his own shadow. He would be called everything from a philosopher and sage to a charlatan and fraud. In the last analysis, there may have been a good deal of truth in all of these attributions. No doubt exists that Gurdjieff, at a minimum, was gifted with both creativity and wit. We turn to a study of him, not because of his more occult and suspect beliefs, but because Gurdjieff developed a remarkably modern view of human psychology, much of his thinking focusing on the interpersonal matrix as well as man's abilities to develop increased self-awareness.

He felt that most people operated, during their moment by moment existence, in a habitual fashion, seldom "awake" to both what they were doing and why they were doing it. In such a state, he postulated that it was impossible to effectively alter behavior or patterns of thought, owing to habit acting as a protective shell against self-growth. Consequently, Gurdjieff attempted to help people gain an awareness of their spontaneous thoughts, emotions, and body movements.

In one famous exercise, as his dancing troop performed a strenuous routine, he would intermittently clap his hands. At the sound of the clap, all dancers were to hold their positions no matter how complex. With this exercise Gurdjieff attempted to instill in his dancers an immediate awareness of the normally unconscious movements and positionings of their bodies.

Although quite serious about his beliefs, Gurdjieff had a knack for making sure that neither his students nor those who came to observe his training programs took themselves too seriously. With regard to the above exercise, it is said that during one performance, he sent his dancers racing towards the audience. Gurdjieff clapped, rather late it would seem, and his dancers froze into human statuettes as they soared into the front rows of the audience. The startled audience had clearly expected the dancers to be halted before take-off, as did the dancers. But then Gurdjieff did not generally work from the realm of the expected.

Of more importance to us, Gurdjieff further developed his idea of increasing self-awareness into the concept of "self-remembering," a phrase ideally suited for application to the arena of clinical interviewing, as we shall soon see. Periods of self-remembering occur when people suddenly become aware of their own immediate activity and existence. These periods represent the breakdown of mere habit and are frequently accompanied by a sense of awe or wonderment. For interviewers it is that moment when they become aware of their own participation in the interviewing process. An important distinction must be made here. At these moments of self-remembering, clinicians are not just listening to the patient, they are aware that they are listening to the patient. This ability to step outside of the process itself is similar to the analytic concept of developing an observing ego, the ability to look at one's own actions as they are unfolding.

Now we can see why it is worthwhile examining the beliefs of Gurdjieff, because during periods of self-remembering, the clinician can consciously choose varying vantage points, at times with an amazing rapidity. The ability to insert periods of self-remembering into the interview itself provides the solvent that loosens the ties of habit binding many untrained interviewers. In this regard, several times during the scouting period, the clinician should consciously move into interludes of self-remembering during which various vantage points may be explored. During the remainder of the interview it is wise to insert at least four or five other periods of self-remembering.

In the early stages of training, clinicians generally must consciously insert periods of self-remembering while consciously utilizing differing vantage points. Eventually interviewers become adept at entering them facilely. Soon enough, these periods of increased awareness appear spontaneously as well. For skilled interviewers, there is a feeling of being at home during these periods, as if all their resources were suddenly at hand, which is indeed the case. It is a moment of balance, the natural poise that marks the style of a veteran clinician.

These moments of self-remembering are at the very heart of psychotherapy. Through them the therapist changes vantage points, utilizing various conceptual frameworks or shifting into a purely intuitive mode. At these interludes the therapist's own fantasies are transformed from distractions into avenues of insight. These interludes of self-remembering, through which the clinician flexibly adopts various vantage points, represent true bridges into the psychotherapeutic process itself. To the degree that the clinician can develop an ability to frequently experience periods of self-remembering this will, in some respects, determine the clinician's ultimate potential as an interviewer or a psychotherapist.

It sounds simple, but this ability remains one of the most elusive skills for the beginning clinician. Some clinicians never obtain it. To further our understanding of the uses of self-remembering, in the remaining sections of this chapter we shall examine in detail the four attentional vantage points and the three conceptual ones mentioned earlier. With these discussions providing an operational framework, it is hoped that the reader will then apply these vantage points in the actual interview situation during periods of self-remembering, for only experience can act as the real mentor at this stage of development.

EXPLORATION OF THE ATTENTIONAL VANTAGE POINTS

Looking at the Patient

We will begin by examining the vantage point that some may view as the most obvious and simplistic, looking at the patient. But this vantage point is deceptively simple. It requires a true discipline in order to utilize it effectively. Sensitive clinicians are frequently drawn toward the vantage point of looking *with* the patient in an empathic sense. Naturally this empathic perspective is extremely valuable and, in a sense, is critical for success. But it can be a trap if the clinician overutilizes it to the detriment of other vantage points, such as looking *at* the patient. In this context I observed a clinician empathizing with a subtly psychotic patient to the point that the clinician did not recognize that the patient was displaying a loosening of associations and other soft signs of psychosis. In this instance sole reliance upon empathic listening blocked the clinician from establishing enough distance to observe with an objective compassion. The clinician was drawn into the patient's world view, with the result that the patient did not receive the appropriate recommendation for antipsychotic medication.

Two slightly different approaches are useful when attempting to observe the patient with a sensitive eye—the "impact status" and the mental status. The impact status refers to the immediate behavior and affect of the patient at any single moment of the interview. Thus, the impact status represents a quick mental snapshot of the patient, in which the clinician focuses upon the immediate impact on the patient of both the patient's inner world and of the behaviors of the clinician. In contrast, the mental status is a composite of all the observations or "snapshots" made during the course of the interview. It is more a time-lapse film as opposed to a single exposure.

In many respects the impact status was discussed in length in the chapter on nonverbal behavior, but this area is worth a second look. The skilled clinician keenly observes all aspects of the patient's behavior, including mode of dress, hygiene, motor activity, affect and facial expression, mannerisms, and attitude. It is valuable, during the course of the interview, to periodically note the immediate affect of the patient, while asking oneself whether one's own behavior may be affecting the patient negatively, as evidenced by a decrease in the blending process. If such negative interactions are recognized early, one can quickly act to alleviate the stress before significant disengagement has occurred. At other times one may opt to explore with the patient the reasons behind the change in affect. In this fashion the clinician may uncover projective defenses or parataxic distortion, as described by Harry Stack Sullivan.

The clinician may also uncover significant unconscious material or attitudes betrayed by the patient's mannerisms. In this regard it is also useful to consciously make a note of the baseline nonverbal activity of the patient, so that subtle variations can be reflected upon. I am reminded of a young woman who had been in psychotherapy for roughly a year and a half. In one of her sessions she described an upcoming meeting with a supervisor in her graduate program. While she commented, "I guess I better go in and find out what my future is gonna be," she gave a child-like grin, accompanied by a helpless tone of voice. Apparently, at that moment in time, the thought of meeting her supervisor produced an attitude of child-like subservience. This impact status observation could be immediately put to use. I asked her what she had been feeling while discussing her upcoming supervision. I also shared some of my observations on her appearance at that time. This led to a rich exploration of her tendency to not take herself seriously. As she became more aware of her facial expressions, she was also able to successfully role-play meeting this supervisor while displaying an adult affect and attitude.

Throughout the book much has already been discussed with regard to nonverbal behavior, the behavioral indicators of blending, and other aspects key to the concept of the impact status. Consequently, it may be of value to shift our emphasis to the numerous considerations involved in uncovering a sound mental status.

The Mental Status

The mental status represents an attempt to objectively describe the behaviors, thoughts, feelings, and perceptions of the patient during the course of the interview itself. These observations are usually written as a separate section of the patient's evaluation. The general topics covered by the mental status are categorized as follows: appearance and behavior, speech characteristics and thought process, thought content, perception, mood and affect, sensorium, cognitive ability, and insight.[2] Clinicians may vary on the exact categories that are used, and some clinicians collect all of these observations into a single narrative paragraph (although I find this somewhat confusing). In any case the clinician attempts to convey the state of the patient during the interview itself, as if a cross-section was being taken of the patient's behavior for 60 minutes.

Here an intriguing phenomenon is encountered, because it is difficult to discuss the gathering of the mental status without carefully considering the process of preparing the written evaluation. The written document frequently reflects the clinician's activities during the interview itself. For example, if the clinician has a difficult time moving into a relatively pure vantage point of observing the patient, then the mental status frequently reflects this inability with omissions, premature assessment opinions, or misplaced bits of the history of the present illness that "explain the patient's psychopathology." In this light a disorganized or confusing written document is usually a reflection of an equally disorganized interview.

Assessment opinions and other conceptual perspectives do not belong in the mental status. They represent contaminants of this vantage point that were probably also present during the interview itself and may have hindered the clinician's ability to observe accurately. The mental status should represent an earnest attempt to describe objectively what is being encountered during the actual clinical interview. It therefore represents a unique and highly valuable aspect of the psychiatric record, because it serves as an area in which the clinician can read about the appearance of the patient, as recorded by a fellow mental health professional at a given point in time. The clinician can then compare the patient's current presentation with the past in an effort to determine evidence of improvement or decline. The use of the mental status in this more disciplined fashion trains clinicians to effectively utilize the vantage point of looking at the patient with as clear an eye as is possible.

The mental status complements other aspects of the written evaluation and is relatively distinct from them. By way of example, the History of the Present Illness (HPI) describes the pertinent historical aspects of the patient's behavior up until the interview itself. The HPI is frequently a compilation of reports from the patient, the patient's family, previous clinicians, written documents, and other sources of information. The mental status only includes information gathered from the patient, in the same sense that the physical examination only includes the immediate blood pressure reading of the patient, not the history of blood pressure readings taken by previous clinicians.

In a similar vein the narrative assessment, a different section of the written document, allows the clinician to piece together the patient's history and immediate presentation into a cohesive whole, utilizing the added perspective of the clinician's opinions and knowledge base. Neither the history of the present illness nor the mental status should include the clinician's assessment opinions, because these are confined primarily to the narrative assessment.

On a practical level, one of the reasons why it is important to emphasize these distinctions is the fact that clinicians frequently waste an inordinate amount of time repeating themselves in the written document. If a good description of the patient's delusions appears in the history of the present illness, then the mental status need only refer to this material as opposed to repeating it, because the focus should be the current thought content of the patient as illustrated below.

Thought Content

The patient has a history of an extensive delusional system regarding communist infiltration (see HPI). In the interview itself he continues to believe that his place of work is teeming with communists. He even believed that the psychiatric nurse he had just met was also a communist. Upon asking whether his mind might be playing tricks on him, he reported, "I'm not crazy. I know for a fact that the invasion has begun, will you help me?" He denied the belief of an alien invasion reported in the HPI.

Note that the clinician does not go into detail about the specifics of the delusional system, because those details had already been related in the HPI. Moreover, the clinician does not discuss his assessment of the patient's distance from his delusion with a statement such as, "This patient clearly remains very delusional and psychotic," for such an appraisal is most effectively made in the narrative assessment, where the clinician provides clinical opinions. Instead, the clinician carefully records the exact words of the patient, which demonstrate the patient's adamant belief in his delusional system. The focus is once again where it belongs in the mental status, on the actual behaviors and thoughts of the patient during the interview itself.

To become an accurate observer, the clinician must learn how to look, in a relative sense, without the contamination of previous beliefs and theoretical assessment issues. This objective stance represents one of the prerequisites of a sound mental status and of the vantage point of looking at the patient. To convey one's observations accurately, it becomes critical for clinicians to utilize a common language. There is no room for a sloppy use of terminology, because such a practice can clearly confuse other clinicians, potentially biasing them towards faulty observations themselves.

Consequently, we shall now examine each segment of the mental status as it might appear in a standard written evaluation. An effort will be made to summarize commonly utilized descriptive terms, to clarify confusing terms, to point out common mistakes, and to provide an example of a well-written mental status. As the clinician becomes adept at writing the mental status, the clinician will also be developing improved skills at using the vantage point of looking at the patient with a highly skilled focus and increased awareness.

Appearance and Behavior

In this section the clinician attempts to accurately describe the patient's outward behavior and presentation. One place to start is with a description of the patient's clothes and self-care. As Wallace suggests, it is probably best to avoid interpretations when describing the patient's clothing and presentation. Instead the clinician records the exact data that ultimately led to the opinions written in the subsequent narrative assessment. In this regard the clinician should describe the patient's apparel as opposed to relying solely on subjective terms such as "stylish," because not everyone would agree upon the meaning of the word "stylish."[3] Striking characteristics such as scars and deformities should be noted, as well as any tendencies for the patient to look older or younger than his or her chronological age. Eye contact is usually mentioned. Any peculiar mannerisms are noted, such as twitches or the patient's apparent responses to hallucinations, which may be evident through tracking movements of the eyes or a shaking of the head as if shutting out an unwanted voice. The clinician should note the patient's motor behavior; common descriptive terms include restless, agitated, subdued, shaking, tremulous, rigid, pacing, and withdrawn. Displacement activities, such as picking at a cup or chain smoking, are frequently mentioned. An important, and frequently forgotten characteristic, is the patient's apparent attitude toward the interviewer. With these ideas in mind, let us first take a look at a relatively poor description.

Clinician A

The patient appeared disheveled. Her behavior was somewhat odd and her eye contact didn't seem right. She appeared restless and her clothing seemed inappropriate.

Although this selection gives some idea of the patient's appearance, one does not come away with a feeling for what it would be like to meet this patient. Generalities are used instead of specifics. Let us look at a description of the same patient that captures her presence more aptly.

Clinician B
The patient presents in tattered clothes, all of which appear filthy. Her nails are laden with dirt, and she literally has her soiled wig on backwards. She is wearing two wrist watches on her left wrist and tightly grasps a third watch in her right hand, which she will not open to shake hands. Her arms and knees moved restlessly throughout the interview, and she stood up to pace on a few occasions. She did not give any evidence of active response to hallucinations. She smelled badly but did not smell of alcohol. At times she seemed mildly uncooperative.

This passage clearly presents a more vivid picture of her behavior. The reader now has an idea of what her odd behaviors consist of. The clinician has included pertinent negatives, indicating that she shows no immediate evidence of hallucinating, as might be seen in a delirium. In this example one can almost intuit some of the thinking processes of the clinician with regard to the development of a differential diagnosis. This is a hallmark of a well-organized mental status. Each section adds a new series of pieces to the puzzle, suggesting certain diagnoses and making others less likely. For instance, this patient's agitation may be suggestive of a manic picture.

Speech Characteristics and Thought Process
The clinician can address various aspects of the patient's speech, including the speech rate, volume, and tone of voice. At the same time the clinician attempts to describe the thought process of the patient as it is reflected in the manner with which the patient's words are organized. The term "formal thought disorder" is utilized to suggest the presence of abnormalities in the form and organization of the patient's thought, as discussed in this section of the mental status. The less commonly used term, "content thought disorder," refers specifically to the presence of delusions, and it is addressed in a different section of the discussion of mental status. The more generic term "thought disorder" includes both the concept of a formal thought disorder and of a content thought disorder. In this section the emphasis is on the process of the thought (presence of a formal thought disorder), not the content of the speech. Frequently used terms by clinicians include the following:

- **Pressured speech:** Refers to an increased rate of speech, which may possibly best be described as a "speech sans punctuation." Sometimes it is only mildly pressured, whereas at other times, the patient's speech may virtually gush forth in an endless stream. It is commonly seen in mania, agitated psychotic states, or during extreme anxiety or anger.
- **Tangential thought:** The patient's thoughts tend to wander off the subject as the patient proceeds to take tangents off his or her own statements. There tends to be some connection between the preceding thought and the subsequent statement. An example of fairly striking tangential thought would be as follows, "I really have not felt very good recently. My mood is shot, sort of like it was back in Kansas. Oh boy, those were bad days back in Kansas. I'd just come up from the Army and I was really homesick. Nothing can really beat home if you know what I mean. I vividly remember my mother's hot cherry tarts. Boy, they were good. Home cooking just can't be beat." "Circumstantial thought" is identical in nature but differs in the fact that the patient returns to the original topic at hand.
- **Loosening of associations:** The patient's thoughts at times appear unconnected. Of course, to the patient, there may be obvious connections, but a normal listener would have trouble seeing them. In mild forms, loosening of associations may represent severe anxiety or evidence of a schizotypal character structure. In moderate or severe degrees, unless the loosening is a product of malingering, it is an indicator of psychosis. An example of a moderate to severe degree of loosening would look like this: "I haven't felt good recently. My mood is shot, fluid like a waterfall that's black, back home I felt much better, cherry tarts and Mom's hot breath keeps you going and rolling along life's highways." If loosening becomes extremely severe it is sometimes referred to as a "word salad."
- **Flight of ideas:** In my opinion this is a relatively weak term, because it essentially represents combinations of the above terms, which is why most trainees find it confusing. For flight of ideas to occur, the patient must demonstrate tangential thought or a loosening of associations in conjunction with a significantly pressured speech. Usually there are connections between the thoughts but, at times, a true loosening of associations is seen. A frequently but not always seen characteristic of flight of ideas is the tendency for the patient's speech to be triggered by distracting stimuli or to demonstrate plays on words. When present, these features represent more distinguishing hallmarks of a flight of ideas. Flight of ideas is commonly seen in mania but certainly can appear in any severely agitated or psychotic state.

- **Thought blocking:** The patient stops in mid-sentence and never returns to the original idea. These patients appear as if something had abruptly interrupted their train of thought and, indeed, usually something has, such as a hallucination or an influx of confusing ideation. Thought blocking is very frequently a sign of psychosis. It is not the same as exhibiting long periods of silence before answering questions. Some dynamic theorists believe it can also be seen in neurotic conditions, when a repressed impulse is threatening to break into consciousness.
- **Illogical thought:** The patient displays illogical conclusions. This is different from a delusion, which represents a false belief but generally has logical reasoning behind it. An example of a mildly illogical thought follows: "My brother has spent a lot of time with his income taxes so he must be extremely wealthy. And everyone knows this as a fact because I see a lot of people deferring to him." These conclusions may be true, but they do not necessarily logically follow. Of course, in a more severe form, the illogical pattern may be quite striking as with, "I went to Mass every Sunday, so my boss should have given me a raise. That bum didn't even recognize my religious commitment."

Let us take a look again at the woman we have already begun to describe. The first example once again could use some improvement.

Clinician A
Patient positive for loosening of associations and tangential thought. Otherwise grossly within normal limits.

This clinician has made no reference to the degree of severity of the formal thought disorder. Specifically, does this patient have a mild loosening of associations or does she verge upon a word salad? Moreover, the clinician makes no reference to her speech rate and volume, characteristics that are frequently abnormal in manic patients. The following brief description supplies a significantly richer database:

Clinician B
The patient demonstrates a moderate pressure to her speech accompanied at times by loud outbursts. Even her baseline speech is slightly louder than normal. Her speech is moderately tangential, with rare instances of a mild loosening of associations. Without thought blocking or illogical thought.

Slowly one is beginning to develop a clearer picture of the degree of this patient's psychopathology. More evidence is mounting that there may be both a manic-like appearance and a psychotic process. In any case, coupled with her strikingly disheveled appearance, the clinician may be increasingly suspicious that the patient is having trouble managing herself.

Thought Content

This section refers primarily to five broad issues: (1) ruminations, (2) obsessions, (3) compulsions, (4) delusions, and (5) the presence of suicidal or homicidal ideation. Ruminations are frequently seen in a variety of anxiety states and are particularly common in depressed patients. Significantly depressed patients will tend to be preoccupied with worries and feelings of guilt, constantly turning the thoughts over in their minds. The thinking process itself does not appear strange to these patients, and they do not generally try to stop it. Instead, they are too caught up in the process to do much other than talk about their problems. In contrast, obsessions have a different flavor to them, although they may overlap with ruminations at times.

An obsession is a specific thought that is repeated over and over by the patient, sometimes as if seeking an answer to some question. Indeed, the patient frequently obsesses over a question and its answer. As soon as the question is answered, the patient feels an intense need to ask it again, as if some process had been left undone. The patient may repeat this process hundreds of times in a row until it "feels right." If one interrupts the patient while this process is occurring, the patient will frequently feel a need to start the whole process again. Unlike the case with ruminations, patients generally find these obsessive thought processes to be both odd and painful. They frequently have tried various techniques to interrupt the process. Common themes for obsessions include thoughts of committing violence, homosexual fears, issues of right and wrong, and worries concerning dirt or filth. Obsessions may consist of recurrent ideas, thoughts, fantasies, or images. If one takes the time to listen carefully to the patient, bearing the above phenomenological issues in mind, the clinician can usually differentiate between ruminations and obsessions.

Compulsions are strong urges to perform an activity, which the patient often recognizes as silly or unnecessary. Nevertheless, it is very difficult for the patient to resist a compulsion. Common compulsions include repeated hand washing, repeatedly counting, repeatedly saying a phrase or prayer, checking to see if one has left something unlocked or turned on, returning to see if one has hit somebody with a car, and cleaning something like a plate or table counter repeatedly. Compulsions are often, but not always, coupled with obsessions.

Obsessions and compulsions are seen in obsessive-compulsive disorder, an extremely painful and disruptive condition, that is surprisingly common and amenable to treatment. Patients are so embarrassed by these symptoms that it is rare for them to share these symptoms with a therapist (sometimes even after years of therapy). Consequently, it is critical in the initial diagnostic assessment to ask every patient about obsessions and compulsions.

Delusions represent strongly held beliefs that are not correct or held to be true by the vast majority of the patient's culture, as described in detail in the chapter on psychotic process.

The fourth issue consists of statements concerning lethality. This is a complex area, as noted in Chapter 8. Since all patients should be asked about current lethality issues, these issues should always be addressed in the mental status write-up. In general, the clinician should make some statement regarding the presence of suicidal wishes, plans, and degree of intent to follow the plans in an immediate sense. If a plan is mentioned, the clinician should state to what degree any action has been taken on it. It should also be noted whether any homicidal ideation is present and to what degree, in the same fashion as with suicidal ideation.

Let us return to our patient with two sample excerpts concerning thought content.

> Clinician A
> The patient is psychotic and can't take care of herself. She seems delusional.

This excerpt is just simply sloppy. The first statement has no place in the mental status, because it is the beginning of the clinician's clinical assessment. The description of the delusion is threadbare and unrevealing. The clinician has also omitted the questioning concerning lethality. Assuming that the clinician asked but forgot to record this information, the clinician may sorely regret this omission if this patient were to kill herself and the clinician was taken to court. A more useful description is given below.

> Clinician B
> The patient appears convinced that if the watch is removed from her right hand, the world will come to an end. She proceeds to relate that consequently she has not bathed for 3 weeks. She also feels that an

army of rats is following her and is intending to enter her intestines to destroy "my vital essence." She denies current suicidal ideation or plans. She denies homicidal ideation. Without ruminations, obsessions, or compulsions.

Now we have evidence of someone who is clearly psychotic with concrete delusions. The next question is whether hallucinations play a role in her psychotic process.

Perception

This section refers to the presence or absence of hallucinations or illusions, which were described in detail in Chapter 6. It is of value to note that there sometimes exists a close relationship between delusions and hallucinations. It is not uncommon for the presence of hallucinations to eventually trigger the development of delusional thinking, but the two should not be confused. Let us assume that a patient is being hounded by a voice screaming, "You are possessed. You are a worthless demon." If the patient refuses to believe in the reality of the voice, then one would say that the patient is hearing voices but is not delusional. If on the other hand the patient eventually begins to believe in the existence of the voice and feels that the devil is planning her death, then the patient is said to have developed a delusion as well as to be experiencing auditory hallucinations. We can now turn to our two clinicians.

Clinician A
Without abnormal perceptions.

The question arises as to whether it is appropriate in the mental status to use phrases such as, "grossly within normal limits" or "without abnormality." Generally speaking the mental status is improved by the use of more precise and specific descriptions, but sometimes clinical situations require flexibility. For example, if the clinician is working under extreme time constraints, then such global statements may be appropriate, but in most situations it is preferable to state specifically the main entities that were ruled out, because this essentially relays to the reader that the clinician actually looked for these specific processes. Stated differently, with these global phrases, the reader does not know whether they are accurate or the end result of a sloppy examination. If one has performed a careful examination, it seems best to let the reader know this fact.

Another problem with the phrasing used by Clinician A is the fact that he has stated that the patient does not, in actuality, have hallucinations, but perhaps this patient is simply withholding information for she fears that the voices represent a sickness. Numerous reasons exist for a patient to not share the presence of hallucinations with a clinician, including the fact that the voices may have told the patient not to speak to the clinician. Thus, it may be more accurate to state that the patient denied having hallucinations rather than stating categorically that the patient is without them. With these ideas in mind a slightly more sophisticated report would be as follows:

Clinician B
The patient denied visual, auditory, and tactile hallucinations and any other perceptual abnormality.

Mood and Affect

Mood is a symptom, reported by the patient, as to how the patient has been feeling recently in general and tends to be relatively persistent. Affect is a physical indicator noted by the clinician, as to the immediate feelings of the patient. It is demonstrated by the patient's facial expressions and other nonverbal clues during the interview itself and frequently is of a transient nature. Mood is a self-reported symptom; affect is a physical sign. If a patient refuses to talk, then the clinician can say essentially nothing about mood in the mental status itself, except that the patient refused to comment on mood. Later, in the narrative assessment, the clinician will have ample space to describe the clinician's impressions of what the patient's actual mood has been. In contrast to mood, in which the clinician is dependent upon the patient's self-report, the clinician can always say something about the patient's affect.

Thus it is conceivable that a patient who is quite depressed could deny his or her depression, while still appearing sad during the interview. Such a situation would be reported as follows, "The patient demonstrated a sad affect throughout most of the interview, including several short episodes of tearfulness. However, when questioned as to her mood she reported, 'I'm feeling just fine, really I am.' " Later, in the narrative assessment, the clinician would note that the patient's reported mood was inconsistent with both the history and the mental status, perhaps suggesting the presence of active mechanisms of denial or repression. In this situation, some clinicians are tempted to ignore what the patient states, persisting in relaying in the mental status that the patient is depressed. But this prevents the reader from seeing the patient's denial mechanisms. It is much better to let the story speak for itself, while providing one's final assessment in the proper section of the written report. Let us now return to our patient.

Clinician A

The patient's mood is fine and her affect is appropriate but angry at times.

This statement is somewhat confusing. In which sense is her affect appropriate? Is it appropriately fearful for a person who believes that rats are invading her intestines, or does the clinician mean that her affect is appropriate for a person without a delusional system? The clinician should always first state what the patient's affect is and then comment upon its appropriateness. Typical terms used to describe affect include normal (broad) affect with full range of expression, restricted affect (some decrease in facial animation), blunted affect (fairly striking decrease in facial animation), a flat affect (essentially no sign of spontaneous facial expression), bouyant affect, angry affect, suspicious affect, frightened affect, flirtatious affect, silly affect, threatening affect, labile affect, and edgy affect. The following description gives a much clearer feeling for this patient's presentation:

Clinician B

When asked about her mood, the patient angrily retorted, "My mood is just fine, thank you!" Throughout much of the interview she presented a guarded and mildly hostile affect, frequently clipping off her answers tersely. When talking about the nurse in the waiting area she became particularly suspicious and seemed genuinely frightened. Without tearfulness or a lability of affect.

Sensorium, Cognitive Functioning, and Insight

In this section the clinician attempts to convey a sense of the patient's basic level of functioning with regard to the level of consciousness, intellectual functioning, insight, and motivation. It is always important to note whether a patient presents with a normal level of consciousness, using phrases such as "the patient appeared alert with a stable level of consciousness" or "the patient's consciousness fluctuated rapidly from somnolence to agitation."

It should be noted that this section may have evolved from two processes, the informal cognitive examination and the formal cognitive examination. The informal cognitive examination is artfully performed throughout the interview in a noninvasive fashion. The clinician essentially "eyeballs" the patient's concentration and memory by noting the method by which the patient responds to questions. If the clinician chooses to perform a more formal cognitive examination, it can range from a brief survey of orientation, digit spans, and short-term memory to a much more comprehensive examination, perhaps lasting 20 minutes or so. Clinical considerations will determine which approach is most appropriate. Let us examine the report, which could use some polishing, by Clinician A:

Clinician A
The patient seemed alert. She was oriented. Memory seemed fine and cognitive functioning was grossly within normal limits.

Once again this clinician's report remains vague. Most important, the reader has no idea exactly how much cognitive testing was performed. No mention has been made regarding the patient's insight or motivation as well. The following excerpt provides a more clarifying picture:

Clinician B
The patient appeared alert with a stable level of consciousness throughout the interview. Indeed, at times, she seemed hyperalert and overly aware of her environment. She was oriented to person, place, and time. She could repeat six digits forwards and four backwards. She accurately recalled three objects after 5 minutes. Other formal testing was not performed. Her insight was very poor as was her judgment. She does not want help at this time and flatly refuses the use of any medication.

At this point we are almost at the end of our discussion on the mental status. A simple exercise can demonstrate the power of a well-written mental status. Simply go back and read in a consecutive fashion the excerpts written by Clinician A. One is left with a rather bland and nebulous picture of the woman in question. Afterwards, read the model excerpts in succession by Clinician B. A strikingly more vivid picture of the woman appears. She suddenly seems more human, and the reader can easily picture her warily stalking the room. This then is the goal of the mental status, to ultimately provide a fellow clinician with a reliable image of the patient's actual presentation over the course of the interview.

It should be openly acknowledged that, in actual practice, the written mental status may need to be significantly briefer, but the principles outlined above remain important and can help prevent the briefer mental status from being transformed into an inept mental status. (For more tips and strategies on the written document, please see Appendix III: Guidelines and Strategies for the Written Document, which also includes quality assurance guidelines and a sample written assessment.)

Even more important, the mental status and the impact status create in the clinician a sharpening of the mind's eye. With time these observational skills become more and more keenly honed, allowing the clinician to quickly and gracefully learn from observing the patient, to successfully utilize the vantage point of looking at the patient. The slightest smile becomes an opening into the world of the patient. Without these observational skills, the clinician may be at the risk of being swallowed by the patient's world as opposed to learning from it. In the next section we shall examine in more detail the methods that help one to see with the patient's eyes.

Looking with the Patient

Looking with the patient, the second attentional vantage point, is frequently viewed by many clinicians as the most natural. It is the perspective of empathic listening. Its importance cannot be overstated. I have never seen an accomplished interviewer who was not adept at it. This vantage point remains so integral to the interviewing process itself that we have already discussed many aspects of it in the previous sections of this book.

Pertinent concepts discussed thus far include the engagement process, blending, unconditional positive regard, empathic statements, the empathy cycle of Barrett-Lennard, the phenomenological perspective, tracking, the use of natural and referred gates, and the numerous nonverbal techniques utilized for conveying empathy to the patient. In this section we will not emphasize these concepts again. Instead we shall look at some new ideas, which provide further avenues for understanding the patient's experience of living. These concepts include somatic empathy, the linguistic techniques of Grinder and Bandler, and counterprojective techniques as described by Leston Havens.

Somatic Empathy. Somatic empathy was alluded to in the chapter on nonverbal techniques. It is based on the precept that the posturing of the patient's body not only reflects the defenses and feelings of the patient but also serves to foster a way of experiencing the environment itself. For example, a tight-fisted man who sits persistently grinding his jaw will, by the very act of grinding his jaw, experience the world in a "tight-jawed" fashion. One is reminded of the work of Wilhelm Reich, who discussed the term "body armor," a term suggesting that body positioning may itself represent a type of defense mechanism or manner of coping with the stresses of the environment.[4]

In its most effective form, somatic empathy is fostered by literally assuming the position of the patient. Thus, it is usually done not in the presence of the patient but between therapeutic sessions. By assuming the patient's posture or mannerism, the clinician obtains an actual feeling for what the patient was experiencing in the session itself. Clinicians can allow their imaginations to wander freely in the assumed position, noting everything from spontaneous fantasies to muscle tensions. It is sometimes quite surprising to experience the peculiar sensations of rigidity and tension that many patients literally carry around with them. This simple exercise, if carried out in an uninhibited fashion, can provide a powerful experience for the clinician, producing a peculiar sense of closeness with the patient as if suddenly understanding, for the first time, what the patient had been saying.

I am reminded of one woman who spoke with a flutter of gesticulations, as if her wrists were floppy hinges. At times during the initial interview, she would hang her arms down over the arms of the chair. From this position they would jerk around, banging loosely against the arms of the chair as she spoke, a human Raggedy Ann. After the session, when I actually attempted to mimic these movements, I was surprised at the unsettling sensation of being out of control that such posturings could produce. The patient's world was just such a "theater of the helpless." At times during the session itself the clinician may note a small gesture of the patient, perhaps a way of holding his or her hand, that can be mimicked immediately without the patient's awareness. This exercise may help move the clinician into a more empathic understanding of the patient at that moment in time.

Deep and Surface Structure. Leaving the world of nonverbal behavior, the focus can move to a method of increasing an understanding of the patient's world, determined by the patient's language itself. Grinder and Bandler have developed a conceptual model that can help the clinician to move more effectively into the world of the patient. The following description provides a brief introduction to these techniques, and I urge the reader to look at the original work itself.[5]

At one level, language results from the experience of the human organism as it attempts to translate information into a code, which can be immediately understood by other organisms. But the code itself may ultimately begin to determine the manner in which the organism experiences the surrounding world. In a sense, humans begin to limit their interpretations of their experience to those that can be encoded by the language. Unfortunately, as this process unfolds, the language begins to limit experience as opposed to describing it. Stated somewhat differently, the range of actual human feelings and perceptions is vastly more complicated than the language can describe.

For the sake of clarification, if there exist only two words to describe snow, then the person will probably pay little attention to the numerous variations among different types of snow. On the other hand, if there existed 10 nouns to represent snow, the human would, by the nature of the language itself, need to pay more attention to what type of snow was encountered in order to communicate the experience clearly. A person armed with 10 words may experience the nuances of the snow much more intensely than a companion limited to two words. Experience can literally be determined by language. In this sense it becomes crucial for the clinician to listen to the language utilized by the patient, for the possibility exists that the patient's language may be creating a framework that is detrimental to the patient, because it limits or distorts the patient's view of actual circumstances.

The language used in daily conversation tends to represent a "shorthand" of what the person is actually thinking. Large amounts of the actual message may be left unstated and lost to the receiver of the message, in this case the clinician. Even more disturbing is the possibility that the patient will begin to conceptualize the situation via the limiting framework of this shorthand message. At first, these ideas may appear somewhat abstract, but they become clearer if one views language as having two different levels of meaning, depending on the completeness of the message communicated. Based on the study of transformational grammar, Grinder and Bandler describe these two levels as deep structure and surface structure. A very simple and effective method of seeing the world more clearly through the patient's eyes consists of gently probing the patient's surface statements until both the patient and the clinician discover the deleted deep structure.

An example may serve to clarify. Suppose the patient makes the following statement:

People constantly hurt me.

This statement has emerged from a specific substrate that is potentially ripe with powerful information to the clinician but is currently unavailable. There must exist a deep structure, as illustrated below from which the patient's comment was transformed:

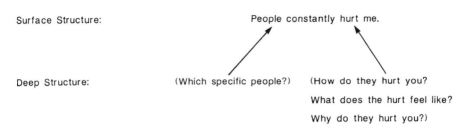

Surface Structure: People constantly hurt me.

Deep Structure: (Which specific people?)   (How do they hurt you?
                                                      What does the hurt feel like?
                                                      Why do they hurt you?)

The deep structure holds many important secrets. Is the patient referring to all people, people at work, his parents, his siblings? Is the pain the "hurt" of rejection, shame, inferiority, abandonment? Grinder and Bandler maintain that by gently seeking answers to such questions, the clinician will gradually uncover progressively more important material, and, at times, the patient may be surprised by the implications of the deep structure. For instance, the patient may have been unaware of feeling rejection or the pain of sibling rivalry. Such discoveries may eventually change the patient's perception of the related experience itself. In any case, at the very least, the clinician gains a better view of what the world looks like to the patient. Let us see the technique in action.

Pt.:   People constantly hurt me.

Clin.:   Exactly which people are you talking about?

Pt.:   Oh, my wife and her brother, I hate him so much.

Clin.:   What other people are you referring to?

Pt.:   Well I . . . Let's see, her sister is pretty nasty too.

Clin.:   What about your own family?

Pt.:   Well, my brother is hard to get along with, but my parents are actually pretty supportive. (pause) You know, come to think of it, my parents really have been pretty nice to me recently.

Clin.:   It sounds like that seems different to you than in the past.

Pt.:   (Patient chuckles) To tell you the truth, a year or so ago I'd have been telling you how much I hated my parents, but they really seemed to change back then. (Undoubtedly the patient, either consciously or unconsciously, is referring to a specific time or event by the word "then," so the clinician probes for the deep structure.)

Clin.:   When did you notice the change?

> **Pt.:** Back when Jan and I moved out of their house. I don't know, maybe living with them was a strain on all of us. It really was too crowded, uh, felt cramped, sort of like a crowded bus station?
>
> **Clin.:** Do you think your parents realize that you appreciate their new attitude?
>
> **Pt.:** Hmmm, I really sort of doubt it. Maybe I ought to give them a call sometime, maybe.
>
> **Clin.:** Let me make sure I have this straight. You're having increased problems with some specific people in your life like your wife. On the other hand your relationship with your parents has matured and is actually stronger?
>
> **Pt.:** Yes, yes that's it in a nutshell.

But what a different nutshell than the patient began with. By uncovering the deep structure, the patient has come upon information that is both revealing and comforting. The original statement, "People constantly hurt me" was a gross distortion caused by generalization. Since the patient came to believe this generalization, the situation seemed worse than it was in reality, because, in truth, some good things were also occurring. By probing for the patient's deep structure the clinician has clearly gained a more accurate perception of what the world looks like to the patient. Yet there is more to the story, because the patient is now viewing the situation in a slightly more positive light. The therapeutic process itself has begun.

These uncovering techniques described by Grinder and Bandler serve as another bridge into the therapeutic process, for the patient may "stumble" upon a more realistic and less threatening perception of reality. These uncovering techniques are similar to the principles behind therapeutic modalities such as cognitive therapy or rational emotive therapy.

In this example the clinician chose to explore the subject of this sentence but could have just as easily chosen to explore the deep structure beneath the verb or the adverb. In fact by exploring what the patient meant by the word "constantly," the patient may very well have discovered that his wife is not *always* mean to him, a realization that may be of some importance.

Grinder and Bandler state that two of the more frequent transformations that occur between the deep structure and the surface structure are deletions and generalizations, as illustrated in the dialogue above. Although this uncovering technique appears at first glance to be almost too simple, it is remarkably powerful. In order to use this technique well the clinician must be able to switch vantage points.

Counterprojective Statements. The next technique, the use of counterprojective statements, yields another method of improving the blending process, as the clinician attempts to see the world with the patient. Counterprojective techniques were developed by Leston Havens for use in psychotherapy itself as well as during the initial interview.[6] Their use is described in detail in his highly informative and entertaining book *Making Contact*.[7]

Counterprojection is utilized when a guarded or actively paranoid patient is beginning to project hostile impulses onto the clinician. At these moments it is very difficult to view the world through the patient's eyes, because the patient's focus is on the clinician, who may appear to the patient as representing an antagonistic "other." For blending to proceed, the clinician must switch the focus of the patient off of the clinician and onto a common "screen" that both the clinician and the patient can look at together. Put more colloquially, the clinician wants the heat off himself or herself.

The goal of the counterprojective statement is to deflect the projection off of the clinician before it becomes stabilized and difficult to defuse. In the specific context of the initial interview, the goal is to immediately deflect the patient's suspicion while subsequently sidetracking the patient to a new topic that is away from a focus upon the clinician. It is hoped that this sidetracking will provide the clinician with enough time to shore up the engagement process, resulting in a more trusting alliance. In a simplistic sense the principle works upon the adage that one should not try to stop two people from arguing, for, soon enough, the two will turn on the newcomer as the common enemy. With counterprojection, one attempts to find a common antagonist or area on which to focus the attention of both the patient and the clinician. Let us watch the technique in action:

> **Clin.:** What were some of the problems that have been particularly upsetting to you, Mr. Hughlings?
>
> **Pt.:** They're really quite specific and relate to the needling behavior of my wife, who has to know everything.
>
> **Clin.:** What are some of the specifics?
>
> **Pt.:** That's rather difficult to say. She's got her own problems, if you know what I mean.
>
> **Clin.:** What are some of the things that are most unsettling to you, that you came here today about?

> **Pt.:** I don't really see why the details should concern you, I don't like it when people ask too many probing questions, if you catch my drift.
>
> **Clin.:** I don't like it when people push me to talk about things that I don't feel like talking about either. Let's back off for a moment. I take it your wife has been pushing and prying recently. Is that correct?
>
> **Pt.:** Yes, she's gone further than she should, if she knows what is good for her.
>
> **Clin.:** She's always on your case then.
>
> **Pt.:** Absolutely, I'm really tired of it.
>
> **Clin.:** Is this a totally new behavior for her or is this sort of a long-standing trait that has gotten worse?
>
> **Pt.:** It's gotten much worse, but I think she's always been part busybody, it's in her genes.
>
> **Clin.:** Her family was also like this?
>
> **Pt.:** You better believe it. In particular her mother was a real busy-body. Right from the start I knew I was heading for some tough times. You know, the problem is that you don't just marry a person, you marry the whole family and this one came from the cheapest level of the bargain basement.

In the beginning of the dialogue, we find the patient answering with the vagueness that frequently typifies a guarded or paranoid patient. As the interviewer attempts to clarify some of the muddy waters, a curious process begins to unfold. The patient's anger towards his wife is beginning to be projected onto the clinician himself. The situation is personalized by the comment, "I don't really see why the details should concern you." Immediately the patient and the clinician are becoming two separate worlds oppositionally staring at each other, in contrast to two people jointly observing the world "out there." An antagonism is rapidly brewing as the paranoid attitude begins to solidify a projection onto the clinician. To make matters worse, the patient proceeds to accuse the clinician of the very same behaviors that the patient perceives in his wife with the comment, "I don't like it when people ask too many probing questions, if you catch my drift." At this point the clinician is rapidly becoming enmeshed in a sticky unconscious flypaper. It is time to make a retreat, to deflect the projection.

To accomplish this task the clinician responds, "I don't like it when people push me to talk about things that I don't feel like talking about either." The clinician reports feeling a very similar emotion to what the patient has expressed. Suddenly, the clinician and the patient are part of the same camp, which is looking out at all those people who are "too pushy." It is very difficult for the patient to continue attacking the clinician for a behavior that the clinician also dislikes and claims to be seeing in others. Subsequently, the outside focus is solidified by the clinician identifying a specific new object for the joint focus of the patient and himself. The clinician moves the focus onto the patient's wife with the statement, "I take it your wife has been pushing and prying recently."

At this point the heat is off the clinician. Both he and the patient focus their attention on the patient's wife, a topic that eventually perks the interest of the patient. The follow-up statement, "She's always on your case then," is also a counterprojective technique that further solidifies the patient's attention on an object removed from the clinician. The projection has been successfully deflected. The interview proceeds on course. Note that the clinician does not accuse the wife but merely reflects back the sentiments expressed by the patient himself earlier. Clinicians must be careful not to join the paranoid process, but rather to deflect it away from themselves.

Havens points out that three elements must be present for a counterprojective technique to function effectively. First, the object that is chosen for the new focus of attention must be "out there," thus ensuring that the patient's projection will move to a new focus of attention. Second, a specific object or concept (as opposed to a vague generalization) needs to be mentioned so that the patient's attention will become firmly focused. And third, the clinician relates feeling an emotion similar, if not identical, to that being felt by the patient. In this fashion the clinician and the patient are plopped into the same worldview, both of them looking out at those nasty objects that upset them. From this more common ground the clinician can then work to establish a more well-grounded alliance.

Counterprojective statements generally are phrased in the third person, such as, "he always seems interested only in himself," or "they never seem to understand you." The third person stance emphasizes the concept of directing the patient's projection away from the interviewer so that there is something "out there" to be discussed and observed by the patient and the clinician. Havens also notes that these statements may convey an empathic quality.

As illustrated above, in some instances, the clinician may opt to utilize first person statements, in which case he or she emphasizes the shared quality of the emotion that the patient is experiencing. On a cautionary level, first-person statements carry the risk of focusing the patient's attention on the clinician, but in some situations this can be highly effective. For instance, a talented psychiatric resident described the following interaction. An actively paranoid woman interrupted a session with an accusatory tone, "Is this office bugged?" The resident responded, "It would upset me greatly if my office were bugged. No it isn't." The patient accepted this counterprojective deflection readily, and the session continued in a fruitful manner.

We have now reviewed three techniques for enhancing the ability of the clinician to move into the vantage point of "looking with the patient." Essentially the two vantage points explored so far, looking *at* the patient and looking *with* the patient, lie at either ends of an axis whose focus is the patient. The same type of attentional axis can be conceptualized using, not the patient, but the clinician as the focus of attention. Just such an axis is the topic of the next two sections.

Looking at Oneself

This section focuses on the vantage point through which the interviewer attempts to objectively look at himself or herself. The ultimate goal is for clinicians to develop an accurate sense of how they appear to the patient. In this sense clinicians search for their own identifying persona. Naturally, the interviewers cannot know for certain in what ways their persona may be affected by the patient's process of parataxic distortion, but clinicians should possess at least a baseline understanding of their own typical appearance and behavior. From this increased self-awareness interviewers may be able to ward off certain aspects of parataxic distortion before significant problems with blending occur. For instance, a clinician who tends to be rather warm and extroverted may purposely tone down his or her style when initially encountering a paranoid patient, because the clinician is aware that the paranoid processes of the patient may predispose the patient toward distorting the warmth into a sinister attempt to "trick me into trusting you."

Two aspects of this vantage point complement each other. First, during the interview itself the clinician needs to be able to utilize periods of self-remembering, which enable one to ask, "How do I appear to the patient at this moment?" As mentioned in the chapter on nonverbal behavior, this "watching attitude" can be facilitated by imagining a mirror dropping in front of oneself during the interview. This concrete exercise can increase the interviewer's ability to rapidly assume this specific vantage point. The second aspect of this vantage point concerns gaining a knowledge of how one appears, not through imaginative techniques but via feedback provided by outside observers.

In this regard the importance of supervision cannot be overemphasized. Three types of supervision are particularly powerful in helping clinicians to gain an understanding of how they come across to patients. These three types of supervision include videotaped supervision, direct in-the-room observation by a supervisor, and feedback obtained from observing peers (collegial supervision). The numerous advantages offered by videotape supervision are well known, but the latter types of supervision are probably equally of value.

Direct supervision, in which the supervisor sits in on the interview itself, provides a chance for the clinician to be directly observed during actual clinical conditions. The supervisor can also immediately demonstrate techniques as resistances or problems confront the trainee. Despite the naturally occurring hesitancies associated with having a supervisor directly observing, trainees frequently request large amounts of this type of supervision once they have experienced it.

Obtaining feedback from peers provides a third avenue through which a wealth of information can be gained, because each observer tends to notice different aspects of style. Naturally the observers learn as well, for each trainee brings fresh techniques that may be modelled by other trainees.

In this light, it should be emphasized that it is also extremely useful to supervise others. Besides providing an opportunity to observe potentially useful techniques developed by others, the act of supervision trains the clinician to accurately observe the interviewing process. If one cannot first learn to astutely observe the styles of others, then it is highly unlikely that one will be able to effectively study oneself. In this sense it is frequently invaluable to find a peer with whom one switches the supervisory role.

In any case, by utilizing the above techniques, clinicians work towards a sophisticated understanding of their own appearances. Interviewers should ultimately be able to describe their styles along a continuum including the following:

responsive	⟵————————⟶	not responsive
spontaneous	⟵————————⟶	not spontaneous
animated	⟵————————⟶	not animated
transparent	⟵————————⟶	not transparent

Each of these four axes focuses on slightly different aspects of interviewing style. The axis of responsiveness refers to the clinician's tendency to show an affective response to the behaviors or statements of the patient. Thus, a responsive clinician may smile or chuckle if the patient attempts a joke, whereas the nonresponsive clinician would show no change in affect. The axis of spontaneity represents the degree with which the clinician conveys spontaneous affect and opinion. It may be demonstrated by the clinician's use of humor, for example. The axis of animation delineates the spontaneous baseline of affectivity and body gesturing of the clinician. With large amounts of animation the clinician will be gesturing frequently, while, at the other end, the clinician will seem immobile; occasionally, one may even find a clinician remarkably like a stone. The fourth axis, the axis of transparency, is similar to the above axes but refers specifically to the degree with which the clinician consciously reveals emotions or personal thoughts to the patient.

As well as these characteristics the clinician should also be aware of other hallmarks of style, including the following:

1. Tendency to express warmth or empathy
2. Displacement activities
3. Self-touching behaviors (e.g., the hand to the cheek)
4. Use of humor
5. Body language when exploring sensitive areas
6. Body language when confronted with resistance or demands
7. Body language around potentially violent patients
8. Typical distance one sits from patients
9. Frequency and content of notes
10. Rate of speech, tone of voice, and volume of voice
11. Hand gestures and head nodding activity
12. Style of clothing and general appearance (does the clinician look liberal, stylish, establishment, sloppy, preppy, rich, sexy, tired? All of these elements can affect both the engagement process and the development of transference characteristics.)

The ultimate goal is the development of a flexible style in which the clinician feels at ease, while realizing the potential ramifications of the various modes of this style on patients of differing temperaments. Each clinician will develop a distinctive style marked by various aspects of the clinician's own personality.

Once the clinician is aware of stylistic characteristics, flexibility can be achieved. For instance, my own style tends to be mildly animated with a fair amount of spontaneous body language, use of wit, and head nodding. When meeting with a paranoid patient, I consciously tend to decrease all of these elements, arriving at a more low-key style, a style that patients experiencing a paranoid process seem more at ease with initially. Then by following cues given by the patient, I can consciously warm up or further cool down the style as seems appropriate.

In order to gain this type of flexibility, the clinician needs to carefully learn to utilize periods of self-remembering during which the clinician takes advantage of this particular vantage point, a vantage point that is frequently overlooked.

Looking Within Oneself

Looking within oneself represents the final attentional vantage point that shall be discussed. Once again the focus is on the clinician as opposed to the patient, only now the clinician attempts to explore his or her own emotions and fantasies. At first glance, it would seem that it should be a relatively easy task to tune into one's own feeling state. The truth of the matter is that many clinicians have more trouble truly understanding what the world looks like through their own eyes than through the eyes of the patient. Many defenses exist that tend to hide emotional responses from the clinician's awareness.

The first step in utilizing this vantage point effectively lies in the ability of the clinician to accurately answer the question, "What am I feeling right now?" It is important that the clinician search for actual feelings, such as sadness, anger, frustration, attraction, excitement, boredom, time pressure, performance anxiety, and fear. One is not hunting for answers such as, "I was feeling that the patient was probably getting upset with me" or "I was feeling that the patient was probably displaying histrionic traits." These statements are not feelings, they are opinions and intellectualizations, and yet most clinicians when asked what they are feeling will offer such answers, just as patients in psychotherapy frequently answer questions concerning feeling in an intellectualized manner. On the contrary, the answers that one is seeking sound like, "I was feeling awkward in there and a little frustrated" or "I was feeling fairly interested, but no more than usual."

As Pilkonis[8] has suggested, one can easily tell when a response is not dealing with a true feeling, because, in such instances, one can use the word "think" as the verb in the clinician's statement. For instance, using the above examples one can replace the statement, "I was feeling that the patient was probably displaying histrionic traits" with "I think the patient was probably displaying histrionic traits." This phrase sounds natural and its meaning is essentially unchanged, because the clinician was actually reporting an opinion not an emotion. On the other hand, a statement truly reflecting the clinician's emotion makes no sense with this substitution, as seen with, "I was thinking awkward in there" or "I was thinking mad." The illogical quality of these transformations suggests that the original statements by the clinician represented true expressions of emotion.

By utilizing periods of self-remembering, through which this vantage point can be entered effectively, clinicians will become progressively more adept at recognizing both subtle and powerful emotional responses in themselves. The next logical question concerns the possible uses of such information. However, in order to understand the uses of this perspective, one must also understand from where these clinician emotions originate. Three broad areas come to mind, including: (1) naturally intuitive responses, (2) associational responses, and (3) transferential responses. Some clinician responses can fall neatly under one of these headings. Many other responses evolve from two or more of these areas. Each category will be discussed separately, keeping in mind that the separations may be somewhat arbitrary.

INTUITIVE RESPONSES

Intuitive responses represent emotional states and perceptions arising in the clinician that are both easily accessible to consciousness and frequently represent responses that may be aroused in other people who interact with the patient for any length of time. Intuitive responses are not necessarily indicators of the clinician's own deeper dynamics but represent naturally occurring and relatively spontaneous responses to the patient. Sometimes these gut-level responses seem quite natural to the clinician, and at other times they may be somewhat surprising and insightful. For instance, a grossly insulting patient may quickly spark angry feelings in the clinician. Such reactions may be laden with important information, because they may represent mirrors of the patient's psychopathology or feelings. In essence, the clinician is being provided with an immediate sample of how this patient may affect other people in his family or on the street. As mentioned before, the interview represents a dyadic interaction, and if the clinician experiences anger, one must wonder what the patient may be doing that creates such a response in the clinician. In this sense the clinician's spontaneously occurring emotional responses may serve as a tip-off to important information that is being overlooked because of a preoccupation with other vantage points.

For purposes of illustration let us look at the development of a feeling of fear in a clinician. Such feelings, if recognized, should be given careful attention, because the clinician's intuitive skills may be recognizing a potentially dangerous situation of which the clinician is not totally aware. I am reminded of a story told to me many years ago by a professor that highlights this point. I have sometimes wondered if the story was more apocryphal than true, but nevertheless it makes the point.

Apparently a clinician had been working with a patient for

many months without much difficulty. Unexpectedly the clinician began developing intense feelings of being ill-at-ease and frightened with the patient in a vague manner during the sessions. Convinced that he was suffering from problems with countertransference, he sought several consultations but to no avail. One day, to his surprise, the patient began the session with, "Today is your lucky day, Doc." When asked what he meant the patient sported a wry smile, saying, "Today I decided not to kill you." Although not there, I suspect this subtle aside put an end to any notetaking on the part of the clinician. It is indeed a novel way of getting the attention of one's therapist. On a more serious note, over the past several weeks the patient had been carefully following the therapist. He proceeded to show the therapist his comprehensive notes concerning the therapist's moment-by-moment activities. He also provided in detail the method with which the murder was to take place.

Although rather dramatic in nature, the story has a point to convey. Feelings of fear should be taken seriously, especially in settings in which the client is not known to the system, such as when an intake interview is being performed. The fear may represent the fact that the patient is beginning to lose control.

On the other hand, the clinician's fear may reflect different processes within the patient. For example, it can also be an indication that the patient is demonstrating subtle psychotic signs. In this regard, mild aspects of psychotic process, such as inappropriate affect, may be catching the clinician off-guard leading to an uneasy feeling that has nothing to do with potential violence from the patient but may be the first tip-off that psychotic process is alive and well in the room. At other moments, the clinician's fear can represent an empathic resonance with the fears of a paranoid patient.

Other, less disturbing emotions in the clinician can also represent reflections of the patient's psychopathology that may be worth examining from other vantage points, demonstrating the fact that vantage points tend to complement one another. For example, if the clinician becomes unusually fascinated by a patient's story, it suggests that the clinician is in the presence of a "gifted storyteller," perhaps a storyteller with underlying histrionic traits. It may be the patient's dramatic flair that is triggering the clinician's fascination. If during such an interview the clinician looks inwards, recognizing the unusual degree of attentiveness caused by the patient, then the clinician can switch to a more revealing vantage point. The vantage point of looking at the patient could provide confirming evidence suggestive of a histrionic presentation such as dramatic gesturing or flirtatiousness. Thus one vantage point can suggest the use of other vantage points. The key point remains that interviews represent interactional processes in which the clinician's responses are evidence of the patient's attributes and vice versa.

By way of further example, if clinicians find themselves feeling frustrated by the need to constantly repeat questions, this frustration may be the flip side of the presence of either tangential or circumstantial speech in the patient. Feelings of mild confusion in the clinician may suggest the presence of mild forms of loosening of associations or illogical thought in the patient. Boredom in the clinician may reflect the presence of a patient with a blunted affect or monotone voice to whom quite literally it is boring to listen. Boredom may also suggest a variety of other processes that may be occurring within the clinician. For instance, boredom may represent a defense against specific feelings such as anger or erotic arousal.

ASSOCIATIONAL RESPONSES

At times, the responses generated in the clinician such as boredom or anger may represent, for the most part, normal responses to the behaviors of the patient as discussed above in relation to intuitive responses. However, in other circumstances, the clinician may begin feeling a response that most people would not feel or perhaps not feel as intensely with a specific patient. Such idiosyncratic feelings bring us to the second category of response etiologies, associational responses. In associational responses, the patient reminds the clinician of some other person in the clinician's past or current history. These feelings are not particularly deep. They are either immediately conscious or easily made conscious. Various aspects of the patient from clothing to demeanor may be associated with important people in the clinician's life, including people whom the clinician either likes or dislikes. Thus the clinician may rapidly develop feelings ranging from sexual attraction to distaste or bitterness. It is important for the clinician to become rapidly aware of such associational responses, because they can significantly affect the clinician's ability to make sound judgments and may also affect the blending process itself.

If aware of one's associational responses and their possible negative ramifications, then these responses can frequently be utilized to the clinician's benefit. Suppose that a clinician was raised by highly domineering parents with the result that the clinician developed an uptight feeling whenever the clinician was near the parental dyad. If this clinician begins to feel this uptightness around a patient, it may be a sensitive barometer that the patient is exhibiting domineering traits, perhaps even in a subtle fashion. If aware of these inner responses, the clinician could then more carefully explore for the presence of domineering character traits in the patient. In fact, this clinician may actually be more sensitive to such traits, recognizing them more readily than other clinicians because of an ability to identify this uptight feeling.

TRANSFERENTIAL RESPONSES

Emotional responses in the clinician are not necessarily bad or evidence of psychopathology in the clinician. They are frequently useful both in diagnostic interviewing and in psychotherapy itself. It is more the unawareness of these feelings or an inability to work with them that frequently leads to problems.

The concept of the dangers of unawareness raises the last category, responses created in the therapist through countertransference. Countertransference refers to emotions, associations, and defenses triggered by the patient in the clinician, whose etiologies are in a true sense unconscious or difficult to bring to conscious awareness. When true countertransference feelings have crystallized, the clinician begins to re-experience past relationships in the current relationship with the patient. By way of example, a clinician may have domineering parents but was never fully aware of the impact of this domination. Furthermore, at an unconscious level the clinician dealt with this anxiety by withdrawing from both parents, highlighted by a tendency to display a cool exterior towards them. In this instance, as the clinician encounters the domineering patient, the clinician may begin to handle the patient with an unnecessary curtness and coolness, previously displayed to the clinician's parents.

Probing self-reflection, increased attention to the vantage point of looking within oneself, supervision, and psychotherapy are all mechanisms available to clinicians that will provide awareness of such countertransference reactions and their potential impact. This leads to an important point. Generally speaking true transferential responses are not commonly seen in the initial interview, because it often takes time for the countertransference to crystallize. Instead, in the context of the initial interview, the interviewer is more likely to see the seeds of the countertransference emerging. In actuality, the more typical responses in the initial interview are associational responses and naturally intuitive responses.

I point this out because some clinicians tend to use the term countertransference rather loosely to define almost any response generated in the clinician. This loose interpretation can be somewhat misleading, because true countertransference responses require a more sophisticated exploration and may be considerably more difficult to utilize in a positive sense, although ultimately they too can be of extreme utility in the actual work of psychotherapy. As countertransference issues are made more available to the clinician's awareness, they are essentially transformed into associational responses, which can once again be utilized as sensitive barometers of patient characteristics by the clinician.

Indeed, viewed together, naturally intuitive, associational, and transferential responses can become some of the most valuable tools for the experienced clinician. As they gain experience, clinicians may begin to notice certain types of responses in themselves that typically are generated by specific personality styles in patients or may be relatively field specific to certain clinical situations such as impending suicidal acting out. This vantage point can then point the clinician to hunt for confirmation of these hunches through the use of other vantage points and avenues of interviewing.

FANTASY

Thus far the discussion has focused on the emotional responses of the clinician. Another viable region for exploration consists of clinician fantasy material. At times it may be important for the clinician to essentially curb such fanciful wanderings, if for instance the patient needs an empathic listener. At such points, the clinician may mentally note the fantasy images for future exploration. On the other hand, frequently the clinician may be at a point in the interview in which a few moments can be productively spent silently exploring fantasy material in an effort to determine its possible relationship to the immediate clinical interaction.

The fantasy may be tied in with associational or transferential responses or may simply represent the active workings of the clinician's own intuition. In any case, interesting insights may be gained. I remember working with a woman who was describing her activities while working in the home as a housewife. She was in her mid-20s and had entered therapy following an explosive extramarital affair that now jeopardized her marriage. As she was talking about her work and her time spent with her small girl, I began having memories of a previous co-worker. It seemed odd to be thinking about this previous colleague, so I decided to play with the fantasy a bit. I remembered disliking my colleague because she always seemed self-centered and complained rather constantly about her job. She simmered with an underlying resentment of her work and wished to be in a different position.

I wondered if I had been unconsciously led to feelings within the patient of discontent and anger. I turned to her and asked, "Although you talk somewhat glowingly about your work at home, I wonder if at times you feel some anger about being cooped up all the time." She seemed caught off-guard by the comment and proceeded to enter a long description of her complaints about wishing she was back at her job as a secretary and that, in reality, she just did not know what she wanted to do with her life. Tears welled in her eyes. This vignette represents an instance in which the unconscious of the clinician was productively at work. Fantasies can provide valuable grist for the mill. In this regard, some clinicians jot down fragments of fantasy material and other doodlings as an active aspect of notetaking.

Before concluding the discussion of this particular vantage point, it may be valuable to make brief mention of a topic that requires a much more in-depth discussion than is appropriate for this book. Specifically, the question arises as to what degree the clinician should share his or her emotions and memories with the patient. To what degree does the clinician display transparency and self-disclosure? Differing schools vary regarding this issue, and the answer also varies depending on the clinical situation. Generally speaking, I do not use self-disclosure much during initial interviews, for patients will handle self-disclosure remarkably differently depending on their psychopathology. Paranoid patients and patients with a borderline personality disorder can quickly twist the self-disclosure into damaging distortions or may be frightened by the process of facing a clinician who self-discloses. In a dynamic sense, self-disclosure can also disrupt transference development. Moreover, in the initial interview I seldom need self-disclosure in order to powerfully engage the patient. Thus there seems to be little need to use a technique that can backfire in numerous ways.

On the other hand various clinicians may utilize self-disclosure in certain instances in ongoing therapy. Indeed Val Brown[9] has argued convincingly that during periods of intense affect in the clinician, powerful moments of therapeutic change may occur if the clinician and the patient jointly explore how these emotions appeared in the interpersonal context. Frequently the patient gains insight into the effect he or she has upon others. The issue of self-disclosure remains a complex and controversial topic, which the reader is urged to explore in other readings and in the context of supervision.

One point should be made though. Although I tend not to use self-disclosure in initial interviews, it can be useful both with regard to setting limits and with decathecting hostile patients in certain situations. In some instances, comments to a gradually escalating patient such as, "Mr. Jones, I can see that you're feeling pretty angry at me and to be honest you're scaring me a bit, and I know you don't intend to frighten me. Let's sit down and talk some to see if I might be able to understand better what is upsetting you and perhaps do something about it." I have seen this technique work effectively, but one must learn through experience with which patients it is most appropriate.

As we conclude the discussion of the vantage point of looking within oneself, we are also concluding the exploration of the attentional vantage points. It can be readily seen that these vantage points are intimately related to the transition into the psychotherapeutic process itself. Their effectiveness is contingent on the clinician's ability to "step away" from the interview during periods of self-remembering. These periods of self-remembering allow the clinician to utilize complementary vantage points rapidly and effectively. In the next section we shall begin a study of three different conceptual vantage points: the assessment for psychotherapy, the structural interviewing of Kernberg, and the use of intuition.

EXPLORATION OF THE CONCEPTUAL VANTAGE POINTS

Assessment for Psychodynamic Psychotherapy

One of the most challenging tasks facing the initial interviewer is the tentative determination of the patient's potential for psychotherapy. In the first place, the clinician needs to possess an operationally sound understanding of the basic types of psychotherapeutic interventions, including counseling techniques, behavioral techniques, crisis intervention techniques, cognitive therapies, short-term dynamic therapies, cognitive-behavioral therapies, solution-focused therapies, long-term dynamic therapies, psychoanalysis, couple's therapy, family therapy, and group therapy. Naturally, each clinician will develop biases, hopefully not tunnel-vision biases, as to which therapies are most effective under what circumstances.

In this age of managed care and other time constraints, it is increasingly important to rapidly spot which patients can benefit from brief therapy formats, whether individual or group. Such patients frequently represent individuals who have strong enough ego structures to handle confrontation, the weighing of advice, homework assignments, and who possess a motivation for change.

It is important to realize that the initial interviewer need not necessarily be adept at each form of therapy, for frequently the interviewer is acting as a triage agent, who will refer the patient to others. Instead, the clinician needs to understand the advantages of each form of therapy, thus enabling a fit to be achieved between the patient's needs, abilities for change, and the appropriateness of the therapy for the tasks at hand. At differing points during the interview the clinician will be entering the conceptual vantage point concerned with determining the suitability of the patient for some type of psychotherapeutic intervention.

It is beyond the scope of this chapter to discuss the assessment techniques needed to determine the appropriateness of the patient for each form of therapy mentioned above. Instead, the focus will be on the delineation of the maturational level of the patient in the sense of the patient's ego development and sense of a stable self. The maturational level of the patient is of profound importance in determining suitability for psychodynamic therapies (those therapies derived from analytic theory dealing with the unconscious and transference) but is also of definite relevance in determining the potential for success in all of the therapeutic categories described above. The focus of this section is on a common denominator utilized in considering the use of any of the above techniques.

By the maturation level of the patient, we are simply referring to a commonsense concept that patients will be functioning at widely varying degrees of psychological maturity at varying moments of their lives. At one end of the continuum, the patient may be functioning at a severely regressed and psychotic state, in which reality contact itself is compromised. In the middle of the continuum one finds the psychotic-prone personalities (primitive personality disorders such as borderline personality and paranoid personality) described in Chapter 7. These people generally have better reality contact than grossly psychotic patients but tend to interact with people in highly immature fashions, often accompanied by child-like expectations and equally child-like outbursts when such expectations are not met. In the last category we find the more stable character disorders, the neurotic disorders, and those people with healthy functioning.

During periods of stress, individuals may move backwards along this continuum. Following an automobile accident resulting in the death of his spouse, a well-functioning individual may experience a brief reactive psychosis. On a more subtle level, a business executive who displays some passive-aggressive and narcissistic traits may, if hospitalized for a serious illness, begin to function as if truly representing an unstable narcissistic personality disorder.

This issue of stress represents a crucial consideration for the clinician as an attempt is made to identify the suitability of the patient for psychotherapeutic intervention. In general, the more immature the patient's level of psychological integration, the less likely he is to tolerate stress, especially on an interpersonal level. Specific therapies vary in the degree to which the patient is stressed by the clinician either emotionally or cognitively. The goal of the interviewer is to determine which therapy will be of most value for this patient at this time.

It is not really a determination of whether the patient needs psychotherapy, but what type will be of most benefit, because even the most psychotic patients will benefit from a low-keyed supportive interaction, in which the clinician merely attempts to provide some calming reality contact over time. This same psychotic patient would truly run the risk of therapy-induced damage if the clinician attempted to employ a long-term dynamic approach replete with confrontations and interpretations at the time of the acute psychosis. In a similar fashion a behaviorist would generally not employ a hypnotherapy or relaxation technique at the time of an acute psychotic breakdown, because such techniques may backfire dramatically by furthering the regression of the patient.

Michel Hersen, the noted behavioral therapist, has pointed out that the failures found in patients with certain behavioral techniques may be related to the fact that, in a psychodynamic or maturational sense, the patient or client was not capable of handling the challenges presented by the therapy. For instance, a clinician may encounter a patient who angrily drops out of a homework-utilizing therapy after several sessions. What may have been missed by the therapist is the fact that the patient was presenting with the maturational level of a person with a borderline personality disorder. More specifically, for this particular patient, whose need for approval was pathologically enormous, the tension of having homework reviewed by the clinician was prohibitively anxiety provoking. The anxiety of performing these relatively simple homework assignments literally drove the patient out of therapy. "Homework" assignments are often very useful in patients with a borderline structure; however, to be used effectively, the clinician must be ready to rapidly address any dynamic conflicts that can get in the way. As Hersen states, talented behavioral clinicians attend to the dynamic concerns of the client, tailoring the level of stress in the therapy to the patient's ability to handle stress, as evidenced by the patient's maturational level.[10]

The question becomes one of which techniques allow the initial interviewer to easily assess the immediate maturational level of the patient. Two approaches immediately come to mind. The first approach is the determination of a DSM-IV diagnosis. Diagnoses such as schizophrenia, borderline personality disorder, and an adjustment disorder with depressed mood all suggest specific levels of maturation. A second technique consists of assessing the degree of functioning of the patient along a series of differing ego functions and defense mechanisms. This technique adds to the approach by the DSM-IV because it pushes the clinician to assess specific functions, thus allowing the clinician to spot both strengths and weaknesses. Bellak emphasizes this approach and has developed the concept of the Ego-Function Assessment (EFA).[11]

In the EFA, 12 different ego functions are conceptualized by the clinician. These functions include items such as the following: reality testing, practical judgment, impulse control, object relations, strength of psychological defense mechanisms, and the ability to screen out unwanted stimuli and thoughts. This type of approach, coupled with the diagnostic approach of the DSM-IV, creates a more individualized picture of the patient's current functioning. The first step in assessing the psychotherapeutic fit for the patient is a determination of where the patient sits on the continuum of psychological maturation. It should be noted that these so-called steps actually tend to occur in parallel, the various assessments occurring throughout the interviewing process.

The next step consists of determining the "therapy facilitative" characteristics of the patient. These have been written about and described in great detail by numerous authors. Basically one is referring to those characteristics that bode well for a psychotherapeutic intervention. Once again the search for these qualities represents a no-nonsense practical conceptualization. The three qualities that come to mind as routinely mentioned include: (1) motivation, (2) cognitive skills, and (3) psychological mindedness.

In its simplest form the concept of motivation can be summarized as those who want the help the most tend to do the best (although this is not always the case). This motivation tends to arise from two general areas. First, the degree to which a patient is experiencing pain certainly influences the degree to which the patient is invested in seeking help. Second, the patient's drive for help may be strongly influenced by the belief that help is possible. Both of these influences can be more easily ascertained if the clinician, at some point, asks the patient questions such as the following:

a. What made you decide to come here today at this moment as opposed to several weeks ago?
b. What made you decide to see me specifically, in other words, how had you heard about me?
c. What are some of your expectations about whether therapy can help or not?

A patient who responds, "I came here because my wife wants me to be here, and I have no idea how she got your name" is clearly less motivated than a patient who says, "I think I really need some help with the way I handle people, and you really helped a friend of mine."

The degree of pain does not always indicate a readiness for therapeutic intervention. A patient with a paranoid personality may live a miserable existence, constantly alienated from friends and family, but may not view the pain as being related to anything under personal control. In the same vein, psychotic patients may not perceive a need for intervention. Such considerations lead to the associated concept of insight, because insight generally must accompany pain in order for the patient to voluntarily seek help. This insight need not be sophisticated. The patient merely needs to develop an awareness that psychological pain can be causally related to attitudes and behaviors.

The second therapy facilitative characteristic consists of the patient's intellectual abilities and cognitive functioning, including concentration, memory, abstracting ability, baseline intelligence, and creativity. A patient gifted in all of these areas may have a higher chance for success in therapies requiring a sophisticated use of intellect, such as cognitive restructuring or a dynamic-based therapy.

The third characteristic is referred to as psychological mindedness, a somewhat diffuse term that overlaps with the above characteristics to some degree. In a more specific sense it may be viewed as the patient's belief that psychological processes can affect happiness, coupled with the patient's ability to assume a more objective view of personal behavior, including the impact of his or her actions on the happiness of himself or herself and others.

If a patient does not show the types of facilitative characteristics described above, it does not necessarily mean that psychotherapy is not indicated. It means that the patient may not do well in specific forms of therapy. In this light, therapies can be clustered into three broad categories, ego stabilizing, ego nurturing, and ego challenging, listed in order from least stressful to most stressful.

In order to understand how the initial interviewer can triage patients towards these types of therapies, it is of use to digress for a moment into a brief description of these categories. Ego stabilizing counseling and therapeutic techniques represent gentle approaches utilized to help severely ill patients regain a sense of safe environment and sound reality contact. They are often used with psychotic patients, and the sessions may be very brief in nature, essentially helping the patient to reintegrate, as medications such as antipsychotics begin to decrease the terror of the psychotic process. The major goal is to help the patient to regain a reasonable sense of self-integration, accompanied by some mild insight into practical considerations of the current clinical condition. In other instances, nonpsychotic patients may not want psychotherapy of a more probing nature, may not have the intelligence to benefit from such therapies, or may not have the money or time to benefit from such approaches. If these patients are receiving medications, then the medication evaluations themselves can include simple ego stabilizing work, aimed at guiding patients toward a useful understanding of the significance of their problems as they relate to medication issues and their daily routine. Simple fears and anxieties are handled with a quiet and calming educational support.

In contrast to ego stabilizing therapies, ego nurturing therapies gently, but persistently, push the patient toward increased understanding, while recognizing that the character structure of the patient will demand a firm and consistent approach toward primitive outbursts of anger and fear towards the clinician. Examples of ego nurturing therapies are the reparenting techniques frequently seen in use with patients suffering from primitive personality disorders. In contrast to the limited goals of the ego stabilizing therapies, the ego nurturing therapies attempt to foster insight, hopefully accompanied by true gains in self-esteem and a maturing individuality.

The third grouping, ego challenging interventions, are most useful in patients who can be both confronted by the therapist as well as asked to reflect upon the ramifications of their thoughts and behaviors. These therapies frequently demand that the patient display the therapy facilitative characteristics outlined above. Of course, at times, a patient may begin with an ego stabilizing approach and, if successfully treated with this technique, may be able to benefit at a later time from an ego nurturing approach, ultimately moving on toward ego challenging techniques. Ego challenging therapies include techniques such as time-limited psychodynamic therapies, solution-focused therapies, other psychodynamic therapies, psychoanalysis, more complex behavioral therapies, and more sophisticated cognitive therapies. In specified situations, these therapies can also be beneficial with more primitive personalities, but the clinician must always ensure that the patient is not pushed beyond his or her actual capabilities for change.

The following example demonstrates the need for matching the therapeutic intervention to the psychological maturation of the patient. Suppose that the therapist is faced with headbanging behavior in a mildly retarded adolescent. It is doubtful that an ego challenging technique such as a written self-monitoring technique (which requires motivation and a good ability to observe one's actions) will have any chance of success. Even some ego nurturing techniques, such as very simple cognitive techniques, will probably be too demanding for such a patient. On the other hand, an ego stabilizing technique, employing the simple principles of positive reinforcement, may be much more promising. In this regard, counseling techniques and dynamic therapies all tend to vary in terms of how much stress they place on the patient for success. The astute clinician considers these variables while working from the vantage point of assessing potential for psychotherapy.

Returning to initial interview techniques for determining which category of psychotherapy may be most valuable for which patient, one method of assessing the presence of therapy facilitative characteristics was hinted at in the chapter on the structure of the interview. Specifically, the clinician can choose to enter psychodynamic regions during the course of the intake interview itself. In such regions the clinician focuses on the manner in which the patient handles interpretative questions or statements. In particular, the clinician can purposely ask an interpretative question or two in an effort to observe the method by which the patient handles such questions, which may suggest the ability of the patient to work in more ego challenging therapies. At the same time the clinician will carefully note the patient's motivation to look at psychological material as well as the patient's ability to look inward.

An ideal response to an interpretative question consists of the presence of a probing self-reflection followed by the production of new and spontaneous material from the patient.[12] The material may consist of newly recalled memories, associations with current life situations, associations with the relationship with the therapist, or newly recovered unconscious material such as dreams. If this pattern does not emerge, it suggests either that the patient is not ready to accept the interpretation or is not capable of making the self-reflective connections or that the therapist may have missed the mark, having made an inaccurate interpretation or asked a poorly conceived question.

But the response described above is an ideal one. It does not typically occur in the initial interview, because many patients require more experience in therapy before understanding how to respond to interpretative questions. If a patient does respond in this type of reflective and creative fashion, then the chance that the patient represents an excellent candidate for a more ego challenging therapy is high.

A more typical response in an initial interview, but also a good one, is the tendency for the patient to show a sincere attempt to reflect upon the question, accompanied by some response, albeit one with minimal insight. But at least this type of response suggests that the patient is willing to engage in an active therapeutic exchange. On the other hand, if the patient becomes strikingly defensive, hostile, or markedly anxious, then one can suspect that this patient may benefit from a less threatening approach such as an ego nurturing or ego stabilizing therapy. The clinician is learning about the patient's psychological maturation by the method in which the patient responds to the interpretative question. The clinician is also obtaining an on-the-spot look at the patient's motivation, cognitive functioning, and psychological mindedness.

Let us look at the use of such a question during an initial

interview. The patient was a nicely dressed man in his mid-30s. He had been referred for possible psychotherapy. Upon first presenting he appeared anxious and quite distressed, as well he should be, because he was in the midst of a situational crisis. He was married and had four children, all of whom he loved. He also happened to have a homosexual orientation and his long-standing homosexual partner was threatening to leave him if he did not end his marriage.

As he spoke he appeared articulate and seemed to be of above-average intelligence. During the later phases of the body of the interview he began describing some of the actions of his partner that he resented. The dialogue unfolded as follows:

Pt.: I don't know, he's just problematic at times but I think all good relations are that way. But I do hate to bicker.

Clin.: Can you give me an example of the type of thing that you bicker about?

Pt.: (pause) Yes, I can. The other day was a perfect example. We were driving out towards the country and I was enjoying the quiet of the countryside. Next thing I knew he plops a tape into the tape deck and nearly blasts me out of the car, really. I mean really. So I reached over and yanked the tape out of the deck. He must have pouted for over an hour. (The patient seems absorbed in his belief that his partner's behaviors are inappropriate. On the contrary, the clinician is struck by the controlling quality of the patient, and the patient's relative inability to empathize with his lover. The question becomes one of determining whether the patient is capable of reflecting upon his own behavior with any degree of objectivity. The clinician sees an ideal opening for an interpretative question.)

Clin.: Do you feel that you are sometimes a fairly controlling person?

Pt.: (Patient looks away for a moment as he frowns) Controlling? I don't think so, uh . . . what do you mean?

Clin.: I was just wondering if you viewed your yanking the tape out as being somewhat controlling?

Pt.: Oh (raises his eyebrows) I don't really know, uh, I mean I guess at some level I am. Not all the time mind you. But sometimes. (long pause) Hmm, I guess it is sort of controlling to pull the tape out on him, but he didn't ask me if I wanted to listen. (slight smile) Perhaps I was a bit drastic at that. I do tend to tell him what to do pretty frequently. For instance, I almost always choose the restaurant that we will go to, yes almost always.

The patient's response bodes well for the use of an ego challenging form of therapy. We see him balking at first in a natural fashion, but he possesses the ego strength to explore further. Upon further exploration he seems to run material through his mind that the clinician has not mentioned. After a moment of reflection he begins to produce new material. This patient went on to benefit from a dynamic based therapy in which issues of control would play a recurring part.

It is important to realize that the initial balking at the clinician's interpretative question represents in many respects a good sign. Most people will balk when first confronted with an aspect of their behavior that is new to their awareness. The patient who immediately nods his or her head in full agreement, adding phrases such as, "Now I never thought of that but it really is true," may not be such a bargain for the would-be ego challenging therapist. These patients may be attempting to please the therapist and can be excruciatingly frustrating. Later in therapy, when it is eventually pointed out by the therapist that the patient seems to have a need to please, one can almost count on the patient to suddenly smile saying, "My goodness, I never thought of that, but your're absolutely right." Therapists are frequently tempted to return to their own therapy at such moments.

Another method of assessing the presence of therapy facilitative characteristics is provided by the use of "the miracle question." In this technique the clinician asks something along these lines, "If a miracle occurred while you were asleep, what would be different when you awoke?" The miracle question forces the patient to reflect, offering the clinician a glance at the patient's observing ego. By following up with a series of questions, concerning how these changes could perhaps be pursued in real life, the clinician may get a powerful look into the patient's motivation, problem-solving abilities, and strengths. It cannot be emphasized enough that the initial interviewer should carefully search for strengths, with an eye for capitalizing upon them in the subsequent therapy. By the way, the "miracle question" can sometimes be used as an interesting bridge into the closing phase of the interview.

We have reviewed some of the basic principles behind assessing those characteristics that may suggest suitability for therapeutic success. Before ending the discussion of psychotherapy assessment a few odds and ends should be addressed, which for want of a better name can be referred to as practical systems issues.

While making an assessment for psychotherapy, the clinician can ill afford to view the patient in a vacuum. The clinician must consider practical, and at times determining factors, such as the patient's financial resources, managed care limitations on number of sessions, time availability, and the resources of the mental health system itself. For example, the staff therapists at mental health centers are frequently overwhelmed with case loads. Such loads may preclude the chance for most patients to be seen in more demanding types of therapy that require frequent sessions. In such instances it becomes even more important for the assessment clinician to spot candidates who are more likely to benefit from such ego challenging therapies, so that these patients may come to the attention of the interested clinicians.

In a similar vein, the clinician needs to become aware of the types of therapy available in the area as well as a recognition that some clinicians do well with certain patients and poorly with others. In fact, some clinicians may have relatively serious psychological problems themselves, which may make it less advisable that they work with more severely impaired patients such as schizotypal personalities or borderline personalities. In this sense, before doing a consult, it is often rewarding to obtain an idea of what types of approaches are available or popular in the given center. In this sense clinicians can save themselves the embarrassment of suggesting "ivory tower" treatment recommendations that only serve to alienate the consultee.

At this point we can move on to another conceptual vantage point that has some direct connections with our current discussion.

Structural Interviewing of Kernberg

In the discussion of the vantage point of assessing the patient for psychotherapeutic intervention, it was noted that one of the major tasks was a determination of the patient's maturation and ego strength. Moreover, it was pointed out that two complementary methods of addressing this area included formulating a DSM-IV diagnosis and assessing ego strengths in a more systematic fashion. Otto Kernberg[13] has developed an interviewing technique that seems to offer another avenue for looking at both the diagnosis of the patient and the degree of ego strength from a slightly different perspective.

Stated in a highly simplified form, Kernberg suggests that each person can be characterized along a maturational continuum, much as we have already described. Depending on where the person sits on this continuum, the patient will handle stress differently. Specifically, patients will tend to handle questions that challenge them with differing degrees of facility. In this line of thinking the interviewer attempts to delineate the underlying character structure of the patient by noting the process by which the patient handles the interviewer's questions, hence the name "structural interviewing."

Before examining the technique in more detail, several points are worth mentioning. This approach to diagnosis complements the DSM-IV, because the DSM-IV approaches diagnosis by looking at the content of the patient's history and presentation in an effort to determine whether specific content-oriented criteria are satisfied. In contrast, structural interviewing attends not so much to what the patient says but how the patient says it. The process of the response, to a large degree, determines the diagnosis as opposed to the content. In particular, the clinician looks for processes such as the degree of anxiety created in the patient by the question or the resultant hostility or cooperativeness. Consequently, this style of interview can be particularly useful if the validity of the patient's answers are in question, perhaps related to guardedness or even purposeful deceit. In such circumstances it may be difficult to uncover DSM-IV criteria. Another use of the technique is the fact that by utilizing this conceptual vantage point, the clinician may uncover evidence that a more primitive personality style may be present. The clinician can then pursue the expansion of the appropriate diagnostic region by DSM-IV criteria.

The actual technique of structural interviewing is delineated by Kernberg as a specific format of diagnostic interview. In this more formalized approach, the clinician tends to explore various types of psychopathology starting with neurotic dysfunction and moving progressively through characterologic disorders, functional psychoses, and organic brain syndromes. Throughout this process various aspects of the DSM-IV and the more traditional psychiatric mental status are employed, but the interview continuously swings back to observations concerning the methods by which the patient handles the questions, even if the questions pertain merely to a description of symptomatology.

During this process the clinician utilizes three major types of interactions with the patient: clarification, gentle confrontation, and interpretation. In the last section we have already seen the manner in which a clinician may learn about the patient's level of functioning by the fashion in which the patient responds to an interpretative question. Kernberg adds to this process, suggesting various avenues of understanding the dynamics of the patient even as the patient clarifies the history of the present illness. In a sense the whole interview is transformed into an exploration of the processes by which the patient handles environmental stress as reflected in the manner in which the patient responds to the clinician.

In everyday clinical work, the more formalized structural interview is not particularly effective for gathering large amounts of material within the time constraints facing the clinician functioning as an intake interviewer. But the clinician can utilize this vantage point intermittently throughout the assessment interview as it naturally unfolds. For example, the clinician may consciously utilize clarifications, confrontations, and interpretations during the expansion of what we referred to earlier as psychodynamic regions. Sensitive observation by the clinician of even a few responses by the patient can provide surprisingly large amounts of data concerning defense mechanisms and the underlying character structure of the patient.

On a cautionary note, I do not believe that one should rely solely on techniques such as the structural interview in order to obtain a diagnosis, because these techniques are far too dependent upon the subjective opinions and skills of the interviewer to provide a reliable system of diagnosis. Instead, used creatively and with good timing, structural interviewing can provide powerful insight into the underlying character structure of the patient in a fashion that complements the DSM-IV in an immediately practical sense.

With this background, let us look more specifically at the model proposed by Kernberg. Three broad categories of development are delineated, moving from the least stable sense of self to the most stable sense of self. These three categories are the psychotic structure, the borderline structure, and the neurotic structure. Of particular note is the fact that Kernberg's category of the borderline structure is not used in the sense of only including the borderline personality as described by the DSM-IV. Instead, he seems to be referring to a variety of DSM-IV disorders, which earlier we had grouped as the psychotic prone or primitive personality disorders. These disorders include the schizotypal personality, the borderline personality, and the paranoid personality. When poorly integrated, the histrionic and narcissistic personalities may also be included.

These three broad categories (neurotic, borderline, and psychotic) are believed to vary with regard to three structural components, which Kernberg refers to as degree of identity integration, level of defensive operations, and reality testing. By way of example, the patient with a neurotic character structure tends to use relatively high-level defenses such as rationalization, intellectualization, reaction formation, and undoing. The more primitive borderline states rely more on lower-level defenses such as denial, splitting, magical thinking, and inappropriate idealization. Finally, people with a psychotic structure will tend to utilize more psychotic adaptations such as delusions and hallucinations, although higher-level defenses may be intermittently present as well.

Since these different defense mechanisms are at the very core of protecting the patient from anxiety, one would expect each category of patient to respond to stress with the appearance of the structure-specific defenses available to the patient. And here we approach the underlying premise of structural interviewing. The clinician utilizes processes such as clarification, confrontation, and interpretation to trigger various levels of anxiety, noting which style of defenses arises to alleviate the stress. The resultant styles of defense suggest the possible underlying character structure.

For illustrative purpose we shall focus on the use of mild confrontation. In this technique the clinician looks for an area of self-contradiction made by the patient during the course of the interview. The patient is then presented with the contradiction, not in an accusatory sense, but from the clinician stance that, "I am a little confused by some of your statements for they seem to contradict themselves." Having provided a somewhat stressful situation, the clinician sits back to observe the manner in which the patient handles the stress with regard to the appearance of underlying defensive mechanisms. From the constellation of defenses that appear, the clinician gains an understanding of the patient's core character structure.

The use of gentle confrontation in the context of structural interviewing will be clarified through the use of three examples. In each patient it will be assumed that similar content has been discussed but that the patients differ in the level of their structural development. In each case it will be assumed that the patient is a male in his mid-30s who presents feeling dissatisfied with his personal relationships. Earlier in the interview the patient had stressed that, "I'll tell you one thing, I'm sure not a male chauvinist like my brother. Now he and I don't see eye to eye when it comes to the roles of the sexes." In each of the subsequent illustrations we will see the patient eventually contradict this earlier statement, and the clinician will present this discrepancy to the patient. The responses of the patients will then be examined with regard to the underlying structural style that they belie:

ILLUSTRATION I

Pt.: Things haven't been going all that good at home. I've got some problems with the little woman. She seems to feel that I don't spend enough time with the kids, you know, like I should stop going out for a drink with the guys after work or something like that.

Clin.: I was just struck by something you said. You referred to your wife as the "little woman" and yet earlier you said that you were a far cry from a chauvinist. I guess what puzzles me is that the term "little woman" would be viewed as quite chauvinistic in most circles, wouldn't it?

Pt.: Uh (pause) uh (pause) I guess in some circles that would be true. I (pause) I didn't really mean it to be chauvinistic. You see my wife and I joke around a lot and sometimes I call her pet names and she does the same with me. I sort of meant that like a pet name. I didn't mean it to be chauvinistic, at least I didn't think I did.

Clin.: How do you think you actually view your wife?

Pt.: I've always thought that we had a pretty good relationship. And don't get me wrong, I think we do. We have our spats, but we work things out.

Although this patient may not be demonstrating the most profound insight in the world, one would not expect him to exhibit striking insight during an initial interview. But what his answer does suggest is that he possesses an ability to handle the tension of the moment reasonably well. He has been confronted with a contradiction. Like most normal or neurotic people he is disturbed by the apparent contradiction, a contradiction that he admits, albeit reluctantly. The person with a neurotic or normal structure (as this patient represents) will want to resolve this contradiction, for the patient is disturbed by the incongruity, which had been hidden from conscious awareness before. Moreover, the patient does not wish to be viewed as illogical or hypocritical.

In this particular patient, the defense of rationalization has allowed the patient's anxiety to be dissipated, as the patient rationalizes that the term "little woman" was just another example of a pet name, and his wife calls him pet names too. Following his rationalization the patient is then able to proceed with the conversation with relative ease, although one gets the flavor that the point of the clinician was not totally missed. Now let us see how a patient with a different underlying structure might respond.

ILLUSTRATION II

Pt.: Things haven't been going all that good at home. I've got some problems with the little woman. She seems to feel that I don't spend enough time with the kids, you know, like I should stop going out for a drink with the guys after work or something like that.

Clin.:   You know, I was just struck by something you said. You referred to your wife as the "little woman" and yet earlier you said that you were a far cry from a chauvinist. I guess what puzzles me is that the term "little woman" would be viewed as quite chauvinistic in most circles, wouldn't it?

Pt.:   So what if it is. I can call my wife anything I feel like calling her.

Clin.:   I certainly wouldn't challenge your right to refer to your wife in any way you choose. But I was wondering if there was some contradiction between your earlier statement and some of the attitudes you have just talked about?

Pt.:   Look, I'm not here to play word games with you. And I don't think I like your attitude that you're so goody goody, as if you never contradict yourself. And I don't particularly appreciate your insinuation that I'm a bad husband.

This patient has responded to the confrontation in a strikingly different manner than the first patient. He has attacked the clinician, displaying a rather quick-tongued bite at that. The anxiety generated by the clinician's question is being handled with significantly more lower-level defenses. The patient rapidly fires off a salvo of entitlement as he tells the clinician, "I can call my wife anything that I want to." The patient seems to be projecting his angry feelings out onto the clinician, who is subsequently misperceived as having stated that the patient is "a bad husband." The projection is accompanied by a tendency to devalue the clinician and see him as all bad, the early buddings of the primitive defense mechanism of splitting.

In this example the patient has demonstrated a variety of defenses suggestive of a borderline structure as might be seen in a borderline personality disorder or a poorly integrated narcissistic personality disorder. Thus the technique of calmly presenting the patient with one of the patient's own contradictions has resulted in a rather distinctive display of primitive defenses.

Not all people with primitive personalities will necessarily display anger or projection. In some instances, the patient may almost seem to transiently crumble psychologically as if crushed by a feeling of intense abandonment or rejection. In such instances the patient may perceive the clinician as viewing the patient as all bad or inadequate. At other times the patient's splitting defenses may be so powerful that the patient sees no problem with the contradiction, thus experiencing little if any anxiety. I remember pointing out to an adolescent that he had stated earlier a desperate desire to stay in his current remedial placement, yet he had just told me that he would continue to break the rules even if it meant getting thrown out. I pointed this out as appearing somewhat contradictory. He looked me coolly back in the eyes saying, "I do what I feel like doing. I can say both things if I want to. I don't see any problem with that."

In all of the above examples, the defenses of the patient suggest some type of more primitive character structure at the time of the interview. One does not see the initial anxiety seen in the person with primarily neurotic defenses, who feels uncomfortable with the fact that a contradiction has been displayed. Patients with borderline structure do not as frequently attempt to correct the discrepancy with defenses such as rationalization or intellectualization. Thus we see that the type of response does indeed seem to belie the underlying dynamic structure. It should be remembered that these inferences are broad generalities, and any patient may provide a range of defensive styles. What the clinician is looking for is the preferential style of the patient or any hints that more primitive processes may be present, perhaps suggesting the need for a more thorough diagnostic expansion of the various primitive personality disorders. In the following example the clinician will see evidence of an even more primitive process in the fashion in which the patient responds:

ILLUSTRATION III

Pt.: Things haven't been going all that good at home. I've got some problems with the little woman. She seems to feel that I don't spend enough time with the kids, you know, like I should stop going out for a drink with the guys after work or something like that.

Clin.: You know, I was just struck by something you said. You referred to your wife as the "little woman" and yet earlier you said that you were a far cry from a chauvinist. I guess what puzzles me is that the term "little woman" would be viewed as quite chauvinistic in most circles, wouldn't it?

Pt.: Oh uh . . . I I don't really know, I guess somewhere someone would say that (patient looks quite flustered and tense). I guess they could get mad at me, I guess they really could get mad, but chauvinists aren't all

> that bad. My brother is chauvinistic and he's a
> reasonable guy. I mean we don't see eye to eye but he
> is reasonable.

Clin.: Well, how do you feel you view women in general?

Pt.: (long pause, as if having a difficult time sorting his
thoughts) I view them, let me see. I like women, I do.
But sometimes they can be real difficult. But not
usually, my mother and my sister are both very nice
and very intelligent. I think intelligence is very
important in a person. I admire it a lot. One of the
things that has always been a strong trait in my family
is intelligence. We have always prided ourselves in
being up with the times and sometimes ahead of the
times.

In this illustration the clinician may find himself experiencing a
brief period of confusion, because the patient's answer is somehow
lacking in clarity. There are plenty of words, but they seem to have
been forged without meaning. This empty quality is the result of a
regressive disorganization of the patient, as witnessed by actual
problems in organizing his thinking. The thought process seems
subtly disturbed with a tangential flow, which eventually allows the
patient to not answer the question as to how he actually views
women. One can also see the patient's ambivalence as he swings
back and forth between viewing women as difficult or "good
mothers." In short, the patient's response to the stress of the
clinician's question is represented by the surfacing of soft signs of
psychotic process. He shifts rather radically from a speech pattern
suggestive of a fairly level-headed individual to speech suggestive
of someone quite unsure of himself. At the tail end of the dialogue
he begins to regain his composure.

This type of pattern is more frequently seen in people with an
underlying psychotic process. If the psychosis is closer to the surface, the clinician may find more and more dramatic disorganization
as the patient's defenses are overrun by anxiety. Perhaps even harder
signs of psychosis may eventually emerge, such as delusions or
ideas of reference.

The above illustrations demonstrate the manner in which structural interviewing can provide valuable insights into the level of
functioning of the patient at the time of the initial interview. Of
course, to utilize this conceptual vantage point, the clinician must
be able to "pull back" from the interview itself, adopting, for a
moment, a period of self-remembering. Once again these periods of
self-remembering provide the portals through which the clinician

can utilize both attentional vantage points and conceptual vantage points, in this case viewing the patient from the theoretical background envisioned by Otto Kernberg.

Intuitive Vantage Point

*I*n particular he [a medieval alchemist] approached matter with a passionate conviction that it held a mystery, a "mysterium magnum," the nature of which was different in quality and in essence from its material container . . .

A. McGlashan
Savage and Beautiful Country

We have come to the last vantage point to be discussed in this chapter. Curiously, it is a conceptual vantage point that arises without any conscious attempt by the clinician to apply a conceptual framework. It simply happens. To be aware that one is employing intuition would signal an immediate end to its presence. Elusive and difficult to describe, intuition is both a vital and vitalizing ingredient in the clinical interview. In actual practical terms, its worth is essentially impossible to overvalue. Every experienced clinician can relate times that the clinician just "felt something" such as "this patient is contemplating suicide" or "I have a feeling that this child is being abused." These hunches, if listened to, can then be followed by skillfully guided explorations. Indeed, hunches, guesses, and feelings represent the stuff of which intuition is born. Gifted interviewers are at home here.

But the question remains, "What is intuition and can it be taught?" In the first place, intuition remains difficult to define, thus decreasing to some degree the practicality of the first part of the question. Concerning the second part, it is probably next to impossible to teach intuition didactically. With regard to intuition, one then wonders whether clinicians should hopelessly throw up their arms while praying that somehow or other they have been given the gift? I do not think so, because intuition is not really a gift. It is more of a beneficent habit of sorts, a valuable habit that is ironically often ground out of humans by the educational process itself.

Consequently, in this closing section we shall look more closely at this most peculiar and beneficial of habits, in the hope that our explorations will help us to cultivate it, for intuition is not so much something that originates from something gained as it arises from something lost. More specifically, clinicians must lose the enculturated rules and rigid conceptualizations that block intuitive functioning. Most clinicians begin their work with a healthy abundance of intuition. A misguided education can quickly lay this abundance to rest.

Those clinicians who seem to utilize intuition effectively frequently share a triad of qualities. This triad consists of fascination, openness, and playfulness. All of these qualities depend on the clinician's ability to become involved in the moment at hand while analytical thinking recedes for a moment. The vacuum is replaced by feeling. Clinicians who cannot give way to the moment in this fashion are seldom intuitive. The interview becomes all thought, no feeling, just another matrix to be solved.

But where does the mystery originate that leads the clinician into moments of fascination? Apparently the mystery frequently arises much in the same fashion that it arose for the medieval alchemist, for the clinician realizes that no human can ever be fully fathomed by another human. The clinician's "mysterium magnum" is the innate complexity of the human organism itself. An immersion in this type of wonderment predisposes the clinician to all three of the qualities conducive to the appearance of intuition.

Indeed, this book is an attempt to increase the clinician's sense of wonderment, as the interviewer finds layer after layer of processes at work during any meeting between patient and clinician. A practical knowledge of the principles behind interviewing sets the stage for the birth of intuition. But there exists an even greater bond between intuition and knowledge. Intuition is essentially the spontaneous appearance of past knowledge whose acquisition the student has forgotten. The lessons gained by experience become so ingrained that the student not only consciously evokes them, but they unconsciously arise into awareness. In some instances, the student may have never been aware that a lesson was learned in the first place.

For example, an interviewer may suddenly feel that a patient is deeply saddened but have no awareness as to why this empathic realization has occurred. In actuality, as the clinician grew up, he or she probably became aware of numerous facial mannerisms, inflections of voice, and word choices that came to be associated with sadness. It may very well be an unconscious awareness of such nonverbal signals that have resulted in the intuitive feeling of the clinician. It is the subliminal level and the spontaneous application of this knowledge that leads us to call it intuition. But the intuition itself is based on a knowledge base, not on an ill-defined emanation. This does not suggest that intuition can fully be explained, but it does suggest that intuition may be more accessible than it is magical.

The explanation advanced thus far has been given to support the notion that one can develop intuitive skills in a positive sense. In this regard, as alluded to in Chapter 2, the principles discussed in this book will, with increased familiarity, begin to spontaneously cue the clinician into numerous subtleties and intuitive flashes. In addition, if one surrounds oneself with enthusiastic clinicians who share their ideas and observations, one eventually begins to incorporate the material both consciously and unconsciously. The struggle to learn how to tap this conscious reservoir, while not damming up the spontaneous messages of the unconscious reservoir, is a pivotal developmental task facing all clinicians.

On one hand, clinicians can rely far too much on intuition, feeling, "I already know how to interview. I really have a great feeling for people." As we have clearly seen, such a pompous attitude is the key to ignorance. On the other hand, some students can apply the principles of interviewing in a fashion that can stifle, as opposed to encourage, the growth of intuition. An example will clarify this point and stand as an important process for supervisors to alertly attend to if it appears.

I am reminded of a social work student who was both innately gifted interpersonally and also enthusiastic and dedicated. After about 3 weeks in our training program, I began to notice a rather disquieting development in her interviewing style. She was becoming progressively cooler during her interviews, with seldom a smile or sign of spontaneity. She did not seem to have a "feel" for the patient. To my surprise, as soon as she was out of the interview situation, she returned to her engaging and pleasant persona.

As this process was discussed with her, she noted that she was feeling very strained during her interviews saying, "I've just got to get better at this. I know I can be a much better interviewer!" When asked what she was thinking about during her interviews, she began to produce the 600 pages of this book verbatim. No wonder her interviewing was deteriorating. She was a "superego junkie." Her intensity and zeal for perfection were rapidly destroying her intuitive abilities. The prescription for the illness was simple: "Forget everything you've learned and just go in there and interview." Within a few days she returned with a smile on her face, stating that her interviews were going much better. Much of the material taught in the class was spontaneously becoming available to her during her interviews. She proceeded to develop an engaging and effective style, which reflected both her personality and her prospering knowledge base.

She represented a rather extreme form of intuitive shut-down, but supervisors should carefully look for this type of response in trainees, as well as the trainee looking out for the same process within himself or herself. The surest sign that one is thinking too much or trying too hard is the feeling that the interview is strained. Good interviewing is, for the most part, fun. In an effort to actualize

572 Advanced Techniques of Interviewing

the goal of creatively developing specific techniques while not inhibiting intuitive functioning, it is often useful to pick a single or perhaps a small number of techniques to focus on during any given interview. In this fashion the student's mind does not become cluttered and overwhelmed. Different clinicians can focus on varying numbers of skills without interference with their natural abilities. In actual practice, we have found that clinicians can frequently monitor and explore around two to five characteristics during an interview.

Gradually the student gains increasing proficiency in numerous techniques. Interviewing becomes progressively more intriguing as a new sense of balance and confidence arises in the clinician. And here we return to the idea of intuition, for as the clinician gains confidence, the appearance of intuitive moments seems to increase. This increase is probably easily explained by the fact that the openness and playfulness, described earlier as prerequisites for intuition, are greatly dependent upon the clinician's level of confidence. Clinicians are willing to be open and flexible if they feel that they will be able to handle whatever situation faces them. In this more indirect fashion, the knowledge gained from a text such as this one should further increase the intuitive skills of the clinician.

This willingness to experience the interview in a spontaneous fashion is pivotal in the clinician's ability to develop an intuitive eye. This type of seeing and experiencing is gracefully described by the writer Annie Dillard as she discusses her wanderings in nature.

But there is another kind of seeing that involves a letting go. When I see this way I sway transfixed and emptied. The difference between the two ways of seeing is the difference between walking with and without a camera. When I walk with a camera, I walk from shot to shot, reading the light on a calibrated meter. When I walk without a camera, my own shutter opens, and the moment's light prints on my own silver gut. When I see this second way I am above all an unscrupulous observer.[14]

It is from just such a mode of seeing, what we can call the intuitive vantage point, that the clinician will be most open to intuitive insights. As the interviewer develops the delicate art of intermixing this vantage point with more theoretical vantage points, the interviewer becomes increasingly more flexible and sensitive. This open fascination with both learning and the clinical interaction itself is an ongoing process for the clinician. Hopefully, the clinician will still possess this sense of creative naiveté during the last interview of his or her career. Learning becomes not a goal but a way. This approach to learning is powerfully stated by the Zen Master Shunryu Suzuki in his book *Zen Mind, Beginner's Mind.*

So the most difficult thing is always to keep your beginner's mind. There is no need to have a deep understanding of Zen. Even though you read much Zen literature, you must read each sentence with a fresh mind. You should not say, "I know what Zen is," or "I have attained enlightenment." This is also the real secret of the arts: always be a beginner. Be very very careful about this point. If you start to practice zazen, you will begin to appreciate your beginner's mind. It is the secret of Zen practice.[15]

It is also the secret of interviewing.

References

1. Speeth, K. R.: *The Gurdjieff Work*. New York, Pocket Books, 1976.
2. Mezzich, J. E., Dow, J. T., Rich, C. L., et al.: Developing an efficient clinical information system for a comprehensive psychiatric institute. II: Initial Evaluation Form. *Behavior Research Methods and Instrumentation* 16 (4):464–478, 1981.
3. Wallace, E.: *Dynamic Psychiatry in Theory and Practice*. Philadelphia, Lea & Febiger, 1983, p. 157.
4. Elkind, D.: Wilhelm Reich. In *Comprehensive Textbook of Psychiatry III*, edited by H. I. Kaplan, A. M. Freedman, and B. J. Sadock. Baltimore, Williams & Wilkins, 1983, pp. 833–838.
5. Bandler, R., and Grinder, J: *The Structure of Magic I*. Palo Alto, CA, Science and Behavior Books, 1975.
6. Havens, L.: Experience in the uses of language in psychotherapy: Counterprojective statements. *Contemporary Psychoanalysis* 16:53–67, 1980.
7. Havens, L.: *Making Contact*. Cambridge, MA, Harvard University Press, 1986.
8. Pilkonis, P.: Personal communication.
9. Brown, V.: *Psychotherapists' Strong Reactions: An Empirical, Phenomenological Investigation*. Doctoral dissertation from Duquesne University, 1986.
10. Hersen, M.: Personal communication.
11. Bellak, L., and Small, L.: *Emergency Psychotherapy and Brief Psychotherapy*, 2nd ed. New York, Grune and Stratton, 1978.
12. Wallace IV, E. R.: *Dynamic Psychiatry in Theory and Practice*. Philadelphia, Lea & Febiger, 1983.
13. Kernberg, O.: "Structural Interviewing" from *The Psychiatric Clinics of North America, Borderline Disorders*, edited by Michael Stone. 4 (i):169–195, 1981.
14. Dillard, A.: *Pilgrim at Tinker Creek*. New York, Bantam Books, 1975.
15. Suzuki, S.: *Zen Mind, Beginner's Mind*. New York, Weatherhill, 1984.

10

The Art of Moving with Resistance

"*A*nd how exactly like an egg he is!" she said aloud, standing with her hands ready to catch him, for she was every moment expecting him to fall.

"It's very provoking," Humpty Dumpty said after a long silence, looking away from Alice as he spoke, "to be called an egg—very!"

"I said you looked like an egg, Sir," Alice gently explained. "And some eggs are very pretty, you know," she added, hoping to turn her remark into a sort of compliment.

"Some people," said Humpty Dumpty, looking away from her as usual, "have no more sense than a baby!"

Alice didn't know what to say to this.

Lewis Carroll
Through the Looking Glass

*O*ne can easily empathize with the plight of young Alice. She is encountering the unpleasant slap of resistance, and she does not know where to move next. She is probably wondering if she should rebuff the cantankerous egg or politely retreat, admitting her gaffe. The answer, ironically, is that there is no single correct answer.

Clinicians will frequently meet resistance during the initial interview, and indeed throughout the course of therapy itself. Attempts have been made to provide steadfast rules with which to handle these resistances, such as "Always address process" or "Never answer directly." Such statements may provide valuable suggestions for action, but when they become rules, they become traps. These traps are littered with the remains of frustrated interviewers. As opposed to rigidity, creativity and flexibility represent the keys to handling resistance.

More specifically, in this chapter, the focus is not upon rules; it is upon the development of a language with which to discuss resistance as it occurs in a clinical setting. This language will provide a clarifying foundation for understanding the underlying principles at work during periods of resistance. By understanding these principles, a variety of methods of transforming resistance will suggest themselves.

In a practical sense, an appreciation of the language of resistance can help an interviewer review a problematic interview with the hope of figuring out what happened in the interview while discovering methods of handling the situation differently the next time it presents itself. At other times the clinician may actually be helped during the interview itself, for specific principles may be recognized and possible courses of action immediately undertaken.

As the clinician becomes more adept at transforming resistance, it becomes correspondingly less threatening. Indeed, a seasoned clinician eventually recognizes resistance not as a demon but as an odd ally of sorts, offering an opportunity for insight. The presence of resistance serves to alert the clinician to the fact that the anxieties and defenses of the patient are near the surface. If attended to sensitively, resistance is a pathway to understanding.

During the moments of interpersonal tension stoked by resistance, a curious process frequently occurs. The clinician's own defenses and insecurities are triggered. In this sense few areas of the initial interview provide a better window into the psyche of the clinician than watching the clinician's natural responses to resistance. As Harry Stack Sullivan has suggested, the self-system of the therapist quickly comes to the fore, staunchly defending the therapist from the affronts cast by the patient. This point brings us back to Alice, who has clearly been insulted by Mr. Dumpty. The rest of this chapter will attempt to show that Alice has a variety of viable pathways to follow, any one of which may help her to both engage and understand her would-be antagonist. Even for Alice, innocence and good intentions are not enough.

In order to accomplish this task, the chapter is divided into two sections. In Part 1, the language of resistance is examined. In Part 2, common types of resistances encountered in the initial interview are discussed, providing a variety of different approaches that can be utilized.

As a last note before beginning, it should be remembered that the goal is not to remove resistance: The goal is to make use of it.

PART 1: THE LANGUAGE OF RESISTANCE

In this section we shall attempt to delineate a method of examining resistance as it unfolds. As has been the case in the past, one of the best ways to begin the exploration is to look at a piece of dialogue itself.

In this particular situation, a woman in her mid-30s had been brought to the evaluation center by the police. Apparently her neighbors had become concerned when they heard angry screams pouring out of the screened windows of her living room. When the police arrived, they found the patient, whom we shall call Mrs. Weston, savagely destroying her furniture. She claimed that, "the witches have my furniture, it's no longer mine!" She was brought to the center on an involuntary commitment.

Mrs. Weston was somewhat unkempt and a little rotund. She frequently looked away with an air of disgust. She adamantly claimed that nothing was wrong with her, but that her neighborhood was teeming with witches and warlocks. These people had been invading her house, planting evil things in her furniture. She was also very proud that she had joined a Pentecostal religion, and she did not want any of those "bad drugs" that were given to her in the past during a hospitalization.

She had been treated for schizophrenia for about 10 years but had not taken any medications or been seen for follow-up in the last 2 years. She also admitted to hearing voices and being "hit by demons." She vehemently denied homicidal or suicidal plans. The clinician was about to explore her psychotic ideation in an effort to determine whether potentially dangerous psychotic processes such as alien control or command hallucinations were present.

It was at this point that the interviewer made a rather significant error, for which I take full credit, since I happened to be the unfortunate clinician. The error consisted of relaying a subtle self-disclosure, which was said with the intention that the patient might take an interest in educating me about her experiences with demons. To my surprise, the plan resoundingly backfired, plopping me smack into Wonderland, as Alice might say. Let us look at both this point of disengagement and the resulting attempts to rekindle the blending process.

> **Pt.:** I don't know what I'm gonna do about those people, disgusting that's what they are. No right being in my living room, no right at all ruining my furniture, giving it to the devil, his dues alright!

> **Clin.:** Mrs. Weston, one thing that you could help me to

understand a little better is what it's like to be hit by a demon. I've never had that experience and I'm wondering what it feels like to you.

Pt.: You never been hit by a demon? (said with surprised indignation)

Clin.: Well . . . I've never had that exact experience.

Pt.: Then what are you doing talking to me! (She sits bolt upright, shaking her finger brusquely.) You ought to know all about this stuff, and you're telling me you ain't been hit by a demon. Who are you anyway? I ain't talking to you no more (mumbled angrily beneath her breath).

Clin.: Mrs. Weston, it looks like you're concerned about my lack of knowledge about being hit by demons. What specifically about that is upsetting you?

Pt.: It would mean you ain't no doctor, that's what it would mean.

Clin.: And how would it mean that I wasn't a doctor?

Pt.: Because to be a doctor you got to deal with demons all the time, any idiot knows that . . . I just don't know what is going on here, I just want help with these demons, and they send me to a moron.

Clin.: I'm going to be honest with you because I think that is very important. I must admit I may not know everything about things that are important to you, but I am honestly trying to understand better, and you can help me to do that. And I didn't mean to upset you. If other things I say upset you, please let me know. I'm wondering if the demons have tried to hurt or enter your daughter?

Pt.: Yes they have, and I ain't gonna let it happen.

Clin.: What have you done to protect her?

Pt.: I put extra locks on her doors.

Clin.: And where does she live?

Pt.: She lives down on the East Side.

Clin.: Roughly how far away from you?

Pt.: Too far for her own good.

Clin.:   In what way?

Pt.:   She doesn't have a good head on her shoulders, she thinks she knows everything, but she'll learn, she'll learn the hard way. She's just growing up and don't know no better.

Clin.:   What are some of the things you've been trying to teach her?

Pt.:   To learn to be more careful with men. She don't know what is going on. They're with the devil I tell her. She's been hit, that I know.

Clin.:   How does she act when she's been hit?

Pt.:   She gets that dazed look in her eyes, talks real funny. A mother can tell she can, and I know she's got demons in her.

Clin.:   Have you thought of any ways to get them out?

Pt.:   Praying with the Lord, that's all I know.

Clin.:   Do the demons in her ever ask you to hurt her or try to trick you into killing her?

Pt.:   They ask me to do things like that. They told me to cut off her eyelids, but I know that's the devil talking. And I seen him in her eyes. Somehow I've got to get him out.

At this point it looks as if the interview is back on track. The blending, although still tenuous, is certainly a good deal better than it was when the patient mumbled, "I ain't talking to you no more." Besides the improvement in the blending, the patient is providing the exact type of lethality material that is of interest.

In this interaction, I made the mistake of sharing personal material with a paranoid patient when I related that I had never been possessed. I would never have thought that the patient would find this fact unsettling or odd. But it goes to show that paranoid patients can frequently twist any personal piece of information. Consequently, it is generally best not to self-disclose to such patients. The subsequent situation was a little bit like Alice referring to Humpty Dumpty as an egg. She had no idea she was putting her foot in her mouth, but somehow it found its way there. Resistances may arise from such awkward clinician maneuvers, or they may arise spontaneously without any error on the part of the clinician.

Recognizing Observable Resistance

In order to analyze the appearance and handling of a resistance, the clinician must first determine the observable form with which the resistance manifests itself. This observable resistance may appear with a verbal, nonverbal, or mixed presentation. The latter form appears the most frequently. In this example, the resistance was mixed. The patient verbally resisted by challenging my identity as a doctor, culminating in a statement of her intention to no longer talk. I had, in a sense, been dismissed.

The patient made her point nonverbally as well. For instance, her tone of voice became undeniably irritated, and she wagged her hand with the unmistakable gusto of an Inquisitor General. In this case, the nonverbal resistances were quite obvious, complementing her blatant verbal resistance.

Unfortunately, spotting resistance is not always this easy. A problem may arise if the patient conveys resistance only through subtle nonverbal cues. Clinicians can easily miss these unintentional messages. To avoid missing such cues, it pays the clinician to develop a habit of periodically reviewing the blending of the interview. A sudden drop in the blending process is usually indicative of resistance and can be picked up during periods of self-remembering.

Here we have stumbled on one of the major principles of working with resistance. If resistance is building, it is generally best to deal with it. If it is not dealt with during the interview, the patient may never return.

It is also worth keeping in mind that in the same sense that a patient may demonstrate resistance both verbally and nonverbally, the clinician may choose to respond, utilizing either or both of these channels. For example, in the above interview, as the patient became more hostile, the clinician could nonobtrusively push his chair further away, so as to provide the patient with more interpersonal space. Small changes, like this one, can sometimes have surprisingly powerful effects on an interview. Similarly, an interviewer may choose not to take notes if a patient appears guarded or paranoid.

Recognizing Seed Resistances

After noting the observable resistance, it is worth considering the possible presence of nonobservable resistances or what can be called "seed resistances." Most, if not all, observable resistances arise as a defense against some form of patient discomfort, a discomfort that can be called a seed resistance. These seed resistances are none other than the core pains discussed in detail in Chapter 4.

For the purpose of review, these core pains include processes such as the intense pain of isolation, self-loathing, fear of the unknown, fear of an impending loss of internal control, fear of an impending loss of external control, the loss of meaning, or the actual fear of physical pain. An ability to understand and eventually sense the presence of these pains lies at the very root of mastering resistance, because if the interviewer ignores the underlying seeds of resistance, new observable resistances may emerge. This tendency for displacement is not always the case, but it reminds the clinician that one always has the choice of addressing the observable resistance, the seed resistance, or both. As a basic principle, if the clinician finds that resistances repeatedly arise during an interview, then it is often best to consider the notion that underlying seed resistances may be at work. These seed resistances may need to be addressed more directly.

To better understand the concept of seed resistance, an illustration may be useful. In the following example the patient is a young woman in her early 20s. She presents with a sense of agitation, her fingers picking vociferously at each other. She is neatly dressed in a business-like blouse and skirt. During the interview she seems quite distracted, and at one point she asks for an ashtray to be brought to her. Her tone is somewhat demanding. In a few minutes she stands, moving toward the window. Throughout the exchange she has seemed hesitant, resulting in the development of a shut-down interview. After she stands up, the interviewer gently says, "You might find that in the long run you'll feel a little more comfortable sitting." She tersely responds, "I prefer standing."

She continues to appear unsettled and anxious. After a few more terse responses, the interaction continues as follows:

Clin.: What are some of the things that have been concerning you recently?

Pt.: You know, I really need to take a break. I'm going to sit out in the lobby. If you want to continue the interview there that's fine with me.

Clin.: Before you step out, why don't you and I talk frankly for a moment. I guess that both you and I realize that this is an anxiety-provoking situation. It's difficult sharing important and personal material with a professional, who is also a stranger. I'm wondering what you thought was going to happen today?

Pt.: I don't know, I guess you're going to "shrink my head," isn't that what shrinks do?

Clin.: Well, I guess that depends upon what you mean. In all seriousness, what were you actually expecting today?

Pt.:   (said with some exasperation but with less tension) I don't know. I just don't know. I thought I would be layed out on some couch and analyzed. I also thought that some students would probably be brought in to "see the nut."

Clin.:   Well, I'm not surprised that you were feeling a little anxious. I can fill you in a little better on what's going to actually happen. Would you like that?

Pt.:   I guess so.

Clin.:   There is no promise that you'll feel better, but it might help.

Pt.:   Sure.

Clin.:   First of all, there won't be any such couch or any students. As I said earlier we will talk for about 40 more minutes. But we will talk about what you feel is important. If something is too difficult to talk about, I want you to tell me. You don't have to talk about something that is too painful at present. I leave that up to you. We need to move at your pace. Is that all right with you?

Pt.:   Yeah, that will be fine.

Clin.:   By the way, one thing you said concerned me. You had said that you felt students would be brought in to see "the nut." Are you worried that I'm going to see you as unstable or "nuts," as you said?

Pt.:   I must say the thought crossed my mind.

Clin.:   What exactly are you worried about?

Pt.:   My boyfriend thinks I'm crazy. He's convinced of it, and I'm beginning to wonder myself.

From this point onwards the interview could proceed more smoothly and with a significantly stronger blending. The observable resistance consisted of repeated requests by the patient, eventually highlighted by the request to leave the room, a not-so-veiled invitation to end the interview itself. The interviewer could have addressed these observable resistances directly and even bluntly denied them, but instead the seed resistances were explored.

This patient appeared to be struggling with both a fear of the unknown and a fear of an impending loss of external control. To counterbalance these fears, she began to "take control" of the interview by making demands on the interviewer. Her requests were merely manifestations of her seed pains or fears. If the interviewer would have ignored these seeds, perhaps by following the patient out the door, then new observable resistances would most likely have emerged.

At the moment that the patient requested to walk out, the clinician did not address the observable issue of whether the patient should leave or not. Instead, an inquiry was made as to what the patient was feeling about the entire situation. In this fashion the clinician was able to explore some of the seed resistances. Not only did the clinician explore these seed resistances, the clinician relieved them. For instance, concerning the patient's fear of the unknown, the clinician described what would be happening. With regard to the patient's feeling that she had no control in the interview, the clinician literally gave her control with phrases such as, "If something is too difficult to talk about, I want you to tell me."

In this fashion an interview that could have become quite an exercise in antagonism resolved itself. This example illustrates the concept of seed resistances. The interviewer can choose to address either the observable or the seed resistances. Different situations require different techniques. Generally speaking, as mentioned earlier, if the clinician finds that resistances keep popping up or returning, it is often a good idea to consider the possibility that a seed resistance is not being adequately addressed. For example, this woman may also have been coping with a fear of an impending loss of internal control, as suggested by her statements about going "nuts." The interviewer was wisely beginning to explore this issue, because if it had been left unattended, new resistances may have eventually arisen.

Direction of Clinician Response to Resistance

This example introduces another basic piece of language concerning resistance. In the handling of any resistance, one can delineate whether the clinician went "with" the resistance or "against" it. Of course, in many instances, the clinician moves somewhere between these two poles. The task consists of determining where on this continuum the clinician acted. In the above example the clinician would have been fully going with the resistance if he had said, "Sure, why don't we both step outside to finish the interview."

The clinician could have directly opposed the resistance by saying, "I'm afraid that it is impossible to go outside, I never interview in public like that. We'll just have to stay here." Both of these responses would also represent attempts to address the observable resistance itself without addressing the seed. In our actual example, the clinician tended to avoid committing himself in either direction, because he chose to address the seed resistance instead. To some degree his willingness to address the patient's concerns probably also supplied an important metacommunication, that he was not strongly opposed to the patient's views in general and was certainly willing to listen. In this sense, he moved subtly with the resistance.

One might ask what is the best track to take, moving with or against the patient's resistance. However this is the wrong question, because no single answer exists. Once again, flexibility remains critical for success. In some instances the clinician must eventually oppose certain resistances. Certainly, in ongoing therapy, people with specific personality disorders, such as the borderline personality disorder, benefit from the consistent application of appropriate limits. And in the initial interview, limit setting is sometimes needed. In general, however, the more the clinician conveys a willingness to move with the patient, the more likely it is that the resistance will resolve. The more intensely the clinician attacks the requests of the patient, the more likely it is that the patient will "dig in."

Strongly opposing a resistance is asking for a fight from the patient, and the clinician will usually get it, if the clinician authoritatively denies the patient's needs. If a clinician discovers a need to consistently and rapidly oppose patient requests by laying down the law, then the clinician should explore his or her own psychological dynamics. Seed pains are not always found only in patients.

Let us review for a moment (Fig. 15). Thus far we have determined that in any given resistance, one can examine the following points: what was the observable resistance; how was this resistance manifested (was it verbal or nonverbal?), what were the seeds of the resistance; and did the clinician move with or against the resistance? This basic language allows one to discuss and learn from any example of patient resistance. At this point a few more terms will complete the tools necessary for understanding resistance. These terms deal directly with techniques of transforming resistance.

Specific Approaches for Transforming Resistance

Three basic approaches appear most frequently (Fig. 16). The clinician can attend to the content of the patient's comment or to the

seed resistance ⟶ observable resistance ⟶ verbal / mixed / nonverbal
(core pains)

Figure 15

Forms of resistance.

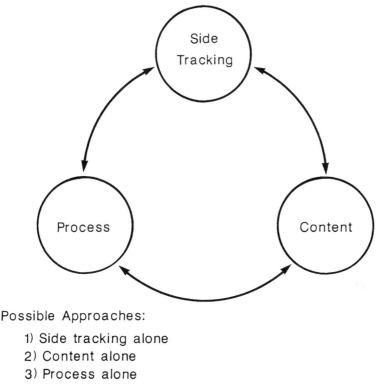

Possible Approaches:

1) Side tracking alone
2) Content alone
3) Process alone
4) Combination of two or three of the above

Figure **16**

Methods of handling resistance.

process of the patient-clinician interaction, or the clinician can side-track the patient away from the area of resistance. Each technique has its pros and cons.

CONTENT RESPONSES TO RESISTANCE

One of the most common approaches consists of directly responding to the content of the patient's statement. In other words, the clinician answers the question. This approach is common, because it represents the natural manner in which people in an everyday situation respond. If a spouse asks, "Why didn't you tell me we were supposed to be dressed up?" the queried partner generally responds directly to the content of the question. The partner might say, "I'm sorry, I simply forgot." This alibi should probably not be relied on too frequently, but in a pinch it will do. A clinician is answering the content of a resistance whenever the clinician provides a specific answer to the actual question of the patient. It should be kept in mind that if one responds to the content, then one is automatically placing oneself on the continuum of going with or against the patient's intentions, in which case the patient may either like or dislike the clinician's stance.

For clarification purposes let us take another look at the dialogue used to introduce this chapter, in which the paranoid woman suspected that I was not a doctor, because I had never been possessed. Instead of handling it in the fashion shown, we shall imagine what might have happened if I had attempted to respond solely to the content of the patient's accusation.

> **Clin.:** Mrs. Weston, one thing that you could help me to understand a little better is what it's like to be hit by a demon. I've never had that experience and I'm wondering what it is like.
>
> **Pt.:** You never been hit by a demon? (said with surprised indignation).
>
> **Clin.:** Well . . . I've never had that exact experience.
>
> **Pt.:** Then what are you doing talking to me? (She sits bolt upright, shaking her finger brusquely.) You ought to know all about this stuff, and you're telling me you ain't been hit by a demon. Who are you anyway? You can't be a doctor. I ain't talking to you no more (mumbled angrily beneath her breath).
>
> **Clin.:** I assure you that I am a doctor. You see, not all doctors are familiar with demons and possession. It depends on what your own beliefs happen to be. One does not have to believe in demons in order to be a good doctor. What remains important is that one cares.
>
> **Pt.:** Are you telling me that you don't believe in demons?
>
> **Clin.:** I guess at some level that's true. What I'm trying . . .
>
> **Pt.:** (Patient cuts off clinician) What you're trying to tell me is that you ain't no good Christian. You're with the devil, aren't you?
>
> **Clin.:** No, I'm not with the devil.

And here we see aptly illustrated one of the main hazards of responding to the content of the patient's resistance. The clinician can rapidly be drawn into a never-ending debate. As the debate thickens, the interviewer may quickly find the patient becoming progressively more hostile. The clinician may find it difficult to know how to respond. It is just this tendency to respond to content that places Alice into such difficult situations in Wonderland, because she frequently responds to the content of what she is asked. This tendency is also extremely common among therapists, for it is a natural response to explain oneself if one feels misunderstood.

One of the other problems with responding to content is the fact that such immediate responses tend to eliminate the chance of learning about the patient's defenses—in short, learning why the patient needed to ask the question in the first place.

On the other hand, in some cases, it may be expedient to directly respond to the patient's content. At times it is the best way to handle a particular situation. Clinicians who develop the rigid habit of always avoiding the content of the patient's inquiries, by addressing the process with questions such as, "What made you ask?" can dig themselves into a deep pit of trouble. With certain patients such process responses may be simply ill-timed and very frustrating.

For example, one can well imagine the response from the psychotic woman just described if the clinician had made a process statement such as, "You seem to be angry that I'm not familiar with demons. I'm wondering why you have such a need to present yourself so hostilely?" If the clinician is lucky, the patient will not have any idea what he just said so obtusely. If unlucky, and the point strikes home, then one hopes this clinician has his running shoes on. A rigid need to never answer questions directly probably represents an error in training or a need for control on the part of the clinician. Later we shall see examples in which content responses seem quite effective.

PROCESS RESPONSES TO RESISTANCE

We have already hinted at the basic mechanics of the second major method of handling resistance, namely to address the process of why the question is being asked. This is not the manner in which one is raised in our culture to respond to questions. As an adolescent one does not turn to the school principal and ask, "Gee Mr. Claybourne, I'm wondering why you have such an urgent need to know why I was smoking in the bathroom, and I might add that you are wearing a very handsome suit today." An obsequious Eddie Haskell from the "Leave It To Beaver" show might have said something like this, but few principals would be impressed. The point of this excursion remains the fact that because process responses are not natural, their effective utilization can be difficult to learn.

What a shame it would be not to learn the nuances of such a powerful technique. In the long run, effective process responses are essential elements of intensive psychotherapy, and they can also guide the clinician out of many a difficult situation in the initial interview.

In an operational sense, process is addressed whenever the clinician asks the patient to reflect upon what is happening in the interview itself, within the patient, or within the clinician. The clinician does not attempt to directly answer the specific question of the patient, but rather attempts to shift the focus of the patient to the actual process of the interaction itself, the feelings generated by the interview, or the thoughts that led to the patient's question in the first place. Various methods of attending to process are available to the clinician. Let us make a quick review of some of these techniques, which we shall see in more detail in the second part of this chapter. It is valuable to be familiar with all of these techniques, while discovering new ones from experience.

To begin the survey, one of the most basic methods of focusing on process consists of pointing out to patients their own behaviors. For instance, the interviewer may notice that an interview is becoming shut down after an animated beginning. The clinician could turn to such a patient and say, "You know, during the last couple of minutes I've noticed that you've become pretty quiet. I'm wondering what you are feeling."

At times the interviewer may choose to be more specific about the exact change in behavior. A patient may begin asking a variety of questions as the interview proceeds such as, "What do you think I ought to do?" At such a point the clinician may ask, "In the past couple of minutes you've asked a lot of questions. You weren't asking many questions earlier. I'm wondering what has changed so that now you seem to want some answers from me?"

The interviewer could also explore process by directing attention to the immediate effect of one's actions upon the patient. For instance, with the previous example one could say, "I guess you've noticed that I'm not directly answering many of your questions. I'm interested in how you're feeling about my apparent reluctance to answer directly." A response to this question may reveal some important traits in the patient, such as an ability or inability to be appropriately assertive. By way of example, a patient exhibiting many dependent traits may feel quite awkward at this point, saying, "Oh don't worry about it, I guess that's just your job." A person with narcissistic traits, on the other hand, may snarl a sarcasm such as, "Shrinks are too afraid to deal with people like people, isn't that right?" In any case the process question has provided significant material for exploration.

In other instances, the clinician may choose to address the patient's affect as opposed to the patient's behavior per se. A patient may begin to appear sad. The clinician may directly point out the affect with, "You're looking sort of sad right now, what's going on?" Or the interviewer may inquire at a more general level such as, "I was wondering what you were feeling just a moment ago, when you spoke about your dad?"

In a somewhat similar vein, if the clinician senses a growing hostility from the patient, the clinician may choose to note the affect itself. "Mr. Jason, it looks like you're feeling a little angry, what's going on?" In some instances, the clinician can directly point out the problems arising in the blending process. An angry patient may say, "Look, there's nothing wrong with me that a little time won't cure, get the picture!" To this the clinician may respond, "I'm sorry if you are starting to feel some anger, let's see what's happening here. It looks like some of my questions are irritating. What am I asking that seems uncalled for?"

At this point one of the characteristics of process interactions seems more apparent. Specifically, when addressing process, the clinician cannot afford to be afraid of exploring the resistance itself, no matter what emotions are being aroused. Instead, the clinician moves into the "eye of the storm," while carefully trying to understand what is actually being experienced by the patient. Many times patients appreciate this honest attempt of the clinician to "uncover the real problem here."

In an interview in which a patient is becoming more distant, but is unable to verbalize anger, the logjam can sometimes be broken by personalizing the interaction, as with, "Mr. Wilkins, are you feeling a little angry with me?" Once the patient becomes engaged in talking about his or her own anger, some of the anger may actually dissipate. It is somehow harder for patients to be angry with someone who can openly acknowledge true feelings. At such moments the interviewer seems more human and less like a sterile clinician. In general, one of the best manners with which to make covert resistance less obstructive is simply to make it overt, put the cards on the table so to speak.

Another fruitful method of addressing the process consists of asking patients what answer they are expecting. The patient may ask, "Do you believe in God?" The clinician may respond, "That's a tough question, John. What kind of difference would it make to you if I said yes or no?" In this fashion the clinician may get a good warning as to what results may follow if the clinician would choose to respond to the actual content of the question. But in many cases, once the patient begins answering what difference it would make, the original question never returns.

Herein lies another hallmark of process responses in general. Process responses provide clinicians with time to think and re-collect themselves. They are punts of a sort, which clearly put the ball back in the patient's hands. During the time in which the patient must come up with a response, the clinician can get a better idea of how to ultimately respond to the resistance in question.

In a behavioral sense, process comments may also serve as punishing reinforcers to patients who are simply trying to needle the clinician with tricky questions. Each time these patients ask a bothersome question, the process comment turns the focus back upon themselves. Soon enough they tire of being put on the spot. By way of example, one might say to such a patient, "You seem to get a charge of putting me on the spot. Any ideas why you like to do that?" If the patient persists, the clinician can continue to pursue the point, "There's another one of those pointed questions. What are you feeling when you ask questions like that?" Done with a calm and nonvindictive tone of voice, these questions serve the dual purpose of helping the patient to look at himself, while simultaneously decreasing the frequency of such barbed questions.

A final process technique, which we have not yet discussed, is the judicious use of self-disclosure. If one feels frustrated by the appearance of repeated resistance, one may turn to the patient saying, "You know, I'm feeling a little puzzled right now. We don't seem to be getting anywhere. Do you have any ideas about what is going on between us?" A more interpretative variant of such a response may be, "Do you have any ideas why we are getting into a debate here? Is this the same type of argument that you find yourself in with your wife, or with your boss?"

As a final example, one of the most common process techniques is to respond to a patient's question with a simple, "Why do you ask?" To me this question is occasionally useful, but, in actuality, it is often not fully understood by the patient in an initial interview, because these patients are not yet trained to understand process as opposed to content. In short, they wonder, "What does he mean, why do I ask?" Moreover, I have noticed that many supervisees automatically snap off this response any time a patient asks a question. More often than not, the accompanying tone of the clinician's voice has a defensive quality to it. Utilized in this fashion, this question can be malproductive. If the clinician keeps these potential problems in mind, this standard example of a process response remains a viable option.

Now that we have delineated various methods of responding to process as opposed to the content of the patient's statements, the question becomes one of uncovering the possible advantages of such process responses. Several advantages come to mind. Process statements and questions provide time in which the clinician can reorganize, as stated earlier. They also push the patient to begin a self-exploration, which will hopefully continue if the patient proceeds into psychotherapy. Moreover, as the patient responds, the clinician gains a chance to understand the patient's defenses, fantasies, and interpersonal style. If a question is answered on a content level by the clinician, much of this opportunity may be lost. Finally, when clinicians respond to process as opposed to content, the issue of going against the resistance is somewhat muted, because no opinion has actually been offered. Consequently it becomes less likely that the clinician will put his or her foot in his or her mouth.

All in all, process comments and questions appear to have many advantages. It is probably not too risky to state that process responses are generally better than content responses. But there are times when content responses may be superior, and one should be familiar with both methods. Another very important point remains the fact that the clinician may frequently find it useful to combine process and content techniques.

Let us take a look at some process maneuvers in an actual clinical situation. Although this particular dialogue was not in an initial interview, it illustrates the advantages of a process approach when it hits its mark. The patient was a young man, whom we have discussed before. He had a long history of a compulsive drive for success, which had brought him many societal rewards but left him feeling empty and unloved. He appeared to benefit significantly from psychotherapy as well as the interim use of a tricyclic antidepressant.

In the termination phase of his psychotherapy the following exchange occurred generally as follows. In it we shall see the patient ask a specific content-oriented question. Rather than respond to the content of the question, a series of process questions provided an entrance into a wealth of psychodynamic material.

Clin.:   What was the last session like for you?

Pt.:   It was uh, pretty upsetting. I don't like thinking about the death of my parents. And I was a little surprised at how upset I was feeling. I've been thinking about the ending of the therapy a lot. I think I'm ready, but uh, it's, it's a little scary . . . I don't like saying good-bye and you had asked what I'd do if my father was dying . . . I really don't know. But there has to be something more than death. There has to be a life after death or else all this would be so senseless . . . What do you think, do you think there is life after death?

Clin.:   When you ask that question, what do you picture me answering?

Pt.:   Oh I don't really know. I guess I hope you'll say yes, because, because that's what I think too.

Clin.:   Well what would it mean to you, and this isn't necessarily my answer, but what would it mean to you if I said, "No"?

Pt.:   Uh, hmm, I think that would upset me.

Clin.:   In what way?

Pt.:   Because it would mean that you disagreed with me and I wouldn't like that. That would bother me, that would bother me a lot.

Clin.:   Why?

Pt.:   I don't know. I, I, guess it's important to me what you think of me.

Clin.:   So let's get back to your question, because what seems important about it is the fact that you are hunting for me to agree with you, as if you need my approval to be "good." What do you make of that?

Pt.:   (slight smile) It reminds me of earlier in the therapy, when I needed you to praise me in order to feel good. Like when I got mad at you because you hadn't read the newspaper articles about my ball games. That upset me, it was like I needed your approval to be O.K. And I know that I've felt that need about my father for years. He was the reason I played ball . . . I felt I had to play ball or he wouldn't love me. But I thought I got over that need.

Clin.:   I guess not entirely. You did it just now with me again. You wanted my approval of your answer. But the point is that you don't need an answer from me. You don't need my approval. It would be fine for us to disagree. You won't be destroyed. Our relationship will not end simply because we disagree or because I wouldn't approve of one of your beliefs.

Pt.:   I know that, but sometimes I have a hard time feeling it. I thought I was totally over that feeling, but I guess there is a part of me that still demands approval, perhaps too strongly. (pause) I was very upset with something my sister said to me a couple of days ago. She told me that I'd better stay in therapy a little longer, 2 years wasn't enough. And that really bothered me . . . but I eventually realized that it didn't really matter what she thought. I know that I've made a lot of progress. And I may not be perfect, but I'm not so bad either. And she doesn't really know me. I am cautiously optimistic about the future. I really think that I am ready to end therapy. It won't be easy, but I don't think it ever would be.

In this excerpt, the focus was turned back upon the reason why the patient asked the question. No effort was made to actually answer his question directly on a content level. The approach, via process, led the patient into a rich area of reflection, which cut directly to one of the main themes of the therapy as it related to the issue of termination. Eventually the patient achieved a deeper understanding of why he "needed" an answer, a need that was gradually decreasing as his sense of self-esteem improved. To have responded with a content approach would have completely short-circuited this powerful therapeutic interlude.

We can see the power inherent in responding to the process as opposed to the content. When done effectively, the patient and the clinician are often moved inward. Although this excerpt originated from an exchange during the termination phase of therapy, it nicely illustrates the basic principles and strengths of a process-oriented technique.

At this juncture, one might argue that if process responses can provide such insight, then why would a clinician ever use anything but a process-oriented approach. And here lies an important but often underplayed point. The immediate goal of the clinician, when transforming a resistance, is not necessarily to provide insight. Let us backtrack for a moment in order to explore this issue in more detail.

When working with resistance, the clinician may choose to achieve any of the following three tasks: (1) to decrease the resistance itself, so that communication is improved in the setting of a strengthened engagement process, (2) to learn about the patient's defenses, while uncovering the anxieties that stirred these defenses, and (3) to help the patient learn a method with which to explore the patient's own dynamics. Each of these goals is important; however, the emphasis placed on each goal by the clinician may vary considerably, depending on the stage of therapy. Once again, as with the interview itself, goals and tasks change with each phase of the therapeutic encounter.

In the above excerpt the patient was in the closing phases of a long-term, dynamically oriented therapy. At this stage of therapy the alliance is generally extremely strong. Consequently, the first task listed above is of little relevance, the alliance having been secured much earlier in the process. Indeed, during this stage of therapy, I was able to be fairly confrontational with this patient without endangering my alliance with him. On the other hand, while in the termination phase of therapy, both participants should be concerned with recognizing and understanding the patient's anxieties and defenses. If the therapy has proceeded well, the patient should be nearing a phase in which he progressively functions as his own therapist. The last two tasks mentioned above are of prime importance. Process questions and interpretations remain the best method of accomplishing these tasks.

Let us look at the needs associated with an initial interview as compared with later stages of therapy. The main goal is not to uncover defenses in detail or to help the patient gain insight. Instead the most important task is the establishment of a sound alliance, while gathering the most valid information available in order to determine the treatment options available for the patient. Patients may gain psychotherapeutic insight in the process, but there will be time in the subsequent therapy for a focus upon the acquisition of insight.

In this light, it becomes apparent that the last two potential tasks associated with handling resistance, mentioned earlier, are not of major importance in the initial interview. The first task of decreasing the resistance in order to allow the gathering of valid data becomes paramount. In this sense process maneuvers are frequently valuable, but other methods of handling resistance may also be valuable, and in some cases more useful for the task at hand. This is why we mentioned earlier that content responses to resistance have a real place in the initial interview, because the task of the initial interview is a unique one. This distinction between the goals of the initial interview as opposed to ongoing therapy is further highlighted if the initial interviewer is functioning as a consultant or triage agent, who may never see the patient again.

SIDE-TRACKING RESISTANCE

While considering the above line of thinking, it is worth mentioning another method of handling resistance besides the previously described techniques of addressing content or process. This other technique is much more commonly utilized during initial interviews rather than in ongoing therapy, because it certainly provides no insight for either the patient or the clinician. Yet it can work surprisingly well in breaking up a logjam of resistance. The technique is called side-tracking the patient, which in less euphemistic terms one might call ignoring the resistance.

At first glance this sounds like an unsavory undertaking. But let us see it in action before passing judgment. Imagine a mildly angry man of about thirty, brought in for an evaluation, somewhat against his will. His family describes symptoms suggestive of incipient mania, and he indeed displays both a pressured speech and tangential thought, accompanied by a labile affect. We will pick up the interview somewhere in the opening phase.

Clin.: Mr. Preston, a little earlier you had mentioned that you had been thinking of hurting yourself . . . (patient cuts off clinician).

Pt.: What is it with you shrinks, you're always talking about people killing themselves, can't a man kill himself if he wants to? Can't a man control his own destiny?

Clin.: Who else has been trying to control your life?

Pt.: Who hasn't! You name them, the President, the Pope, and all the saints in heaven. My wife is the big know-it-all. She's the boss. To her everything makes sense but me. But she don't know it all, trust me.

Clin.: Besides feeling angry with some of these people, have you been feeling sad at all?

Pt.: You know it's the strangest thing but I do get sad sometimes real sudden-like (tears well-up in eyes).

This example nicely illustrates the successful use of a sidetrack. The patient's anger at the clinician has subsided, and the interview is proceeding into a data gathering phase. But the patient's questions concerning "shrinks" and their generic interest in suicide has been sidestepped. The clinician will reapproach suicidal ideation at a later point in the interview, but for now the flow of the interview has been restored. An attempt to respond either to the process or the content of the patient's question may have been considerably less productive in moving through this resistance.

Sidetracking is frequently useful with hypomanic or manic patients, because it takes advantage of the patient's inherent tendency to jump from topic to topic. A few other points concerning sidetracking are relevant. If the clinician uses a sidetrack, the clinician needs to carefully watch the patient's response. If successful, the patient will quickly follow up on the new topic. If the patient returns to the patient's original question, then sidetracking is probably not going to work and a content or process response will be needed. It is generally not wise to continue side-tracking an issue, for such persistence is often irritating and rightfully so to a patient. If a sidetrack fails, try a different technique.

Another point to keep in mind is that sidetracking frequently works best when the interviewer changes the topic to an area of high importance or affect for the patient, as was demonstrated in the excerpt above. It is also useful to side-track the topic away from oneself if the patient is expressing anger towards the clinician.

Direct Application of the Language of Resistance

Thus far we have discussed three methods of handling resistance: addressing the content, addressing the process, and sidetracking. These techniques complement each other and may be used singly or in conjunction with each other. We have also seen that depending on the phase of therapy or the patient's clinical state, different techniques may be more or less useful. Combined with the concepts of observable resistance, seed resistance, and direction of the clinician's response (either with or against the resistance), we have developed a language that can allow us to explore essentially any example of resistance encountered in clinical work.

For instance, these terms can be readily applied to the striking piece of resistance illustrated in the beginning of this chapter. It may be of value to review this piece of dialogue as viewed with the concepts delineated above. The patient was the 30-year-old woman escorted by the police into the emergency room on an involuntary commitment after she had been found destroying her "demon-possessed" furniture. The dialogue had proceeded as follows:

Clin.: Mrs. Weston, one thing that you could help me to understand a little better is what it's like to be hit by a demon. I've never had that experience and I'm wondering what it feels like to you.

Pt.: You never been hit by a demon? (said with surprised indignation).

Clin.: Well . . . I've never had that exact experience.

Pt.: Then what are you doing talking to me! (She sits bolt upright, shaking her finger brusquely.) You ought to know all about this stuff and you're telling me you ain't been hit by a demon. Who are you anyway? I ain't talking to you no more (mumbled angrily beneath her breath).

It is rather easy to pick out the observable resistance at this point, as mentioned earlier. On a verbal level the observable resistance begins with the accusatory question, "You never been hit by a demon?" This is quickly followed by a deeper pit of resistant statements, culminating in a refusal to talk anymore.

All of these verbal antagonisms were accompanied by many observable signs of nonverbal resistance. Her tone of voice became acrid, accompanied by an angry stare. The stare itself was waved in by a hostile wagging of her finger. In short, the observable resistances, on both a verbal and nonverbal level, were openly displayed.

But what of the potential seed resistances? Which core pains may have been at work with this particular woman? One must remain somewhat speculative in this regard. And yet the seeds of her resistance seemed fairly apparent. In the first place, the situation itself, of being brought in by the police involuntarily, suggests the likelihood of a great deal of fear and anger concerning the issue of a loss of external control. Earlier in the interview she had animatedly discussed the need for all people to convert to her religious beliefs. Beneath her intensity one could sense a feeling of inferiority, which she guarded by putting all other faiths down. In this sense another possible seed resistance was a feeling of low self-esteem. These two core pains seemed most acutely active, but other tensions such as a fear of the unknown or a fear of a loss of internal control (ergo violence) may also have been at work.

It appears that the actual resistances, both overt and covert, can be categorized nicely by the language developed so far. The next question becomes one of delineating the actual attempt to resolve the resistance, for this interview had potentially reached a dead end.

In the first place, the resistance is addressed by my immediate reply, "Mrs. Weston, it looks like you're concerned about my lack of knowledge about being hit by demons." This statement represents a process response, in which the patient's affect is being acknowledged. This pathway is furthered by my next question. "What specifically about that is upsetting you?" Once again this statement focuses on the process of what is disturbing to Mrs. Weston. It acknowledges her right to be angry, and it suggests a willingness on the part of the clinician to find out how he is upsetting her. The metacommunication is clear and reassuring to the patient: "I would like to find out what I'm doing to upset you, and I may be able to change it."

The tone of voice used was a gentle one. In this regard a nonverbal as well as a verbal medium was utilized to respond to the patient's resistance. Both the verbal and the nonverbal response were nondefensive. They represent a moving with the resistance. No attempt is made to contradict or block the patient's anger, as would have been displayed with a clinician response such as, "Now there's no need to be angry here" or "You're going to have to talk to me so that this can be straightened out." Both of these statements represent content responses, because they immediately address the patient's stated demands. Such statements would probably have served to anger this patient even more, because in essence they strip her of even more control.

The process techniques actually used began to soften the patient's resistance, as shown below.

> **Pt.:**   It would mean you ain't no doctor, that's what it would mean.
>
> **Clin.:**   And how would it mean that I wasn't a doctor?
>
> **Pt.:**   Because to be a doctor you got to deal with demons all the time, any idiot knows that . . . I just don't know what is going on here, I just want help with these demons and they send me to a moron.

Clearly the patient remains hostile, but her admission of feeling confused is suggestive that the hostility is residing. One may be able to reach her on a more cooperative level. In general, once a clinician acknowledges a patient's anger in a nondefensive fashion, it is not unusual to see the beginning of a de-escalation of affect.

In the next few statements I employed a slightly different approach with, "I'm going to be very honest with you because I think that is very important. I must admit I may not know everything about things that are important to you, but I am honestly trying to understand better, and you can help me to do that." This represents a content response, which directly acknowledges the patient's statement that I essentially do not know what I am doing. There is a toned down admission that the clinician is "guilty as charged," but this is turned to advantage by asking for the patient's help. Here we see a seed resistance being addressed. The patient has a need to feel superior, and the clinician responds to this need by taking a one-down position.

The next two statements, "And I didn't mean to upset you. If other things I say upset you, please let me know," address the other seed resistance discussed earlier. More specifically, these statements give some control to the patient, thus decreasing the tensions surrounding her fear of a loss of external control while conveying a sense of respect.

Directly on top of these efforts to decrease the patient's core pains, a sidetracking technique was employed. The patient was asked, "I'm wondering if the demons have tried to hurt or enter your daughter?" As mentioned earlier, an effective sidetrack tends to move the patient into an area of high affect or interest. In this case the area involved the patient's daughter and completely moves the discussion away from the immediate interviewing situation.

Fortunately the patient accepted this sidetrack, probably because her anger towards the clinician was resolving. It is frequently useful to piggyback sidetracking statements onto other techniques as shown above. The trick is to quickly move the topic of discussion, thus decreasing the likelihood of the patient's anger rekindling.

At this point a series of closed-ended questions was used to keep the patient in the new area of discussion, thus cementing the sidetrack. A decision was then made to continue using the daughter as a focus of discussion, because the patient seemed to increase her blending around this topic. Eventually the further expansion of the psychotic region and the lethality region was accomplished utilizing this new focus of discussion. The interview proceeded more smoothly, the resistance having fallen away.

By examining this particular resistance in detail, it is apparent that we have indeed developed a language with which to explore the subtle nuances of the complex phenomenon known as resistance. In the next section, this language will allow us to directly address specific resistances commonly encountered during the initial interview.

PART II: HANDLING COMMON RESISTANCES

That the yielding conquers the resistant and the soft the hard is a fact known by all men, yet utilized by none. . . .[1]

Lao Tzu
(Chinese Sage)

Resistances Concerned with Clinician Competence

Certainly one of the more common forms of resistance is illustrated by questions such as, "What type of training have you had?" or "Are you a student?" Patients may be concerned about a variety of issues such as training, professional affiliation, age, sex, and race. The issue becomes one of to what degree should the clinician directly respond, and whether the response should be on a content or process level. As one would expect, there exist no perfect answers, but some guiding principles can be discerned.

In the first place, these types of questions commonly arise from a single seed resistance, the fear of the unknown. In this case the specific fear can be succinctly stated as, "Can this particular clinician help me?" With this idea in mind, the goal becomes one of helping the patient to recognize the nature of the question actually being asked, to help the patient see where such a question may be coming from in a psychological sense, and to decrease the patient's anxiety.

It is also relevant to realize that such questions may not actually always represent resistance. They may represent intelligence. It is not inappropriate, when seeking a professional, to want to know if the supposed professional is any good. Many patients have no way of prescreening and simply end up choosing a number from the telephone book or receiving a referral to their local mental health center.

Around this issue of whether these requests represent resistance or not, two schools of thought have evolved. For those who view it as a form of resistance, an argument is generally advanced that only a process response is appropriate from the clinician. According to this school of thought, the clinician should find out why the question is being asked. To answer directly will short-circuit the opportunity to uncover important psychodynamic information. The clinician also runs the risk of providing an answer that will unsettle the patient. For example, the clinician might quickly respond that the clinician's training has been in behavioral techniques. If the clinician is unlucky, the patient may possess all sorts of distorted views about behaviorism, resulting in an immediate wariness of the clinician.

The second school views these questions as a legitimate aspect of the contract and leans towards answering them directly, utilizing a content-oriented response. One does not go to a surgeon without finding out whether the surgeon is skilled. With something as sensitive as one's personal memories, it makes sense to find out if the clinician is talented and trustworthy. This argument is strengthened by the fact that many unskilled and poorly trained people can label themselves as therapists without ever having spent a single day in a legitimate school of counseling.

Both of these arguments seem to hold water as one reads them. This somewhat contradictory situation arises because both of these arguments are, in reality, quite legitimate. The wisest resolution may be to incorporate both arguments, utilizing both a process and a content response. For instance, the clinician may respond as follows, "I think your question about my training is a very good one. In just a little while, I'll answer any basic questions you have about my training, but first I'd like to get an idea of what some of your concerns may be. For instance, what type of clinician were you hoping to find here today?" As the patient begins to describe specific concerns, a variety of followup questions can be asked, including the following:

a. What was it like coming here today?

b. What types of concerns did you have about coming to the appointment today?
c. What had you imagined it would be like talking with a psychiatrist?
d. What are some of your specific fears about my training or background?
e. Did you have any dreams or fantasies about coming to see a psychologist?
f. What have you heard about social workers or other mental health professionals?
g. What does seeing a psychiatrist mean to you?

All of these questions are process oriented in nature, allowing ample room for the clinician to explore some of the dynamic issues behind the original question. The information provided by the patient may also help the clinician to choose a better method of responding on a content level. For instance, if the patient relates distorted information about therapy in general or specifically, then the clinician can gracefully acknowledge the patient's anxiety, while hopefully decreasing it through appropriate education. The clinician may say something such as, "I can understand why you would have concerns about behavioral therapy. Let me clarify some issues, and I think you'll find that the therapy we are discussing, although behavioral in nature, is quite different from what you've heard."

Other methods of returning to the content response, which was promised to the patient, may be as simple as saying, "I appreciate your sharing some of your concerns, let me tell you a little about my background as I said I would." Besides providing appreciated information, this comment conveys the metacommunication that "this clinician keeps his or her word" and respects the needs of the patient.

To me, the combined process/content technique described above allows the clinician to gather a substantial amount of pertinent information, while also answering the legitimate questions of the patient. Once again, in an initial interview, as opposed to ongoing therapy, the premium is on engaging the patient, not on providing insight. The above technique is strongly engaging while providing an appropriate degree of dynamic exploration.

Some clinicians use the above approach but switch the order of the techniques. First, the clinician simply answers the question as with, "Oh, I received my medical training at the University of North Carolina at Chapel Hill and then did my psychiatric training right here at Western Psychiatric Institute and Clinic. This immediately "moves with" the patient's resistance. But the clinician does not ignore the core pain beneath the resistance. The second step is now to address the process with the types of exploratory questions listed above such as, "I'm wondering what types of fears you may have had about seeing a psychiatrist?" Another useful follow-up question is, "Have you had some bad experiences with psychiatrists in the past?"

With regard to issues such as sex, age, and race, a similar approach may be taken. The trick is not to become defensive. The clinician attempts to provide a safe milieu within which the patient can discuss concerns. The clinician might ask, "I noticed that you mentioned that I seem young, I'm wondering what some of your concerns are about my youth." The nondefensiveness of such a response probably conveys more professionalism than a string of diplomas hanging on the office wall.

After hearing the patient's concerns, the clinician will have a better idea of where to move next and whether to directly respond to the content of the patient's questions. Once again, content responses can be valuable. In the next illustration the clinician will follow a process response with a content-oriented technique, in which an attempt is made to acknowledge the inherent differences between the patient and the clinician, raised by the patient herself.

Clin.: What I'd like to do today is spend the next 40 or so minutes trying to gather from you what you see as the major problems. Perhaps we could start with what brought you here today.

Pt.: You know, before we start I need to say something.

Clin.: Sure, what did you want to say?

Pt.: Well, I don't know how to put this, uh, well, I might as well just say it. I really would strongly prefer talking with another woman. I don't feel comfortable talking to a man. You know, I had requested a woman as a therapist.

Clin.: I must have been quite a shock (smiles gently).

Pt.: No kidding! But you, you seem nice and all that, but I really would prefer talking with a woman.

Clin.: Sometimes that can be important. Before we decide what to do, tell me a little bit about what your concerns are about talking with a man, in this case me.

Pt.: Well, there is no way that a man can know what I've been through. A lot of my problems have to do with guys and some of the sexist things they do. Every man I meet seems to want something from me and I resent that. And so, well, I need a woman who will understand, because she has experienced the same things as I have.

Clin.: Hmmm, I see what you mean. First let me state that I agree that I can't know exactly what you are feeling. Only a woman can know exactly what it is like to be a woman. Moreover, even if I was a woman, I couldn't know exactly what you are feeling, because each person's feelings are unique. But in therapy the goal is not for me to know exactly what you are thinking, but to help you to explore your own thoughts and feelings. And I have had considerable experience with people of both sexes who have felt put down and abused. For each person I've worked with, I've learned something, and some of the things I've learned may be helpful to your own understanding.

Pt.: I understand what you're saying and actually it makes sense, but somehow I think I would feel more comfortable with a woman.

Clin.: Well that brings up another important point.

Pt.: What's that?

Clin.: Perhaps you'll miss an opportunity if you avoid a male clinician.

Pt.: In what sense?

Clin.: The very thing you want to learn about is how you react and respond to men. With a male therapist you may have a better chance to see what your natural responses, fears, and expectations are like. Does that make any sense?

Pt.: Yes it does, and I never thought of it that way.

Clin.: I'll tell you what. Let's try to work together and if problems arise I want you to tell me immediately. O.K.?

Pt.: O.K., you got yourself a deal.

In this example the clinician discussed in a matter-of-fact manner the specific resistance voiced by the patient. The resistance was, at that moment, dealt with on a content level. The patient was convinced of the usefulness of at least trying to work with the male clinician. The clinician also tended to move with the patient's resis-

tance by acknowledging that he could not know exactly what she
was feeling. To move against the resistance, with a statement such
as, "Even though I'm a man I think I have a good idea of what
you are feeling," would probably have disengaged the patient. In
response, she might have proceeded to further argue her point.

With the phrase, "I must have been quite a shock" the clinician
utilized humor effectively to break the tension. Well-timed humor
can be very effective in this regard. The clinician also utilized another sound technique, a trial agreement when he said, "Let's try to
work together and if problems arise I want you to tell me immediately. O.K.?" This concept decathected the situation by not forcing
the patient to make an immediate decision.

Perhaps more than the issue of sex, the inexperienced mental
health professional is in fear of questions such as, "Are you a
student?" Most students are naturally sensitive to their lack of
experience. At some level this is an appropriate realization. But a
lack of experience does not imply incompetence. To the contrary, if
the clinician listens carefully, the interview will probably proceed
well, resulting in the collection of a useful database from which to
help the patient. An interview can be very useful without being
perfect. There exists no need for a young clinician to become defensive over such a question. The very act of calmly responding to such
challenges often conveys a reassuring sense of competence to the
anxious patient, as shown in the following:

> **Pt.:** You know, just looking at you, I'm getting a little
> concerned, I mean are you a student or what?
>
> **Clin.:** Yes, I am a student, I'm in my second year of graduate
> training. You look like it is a little unsettling to be
> working with a student. What are some of your
> concerns?
>
> **Pt.:** Oh, I, I, well, I just think that someone with more
> experience might be more able to understand what is
> going on here. I mean this is pretty complicated.
>
> **Clin.:** It certainly seems to be very complicated. And if I were
> you I might also be concerned about my age, but I'll
> tell you what, the most important thing for a clinician
> to do is to listen carefully and with a sensitive ear. And
> that is something that I do well, in fact it is one of the
> main reasons that I entered this field. And I'd like to
> try to help you today. If there are specific problems that
> arise as we go along just let me know. We'll get an idea
> soon enough whether we will work well together or

not. Let's start with why your wife sent you here. Do
you agree with her views on the problem?

Pt.: No. She's got it backwards. I haven't been depressed,
I've been angry and she should know that.

Clin.: And how should she know that?

Pt.: Because she's the one who is causing all the friction,
what with her stupid meddling into my business
affairs. She should know better. I know what I'm
doing, I don't need her 8-foot nose in my way, sniffing
around my office.

In this example the clinician has used both process and content
techniques to move through the resistance. Without appearing defensive the clinician has reassured the patient that the clinician
himself feels confident in a realistic fashion. A sidetracking technique was then utilized to get the conversation moving.

Along these lines, the clinician should feel perfectly safe mentioning the fact that supervision is also going to be utilized. These
statements may actually calm the patient. By way of example, the
clinician may say something like, "Your point is a good one, which
is one of the reasons that we are always closely supervised in our
work. In fact as soon as we are done talking I will be discussing
what we learned with a very talented supervisor, Dr. Jones. We
work well as a team. So let's try to get at least a start in understanding what is going on here. Now what was it your husband said he
didn't like about the way you handled your son?" Once again the
trick is in not becoming defensive. In the last analysis, the enthusiasm and willingness to listen carefully, which is so common in the
young clinician, sometimes counterbalances the lack of experience
that comes with the turf of being a trainee.

Before leaving the topic of challenges to the clinician's competence, another point is worth mentioning. In situations in which
race may be an issue, it is wise to carefully attend to nonverbal as
well as verbal clues that the patient is ill-at-ease. Unlike the woman
above, some patients will not spontaneously bring up their discomfort. But if it is not addressed, the patient may never reappear for a
second appointment. If I feel that a patient of a different race or
culture is looking uncomfortable, I may raise the issue myself in a
gentle fashion with phrases such as, "Mr. Macken, one thing I'm
wondering about is what it's like for you to be working with a
white clinician?" This may bring the covert resistance to the surface
where it can be examined and hopefully worked through.

Many of the above ideas concerning challenges to the clinician's
competence are excellently discussed by Anderson and Stewart, two

family therapists who have carefully examined the entire range of resistance behaviors. Their book stands as an outstanding introduction to the issues of resistance in various aspects of therapy.[2]

Attempts to Gain Personal Information About the Clinician

This type of situation represents a more invasive extension of the issues just discussed. Instead of wanting to know appropriate information about the clinician's background, the patient wants "the scoop" or "low-down" on the clinician. This type of situation can be truly more threatening. Probably because of this threat, clinicians frequently over-react by abruptly going against the resistance with phrases such as, "I'm afraid that is not what is important here, we are here to talk about you, not me." This curt oppositional approach may lead to problems, as shown in the following:

> **Pt.:** Yeah, so I've been out of sorts since I began having this affair, you know how it is, you've had an affair haven't you?
>
> **Clin.:** Mr. Raphael, I fail to see how that is relevant. Let's get back to your problems.
>
> **Pt.:** But it is important, if you haven't had an affair how are you going to know what I'm talking about?
>
> **Clin.:** Well, I guess you'll just have to deal with that, because psychiatrists don't discuss their personal lives with patients.
>
> **Pt.:** I guess that settles that.
>
> **Clin.:** I guess so.

With such an antagonistic exchange, there exists a very good chance that the rest of this interview will be of little consequence. An initial attempt, utilizing a process response, may have been more rewarding, as demonstrated in the following:

> **Pt.:** You've had an affair, haven't you?
>
> **Clin.:** You make it sound like it would be odd if I said I had never had an affair.
>
> **Pt.:** I think that would be sort of odd, I thought all men had affairs at some point or another.
>
> **Clin.:** Do you think that you make a lot of assumptions about what the people around you are thinking, for instance what you think your wife is feeling?

Pt.: That's hard to say. I never really gave it much thought.

Clin.: Suppose for a moment that I told you that I had never had an affair. How would that affect you?

Pt.: Uh, it would make me think that we were pretty different people, and I don't know how comfortable I'd be.

Clin.: So then you feel uncomfortable if someone seems different from you?

Pt.: I suppose that at some level, I do.

Clin.: In what sort of ways?

In this example the clinician has moved around the resistance, and the process questions serve to guide the patient toward self-reflection. But what if the patient were more stubborn? How might one proceed?

Pt.: You've had an affair, haven't you?

Clin.: What makes you ask?

Pt.: That's for me to know and you to guess (patient smiles); you're a doctor, surely you've had an affair?

Clin.: Looks like you're going to keep at it until you get an answer of some sort.

Pt.: That's right.

Clin.: Well, I'll be honest with you. In the past I've found that my sharing of personal information always gets the therapy into trouble. And if you wish, I can go into detail later about how such information hurts the therapy itself. But in any case I won't be supplying those types of answers. On the other hand something has just happened that is of interest. Do you know what it is?

Pt.: No, I don't think so.

Clin.: Well, I was feeling put on the spot by you. And while you did it, you were smiling to yourself, it seemed sort of pleasurable for you. Are there other instances in your life where you purposely put people on the spot?

Pt.: I got to admit, I've been known to do that on occasion. Like, it's just sort of a way to tease, you know what I mean (smiles).

This example illustrates that at times the clinician must set limits. But limit setting is not the immediate response of this clinician, nor his only response. Also of interest is the fact that the reason for the limit was conveyed. The clinician did not merely pass on an authoritative proclamation to the patient.

Patients may make inquiries concerning a broad range of areas, including marriage, dating patterns, sexual activity, children, financial situation, religion, and many others. The clinician must decide what type of information is appropriate to disclose. Clinicians will vary on this issue, but I think that most clinicians would state that in an initial interview little if any background personal information should be disclosed. Many clinicians disclose little personal information even later in therapy. Such self-disclosure opens the clinician up to personal attack and loss of respect from the patient, and also short-circuits the projection of the patient's issues onto the clinician.

Another point is of interest here that can affect the manner in which the clinician chooses to respond to such personal inquiries. The seed resistance represented by such inquiries tends to fall into two different camps. In one camp these personal inquiries represent yet another fear that the clinician will not be able to help. For instance, a patient may ask whether the clinician has children or not. This request may arise from the patient's fear that a childless clinician could not possibly understand. In these instances, as shown before, the clinician will want to help the patient to bring this fear into the open.

But the patient above, who kept pushing the clinician to talk about affairs, represents a different camp. This hounding of the clinician probably represents a characterological display of sorts, like a peacock fanning its plumage. In the case just shown, the patient demonstrated a rather curious pleasure in watching the clinician squirm. Perhaps his mild sadism represents a counter-reaction to some deep-seated core pains, such as feelings of inferiority. The clinician can file this information away, while later stroking the patient, so as to decrease the patient's need to attack. On a more immediate level, these characterological patients may need limits set, while being helped to look at the reasons that limit setting was needed. This type of reflection must be done in a noncritical fashion and without any angry countertransference response. When done well, the patient does not feel confronted. Once again the technique is flexibly matched to the needs of the patient and of the clinician.

Resistance in the Form of Patient Requests

It is not uncommon, during an initial interview, for a patient to make a request of the clinician. These requests can range from innocuous issues such as wanting a glass of water to more extravagant requests such as wanting a date. Once again the key lies in attempting to understand the reasons behind the requests. Does the request for water represent a need to control the interview, a manifestation of oral needs, or simply a thirsty patient? In a similar fashion, is the request for a date a defensive posturing or the workings of a manic process?

If a request is made for a simple physical issue such as a glass of water or a trip to the restroom, it can often be accommodated by the clinician. Unfortunately, especially if repeated, these requests may, if granted, use up valuable and limited clinical time. In such instances, I have found that a simple explanation of the situation will often satisfy the patient. One might say, "Mr. Miller, we've got a little bit of a problem with time. Let's try to go on with the interview without any breaks, because you're bringing up a lot of important information that I need to hear. If you feel later that you must get another drink of water, please mention it again."

Probably a more frequent request, as opposed to asking for an activity or an object, is an attempt to procure an opinion from the clinician on a topic on which the clinician should not be offering his or her two bits.

> **Pt.:** The bottom line of all this remains the fact that I'm a hard-working single mother. Trust me, it isn't easy and my sister thinks that I should also be taking care of my sick father. Now you're a professional, what do you think of that?
>
> **Clin.:** I think that it upsets you a lot. What do you say to your sister when she brings up the topic?
>
> **Pt.:** I tell her to forget it; sometimes, sometimes I, I would just like to belt her!
>
> **Clin.:** What do you do with your anger?
>
> **Pt.:** I let it out, and I've got a right to let it out. She's lucky I just don't burn her house down.

In this example the clinician moves past the resistance by offering an opinion, not on the patient's question, but on what the question signifies about the patient. In essence, this is a variant of sidetracking.

At times patients may be a bit more persistent.

> **Pt.:** Then my mother had to put her two cents in. Nothing new about that. Believe it or not she had my phone

	tapped. Now tell me the truth, she's way out of line, right?
Clin.:	Well she certainly has made you very angry.
Pt.:	No joke! But seriously, don't you think she's way out of bounds?
Clin.:	What would you like me to say?
Pt.:	I don't know . . . agree with me I guess.
Clin.:	I don't think that my agreeing would do that much for you, but have you found much support among your friends or family?
Pt.:	I haven't found much support from anyone at any time. Everyone views me as a loser.

Here the clinician first tried a sidetrack similar to the one just demonstrated, but this time the patient persisted. Then the clinician used a process question that bought some time and resulted in a new line of response. The patient was successfully side-tracked using this new avenue. Flexibility remains critical for success.

Awkward Situations Encountered with Psychotic Patients

There are many unusual situations that can arise for the clinician when dealing with psychotic patients; however, two reappear fairly frequently. Both interactions once again involve patient requests for the clinician's opinion. The first occurs when a delusional patient asks a clinician whether the clinician believes in the patient's delusion. The second potentially awkward moment arises when a psychotic patient asks whether he or she is crazy. The frankness of this question frequently catches interviewers off-guard. Let us begin with the first situation.

It is not unusual for a delusional patient to wonder whether the clinician believes the patient's story. In one sense this represents a healthy attempt by the patient to check with reality. It also places the clinician in a rather unsettling spot. If the clinician goes along with the patient, then the patient is being given a false verification of delusional material. On the other hand, if the clinician flatly disagrees with the patient, then the patient has only one of two conclusions to reach. First, the patient can feel that the clinician believes the patient is lying. Second, the patient can feel that the clinician believes that the patient is "crazy." Needless to say, neither of these perceptions by the patient is likely to increase blending.

In general, I feel that it is seldom appropriate to agree with the patient's delusional system. There may be exceptions, which will be discussed below. To agree with the delusional material is risky business. By way of illustration, if the clinician would agree with a paranoid patient that someone is "out to get me," there is always the risk that the clinician will eventually be included as one of the persecutors in the evolving delusional system. At such a point the clinician, who is now being accused by the patient, cannot suddenly change his opinion, telling the patient that he was kidding earlier. Furthermore, it can make it very difficult for the subsequent treatment team if the patient keeps saying, "But Dr. Blake believed me, why don't you?" Dr. Blake will not be popular with his fellow mental health workers.

To me, the best method of handling such a situation so that one does not antagonize the patient is an honest approach, coupled with a suspended judgment, as illustrated in the following:

> **Pt.:** The entire string of circumstances terrifies me. I am convinced that my husband has been contacted by aliens.

> **Clin.:** And how do you know that?

> **Pt.:** Oh, I've been keeping tabs on him for months. Every night when he comes home he has a funny smell to him. It's the smell of aliens. And, I have seen him sneaking out at night. I believe he is planning to give our boy to the aliens for experimental reasons. Oh you've got to believe me, tell me you believe me and will help me.

> **Clin.:** Mrs. Jason, I'm not at all surprised at your concern. I'll be very honest with you, as I'm sure you are aware, what you are saying is so unusual that it is hard to believe. But I want to learn more. When do you think he made contact with the aliens?

> **Pt.:** I'm not certain, but I think it was at least a month ago. It is also possible that he intends to get rid of me.

> **Clin.:** Have you done anything to protect your son and yourself against him?

> **Pt.:** . . . Yes . . . yes, I have gotten the gun out of the attic. And I bought some new bullets for it; oh I can't believe this is happening.

The approach taken by this clinician has conveyed a feeling of unconditional positive regard, while indicating that the clinician has some doubts about the validity of the story. Despite these doubts, the clinician conveys an active interest in hearing more. This clinician interest frequently appeals to delusional patients, who seldom find anyone who will listen to their story attentively. The clinician caps off the movement through this resistance point by quickly side-tracking the patient with a specific question.

In the initial interview the goal is to build an alliance strong enough that important information will be conveyed to the clinician. To have told this woman that her story makes no sense or as some clinicians phrase it, "I can see that you believe your story, and that's what counts," runs the risk of jeopardizing the tenuous blending so characteristic of paranoia. At an early stage of the interview, there is seldom a need to tell the patient point blank that you do not believe the patient's story.

This excerpt demonstrates the need to continue the interview in an effort to determine the potential dangerousness of the patient. This particular woman has already taken a striking action towards violence. If she reaches a point in which she truly feels that her husband is about to harm her child, a shooting would not be out of the question. If she had felt disbelief from the clinician, this critical material may never have been shared.

In the closing phase of the interview, clinicians can more appropriately bring up their feelings of disbelief in a fashion that is not overly confrontational such as, "Mrs. Jason it is a very frightening story. Once again, I'm going to be very open with you. It's still very difficult to believe, but I realize that it is very real in your opinion. Sometimes, and I'm not necessarily saying that this is the case, but sometimes one's mind can perceive reality in a slightly distorted fashion, for instance when a person clearly sees water in a desert when no water is around. Do you think that this might be the case with you?"

If the delusion is fixed, the patient will probably say something like, "No way, this is not a trick of my mind." With a less fixed delusion the patient may be more open to considering the possibility. But, in any case, by this time the clinician has gathered the critical information needed for triage, while still providing some reality contact for the patient.

Earlier I stated that on rare instances it may be appropriate to go along with the patient's delusion temporarily. This may be the case if the patient is rapidly escalating towards violence and any antagonism from the clinician could set him or her off. I am reminded of a humorous example of this process.

A young and agitated woman about 30 years of age was brought into the emergency room on an involuntary commitment. She was terrified that "the lesbians are all around me. They want to kill me, they want to kill me!" She had already attacked one person, and it was soon clear that she would need admission. Unfortunately, a former male partner of hers had been brought into the emergency room, close to the same time, also on an involuntary commitment. The charge nurse felt that he was "ready to blow." He also happened to be acutely intoxicated. Needless to say the charge nurse thought that it would be a very bad idea for the two patients to meet.

As the fates would have it, the first patient decided that now was the time to escape, and she headed for the door leading to the receiving area, where her past partner was stomping about. Not feeling that it was safe to try to physically stop her by myself, I stood aside. But for whatever it was worth, an idea crossed my mind, and I told her, "I wouldn't go out in that waiting room if I were you, it's packed with women." I don't think her eyes could have gotten much wider. It took her about 2 seconds to run back into the safety of the interviewing room.

The other problem mentioned earlier arises when the patient pointedly asks for a judgment on his or her sanity. Early in an interview a patient may ask, "Look, I need to know, am I nuts?" If the patient has been animatedly discussing a recent lunch with Neptunians, the clinician may have a perverse desire to say something like, "You're not nuts, you're very nuts." Clearly this is totally inappropriate, and it must be locked away in the recesses of the clinician's id. But all humor aside, what can the clinician say?

Probably a variety of techniques are useful. I tend to reframe what the important point is while proceeding with a rapid sidetrack to this new point, as shown in the following:

Pt.: I just don't know what to do. I honestly think I'm losing my mind. Am I crazy?

Clin.: Mr. Bach, I'm not really certain what people mean by that term. And I don't think that's the major issue for us. Rather it is obvious to both of us that you are not feeling yourself, and that's what we need to look at. How long have you been feeling depressed?

Pt.: Oh about 3 or 4 months. I know that, because 4 months ago I visited my son and his family, that's when the trouble began.

The clinician can also tell the patient about misgivings concerning such a term as "nuts" or "crazy." Or the interviewer can utilize a process maneuver by asking the patient questions such as, "Have you been thinking that you are crazy?" or "What exactly have you been worried is happening to you?" Naturally, if the clinician has gathered enough data in order to feel comfortable that the patient is not psychotic, then one can share this opinion with the patient. This simple gesture can be remarkably calming for some nonpsychotic patients, who are dealing with extreme anxiety. For instance, patients with obsessive-compulsive disorder frequently are worried that they are going insane and are often greatly relieved by a clinician's reassurance that this is not the case. Some patients, on the other hand, have not come for an opinion. In fact, they wish that they had not come at all, as the next section illustrates.

Situational Resistance: The Unwilling Patient

There are probably at least three different types of patients who could be considered unwilling: (1) a patient who is self-referred but feels extremely ill at ease, (2) a patient who came only at the insistence of another person, and (3) an involuntary patient on a commitment. The seed resistances may be significantly different with each type, resulting in differing possibilities for resolving the observable resistance of a shut-down interview.

In the first instance, a patient who feels tenuous about the whole idea of seeing a therapist, the seed resistances may be manifold. The patient may have low self-esteem and may consequently be frightened of rejection by the clinician or of being "found out" as a weak person. A fear of the unknown may be actively at work, as the patient imagines all sorts of nasty things that a psychiatrist might do. Frequently, patients are concerned that somehow or other, they will not be in control of what they say, suggesting another possible core pain, the fear of a loss of internal control. The list could go on and on. But the important point remains the fact that there is a reason behind the patient's reticence.

If a patient continues to remain shut-down, despite the use of the many techniques described earlier for opening up such interviews, then the clinician should probably attempt to make the covert resistance overt. In a gentle tone, the clinician may simply say, "Mrs. Ford, I know that it's difficult to talk at first. I'm wondering what some of your concerns are about being here today?" A different tack may be to demonstrate a willingness to help relieve the tension with a statement such as, "Mrs. Ford, it can be hard to talk about personal matters, it certainly is for me. What can I do to make things easier?"

If the clinician obtains a better idea of what the seed resistance is, it can be addressed even more directly. For example, suppose the clinician suspects that the patient is afraid of saying something self-incriminating. The clinician might say, "It's tough to begin talking with a stranger, and it may take time for you to trust me. That's natural, and I don't want you to say anything that you feel uncomfortable with until you're ready."

The above example also brings up the issue of using paradox, in short, telling the patient not to talk, with the hope that this will trigger a desire to continue. When done gently, this technique can be strikingly effective, as was the case with a young man sent by the Army after trying to hang himself. He gave a long history of impulsive behavior and seemed concerned about his tendency for violence. When probed, he began to be resistant, but a gentle paradox quickly resolved the tension.

Pt.: I have had problems with my temper in the past, and I'm afraid of what it all means.

Clin.: What exactly are you afraid of?

Pt.: I've been in some pretty bad fights, uh, I guess that's what bothers me.

Clin.: Have you ever been hurt in one of the fights?

Pt.: Not really, a few stitches here and there, nothing to brag about.

Clin.: What about the other guy, did you ever hurt one of them pretty badly?

Pt.: Yeah, pretty bad, I had a knife on me and it caused some problems.

Clin.: Did you actually knife him?

Pt.: (The patient began moving around in his seat and put his head down.) I, I don't want to talk about it, I don't even want to think about it right now.

Clin.: That's all right. There's no need to go into that right now. It may be of value in the future to talk about it. It might help you to feel a lot better.

Pt.: Yeah, I know that. The funny thing was I didn't really want to hurt him, but when he came at me, I just stuck it in him. I think I might still do the same thing, it really was, uh, self-defense. You see, we was out looking for some action and I was a little drunked up.

In this instance the patient apparently felt a need to talk, although guilt was blocking the way. Paradoxically, when assured he did not have to talk, he proceeded to tell his story in great detail.

Usually the above types of techniques help to resolve the resistance. Just the process of talking about the resistance frequently increases the patient's duration of utterance and gets the ball rolling. Things can be a little more difficult with a patient who is in the office at the request of someone else and who, unlike the Army recruit, does not want help.

Patients may find themselves in a "shrink's office" at the order of their bosses, friends, or family. It is not uncommon for a spouse to threaten divorce unless the patient seeks help. Clearly this is an awkward situation for both the patient and the therapist. To handle it, Herbert Strean provides some excellent guidelines in his book *Resolving Resistances in Psychotherapy.*[3]

He emphasizes several points. These patients, who are essentially psychologically handcuffed, frequently are very angry. They may need a chance to ventilate some of their frustration before proceeding into the body of the interview. They may also view the clinician as somehow "in on it." Consequently, it becomes important to help the patient differentiate between the clinician and the person who pressured the patient to seek help. An open acknowledgment of the situation can help break the logjam, as follows: "Mr. Sanders, it looks like we both feel some tension here. I realize that you don't want to be here, and I respect that. I guess we are both in an awkward position. Let's try to find out if there is anything that you can gain from our talking, and let's leave your wife's desires out of it for a while. Tell me a little more about what your relationship was like at the beginning."

In this fashion the clinician is actually addressing the seed resistance, because the patient is experiencing a loss of external control. With the words, "and let's leave your wife's desires out of it for a while," the clinician has effectively released the handcuffs. The patient is being given a chance to create his own agenda. At the tail end of the statement, the clinician is side-tracking the patient toward an affectively charged topic.

Of course, some patients present with real handcuffs, representing the third category of unwilling patient, those patients who are involuntarily committed. This situation is obviously not ideal for interviewing. One of the keys to successfully navigating it consists of realizing that both the patient and the clinician are uncomfortable. In essence, there is a common enemy, the situation itself. If the patient refuses to talk, it often pays to point out this common enemy, while matter of factly describing the situation more clearly, as depicted in the following:

Pt.: Look we've been talking for 10 minutes and I don't want to talk anymore, period. Got it?

Clin.: Mr. Phillips, I'd be upset if I was in your spot too. In fact, I'm not particularly at ease with this situation to begin with. It's awkward for both of us, but here's the bottom line. I know that you want to get out of here. By law, I'm supposed to determine whether you need to be here or not. If I can't talk with you and get more information, I'll have to act cautiously and consequently continue the commitment, because I can't risk letting you hurt yourself. The only way for me to decide whether you can leave is to talk with you. And I'm not pulling any punches here, I'm not saying that if you talk I'll let you go. I'm just saying that if you don't talk you'll definitely have to stay.

Pt.: Well, what do you want me to talk about?

Clin.: Let's start with your side of the story. What actually happened last night?

Pt.: What happened was that I found out that little innocent Susan wasn't so innocent. She was out getting some action. I loved her and she kicked my face in!

Clin.: Any ideas why she did it?

Pt.: That's what I don't understand, I just don't understand it!

Clin.: What happened after you found out?

In this excerpt the clinician also asks the patient for his opinion on what happened. Most committed patients feel that no one is seeing their side of things. If given an opportunity to tell their story, they often will eagerly accept that opportunity. Of course, all of the previously described principles for resolving resistance are equally applicable to the committed patient as well.

The main point is to avoid a battle for control as instigated by statements like, "You have to talk with me and that's that." With these patients the core resistance is frequently a fear of a loss of external control, which for the most part has been stripped away from them. It is indeed a terrifying feeling. The more that the clinician can offer some semblance of control to the patient, while establishing a common agenda, the more likely that the resistance will settle.

Resistance in the Form of Anger

During the initial interview, anger may arise from a variety of causes. In the patients discussed above, the anger was primarily situational in nature. At other times the anger may stem from character pathology, as seen with the primitive rage of borderline and narcissistic personality disorders. In other instances, the clinician may not find the anger coming from the patient. Instead, the clinician faces the brewing anger of irate family members.

One of the first steps necessary in handling angry patients well has nothing to do with the interview itself. It has to do with the clinician's realization that the patient's anger should not be taken personally. No one likes to have people angry at them, but all clinicians will sooner or later have patients who are inappropriately hostile.

One method of placing the patient's anger in perspective is to view the anger as a reflection of pain. Narcissistic rage is often the end result of intense feelings of inferiority. In a similar light the borderline patient's anger may be an artifact whose roots lie in fears of annihilation or abandonment.

Keeping these ideas in mind, certain principles in handling angry patients (and I am not referring to violent or psychotic patients here) are worth examining in more detail. In the first place, one often needs to offer the angry person a chance to ventilate appropriately. In a curious sense, one could say that the clinician attempts to provide the patient with a safe environment in which to be angry. This safety arises from the fact that the clinician will not counterattack, matching force with force. The interviewer steps out of the way of the patient's anger by not providing opposition. The patient cannot resist if there is nothing to resist against.

The clinician should calmly try to determine what exactly is angering the patient. Patients tend to appreciate an honest effort to sort things out. More important, if the clinician can decipher which seed resistances are driving the rage, then these core pains can be assuaged more directly. Perhaps the key point consists of conveying to the angry patient that the clinician is listening carefully. The interviewer listens to the patient's demands calmly and with fairness. Patients who become progressively angrier almost invariably feel that their needs are being ignored. Such an escalation in hostility can frequently be prevented by attentive listening.

In the following scenario, the father of a girl with anorexia is throwing a fit in the emergency room waiting area. His family has been waiting for about an hour to see the initial interviewer. When the father discovers that the clinician is a psychiatric nurse, the father becomes livid, even though he has been told that a doctor will also see his daughter.

> **Father:** Just what is going on here?! My daughter is not talking with a nurse. We did not drive 100 miles to see a nurse.
>
> **Nurse:** Mr. Landis, I'm sorry that this has caused you to get so angry. That concerns me and I need to find out more about what it is about my seeing your daughter that is so upsetting. By the way, I understand that you've been waiting quite some time. We appreciate

your patience; as you can see, things are very busy here today. I apologize for the delay and will try to move things along for both you and your family. But first, what are your specific concerns about my seeing your daughter?

Father: I don't think that a nurse is qualified to see my daughter. The problem is far too complex. It's nothing personal, we just don't want a nurse.

Nurse: I see. Just to give me a little background, what are some of the main problems that your daughter is having?

Father: She's got this thing called anorexia nervosa, and it's driving us all mad. The last clinician, a psychologist, didn't do beans for her. And the shrink before him didn't have a clue as to what is going on with her. And we heard that Dr. Wilson here is an expert so we set up an intake appointment.

Nurse: I see. Well, it certainly does seem like a complicated problem, and I also see why you were upset when you saw me coming. Clearly you were expecting a physician. And I certainly agree that Annie needs to see a physician. If you could give me just a moment of your time, I'll try to clarify things and once again get things moving so that Annie can see the doctor. The way Dr. Wilson likes to handle all new referrals is through us. He always has a team approach, because he feels that, especially with people who have eating disorders, it is valuable to get several clinicians thinking about the case. I always see the patient first to scout out the information. After I speak with Dr. Wilson he will want to talk with all of you in some detail. Are there any questions so far from any of you?

Father: So she is definitely going to see the doctor?

Nurse: Absolutely, we wouldn't have it any other way. And the sooner that Annie and I get talking the sooner she'll see the doctor.

Father: O.K., let's get rolling then.

Nurse: By the way, while I'm talking with Annie be sure to organize and prepare any questions you may have for the doctor. He'll want to hear them all. It is very important for us to hear your opinions on what is going on. We'll try to make this long trip a worthwhile one for everyone.

Father: Well, it will be if my little girl gets some help.

What could have been a real mess has been resolved gracefully. This clinician earned her pay and then some. By remaining poised and nondefensive, she was able to put her ego aside as she dealt with the bruised ego standing before her. Core pains were quickly addressed, and the clinician gained ground by giving ground. How differently this interview might have gone if the clinician had made content responses such as, "Mr. Landis, you'll have to realize that I am extremely well trained and am more than well qualified to see your daughter" or, "Listen, you're going to have to wait just like everybody else here, I don't care how far you came." Meeting angry statements with more anger is seldom productive.

The clinician also demonstrated several other subtle yet effective techniques. Her opening two statements were as follows, "Mr. Landis, I'm sorry that this has caused you to get so angry. That concerns me and I need to find out more about what it is about my seeing your daughter that is so upsetting." Although a bit convoluted, the statements have personalized the conversation with the use of the word "my." It may be harder for Mr. Landis to be mad at this specific person as opposed to nurses in general. Indeed the desired effect appeared to occur, for Mr. Landis literally made a subsequent point of saying that his concerns were not personal in nature. At this early stage, the resistance had already begun to soften.

Once the clinician realized the father's strong commitment to Dr. Wilson, she took advantage of this fact by aligning herself with the physician. This was accomplished by emphasizing the team approach and by using the word "we." Furthermore, she deflected responsibility for the situational circumstances irritating the father by stating, "The way that Dr. Wilson likes to handle all new referrals is . . ." but of even more significance, she made the father feel important, while listening carefully to both his conscious and unconscious needs. In essence, the clinician does not want to reflect the patient's anger, the clinician wants to absorb it. This process is difficult at times, especially for trainees, but the payoffs are immense.

It seems appropriate to be concluding this chapter by discussing the approach to angry patients, for all of the principles concerning resistance are brought to the forefront in such situations. It also serves to highlight the point, mentioned earlier, that the real goal is not to oppose resistance but to understand it, learn its directions, and move with its tensions. This skill is not always easy to master, but few skills yield more positive rewards.

In putting the final touches to this chapter, dear old Alice comes back to mind. Hopefully our work with patients is a good deal less confusing than Alice's interactions in Wonderland. But who knows? Perhaps even in Wonderland, the principles discussed here would have been of service. It probably would not have taken long to intuit the core pains behind a figure as fragile as Humpty Dumpty. And once Alice understood his needs, perhaps she would not have found herself quite so speechless.

References

1. Brower, D. (ed.): *Of All Things Most Yielding*. San Francisco, Ballantine Books, date of publication unlisted, p. 18.
2. Anderson, C., and Stewart, S.: *Mastering Resistance: A Practical Guide to Family Therapy*. New York, The Guilford Press, 1983, pp. 120–150.
3. Strean, H.: *Resolving Resistances in Psychotherapy*. New York, John Wiley, 1985, pp. 120–148.

SUPERVISION UTILIZING FACILIC ANALYSIS

Helping trainees to understand the nuances of structuring the interview, while actively attending to engagement, represents a challenging task for the supervisor. The concepts of facilic analysis can be graphically employed in a fashion that brings the interview to life for the trainee while presenting an easily understood description of what actually took place. In this Appendix a brief description of this graphic system is presented. It is not meant to fully describe the system but to provide an introduction. This system of "shorthand" can be utilized in direct supervision, class discussion, and videotape supervision.

The system grew out of the observation that modern dancers have developed simple systems of representing their complex movements and choreography. It was felt that the structural choreography of the initial interview may also be amenable to symbolic representation. Two complementary analyses are available. In a longitudinal facilic analysis, the interview and its transition are followed from front to back chronologically. In a cross-sectional facilic analysis, a pie diagram allows the clinician to observe the overall structuring process.

Content regions are depicted as rectangles, with the subject matter abbreviated within the rectangle. The degree of thoroughness in expanding any given content region is depicted by slash marks at the corners of the rectangle. One slash represents 25% of the needed information, two slashes represent 50%, three slashes represent 75%, and four slashes represent a completely expanded region. Process areas such as psychodynamic inquiries are represented by circles. The scouting phase is indicated by a combination of both a rectangle and circle. All transitional gates are depicted as follows:

Spontaneous Gates	∿∿⟶	Introduced Gates	─□─⟶
Natural Gates	⟹	Phantom Gates	─⊠─┤
Referred Gates	----⟶	Manufactured Gates	─○─○⟶
Implied Gates	└↓⟶		

622

With videotape supervision, the supervisor first watches the tape alone and subsequently reviews it with the trainee. When first watching the tape, the supervisor uses the facilic schematic system to note the flow of the interview as well as adding comments concerning any other technical aspects of the interview such as engagement techniques and psychodynamic concerns. The time of the interview in minutes as well as the videotape counter number are noted periodically, allowing the supervisor to quickly turn to illustrative videotape excerpts. The system also provides a permanent outline of the supervision hour, which can be referred to in future sessions of supervision by both the supervisor and trainee. An example of a longitudinal analysis is shown below:

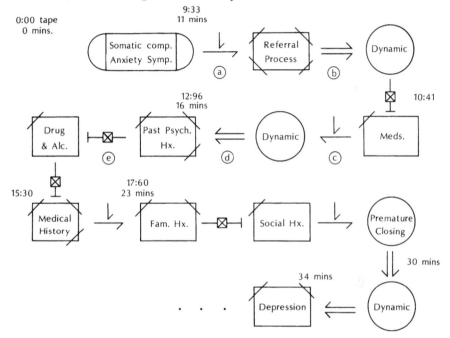

Counter Settings

I. Transitions (Gates)

(a) What made you come to our clinic today?

(b) What were some of your feelings about coming here today?

(c) What role do you think your actions play in some of these problems?

(d) Have you ever seen a psychiatrist before?

(e) Are you a problem drinker?

13:10 *

II. Teaching Points

8:00	1. Scouting phase is appropriately unstructured and free-floating but is too long.
9:50	2. Too much detail and time spent in the referral process region.
10:10 *	3. Good psychodynamic questioning.
10:41 *	4. Decrease use of phantom gates (ask clinician what he was feeling at this point of the interview).
12:96 *	5. Explore use of chronology as a reference framework.
13:00	6. Good use of empathy: "Sounds like the world was caving in on you back then."
14:00 *	7. Use behavioral incidents when delineating the drug and alcohol history. I think this patient was providing invalid information. (Also comment on note taking—too much.)
18:00 *	8. Here's a series of Type A validity errors including multiple questions and negative questions.

The asterisks represent areas of videotape that may be useful to view with the trainee. It can also be seen that this clinician tends to overuse abrupt transitions and to leave content regions prematurely. These errors may result in a weakening of the thoroughness of the database needed in this particular style of intake assessment, in which a complex triage was to be determined and a full diagnostic evaluation was requested. Numerous positive comments were also made in the actual supervision, highlighting the skills of the clinician.

The facilic analysis merely provides a framework for discussion. The actual supervision itself is characterized by spontaneity, humor, and discussions of both dynamic and personal feelings related to the interview. The trainee may request certain areas of the tape to be viewed. Emphasis is also placed on nonverbal interaction.

A second type of facilic analysis, a cross-sectional view, provides an illuminating view of the actual use of time in the interview. Thirty minutes of a cross-sectional analysis are shown on the following page.

In the videotape supervision, a record is also kept of the types of questions asked (e.g., swing questions, open-ended questions, statements of empathy), as used in the opening 15 minutes.

These facilic schematics help to make concrete and manageable some of the interviewing skills that appear nebulous and confusing at first glance. From this common framework of understanding between the supervisor and the trainee, the possibility of actual changes in interviewer behavior arises, leading to both improved skills and a renewed fascination with the interview process itself.

APPENDIX II

ANNOTATED INTERVIEW (FULL 60-MINUTE INTAKE)

Annotation: Mr. Whitman (fictitious name) was referred to me by his outpatient therapist, as part of an outpatient Veterans' Administration (VA) Program. He was an aging man, growing weary with life, particularly upset with VA doctors and administrators over a long-standing disability battle. His therapist informed me that Mr. Whitman had very little desire to see me, probably projecting that I would be just one more "pain in the butt." His therapist commented, "I think you'll like him once you get to know him (pause), that is, if he gives you the chance."

Mr. Whitman had thinning white hair. As he entered my office he avoided all eye contact and said nothing upon my greeting. He moved with an agitated quickness to his chair. As he sat down he leaned forward, crossing his hands over his knees, his feet wiggling nervously.

Dr. Shea: Well, we can go ahead and get started. Do you like to be called Mr. Whitman or Gary?

Patient: Gary. *(No eye contact)*

Dr. Shea: Okay, Gary, let me tell you just a little bit about what we will be doing today, and of course the main thing we are hoping to do is to help you. My name is Dr. Shea, and I am the psychiatrist who works with Phil, whom you have met, and he will be your therapist. I'll be doing a pretty thorough assessment to try to figure out if any type of medication might be of value, or if you are on medication, what we think of that. I also help with trying to decide what types of talking therapies would be most helpful. We always try to fit our work to your needs, because we find that it is the best way to help people. I won't be your therapist. Phil will actually be the person doing the therapy with you.

Our meeting today is probably about 50 to 60

minutes in length. What I am going to try to do is to understand what kinds of stresses and symptoms you are feeling and your perspective of what is working and not working. I also take background information about your family, stresses, and things that you are doing and medical history because sometimes our bodies really can influence what is going on mentally for us. At the end, I will share with you some of my thoughts and we will brainstorm a little bit about how we might be able to help. How does that sound?

Patient: *(nods, no eye contact, still no spontaneous speech)*

Dr. Shea: I want to thank you beforehand for allowing us to videotape. This will be used to help other professionals to be better clinicians and sensitive listeners. So, why don't we start Gary with your telling me a little bit about what brought you in to see Phil and what kinds of things you are dealing with. *(Variant of a Gentle Command, see page 82, Chapter 2)*

Annotation: We have already seen one of the reasons why I chose this interview as my illustration. It wasn't easy. As we have discussed in Chapter 10, Mr. Whitman is displaying some of the nonverbal characteristics of confrontative resistance. At the time, I didn't know whether or not Mr. Whitman would actually display some anger or just be "hard to talk with." Of course it is also possible that we are seeing the early warning signs of a shut-down interview.

As with any scouting phase, the single most important immediate goal was to engage Mr. Whitman. Specifically, I would need to develop a strategy for somehow transforming Mr. Whitman's hesitancy and resistance to seeing me. Right from the beginning the clinician, myself in this instance, was met with the need to focus on the most critical task of the initial interview, to ensure that the patient would return for a second appointment. At present, the patient can barely tolerate sitting still for the first one.

Patient: I have been depressed for quite a while.

Dr. Shea: Okay.

Patient: My kids don't like to listen to nothing. *(pause)* They're off in Arizona.

Dr. Shea: Far away. *(Empathic Statement, see page 85, Chapter 2)*

Patient: We don't see them. We don't hear from them. I don't know where they are. What they are doing. If they are alive or what. We finally heard from them after a year, and it makes you think they don't give a damn about us. You know . . . we write to them. We send them stamps. We do this, we do that for them. They can't write back, and they can't do nothing. Then I tried to get a service connection because I got banged up while I was in the service . . .

Dr. Shea: Okay.

Patient: Like a fool I didn't go into it right off, and now I am having a hard time with that. Everything is just *(pause)* nothing's working, nothing's working for me.

Dr. Shea: Okay.

Annotation: At this point I am just trying to let Mr. Whitman talk. What is interesting is the relatively large amount of talking he is doing. Despite his initial hesitancy, some part of Mr. Whitman obviously wants to talk. He has chosen early on to raise his problems with his kids and with his disability issues. These topics will prove to be core concerns for Mr. Whitman.

Clearly, we are not heading for a shut-down interview. Perhaps we can capitalize on Mr. Whitman's anger and his need to ventilate. Unlike most interviews, in which the clinician heavily emphasizes open-ended techniques during the scouting phase, in this type of interview it frequently pays to funnel the patient towards his or her affective charge. The hope is that once the patient has allowed the clinician into his or her world—a world perceived by the patient as unfair—the clinician will be able to ally with the patient with counterprojective statements *(see page 539, Chapter 9)* and empathic statements, thus transforming the patient's resistance towards the clinician. This "threading" of the patient towards his or her anger is often best accomplished with closed-ended questions and statements of inquiry *(see page 84, Chapter 2)*, some of which will double as counterprojective statements. It's a bit of a gamble, but let's see how it works. If it starts to fail, we can always move back into a more typical reliance on unstructured, open-ended techniques that are more typical of a scouting phase. The key is flexibility.

Also note the cognitive "overgeneralization" and "blackening," which are so common to depressive thinking and are illustrated by Mr. Whitman's comments, ". . . nothing's working, nothing's working for me." Although not apparent at this point, we will discover later that some of Mr. Whitman's comments about his children are also tainted by the destructive cognitive distortion of overgeneralization.

> **Patient:** Like I told Phil *(Mr. Whitman's therapist),* I said way back years ago I was ready to quit. I was ready to put myself out. When he asked me about that I didn't think about it. I was thinking about it the other night. I said it's so easy to just drive a car into a tree and say, "Heh, the hell with it." Let the world take care of itself. Everybody else will take care of them. A couple months ago I was going over the edge. I left the house in a huff, and I don't know why.
>
> **Dr. Shea:** Okay.
>
> **Patient:** Yeh. On the way home I went through the whole thing and actually, I don't know . . . but I was there. That was it, and on the way home, I almost put it off the road. I had that feeling I was all ready to go. I floored the car and I was just waiting to take the wheel.

Annotation: To my surprise, suicide has been spontaneously brought up very early in the scouting phase, hinting at the immense amount of pain that Mr. Whitman is experiencing. This is not the type of man who goes around blithely telling people he is suicidal in a bid to get sympathy. Mr. Whitman is a "tough bug" who normally keeps things close to his chest.

This is an important window in the engagement process, but it is also a window potentially fraught with problems. Mr. Whitman is opening up, but is he opening up too early, necessitating a later retreat into his normal stance of keenly guarded privacy? More specifically, should the interviewer further open the window onto suicidal ideation now, when the engagement is in its birth, or defer to a later point, when the engagement may be a good deal more mature? From nonverbal cues, I intuitively felt that Mr. Whitman seemed almost embarrassed by his "admission" to suicidal ideation, so I decided to wait. My goal was to somehow make Mr. Whitman feel more safe with me, perhaps with some empathic statements and a movement towards a topic that he would feel more comfortable discussing at this early stage of the interview.

Dr. Shea: So you have been in a lot of pain now for months. *(Empathic Statement)* That was several months ago? *(Statement of Inquiry)*

Patient: Yes. Nothing seems to get better. I got a good wife. Wonderful wife.

Dr. Shea: Was that who I just met out there? *(Closed-ended Question)*

Patient: Yes.

Dr. Shea: She seemed very nice. *(An attempt at joining with Mr. Whitman)*

Patient: She is going through hell. She's got diabetes and everything else. Between that, my kids, and all of this stuff building up, I just can't go anywhere. These headaches are . . . I've had all kinds of treatments and everything else. *(Second time that Mr. Whitman has spontaneously brought up his disability issues secondary to headaches)*

Dr. Shea: Just nothing under the sun is helping at all. *(This statement is a variant of a counterprojection)* You look like . . .

Patient: They give me Motrin and stuff like that. If I took it like I should, I'd be eating them like candy.

Dr. Shea: They want you to eat a lot of . . ., *(This is the beginning of a counterprojection, but Mr. Whitman cuts me off again, which is not necessarily a bad sign. I actually think that he is cutting me off because he is so intent on ventilating his frustration. Notice that there is no anger being shown towards me. Our strategy may be paying off. We are being brought into Mr. Whitman's world. As with most scouting phases, there is no structuring occurring into diagnostic regions, and so forth, other than an effort to stay in topics that Mr. Whitman, himself, wants to talk about.)*

Patient: He said take them when it gets bad. Well I wait until I just can't take it any more, then I take them. I lied.

Dr. Shea: Do you think they are migraine headaches or . . .

Patient: No, I blame it on the service.

Dr. Shea: Okay.

Patient: Back when I was in the service, I got hurt three times. I got hit three times in the head. Four years of service and when I came out of the service I was having the headaches. So I went to the doctor and asked him about it and he said well, your blood pressure is up. He said blood pressure will do that.

Dr. Shea: Causes headaches.

Patient: So, I said okay and let it go that way. All this time the headaches kept coming and coming, and I kept taking the blood pressure medicine like the doctor said.

Dr. Shea: So you have been having headaches for decades?

Patient: Yes, and I didn't push it. That's where I made the mistake. Because I was stupid and didn't say well maybe I should go do something.

Dr. Shea: For benefits or something?

Patient: I went to another doctor. He told me the same thing. I went to three different doctors. So I said well they must know what they are talking about. So I took aspirin and stuff like that and then when I got up to Veterans Health, I talked to Dr. Canton and he said no. It can't be your blood pressure. So . . .

Dr. Shea: So you are seeing Dr. Canton now about this?

Patient: Yes.

Dr. Shea: So he is trying to investigate this? (*I've used a series of closed-ended questions and statements of inquiry to keep threading Mr. Whitman into this rich arena for ventilation and joining.*)

Patient: Yes.

Dr. Shea: Well I hope they can sort it out.

Patient: I have had all different kinds of medications and everything else.

Annotation: At first glance this might look like the right time to carefully expand the region of medications. But we are still in the scouting phase, and there is no need for structuring just yet. I would prefer shoring up my alliance with Mr. Whitman first, as shown by the use of an empathic statement.

Dr. Shea: Sounds like you have been going through a rough time.

Patient: I went for a hearing on the disability. And I been wanting to get service connected so that if anything happens I can take care of her. We can save some money to go to the commissary and things like that. I think I am entitled to it because I got banged up. I've got a record . . . *(Mr. Whitman pulls out a piece of paper and starts to look at it.)*

Dr. Shea: Can you show me that? *(Clinician begins to read.)*

Patient: The thing right there is that I wrote out what happened. I got looking at the hearing thing the other night and when I read that I got so mad . . . if that man had been there, I think I would have punched him out, because the hearing papers are wrong.

Dr. Shea: So it's just like nobody is really in your corner here on this thing.

Annotation: Here is another example of a counterprojection. I'm trying to do everything I can to get Mr. Whitman to view me as an ally, who is here to help him. Perhaps my most effective engagement strategy was the effort I made to read his letter. Although this action is time consuming, I believe it paid off very well.

By the frequent raising of his headaches, Mr. Whitman has made it plain that the headaches are a major framework for meaning for him at present. It is a topic that he feels physicians have ignored. So as not to be unconsciously clumped with the "bad guy" physicians, I go out of my way to show an interest, even to the point of taking the time to read the letter. Notice that this entire opportunity for significantly enhancing engagement might have been lost if I had prematurely shortened the scouting phase by exploring medications earlier.

Patient: I got the DAV, what the hell, and the hearing, to me, was a joke.

Dr. Shea: Yeh. Well, I'm struck by the . . . *(Clinician is pointing down into the letter)* steel cover coming

down and hitting you on the neck, that's the
problem. It could have really done something bad.

Patient: It hit me on the head. I got hit right across here,
and there was a scar there. There was a steel
handle that weighs about 5 or 6 lb. That knocked
me down and split me open. I got back up and
went on, and it wasn't even my job. (*In a healthy
way, Mr. Whitman prides himself on a committed work
ethic.*)

Dr. Shea: There are 24 stitches there. You are sort of a tough
guy aren't you? I mean you just keep on going.

Annotation: Here is my response to "Sullivan's Question," directly
addressing his work ethic and past history of psychological strength and grit.
I felt that one of the major blocks to powerful engagement for Mr. Whitman
was the fact that he felt uncomfortable asking for help in the first place
because, in his mind, such an action, combined with his admission regarding
suicidal ideation, might make him appear weak. I believe that the one thing
he most wanted to hear from me, which might increase his sense of safety
(answer to Sullivan's question), would be something that told him that I was
not seeing him as weak. From his subsequent response to my comment, one
gets the feeling that this intervention was "on the mark."

Patient: I mean, I have to keep going. I can't, I raised six
kids and I worked every day. I never missed a day.
I took all the hours I could work. I worked and
worked and worked and it didn't make any
difference. I went to work days, when I thought I
was going to die, but I thought I gotta feed my
family and . . . all this . . . gets to me. (*Tears are
welling up, and his voice is wavering*)

Dr. Shea: Yeh, I bet it does.

Patient: I mean I've done everything I can do to take care
of my family. Now I want somebody to help me
and I can't get it.

Dr. Shea: Yeh, you look like you are almost close to tears.
(*An example of an "observational gate," used to enter
his painful affect. At this point Mr. Whitman began to
cry. His tears, ironically, show us that our interview
strategy has been a success. Instead of anger, which
easily could have been projected onto yet another*

"uncaring doctor," we are seeing pain. Mr. Whitman has opened the door to his world, and it is unlikely that we will be ushered out, unless we make a subsequent engagement error of some sort.)

Patient: It gets you upset . . .

Dr. Shea: Yeh, I bet you're hurt. Putting all those years of helping and, now, you are just looking for help. Let me get you a Kleenex. By the way, would it be alright if I could put a copy of this in my chart later, after this, because I think it is important. *(Good cementing of the alliance by continuing to emphasize a sincere interest in Mr. Whitman's headaches through actions not just words)* Well, you are really going through a lot.

Patient: . . . crying like a baby. *(Looks and sounds like he feels a bit embarrassed)*

Dr. Shea: No, no, no. This is just natural, all of us cry. Trust me. I've cried. You know all that means is, sort of, our souls are telling us that we are in pain. That's all that is. It's like getting a temperature when you are sick. But you have just about had it, huh?

Patient: Yeh.

Annotation: It seemed important to once again reassure Mr. Whitman that his opening up of his emotions was "O.K." I also decided it was time to end the scouting phase, and I will next move into the History of the Present Illness via his recent medication history.

The main task of the scouting phase has been accomplished—the active engagement of Mr. Whitman. Not only is he no longer wary, but also he has actually become fairly open. I think that he senses the presence of a potential ally. For the first time an element of "hope" may be stirring in this, our first encounter.

The upcoming switch of topics will also give Mr. Whitman a chance to distance himself from his pain for just a bit, because I sensed he needed a break. As you will see, the transition here is somewhat awkward and abrupt. Frankly, a natural gate into the topic of depression probably would have been a smoother and more conversational transition, but I didn't see it.

A second potential problem for this interview, which actually transformed into a real problem later on, is worth mentioning here—length. This scouting phase was almost 10 minutes in length as opposed to a more typical 5 to 7 minutes. Because of the complicated nature of Mr. Whitman's early resistance,

I believe that this amount of time was warranted, indeed, it was probably necessary to ensure his return.

The problem is that, as the interview proceeded, I would need to consciously eliminate some of my standard data gathering in order to keep this interview within 60 minutes. As you shall soon see, I will subsequently forget to do this winnowing and hence will run overtime. In any case, let's watch the movement out of the scouting phase.

Dr. Shea: Yeh. Okay. Now, have you been getting some care, have you had a lot of psychiatric care, I mean have they been using medications?

Patient: No, No I just got it. I tried to get it before and . . . it never worked out. And finally Rachel helped me to get it. And I've been on it now since about the first time I come down. I went to a stress clinic.

Dr. Shea: Okay.

Patient: And it relaxed me but it didn't do any good. Well I can't say it didn't do any good. It had to have done some good.

Dr. Shea: Helped calm you down. A little bit of a Band-Aid compared with how much pain you are in. I'll tell you what I would like to do now, Gary. *(Beginning of an "introduced gate," see page 729.)* I would like to get a better handle on what this depression is like, because it is a unique thing for each person. The better I understand it, the better I might be able to figure out how we can help. When do you think that you first started to become depressed, just roughly?

Patient: Well I probably have been for a long time, but basically the worst part hit me now with all of this stuff coming together, then I try this and there is nothing there and . . .

Dr. Shea: When did it start getting worse for you? It might be hard to remember. Let me ask this question, were you depressed at Christmas time? *(Holidays can function as good time frames for pinning down the earliest onset of symptoms.)*

Patient: I didn't have a Christmas to speak of.

Dr. Shea: Okay. Were you depressed at that period of time though?

Patient: Yeh, because I didn't see my kids.

Dr. Shea: Okay and were you depressed at Thanksgiving?

Patient: I mean, I had some kids in Massachusetts that I go and see . . . *(Patient is starting to pivot out of the region of depression here. See Chapter 2, page 114 for a discussion of "pivot points.")*

Dr. Shea: Okay.

Patient: And my other kids I can see, but these kids I can't see.

Dr. Shea: The ones out in Arizona.

Patient: Right.

Dr. Shea: Okay now what about Thanksgiving . . . had the depression started by then? *(Good focusing! It would have been very easy to let Mr. Whitman start to ramble on about his relationship with his kids here.)*

Patient: It's been going on for I don't know how long.

Dr. Shea: Years?

Patient: I see my youngest son once a year *(still starting to wander off the topic of depression itself)*. Of course he calls and everything. He uses the telephone. I see him up here in Chester every year so . . . he calls us and lets us know.

Dr. Shea: Has it been going on for a year at least? *(Good, simple focusing question. We will come back to the role of his children later, perhaps using a well-timed referred gate.)*

Patient: Oh yeh.

Dr. Shea: Okay. Has it been going on for several years?

Patient: *(nods)*

Dr. Shea: Okay. When did it start to get the worst for you? *(By the way, you are seeing an interviewing habit that I'm trying to get rid of in my style—of saying "okay" too frequently. These are meant to be facilitory statements but are probably best replaced with a simple head nod or "Uh-huh." Done too frequently, as I am* *demonstrating, they may sound almost like a cut-off of some sort. Believe it or not, I had almost eliminated this habit from my interviewing style and was rather shocked to see its return in this transcript. One must always keep an eye out for one's bad habits.)*

Patient: Maybe 2 years ago.

Dr. Shea: Two years ago the depression really started to worsen?

Patient: Right, and I decided I was going to . . . 2 maybe 3 years ago . . . and I decided that I had to do something. I got to try . . .

Dr. Shea: So you began having depressed feelings almost 3 years ago? That's a long time. Okay.

Patient: I sit there some nights and I can't sleep. I get up, *(pause)* I just get up and want to get in the car and go somewhere or do something. *(pause)* I can't sleep. *(pause)* I went out and bought a computer figuring that would take my mind off of everything. You know?

Dr. Shea: Okay. Now your depressed symptoms, like your sleeplessness and things like that, have they reached a point now where they are basically with you all the time, day in and day out? And did that start a year ago, 2 years ago? *(This is a cannon question, see page 45, Chapter 1, and may be confusing to the patient. Which question is he to answer? It is better to phrase them as two separate questions and wait for the answer to each question before going on.)*

Patient: I started getting ticked off at everything.

Dr. Shea: But did the symptoms start to be persistent like that as long as a year or two ago? Or is that new?

Patient: About a year ago.

Dr. Shea: About a year ago. Now those . . .

Patient: Now a year ago, I can't sit still.

Dr. Shea: Wound up. You look sort of "wound-up" even as we are talking. That is a very common aspect of depression—that "wound-up" feeling. That is something I can help you with I think. It can be a

real relief if we can get rid of that feeling.
*(Instilling some hope, while acknowledging the
importance of a symptom that is quite disturbing to Mr.
Whitman.)* Now, your depressed symptoms, as I
said, they are different for different people Gary,
and what I am going to do is ask some questions
hoping just to understand what yours look like.
Over the past couple of months, I am going to
focus on that time. You mentioned that your sleep
is off. How long does it take you to fall asleep
usually?

Annotation: I'm looking for evidence of a difficulty in falling asleep.
Also note that I have provided a very simple, but important, explanation for
the reasoning behind my focusing. By sharing this reasoning with the patient,
it allows the patient to "team up" with the clinician on the task of structuring,
as opposed to "fighting it." There are very good reasons for structuring
effectively that will directly help the patient. It makes sense to let the patient
know about them.

Patient: I may fall asleep within an hour, but I'm back up.

Dr. Shea: How many times do you wake up on a given
night? *(looking for a sleep continuity disturbance)*

Patient: I'm up about five or six times a night.

Dr. Shea: Okay. Now when you get up is it hard to fall back
asleep? Do you ever find, Gary, that at say 4 or 5
o'clock you wake up and find yourself worrying
about things and you can't get back to sleep, is
that common? And do you find that this . . .
(looking for early morning awakening)

Patient: Crazy, crazy things in my mind.

Dr. Shea: Such as? *(Well-timed use of an open-ended question,
which also functions as a Behavioral Incident, opening
the door for a better glimpse, phenomenologically, of
what Mr. Whitman is experiencing.)*

Patient: I wake up and think about what is going on for I
don't know . . . it's hard to pick anything . . .

Dr. Shea: Describe one for me . . . what are some of the
thoughts that go through your mind? *(an open-
ended Behavioral Incident)*

Patient: Nothing . . . I think a lot about the kids. *(Once again his relationship with his children seems to be an area of significant pain. Notice that even while delineating specific DSM-IV criteria, important interpersonal and psychodynamic issues will arise that can be re-explored later in the interview when time permits. These same issues may provide immediate tips for engagement or areas for important exploration in subsequent sessions of psychotherapy.)*

Dr. Shea: Okay . . . out there in Arizona? That seems like that is a very painful thing for you. *(Example of a simple but effective empathic statement)*

Patient: Yes, my two grandchildren.

Dr. Shea: Are they way out there?

Patient: *(nods)*

Dr. Shea: Yeh that's tough too. Um, . . . *(some of Leston Haven's empathic grunting, see Chapter 1, page 26)*

Patient: And I know they are going through trouble too because we talked to them about 2 months ago, that's the first time we have heard from them in a year. Maybe 3 months ago . . . we haven't heard from 'em since. She called and they were working and the guy gave her a hard time. I don't know whether the kids went back to their house . . . that's all he would tell us.

Dr. Shea: That sounds like lots of stress there as well, and I know you would like to be helping with that but we want to focus on you for awhile because we are going to try and get you some help right now. You mentioned that . . . your sleep sounds terrible to me. Do you find that your energy is shot during the day? You just don't have the energy? *(Nice focusing statement, simultaneously acknowledging the patient's desire to help his children, while gently guiding him to remain in the expansion of the major depression region)*

Patient: I don't have any anyway. I have respiratory problems. *(Here is another pivot point leading out of the region of depression, but we'll not "bite on it." Instead we'll stay within the region of depression, until we are done exploring it. We'll come back to Mr.*

*Whitman's respiratory problems, when we explore the
Medical History, perhaps using a referred gate. Note
that Mr. Whitman spontaneously changes topics
frequently. Without a careful and sustained attention to
structuring principles, this interview could rapidly
become a classic example of a "wandering interview"
with many errors of omission, see page 90, Chapter 2.)*

Dr. Shea: Okay but do you find that, overall, the past couple
of months your energy is lower than you would
like?

Patient: Yeh.

Dr. Shea: Do you find your concentration is worse?

Patient: I can't, I can't *(pause)*. That is why I set down to do
something on the computer and I play a game or
something just to take my mind off it *(pause)* and
I'll do it for 10 or 15 minutes and I'll shut it off.

Dr. Shea: Do you notice memory problems?

Patient: I sit there watching t.v., and I'll either doze off or
I'll just be looking around. *(Mr. Whitman
demonstrates looking around with his head.)* And,
what the hell did I miss?

Dr. Shea: Right.

Patient: You know.

Dr. Shea: Do you find also that your memory is problematic
for you at all? *(nods agreement)* And how about
your appetite, how has that been affected?

Patient: Up and down.

Dr. Shea: Any weight gain or loss there?

Patient: I had lost weight and back up and back down . . .

Dr. Shea: What about your interests in things? It sounds like
it is hard to pay attention. Do you find that you
are not as interested in things as you used to be,
don't enjoy things? *(In the above segment of the
interview I am continuing to gather diagnostic material
related to the neurovegetative symptoms of depression as
per the DSM-IV.)*

Patient: I'm not enjoying things with my wife like I used

Patient: to. She's the head of the Senior Center, so I go with her every Wednesday to that.

Dr. Shea: What is that like when you are there?

Patient: It used to be a lot of fun. I used to "raise cain" and everything else, and we would go up and Janet and I would set the tables and everything to help her, and I would sit around. I mean, if somebody said something to me, I would talk to them and everything.

Dr. Shea: Is it an effort to talk to people?

Patient: I don't care if you bother me or if you don't bother me any more. *(Said with a demoralized tone of voice)*

Dr. Shea: Okay.

Patient: Then we got a room and a half complex. It's driving me nuts.

Dr. Shea: Okay.

Patient: She has been on my wife's case ever since we moved into the place. And . . .

Dr. Shea: What's she . . .

Patient: *(referring to his landlady)* She is a first-class *(pauses, looks a bit sheepish)* whatever.

Dr. Shea: Problem? *(offering an out)*

Patient: Yeh *(said with emphasis)*.

Dr. Shea: I want to go back for a moment once again to further understand the depression. Your concentration is off. You are not enjoying things. You are not finding that life, like at the Senior Center, that you are not enjoying that as much. *(Note that I'm doing several things here. Once again Mr. Whitman is pivoting out of the depression region, and I am keeping him on track. There will be time to discuss his neighbor later in the Social History. From my earlier explanation, as to why I am structuring, Mr. Whitman seems to understand the reasoning for such structuring and seems quite comfortable with it.*

    The "repeating of the symptoms elicited thus far" serves to check to make sure they are accurate, while also serving to remind me what I've covered, triggering in my mind which criteria remain to be explored.)

Are you finding that there is a change in your sexual drive, that you've lost interest in sex or any other change?

Patient: There's no change.

Dr. Shea: Okay. And what about tearfulness. Are you finding that you feel like crying frequently?

Patient: Some days yes. Some days no.

Dr. Shea: Okay. Would you say that you're crying weekly?

Patient: Yeh . . . once in a while. Sometimes I'll set there and tears will come . . .

Dr. Shea: Is weekly too frequently, or am I overestimating that, or is it at least weekly?

Patient: Yeh.

Dr. Shea: Every 2 weeks?

Patient: Every 2 weeks I'll catch myself.

Annotation: This has been a nice example of the expansion of the DSM-IV diagnostic region of depression. I have attempted to persistently, yet sensitively, help Mr. Whitman to stay focused upon the symptoms of depression, while continuing to foster engagement. In this regard Mr. Whitman appears to have a major depression by DSM-IV criteria. It is time to move on.

Dr. Shea: And you mentioned that you had had some suicidal thoughts. Are you having any suicidal thoughts in the past couple weeks? *(Here is a referred gate into suicidal ideation. As opposed to the early segment of the interview, when Mr. Whitman had first raised suicidal ideation, he is now much better engaged, enhancing the likelihood of valid reporting. He is talking openly about his pain. This seems an opportune time to explore suicidal ideation using the CASE Approach as delineated in Chapter 8.)*

Patient: No.

Dr. Shea: Okay. But in the past you had the one you had described. The driving . . .

Patient: I might have been close. Close on the edge a couple of times but . . .

Dr. Shea: Once again, even over the past couple of weeks any thoughts whatsoever about killing yourself? *(Just double checking)*

Patient: No.

Dr. Shea: Good. But in the past, you said that was a couple of months ago you had the thought about driving the car off the road? *(Entering the region of recent ideation over the past 2 months)*

Patient: I don't know. Like I told Phil *(his therapist)*, I don't know what triggered it.

Dr. Shea: Okay.

Patient: I just . . . I went to the sea this summer, and I came home and got ready to go to the lodge, and was coming down the road headed for the lodge. All of a sudden I just thought about it on the way up. And it hounded me. And I thought about it all the way home. Once I got into Greenfield I was alright.

Dr. Shea: Good. Had you been thinking . . .

Patient: I was close. I was real close.

Dr. Shea: Did you pull off the road? *(Behavioral Incident)*

Patient: I went to go to the edge of the road and, if I had, no one would have found me until the wee hours of the morning.

Dr. Shea: Okay so it was an isolated place? *(Behavioral Incident)*

Patient: I was cranking pretty good.

Dr. Shea: Now had you been thinking about doing that for days or weeks or was this something that came on really rapidly? *(Behavioral Incident. Trying to gauge the degree of premeditation versus impulsivity)*

Patient: It just came . . . it just came on that night and I have no idea in the world.

Dr. Shea: Maybe Phil can help you to sort that out?

Patient: I told him I said I have no idea. I don't remember anything going . . .

Dr. Shea: Particularly bad. *(Empathic Statement)*

Patient: Bad. Just that I came down and I just *(pause)* had that feeling that I wanted to hurt myself.

Dr. Shea: Yeh. It sounds like it was pretty intense. *(Empathic Statement)*

Patient: Here I am all the way up 91. I was handling the wheel and I kept thinking about how easy . . . how easy it would be just to say, "Heh nobody gives . . . any more. The hell with it."

Dr. Shea: Now, Gary, at that time, okay, around that time, what other ways were you thinking about killing yourself, besides driving off the road? *(Gentle Assumption)*

Patient: That was the only thing I was thinking about.

Dr. Shea: Well, did you have any fleeting thoughts of say shooting yourself?

Patient: No.

Dr. Shea: Hanging yourself? *(Mr. Whitman nods "no")* Jumping in front of traffic? *(Nods no)* Jumping off of a building? *(Nods no)* Overdosing? *(Nods no)* Carbon monoxide? *(Nods no. Notice that this is the use of the validity technique of "Denial of the Specific," see page 400, Chapter 7, as per the CASE Approach.)*

Patient: No.

Dr. Shea: So literally the only thought at that time was this impulsive thought about that? *(Behavioral Incident)*

Patient: Yeh.

Dr. Shea: Over the past 3 months, okay, how many times have you thought about killing yourself?

Patient: That once. Serious.

Dr. Shea: Okay. What other ones?

Patient: I guess that is about it. *(Mr. Whitman looks a bit evasive here.)*

Dr. Shea: Well you look like there are a couple in there . . . other thoughts of killing yourself, somehow?

Patient: Well one night I was uptight about something that I had said . . .

Dr. Shea: What did you say?

Patient: I don't know if that had anything to do with it. *(Mr. Whitman doesn't seem to want to share this information, perhaps it was something he feels was mean to his wife. I decided to try again at the specific suicidal ideation.)*

Dr. Shea: What ways were . . . *(Behavioral Incident)*

Patient: Just teed off. I jumped all over her.

Dr. Shea: When was this? *(Behavioral Incident)*

Patient: About a week or so ago. *(Notice that earlier, he had denied any suicidal ideation in the past 2 weeks whatsoever.)*

Dr. Shea: Okay. And did you have some thoughts about killing yourself then? *(Behavioral Incident)*

Patient: I don't even remember. *(Defense mechanisms such as suppression or repression may be kicking in. There is something about this memory that is bothering Mr. Whitman.)*

Dr. Shea: Did you say something to her like I'm going to kill myself or . . . *(Behavioral Incident)*

Patient: No.

Dr. Shea: You thought about this for a minute when I was asking about suicide. What was triggering that? What was the connection between that incident when you got a little angry and suicide? *(Behavioral Incident)*

Patient: I don't know. I . . . it's hard for me to say whether I did or whether I didn't.

Dr. Shea: Are you suspicious that you might have had some thoughts of killing yourself? *(Behavioral Incident)*

Patient: I don't remember. I mean some of these couple of nights here over the past 2 or 3 months.

Dr. Shea: Rough.

Patient: Any other thing we'd huddle together.

Dr. Shea: That's obvious.

Patient: But I do . . . when I get teed off at her I jump all over her. She doesn't deserve it.

Annotation: It's looking more and more like "guilt" is the culprit here. But whatever it is, the recall of the incident and subsequent possible suicidal ideation, or even a gesture, seems to be lost. Notice the power of the CASE Approach to "kick up" hidden suicidal ideation. Although Mr. Whitman's description of this area is quite vague, it suggested the need to speak directly with Mr. Whitman's wife, if he agreed, to see if there may have been some suicidal ideation or behaviors in the past week.

At this point, we are at risk of losing some of our hard-earned engagement with Mr. Whitman. The art will consist of giving him some breathing space from the guilt-producing topic, while providing some psychoeducation related to how depression can stimulate irritability. Part of the goal is to show Mr. Whitman that treatment can help with this unwanted symptom. Even some chit-chat may help give Mr. Whitman some breathing room. Once this is achieved, the trick will be to gracefully finish the CASE assessment, because the CASE regions of past suicidal events and immediate suicidal events remain to be explored.

Dr. Shea: Yeh, you know, sometimes, Gary, I have helped a lot of people with depression and a lot of people were your age. But it doesn't matter whether they are your age, younger, very young, even kids who get depressed, irritability and anger is just a common part of the depression. Frequently people say things they don't mean and wish they had never said. And if we can get this depression under control for you, that is going to go away. I have a feeling that the anger is not "you," but that the anger is something that is being brought on by the depression. Any other times . . .

Patient: I've always been the type of person that was active. I was in the Little League. I was into everything. And I kept busy . . . *(Mr. Whitman is taking the gate to quickly move to an unrelated and less distressing topic.)*

Dr. Shea: Did you coach Little League?

Patient: Yeh. I had a team. All kinds of stuff like that, and I don't do it any more.

Dr. Shea: Yes, well, that's part of the depression too, Gary. I want to focus just a little bit on the severity of your symptoms. I want to make sure I really understand the depth of the suicidal thought. Okay? It sounds to me like you had the real urge the one night, and then again a couple weeks ago during an angry fit, somewhere around there, you might have had some suicidal thoughts. Once again, other than that, what suicidal thoughts have you had in the past say 3 months? *(Gentle Assumption)*

Patient: None.

Dr. Shea: Larry, what about in the past? *(I am now moving into the third region of the CASE assessment, dealing with suicidal ideation and attempts from the more distant past.)*

Patient: The only bad thing is the woman I told you next door. Her and my wife, she called my wife names and everything else. We're going through it with the Housing Association. But here, a week or so ago, she kicked my wife. *(This is a pivot point out of the suicide assessment. The area seems to be emotionally charged for Mr. Whitman and this may be one of the exceptions in which the clinician chooses to follow the pivot into a different area, well aware that the current area, suicide assessment in this case, is incomplete and will necessitate the clinician to return to it.)*

Dr. Shea: Geeze.

Patient: My wife handled it like a trooper. She came in and told me . . .

Dr. Shea: You were ready to throttle her.

Patient: I would kill that woman. I was ready to get up out of that chair and I started towards the door. And I said to myself, "What am I doing?"

Dr. Shea: Glad that your wife was there. *(Mr. Whitman nods agreement.)*

Patient: I said to my wife, "What the hell am I doing?" I could kill her. I just turned around and went back and sat down.

Dr. Shea: Are you having any thoughts about hurting that person now? *(I chose to follow the pivot point with a spontaneous gate into violence assessment.)*

Patient: No. And she's the type of person that I used to help her bring in her groceries up and everything.

Dr. Shea: It's a strange story isn't it?

Patient: Down the stairs. Up the stairs. My wife's in bad shape. She can't walk. And yet she hates my wife. She hates both of us. And I used to do so much.

Dr. Shea: To help her?

Patient: To help her.

Dr. Shea: Does that remind you of any other situation you are in right now?

Annotation: This is a natural gate into a "psychodynamic process region." It's the first time we have seen such a region in this interview. The goal was to ask Mr. Whitman a question that requires him to use his "observing ego." The degree with which he can demonstrate a reasonably robust "observing ego" may provide tips as to how well he will do with a short-term therapy model. It also highlights the importance of the use of psychodynamically oriented questioning, during an initial diagnostic interview, when used judiciously. I still have tucked in the back of my mind that I need to return to the suicide assessment region.

Patient: Nope.

Dr. Shea: Let me ask you again. Think about it. You used to help this person a lot, and now she's not there for you. Does that remind you of any other situation?

Patient: Yeh, the kids. *(Not bad! Mr. Whitman seems to have a reasonably good observing ego.)*

Dr. Shea: Sort of similar isn't it? I imagine that is part of the problem. It's once again someone not being there. Now, Gary, I want to focus again, once again, because I am really trying to understand the depression and that's how I figure I can help with the medicines, have you had any past suicidal . . . ? *Mr. Whitman is coughing)* What's going on there? Are you alright?

Patient: Yeh.

Dr. Shea: Have you had any suicide attempts in the past? *(Nice return to the region in an unobtrusive fashion)*

Patient: I don't think so. *(Generally, if a patient responds to questions about suicidal ideation with an "I don't think so," it is worth pursuing with a simple follow-up such as, "Well, how about any suicidal thoughts at all in the past, even if very brief in nature?" Unfortunately, I don't do this here, and I proceed instead to the region of immediate ideation.)*

Dr. Shea: Gary, right now are you planning on killing yourself?

Patient: No. *(Said quickly, naturally, and with good eye contact)*

Dr. Shea: Gary, can you promise me that if you get suicidal thoughts you'd tell Phil, myself, or the crisis team, 24 hours a day? Promise?

Patient: Promise.

Dr. Shea: Can you shake? It's important? We've got to keep you here, because I think you are a very good person just knowing you this short time. We can get you some help. So 24 hours a day you can call our crisis team. The number is 657–2700. Here you go. Let me write that down for you actually. *(Clinician writes down number and then hands it to Mr. Whitman. Besides ensuring that Mr. Whitman has the number in case of a crisis, this piece of paper, with my handwriting on it, can function almost like a simple transitional object for Mr. Whitman.)* Phil can tell you more about them. They are a great group. That's 24 hours a day. They are supposed to be up at 3:00 A.M., so don't hesitate to call. Hopefully you won't need them though. Gary, you know one of the things . . .

Patient: My wife doesn't know anything about this.

Dr. Shea: About what?

Patient: Suicide. *(I believe this is Mr. Whitman's way of raising concerns of confidentiality, while also indirectly looking*

*for some advice on what to do about his own secrecy.
Rather than address the confidentiality directly, an
approach that would have been a fine strategy as well, I
will opt to address the importance of his opening
communication with his wife about his suicidal
ideation.)*

Dr. Shea: Suicidal stuff. Okay. But she does know about the depression?

Patient: Oh yeh.

Dr. Shea: I would urge you to share at some point with her, maybe after you talk with Phil a little bit later today. Because sometimes it's been so bad for you, that you have had some suicidal thoughts, and it would help you if you could talk to her about them if they come. And then she can say things like, you know, "Are you okay?" and "You can let me know if things are getting tough." When you talk about suicidal thoughts, they are not nearly as dangerous as when you hold them into yourself. By the way, many, many, many people, who have depressions, have suicidal thoughts and just because you have them doesn't mean you have to act on them. So there is a huge difference from having the thoughts to planning them out, to practicing the plan, to actually doing it. You can get help, and we can help with every single step. So the more you can talk about it freely with Phil, we'll be able to help. Now, I have a feeling you're not going to get those again but we'll see. Okay? If we do, we'll deal with them.

Patient: Okay.

Annotation: Mr. Whitman's affect was the calmest of the entire session at this point, and he seemed genuinely relieved. Except for a little weakness in the region of past suicidal events, the CASE approach has been followed pretty nicely, accomplishing its dual goals of a comprehensive and valid database concerning suicidal ideation, while simultaneously improving engagement.

A natural gate will now be used to enter the diagnostic region of bipolar disorder. This is an area that is easily forgotten by clinicians, because it is so easy to get "caught up" in the gestalt of the patient's vivid presentation of his or her depressive symptoms, forgetting that hypomanic or manic symptoms could have been powerful players in the past.

Dr. Shea: This might seem a little strange, Gary, but sometimes people, who tell me they are as depressed as you've been feeling, unexpectedly have the exact opposite feeling. *(Here is an example of Normalization, one of the validity techniques from Chapter 7, see page 402).* It's like a light switch goes off and suddenly they feel very happy, excited, laughing, like giggling. Filled with a love of life. Do you ever have anything like that? It's like a switch.

Patient: Well, sometimes when we go out riding or something, I'm listening to the radio or something, I'm singing or whistling to the radio like I'm in another world.

Dr. Shea: That sounds normal to me. This would be unusual. This is almost like bizarrely being happy and wound up. If you'd had it, you would probably have a feel for it. Do you ever have periods of time where you just stay up at night all the time because you're happy and have tremendous energy, and you're loving the night?

Patient: No.

Dr. Shea: Has anyone ever told you that you had a thing called manic episode in the past or anything like that?

Patient: No.

Dr. Shea: I'm wondering if you have had any other psychiatric history or treatment. Have you ever been hospitalized, for instance, with psychiatric problems? *(This is a natural gate into the region of "past psychiatric history," cueing directly off the exploration of mania.)*

Patient: No.

Dr. Shea: Have you ever had a depression before?

Patient: No.

Dr. Shea: What about psychotherapy? Counseling? Ever been on a psychiatric medication before?

Patient: No.

Dr. Shea: So absolutely no psychiatric history? That must be part of the reason this is so startling to you. It just must seem so odd and out of place for you.

Patient: It all happens . . . it's all bunched together.

Dr. Shea: Yes.

Patient: It's like getting hit with a big ball, and what do I do with it?

Dr. Shea: Yes. Well we're going to talk a little bit about that. What to do with that. Was it like one of those big exercise balls . . . have you ever seen them? They are like huge and heavy, and they bowl people over. That's what depression feels like. Some people tell me it's like a very heavy blackness that settles down over them, and they can't shake it. It is a terrible disease and I think . . . I'll tell you more about how we can help you with it later.

Now, you haven't had any of the manic things. One of the things sometimes people will tell me, Gary, is that they will have periods of time where out of the clear blue sky they are intensely frightened. *(Normalization)* I mean it's literally like someone is putting a gun to their heads and their hearts are racing. They are short of breath and panic stricken. Have you ever had something like that? *(Using an implied gate, I performed a screen for panic disorder.)*

Patient: No.

Dr. Shea: Good. Another thing is sometimes when people are really depressed *(Normalization)* they get so agitated that they start to get worries about strange things like there are germs on their hands, they keep washing their hands repeatedly. Ever have anything like that? *(Another implied gate, moving into a good screening question for obsessive-compulsive disorder [OCD], one of the most frequently missed diagnoses by mental health professionals, despite having a lifetime prevalence rate of close to 2%. Patients very seldom spontaneously describe OCD symptoms, because they are so embarrassing. Instead, patients present complaining of the secondary problems caused by OCD,*

such as serious marital conflict, problems keeping up
with work, or feeling overwhelmed or depressed.
Consequently, an OCD screen should be a routine part
of any initial assessment.)

Patient: No.

Dr. Shea: Another thing is they keep having to check on
things, so they might check on a light switch, 23
times in a row, even though they know it has been
turned off. They keep checking and checking,
anything like that?

Patient: No.

Dr. Shea: Earlier we were talking about the tremendous pain
of your depression. Sometimes people will tell me
that their pain will get so intense, with their
depression, that their thoughts sound almost like
voices to them. Have you ever had anything like
that? *(Referred gate into an exploration of psychosis.*
This is often done with a natural gate directly after a
patient has been describing his or her pain, which is
even more naturalistic and nondisengaging, but the
referred gate worked out good enough here. Also notice
the use of the validity technique of "normalization," yet
again, demonstrated by the words, "sometimes people
tell me that the pain will get so intense . . .", to soften
the entrance into the potentially disengaging region of
psychotic phenomena.)

Patient: No.

Dr. Shea: Hallucinations?

Patient: No.

Dr. Shea: These are all good. You don't want to be having
any of these things. *(Clinician smiles)* Another thing
that happens during depression is people start to
get paranoid. *(Normalization)* People are out to get
them. Have you had anything like that?

Patient: *(Mr. Whitman laughs.)* Well . . . just the regular
old . . . regular things on the road. It almost looks
like everywhere we go somebody pulls out in front
of us. We almost got it twice coming up. *(Note that*
the area of psychosis has been entered so smoothly,
cueing off his pain and using normalization, that Mr.

Whitman's engagement has remained very high. By the way, I remain surprised at how frequently this foray into psychotic symptoms, in people who show absolutely no signs of psychotic process in the interview itself, produces unexpected histories of micropsychotic episodes, offering critical hints that more primitive personality structures, such as borderline personality disorder, need to be looked for.

I will proceed to use a spontaneous gate to move into a pure engagement region in an effort to further establish our growing bond.)

Dr. Shea: I've had similar experiences.

Patient: I told her I said it's getting so it isn't safe to drive anymore.

Dr. Shea: I think people tend to be worse drivers. I don't know what it is.

Patient: I thought it was bad, the time we were in Florida.

Dr. Shea: Have you ever been to New Jersey?

Patient: *(Mr. Whitman laughs.)* Yes.

Dr. Shea: I have to be careful about saying New Jersey. I'll get into trouble. *(Clinician laughs and then jokingly comments)* No, I don't think that is paranoia or anything like that.

Patient: *(Following up on the humor, Mr. Whitman continues the "reversed position" role as interviewer.)* It's an everyday thing huh? *(Without any training whatsoever, he demonstrates a nice example of a gentle assumption.)*

Dr. Shea: Yes. *(Clinician chuckles and then moves on. This brief "engagement region" has seemed to go very well indeed. What a change from the beginning of the interview, in which Mr. Whitman sat guardedly, to this point in the interview, where he is comfortably joking. The major goal of the interview, to ensure a powerful enough rapport that the patient wants to return, has probably already been accomplished.)*

Of course another thing, Gary, that sometimes people will do, we're talking about the paranoia and the pain of the depression at times, is people, to get rid of the pain, they will drink. Do you drink alcohol much? *(Implied gate, bordering on an awkward phantom gate, see page 126, Chapter 2, that seems to work okay because of the use of the validity technique of normalization once again.)*

Patient: I haven't had a drink or a cigarette in over 20 years.

Dr. Shea: Wow, congratulations! That's fantastic. Did you use to drink much?

Patient: Yeh.

Dr. Shea: What was your drinking like in the past?

Patient: I was almost an alcoholic.

Dr. Shea: Okay, tell me a little bit about that. *(Nice example of the open-ended technique of the "gentle command.")*

Patient: On the weekends especially. I could go through a case of beer during the week and in 2 or 3 days I'd get another case of beer and then I'd get another case of beer and on the weekends I'd get two cases of beer, three cases of beer . . . whatever.

Dr. Shea: So two to three cases of beer a weekend? So you were putting it away.

Patient: Yeh. I was putting it away. I would sit there with two cans of beer . . .

Dr. Shea: In each hand?

Patient: At a time, sitting there watching t.v., finish one so I didn't have to get up . . .

Dr. Shea: You were loaded.

Patient: Yeh.

Dr. Shea: Do you mind if I take just a few notes on our . . . it helps me. *(Clinician picks up clipboard.)*

Patient: Okay.

Dr. Shea: So when was it that you were drinking that heavily?

Patient: It's hard for me . . .

Dr. Shea: 30s, 40s?

Patient: It's been um . . . around 20 or 30 years back.

Dr. Shea: How old are you now?

Patient: 63.

Dr. Shea: So in your 20s and 30s?

Patient: Yeh.

Dr. Shea: How long did that last that you drank that much?

Patient: It was like when the kids were young.

Dr. Shea: And you haven't drank for almost 20 years right?

Patient: Yeh.

Dr. Shea: That's wonderful.

Patient: And I quit dead turkey. Just like I did smoking.

Dr. Shea: Wow. Well, one thing is, that it really shows you the strength you have. We are going to try to pull that strength forward to help you with this depression. *(Natural gate into a crisis intervention process region of reminding the patient of past mastery and episodes of handling stress or crisis well.)*

Once again, the drinking was in your 20s and 30s, and you said it was two to three cases per weekend and you were also drinking daily right?

Patient: Yeh.

Dr. Shea: How much were you drinking daily . . . a case? *(Validity technique of "symptom amplification," see page 399)*

Patient: I could go through a six-pack Saturday night.

Dr. Shea: Could you put a case down . . .

Patient: A case every couple of days.

Dr. Shea: Okay. Did you have blackouts back then? What I mean by that is that you wouldn't remember stretches of time while you were drinking. Then when you were done drinking, you'd think well I don't remember what I did at 10:00 last night. I blacked out.

Patient: Once in a while.

Dr. Shea: More than 10 of those?

Patient: I can't remember.

Dr. Shea: Must be having one now, huh? *(Clinician smiles)*

Patient: *(Mr. Whitman laughing)* . . . yeh.

Dr. Shea: Well you had a couple of blackouts you don't remember. Did you find that you were drinking in the morning, sometimes when you would first wake up?

Patient: If I remember right, I didn't touch one in the morning.

Dr. Shea: Okay. Did you ever drink alone at night?

Patient: Too hung over.

Dr. Shea: Well, sometimes when people get up they will drink to get rid of that hangover. Did you ever do that? *(Normalization followed by a Behavioral Incident)*

Patient: No.

Dr. Shea: Do you remember ever drinking in the middle of the night sometimes alone? *(Behavioral Incident)*

Patient: I did most of my drinking at home. I might get up in the middle of the night and have a beer.

Dr. Shea: Okay.

Patient: Something like that.

Dr. Shea: Did you use to have guilty feelings about your drinking?

Patient: No.

Dr. Shea: No. Did you try to cut back . . .?

Patient: I enjoyed it, and I just *(pause)* well, it was just like drinking soda.

Dr. Shea: Yeh, well, yeh, two sodas at once. *(said jokingly)* Did anybody tell you you had a drinking problem? *(Behavioral Incident)*

Patient: No. I had a *(pause)* I'd just come home, and we were going out, we were bowling and everything *(pause)* when I was bowling I'd come home drunk all the time. And I just said to my wife one time, "I'm not going to touch another drink."

Dr. Shea: And you didn't since then?

Patient:	And she says, "I don't believe it." I says, "Well you watch me."
Dr. Shea:	That is remarkable. A remarkable sign of strength. *(Reminding Mr. Whitman of past mastery.)*
Patient:	And I said I don't need this. I said the kids don't need it. You don't need the aggravation that I give you and the crap I put you through. I said "I'm not going to drink any more."
Dr. Shea:	And you stopped the drinking and the smoking . . .
Patient:	People would say, "Come on. We're going out to have a drink," and I said, "Well, I'll go but I ain't drinking."
Dr. Shea:	That's great and you didn't.
Patient:	I didn't. I'd go in the bar with them. Same thing when I quit smoking—they told me the same thing.

Annotation: This has been a nice example of a thorough inquiry into Mr. Whitman's drinking history. It certainly confirms a history consistent with alcoholism in the past, but it's not an example of particularly good interviewing in this particular assessment. The problem is "time management" or, better put, "lack of time management."

Because I had to spend extra time earlier in the scouting phase, appropriately well spent, upon engaging Mr. Whitman, I have lost time concerning data gathering. At this point in the interview, I need to be making some tough decisions about what standard material to leave unexplored in the initial 60 minutes. I won't be able to get it all. From the high level of engagement, I realize that Mr. Whitman will most likely return, consequently this should allow me to defer some less critical data gathering to the second appointment.

In this regard, just one or maybe two clarifying questions on his past drinking would have been sufficient. Keep in mind, it would be different if he was currently drinking, but he is not. With this approach, I could still have emphasized his strength, as witnessed by his recovery process. But most of this past history probably should have been left for future interviewing. I've wasted almost 5 minutes in taking an overly detailed past drinking history. In an interview in which one has already spent an extra 5 minutes to transform resistance, this additional 5 minutes could prove to be costly. With regard to accomplishing the intake in 60 minutes, at this rate of data gathering, I will run the risk of running considerably overtime.

Dr. Shea: You know once again, Gary, that is a sign of real strength, and you are going to pull on that strength. It is going to help you with this. *(Continuing to remind Mr. Whitman of his strengths)*

Patient: I had it, but I don't think I have it any more.

Dr. Shea: Well, depression will sap that feeling for you. And what we're going to do is to get you some reinforcements, because as I explained, your depression, I think, has some real strong biological roots to it. Not just psychological. I told you that stress would be playing a role, and it does. But I think there is a biological depression going on for you as well. The history I'm taking, by the way you've done a great job explaining what's happening *(further indirect stroking of his competence, doing everything I can to bolster his inner reserves)*, you really have hallmarks of a biological depression. I'm going to talk a little bit more about that. The good news about that is that this is something we can help you with. Okay.

Speaking of your health and the biology of your depression, earlier you mentioned migraines and headaches that you think are secondary to the injuries. When did you get those injuries again? *(Referred Gate into Medical History)*

Patient: Service.

Dr. Shea: It was in the service, *(pause)* was that the Navy?

Patient: Yes, in the service, in the Navy.

Dr. Shea: There were three different head blows?

Patient: Yes.

Dr. Shea: Were you knocked out at all?

Patient: Yes.

Dr. Shea: How many times?

Patient: Twice.

Dr. Shea: Okay. And one of them required 24 stitches? I remember that from the sheet that you showed me. And your headaches began then?

Patient: Yes.

Dr. Shea: Have you ever had a seizure?

Patient: No. I had the headaches and I just, you know, what do you say, "Hey, you get rapped in the head, you're gonna have headaches, you're bound to have headaches." I just didn't . . . I just let it go and . . .

Dr. Shea: *(There was no good reason for cutting Mr. Whitman off here. I should have let him finish his thought. Maybe I was feeling some "time pressure.")* Do you know if you lost any memory from the blows to your head?

Patient: No.

Dr. Shea: Okay. So you have had headaches, terrible headaches for years since then?

Patient: Yeh.

Dr. Shea: Okay. Do you have any other medical problem? You mentioned something a little earlier about breathing or something? *(Back to the respiratory problems that Mr. Whitman had mentioned earlier, via a referred gate)*

Patient: I have upper respiratory stuff, which isn't too bad right now.

Dr. Shea: What is it? Emphysema?

Patient: I don't know. All I know is that they classed it as upper respiratory.

Dr. Shea: Upper respiratory breathing problems?

Patient: Yes.

Dr. Shea: Okay. Do you get recurrent infections?

Patient: I haven't had much since I *(pause)* I had pneumonia 3 years in a row.

Dr. Shea: Okay.

Patient: And I almost died.

Dr. Shea: When was this?

Patient: Oh boy!? *(Mr. Whitman shows some light-hearted* *consternation at how hard it would be to remember the date.)*

Dr. Shea: Well was it within 10 years?

Patient: Yup.

Dr. Shea: Within the last 5 years?

Patient: I don't think in the last 5 years.

Dr. Shea: So about 5 to 10 years ago?

Patient: Somewhere in that area.

Dr. Shea: Sounds nasty.

Patient: Yeh, and they put me on medication. I'm on . . . now I take the pneumonia shot. I go and get a flu shot every year. And *(Mr. Whitman knocks on his left armrest)* you knock on wood.

Dr. Shea: Are you on any medications right now?

Patient: Yep.

Dr. Shea: What are you on?

Patient: The breathing .   . I gotta to get another . . .

Dr. Shea: So you are supposed to be taking a breathing medication . . . is it something you spray?

Patient: Yeh. I had ventro something . . .

Dr. Shea: Say that again?

Patient: Ven . . . ventri . . .

Dr. Shea: Ventolin?

Patient: Yeh.

Dr. Shea: Okay.

Patient: But it wasn't doing much, so next time I go up there, I'm gonna ask for something else. I still get winded if I go too fast or I try to hurry.

Dr. Shea: Do you have any other medicines that you are on?

Patient: Like when I come in today and I come up the stairs I sit there and I'm pooped.

Dr. Shea: Okay. *(Looks like he may want some more sympathy on this point, but the engagement is very good and time is* *tight so I opt to move on.)* Any other medications right now that you are on?

Patient: Not for that. I'm on blood pressure medicine.

Dr. Shea: Okay what blood pressure medicine?

Patient: Nifedipine.

Dr. Shea: Nifedipine. Okay. Anything else? Do you know the dosage of that?

Patient: 60 mg?

Dr. Shea: Could you at some point check on the doses and just let us know? Any other medications?

Patient: And I'm on hydrochlorothiazide.

Dr. Shea: Okay and what is the dose on that?

Patient: 25 mg . . . wait a minute it's got to be 50 because it's 25 on each one.

Dr. Shea: So it's one twice a day?

Patient: Yeh, this is a double dose.

Dr. Shea: Okay.

Patient: I think it's one a day. I can let you know.

Dr. Shea: Okay, check on that one too. So you think it might be around 50 mg?

Patient: Yeh.

Dr. Shea: Anything else?

Patient: Piroxicam.

Dr. Shea: Could you spell that?

Patient: P I R O X I C A M.

Dr. Shea: I'm not familiar with that. What is that?

Patient: That's a painkiller.

Dr. Shea: That's for the headaches?

Patient: Headaches and the degenerative arthritis.

Dr. Shea: Okay. Where is your degenerative arthritis?

Patient: In my legs.

Dr. Shea: And how frequently do you take the painkillers?

(Didn't follow the pivot point out of "medication history" into "past medical history." Good move. This is helping to keep Mr. Whitman on track, providing an efficiently flowing interview.)

Patient: One a day. All three of them are one a day. First thing in the morning.

Dr. Shea: And you are supposed to take the Piroxicam every day? Do you take your medication exactly as it is prescribed?

Patient: Yes.

Dr. Shea: Okay, are you on any other medicines?

Patient: Just the Motrin whenever I need them.

Dr. Shea: That is for the headaches. You're not on an antidepressant?

Patient: No.

Dr. Shea: Who is your regular physician? *(Implied gate into medical history)*

Patient: Dr. Canton. Dr. Richard Canton.

Dr. Shea: Where is he based?

Patient: The VA.

Dr. Shea: I'm associated with the VICC program, as is Phil. Any other doctors?

Patient: He's the basic one.

Dr. Shea: And are you allergic to anything?

Patient: No.

Dr. Shea: You mentioned the shortness of breath you get when you are exerting yourself. Do you get any chest pain or anything like that? *(Referred gate into a review of medical systems. Nice type of gate that is not only smooth but conveys careful listening upon the part of the interviewer.)*

Patient: No. Well . . . . I shouldn't say no. Once in a while but nothing bad.

Dr. Shea: Okay and if you have any problems . . . any chest pains . . . when you say "nothing bad" what do you mean?

Patient: I do have a heart murmur. That is something I just learned about.

Dr. Shea: Have you ever talked to your doctor about the chest pain, talked to Dr. Canton?

Patient: A little. We talked about all this.

Dr. Shea: They didn't think that it is a heart attack or anything like that? *(Here is an example of a "negative statement of inquiry," see page 45, one of the most invalid of interview techniques. Moral: Do as I say, not as I do. I think I might have been feeling the heat of time running out and unconsciously hoping there were no significant heart problems, because this could complicate his care. In any case avoid such phrasing, because it is quite leading in nature.)*

Patient: Nope.

Dr. Shea: Have you had an ECG recently? *(Good follow-up question)*

Patient: Yes.

Dr. Shea: When was that?

Patient: Last year.

Dr. Shea: Oh good. And have you ever had your heart functioning tested?

Patient: To be truthful I've had so many things I don't know.

Dr. Shea: Okay. We'll check on that. Do you have any problems getting lightheaded? *(pause)* Dizziness? *(pause)* Constipation? *(pause)* Diarrhea? *(pause)* Shakes or tremors? *(pause)* Any problems with blurred vision? *(Note that these symptoms are typical side effects of some of the more common antidepressants. Consequently, I am trying to get a good baseline on whether or not they are present for Mr. Whitman before starting him on any medications. In this regard, it is often wise to make sure one includes basic side effects as part of the routine medical review of systems.)*

Patient: Yes.

Dr. Shea: Okay, what goes on with the blurred vision?

Patient: Lots of times when I'm driving it's like my eyes close and then they come back.

Dr. Shea: Okay. That's what it feels like.

Patient: Yea, lose sight, and then it comes back.

Dr. Shea: Both eyes?

Patient: Yeh. I went and had my eyes tested, and they told me "there is nothing the matter with your eyes." And I asked them nice like "if there is nothing the matter with my eyes how come I can't see?"

Dr. Shea: How long does that last?

Patient: Snap. Just like that. I'll be watching t.v. or something and then blur. It will go right . . .

Dr. Shea: Have you been tested for things like glaucoma?

Patient: Yeh.

Dr. Shea: And that's negative? *(Mr. Whitman shakes his head)* Have you ever had times when you will lose just part of the vision in one of your eyes—or is it always both eyes?

Patient: Most of the time it is both eyes.

Dr. Shea: Okay. Do you have anything else that looks like you are suddenly losing your ability to function? Your hands, legs, you suddenly get weak?

Patient: Well I have carpal tunnel in my hands.

Dr. Shea: Okay. Do you ever lose sensation or the ability to move the hand or anything like that?

Patient: No. They just don't know.

Dr. Shea: Okay. *(After trying to ferret out the eye symptom, I'm going to continue the review of medical systems. Note that, perhaps because of his age, Mr. Whitman has a fairly long medical history. In most patients, these medical regions can be completed more quickly.)* Do you have any trouble with nausea, vomiting, or anything like that? *(pause)* Any problems with passing your water? *(pause)* Getting your stream started? *(pause)* You mentioned that you do have some arthritis in your legs, any other joint problems?

Patient: No. (*I'll now use an implied gate into "past medical history."*)

Dr. Shea: Do you have any history of venereal diseases? (*pause*) Syphilis? (*pause*) Anything like that? (*pause*) Gonorrhea? (*pause*) Any other infectious diseases? (*pause*) Rheumatoid arthritis?

Patient: I had polio in 1948.

Dr. Shea: Wow, that's a serious illness, but it looks like it didn't leave you with anything . . .

Patient: Nope.

Dr. Shea: You're very, very fortunate.

Patient: Yeh. That's the old fashion . . . that's before they came out with all the medicines and stuff.

Dr. Shea: Now you had mentioned earlier that you have always been a strong person. And it looks from your history that you have actually been pretty healthy except for these headaches and things. How about other people in your family—do they have any medical problems that are significant? (*Sort of an odd combination of a referred gate and a natural gate into "family history." The transition could have been accomplished a lot more easily by just using a natural gate. For instance, I could have simply asked, "How about other people in your family, do any of them have serious illnesses, such as polio or heart disease?"*)

Patient: My dad's got cancer now, but he is 86 years old.

Dr. Shea: Now is your mother still alive?

Patient: Yeh.

Dr. Shea: How many brothers and sisters? (*I'm starting to drift off of the topic of "family history" into the "social history," for no good reason. Let's hope that I return to "family history" later in the interview, because it has been poorly expanded here.*)

Patient: One sister.

Dr. Shea: Who is the oldest?

Patient: Me.

Dr. Shea: How old is she? Roughly.

Patient: I'll say 55.

Dr. Shea: Wow she is much younger. You're what . . . 63 you said?

Patient: Yep.

Dr. Shea: How many children do you have? You mentioned six.

Patient: Six.

Dr. Shea: How many boys? How many girls?

Patient: Five boys and one girl.

Dr. Shea: And now you mentioned that two of them live in this area, is that right?

Patient: My daughter lives here in Pittsburgh.

Dr. Shea: Okay and one of your sons.

Patient: And my son, I have three sons that live in Philadelphia.

Dr. Shea: And then two . . .

Patient: One son in California. And one in Snowflake, Arizona.

Dr. Shea: I noticed, when you began talking, you kept emphasizing that your children don't contact you . . . you know, I was sort of fantasizing almost that you had several children living in Arizona. You were focusing on that earlier. Is there a reason for that?

Patient: Well, he is the one that I worry about the most.

Dr. Shea: Okay.

Patient: Him and Elma and the kids.

Dr. Shea: Are you having contact with your son in California? *(Behavioral Incident)*

Patient: Yeh, yeh. We have a lot of contact.

Dr. Shea: Really. So the son in Arizona is the one out of contact with you? Do your other children spend time with you? *(Behavioral Incident)*

| **Patient:** | Oh yeh. Yeh. I'm up to my daughter's, here in Pittsburgh, quite often. In fact, we just took Josh for the weekend. |

Annotation: Here is a fascinating bit of interviewing. This information sounds so different from what Mr. Whitman spontaneously discussed earlier in the interview, at which time, he seemed to be implying that his children pay little attention to him. Mr. Whitman presented this situation as a major area of pain for him—one of the main reasons why he was depressed. The use of behavioral incidents has uncovered a very different situation.

My guess is that we are seeing the power of his depression to paint the world with disturbing overgeneralizations that can further create depressive mood (see Chapter 5). In a sense the behavioral incident, while being used to simply uncover valid information, is playing a therapeutic role here, allowing Mr. Whitman to uncover a more valid and less depressing world view. By clearing away some of the distorting biases of the depression, the interview is functioning almost like a mini-session of cognitive therapy.

In this regard, it would have been a nice touch if I had said something like, "Oh, that's good news. So in reality most of your children are staying in close contact with you, which is a really nice thing." Such a simple clarifying statement could function to further cement the more accurate, and less depressogenic, world view uncovered by the use of the behavioral incidents. This is a nice example of the point made earlier that the initial interview, although not a session of therapy, should be therapeutic.

Dr. Shea:	How many grandchildren do you have? Probably too many to count! *(Smiles and laughs)*
Patient:	*(Patient smiles warmly)* One, two, three, four, five, six. Six. Wait . . . two . . . five. Five.
Dr. Shea:	By the way, concerning your grandchildren, your own children, siblings, or anybody "blood-related" to you—has anybody else had a depression? *(This natural gate provides a very smooth transition back into the region of "family history.")*
Patient:	No.
Dr. Shea:	Grandparents?
Patient:	No.
Dr. Shea:	Anybody else have a drinking problem?
Patient:	No.

Dr. Shea: Anybody attempt suicide?

Patient: No.

Dr. Shea: Did anybody ever have anything called manic depression?

Patient: No.

Dr. Shea: Schizophrenia, you know, where you hear voices?

Patient: No.

Dr. Shea: Eating disorders?

Patient: Nope. *(Doing a well-rounded search for psychiatric problems in his family, reminded me that I had not asked about eating disorders in Mr. Whitman himself. Flexibly structured interviews, with well-proscribed databases, tend to help the clinician obtain a sound database without errors of omission by this very process of associational cues. It was now easy to cover this forgotten area by the use of a natural gate.)*

Dr. Shea: Have you ever had an eating disorder?

Patient: No.

Dr. Shea: Now earlier you had said that you were in the Navy. How long were you in the Navy? *(Having nicely completed the Family History, I can smoothly move into Social History via a referred gate.)*

Patient: Four years.

Dr. Shea: Four years. Did you see any active combat at all? *(Smoothly flowing natural gate into the history of violence and abuse. Sometimes it is so easy to focus on domestic violence that I find it easy to forget that there are many other arenas in which the seeds of Post-traumatic Stress Disorder can occur, including war, street violence, and exposure to traumatizing events via job occupation, such as an EMT, ambulance driver, and police officer.)*

Patient: No. The closest we got was in the Mediterranean.

Dr. Shea: Have you ever been exposed to any type of violence, whether it is in your own family or . . .

Patient: No.

Dr. Shea: Were you ever abused as a child?

Patient: No.

Dr. Shea: Sexually abused? Has there been any abuse in your family that you know of?

Patient: Nope.

Dr. Shea: Okay good. Outside of the service for the 4 years, what type of work have you done?

Patient: I've done everything.

Dr. Shea: What types of things?

Patient: I have worked in a machine shop for 29 years.

Dr. Shea: Same shop?

Patient: Yeh.

Dr. Shea: Boy, that's loyalty.

Patient: They went out on strike once.

Dr. Shea: Now, what was the company? *(Notice that I have chosen not to follow the pivot point out into the history related to the strike. This is not necessary information, and the interview is already running long. Nice focusing.)*

Patient: Franklin Drill and Tools.

Dr. Shea: What other type of work?

Patient: I've done security work. I had a used car lot. I ran a garage.

Dr. Shea: How far did you go in school?

Patient: Graduated from high school.

Dr. Shea: What were your grades like?

Patient: I got good grades in everything except U.S. history.

Dr. Shea: Okay. When you say good grades—what kinds of grades? *(Behavioral Incident)*

Patient: All Bs.

Dr. Shea: Geeze that's very good. Did you ever fail a course?

Patient: U.S. history!

Dr. Shea: Obviously you were never held back for a year with all Bs. Were you ever suspended or gotten into major problems at school?

Patient: Almost. I happened to go into the principal's office and a friend of mine had just decked the principal. And he took off and I took off because I said if I'm there, I'm going to get nailed.

Dr. Shea: So that wasn't your fault. Did you ever have any problems with the law at all? *(Behavioral Incident)*

Patient: No, I used to work at the police department.

Dr. Shea: Okay, any DWIs? *(Behavioral Incident)*

Patient: No.

Annotation: Typically, the exploration of the social history would be more extensive in an initial intake. But because of the well-spent time lost to extra engagement and the poorly spent time lost to an overlong exploration of past drinking history, I needed to shorten it. On the other hand, this brief foray has been illuminating in its own right, demonstrating little evidence for any significant sociopathy or primitive personality functioning. His approach to both school and work suggests a fairly strong superego and sense of responsibility, both of which we may be able to tap to help him pass through his depression.

We will now see the use of a referred gate to gracefully enter a region of the interview that is traditionally viewed as awkward to approach, but need not be so—the formal cognitive examination.

Dr. Shea: One thing, I did want to touch base with you on, is you mentioned that with the depression your concentration is off. I can vividly picture you in front of the computer just not being able to do much. I would like to do just a little testing to see how your concentration is. Some of these things are very simple. Some of them are a little bit harder. But I'm going to start with some very easy things like "What is today's date?"

Patient: June . . . July . . . no July 2nd.

Dr. Shea: Right. What year is it?

Patient: 1996.

Dr. Shea: And the month?

Patient: July.

Dr. Shea: And the season? What season would you call it?

Patient: Summer.

Dr. Shea: These are the easy ones. What time of day is it roughly?

Patient: About 3:00.

Dr. Shea: Almost exactly. There is a clock right behind you. What town is this?

Patient: Penn Hills.

Dr. Shea: And what is the county that we live in?

Patient: Allegheny.

Dr. Shea: That is exactly right. What state is this?

Patient: Pennsylvania.

Dr. Shea: Obviously the country is?

Patient: United States.

Dr. Shea: Now, those were very simple questions. But every once in a while, you'd be surprised that when people get very depressed, they get flustered and even the simplest of things become problematic. But actually I am impressed that that is not happening for you, and you look like you are thinking clearly. Does your wife think, outside of some problems with concentration, does your wife think you are thinking clearly?

Patient: Most of the time.

Dr. Shea: Depends on what day I'd ask her? *(Said jokingly)*

Patient: Oh, I'll tell you! *(Mr. Whitman smiles and chuckles. Notice that the formal cognitive examination has been introduced into the flow of this interview without any decrease in engagement. The use of the referred gate set the tone by showing that the examination was being done in response to Mr. Whitman's own complaints of poor concentration, looking for evidence of possible impairment due to the depression itself.)*

Dr. Shea: Now let me ask you to remember three things for me—oak tree, a football, and purple. Can you say those back to me?

Patient:	Oak tree, football, and purple.
Dr. Shea:	Okay now say them again, making sure you are trying to remember them.
Patient:	Oak tree, football, purple.
Dr. Shea:	I'm going to ask you for them in just a little bit. I just wanted to check on your concentrating ability, because sometimes depression will throw that . . . I'm going to give you a number, and I want you to say that right back to me when I point to you. Okay. 8,1,4.
Patient:	8,1,4.
Dr. Shea:	Okay. 6,1,2,4.
Patient:	6,1,2,4.
Dr. Shea:	Very good. 7,3,6,8,1.
Patient:	*(Laughs in response to having lost his train of thought)*
Dr. Shea:	Let me try again . . . 7,3,6,8,1.
Patient:	7,3,6,8,1.
Dr. Shea:	That is exactly right. What were those three things I asked you to remember?
Patient:	Oak tree, football, purple.
Dr. Shea:	Great. Now I'm going to give you one more number—8,1,9,6,2,4.
Patient:	8,1,9,6,2,4.
Dr. Shea:	That's perfect. Actually you're sharp. Some people would be missing things by this number. This is called a digit span. It is a way of checking concentration. At this point I'm pretty comfortable with your concentration—you're pretty sharp even though you have been depressed. You know Gary, we've covered . . . *(Just beginning to move into the closing phase of the interview)*

Annotation: I think this was a reasonably good example of a screening cognitive examination in the initial interview. With Mr. Whitman, it was of particular importance because of his age and presentation. The possibility of a mild dementia is quite real and needed to be looked for with some care. In future talks with his wife I will also look for evidence, from her, that might suggest a slowly evolving dementia in Mr. Whitman, but I think it is not likely from his performance on the cognitive examination and his sharpness during the interview itself.

Concerning time management, though, I think I made a mistake here. And it's worth spending some time discussing it. Psychiatrists sometimes have an extra burden in time management in the initial interview, when compared with other mental health professionals, because most agencies expect the psychiatrist to prescribe a medication in the first hour if it is indicated. If the psychiatrist is to do this, then at least 10 minutes will be necessary to discuss the potential use of the medication and jointly decide with the patient whether to try it or not. This will need to be done, in addition to discussing all the other important areas of a good closing, such as education on psychotherapy, joint treatment planning with the patient, and finding out how the session went for the patient. Thus, a psychiatrist often has about 10 minutes less time to gather information than a non-psychiatrist.

In this particular interview I am already running behind. In general, I like to get a good baseline cognitive examination, especially with an older adult, before starting a medication, because the medication could cause cognitive side effects that are hard to "tease out" if one does not have a good baseline.

In this interview though, I probably could get away with a much shorter cognitive examination. This examination "ate up" a lot of time. In hindsight, the engagement was secure, so I could have felt reassured that I would see Mr. Whitman again. At the time, I intended to see him again in 1 to 2 weeks, so I probably could have delayed the more extensive cognitive examination till then. Another option would have been to see if Phil, Mr. Whitman's therapist, would have been willing to do the cognitive examination in the session planned for later in the day.

I basically had the choice of delaying the more thorough cognitive examination, not starting the medication, or doing a terse introduction to the medication. The last alternative is an invitation to medication refusal or noncompliance, and the idea of postponing the medication for another week seems inappropriate considering the intensity of Mr. Whitman's pain.

Even though the 60 minutes allotted to the interview was essentially up, I chose to do all three, which guaranteed a back-up in a busy clinic setting. Sometimes such back-ups are simply unavoidable, but in this case, I think the back-up could have been avoided with a little better time management.

> **Patient:** When I was working on the computer I had to keep looking back at the numbers I was putting in there to make sure I got them right.
>
> **Dr. Shea:** Now, Gary, is there anything *(pause)* we are sort of

coming to the close of the interview at this time, is there anything that you think, I might need to know, that might help me to help you? To understand what you are going through? Anything we haven't covered?

Patient: I don't think so.

Dr. Shea: Well, if something comes to you. . .

Patient: It seems like we have covered most of it but I *(pause)* That's what I mean about "lost," like I go to the doctor or something and we talk like this, I don't remember what I said.

Dr. Shea: That's what you mean by the concentration problems?

Patient: I don't remember what I said before, if I told him what I was supposed to tell him or something like that. I just . . . it's like a black space there.

Dr. Shea: I tell you what . . . I can tell you that what you are experiencing is part of the depression. Why don't I share a little bit now with you before we close. *(I can now follow this naturally arising entrance to fully move into the closing of the interview, which will also include my introduction of a medication.)*

I'm not going to pretend I know you well, by just talking for 50 minutes, but I will share my thoughts with you. The first thing is that I think you have a very clear-cut depression. It is called a Major Depression, and it is a pretty bad one, and I think we can get you some help. *(Presenting the diagnosis in a clear language and in a confident manner helps to decrease Mr. Whitman's anxiety, for he had no framework, other than self-blame, as to why he was functioning so poorly. Now there is some concrete understanding and a message of hope as well.)* I don't think that you are going to need to go to the hospital or anything like that *(prospectively allaying a common fear).*

Basically what we have discovered is that the brain is phenomenally complex. It dwarfs any computer. I mean it is vast, with literally billions and billions of brain cells *(I sound a bit like Carl Sagan here)* with all sorts of connections. Sometimes the transmitters that work between the brain cells don't fire right. What you sometimes get is a lack of some of these molecules that the brain needs. One of them is called "serotonin." It seems to be that in people, who are depressed, it gets low.

What happens is that in most of the areas that you described to me—energy, appetite, concentration, sleep—they are all tucked sort of in the middle of the brain and those depend very much on serotonin. If you get low on serotonin, literally a cell that would normally fire like this for energy *(clinician gestures with rapid tapping of fingers to thumb)*, fires like this *(clinician gestures with slow tapping)*. So to the person, it feels like you just don't have energy any more, and the pleasure centers don't fire right.

Now what we have developed are medicines that really can help with this. What they do is increase the serotonin and sometimes other important transmitters like norepinephrine. Let me just show you. *(At this point I drew out a sketch. Mr. Whitman seemed very attentive during the first part of this psychoeducation. I sensed that the presentation of the science behind his problem was therapeutic for him, probably further providing a framework for understanding that was comforting. Furthermore, many people have a strong faith in science and the background information increases their sense of hope, possibly helping to generate an enhanced positive placebo effect, which can never hurt. Consequently I decided to provide further information, all of which could greatly enhance his interest in taking medications and tolerating side effects. Whether it consists of the hand gestures I used earlier, drawings, or educational posters, many people learn best when visual techniques are implemented. The art of achieving high medication compliance is the art of being a good teacher. This is time very well spent. Note that some people do not want this type of background information, because it may seem overwhelming or too technical, in which case the clinician decreases the amount of psychoeducation or emphasizes different information, always attending to the unique needs of the invidual patient.)*

I'm no artist, but if these are two brain cells, once again, and the energy is trying to go from this brain cell to this brain cell, literally what it does is when the electrical impulse gets here *(pointing to the drawing)*, it fires off these little tiny molecules. In this case, it is called serotonin. They come over here and fit on this next cell like a glove. When enough of them fit, this cell fires. That is how the brain works. Now we are talking 50 or 60 billion brain cells with billions of interconnections.

What I think is going on with you is that you have developed a biological depression. So you are low on this serotonin. So this cell is not firing *(pointing to sketch again).* They are not communicating right, and the medicines, that we have, help with this. We have no way of just giving you serotonin. If it was diabetes, I could give you insulin. It is very much like diabetes. If you have diabetes, you don't have insulin so they give you some. Here, the serotonin, if I give it to you, won't get through your blood to your brain. So instead we have some medicines that do some pretty remarkable things. *(I keep looking and nodding to Mr. Whitman to make sure that he is following and is interested. He appears quite interested indeed. We are on the right path.)*

What happens is, when these things *(pointing to neurotransmitters in the sketch)* are done, they get recycled back into the cell here *(points to presynaptic membrane.)* Basically what these medications do is they slow this reuptake down so that the serotonin gets stuck out here *(pointing to the synaptic cleft in the sketch)*, which effectively increases how much is out there. If you do it long enough, the cells start to "kick over." It's as if we gave you more serotonin. The medicine returns the chemical balance to your brain, giving you the serotonin level, you normally have, when you feel good.

I would like to give you a medicine that can help with this, and it is called Pamelor. It is a very good antidepressant. It has been around for a long, long time *(statements that give validation to the medicine).* It is very good for what you have. You have what we call an agitated depression. There is a lot of agitation in it. That is what you feel in the morning when you are aroused out of your sleep. That is when you feel like this *(clinician makes a tense gesture with face and hands).* So a lot of sort of agitation is almost like too much energy.

What I would like to do is to start you on the Pamelor, and I've had some very good luck with this medicine *(giving evidence of direct success with the medication in my personal practice).* It is very good with older adults. I don't know entirely why, but I think it is one of the best things for people over 50 or 60 *(showing the specialness of the medication and why it has been chosen, all aimed at increasing Mr. Whitman's confidence in the medication).* I will put you on a small dose of it, just 10 mg, twice a day, once in the morning and once at night. I will write you a prescription for that.

It is always important to note if you get side effects, and I will review some of them, for all medications can have side effects. Keep in mind that most side effects go away, not all, but most do. You know, if you just stay on the medicine, your body gets used to it. Your role, and I also want Phil *(Mr. Whitman's therapist)* to be one of the coaches on this, is that you have to watch the medicine and see if the pros outweigh the cons *(actively involving Mr. Whitman and empowering him at the same time).* If they do, you stay on the medicine. If it just takes away that agitation, gives you back your sleep, and gives you back your energy, but it also makes you constipated, that will probably still seem like a fair trade-off to you. If that is the case, then you can stay on the medicine until the depression is gone.

I say that, because one interesting thing, sometimes the side effects come on very rapidly. The improvement may not come for 2, 3, or even 5 weeks sometimes. So we may also need to have a lot of patience, but you are a very tough guy. If you can stop drinking cold turkey, then you can wait 2, 3, or 4 weeks to get the benefit. *(The earlier information, from the alcohol history, pays off unexpectedly here in the form of a convincing and powerful reminder of his strength. Mr. Whitman nodded, showing that he liked the implication of the analogy.)*

Obviously if the side effects are too bad, you

will need to stop the medicine. I am not here to force medicines on you, I'm here to help you find the right one. So if you get bad side effects, let me know. I'm counting on you to tell me. *(Proactively dismantling a common fear of many patients—that physicians are only interested in keeping them on medications and pay little attention to side effects. These statements also empower the patient by asking for his or her help in looking out for side effects.)*

You can get a dry mouth with this. You can get some blurred vision when you read. That is a curious one, but sometimes people get that. Some people do get some constipation. I've seen some tremors at times but that is not common. You get a thing where you get a little lightheaded when you stand up, and that will be something for you to watch out for. That happens because when you go from lying down or even sitting and you suddenly go up like this, gravity pulls on the blood and it literally pulls blood from the brain. The way your brain deals with that is the vessels get very, very small and it sort of increases the blood pressure to the brain, the small vessels. So it is like taking a garden hose and making the nozzle tighter, which causes a stronger stream to squirt out. Well, this medicine will slow that response just a little bit, and that is why some people get lightheaded when they first stand up. All you have to do is get up slowly. What I tell people is if they are lying down in bed, all you do is, when you first get up, is just sit upright in bed for about 1 minute and make sure you are not lightheaded. When you are done, just get up very slowly. *(The clinician stands slowly, demonstrating the technique. Although orthostatic hypotension is not overly likely with this medication, because of his age and the presence of several medications that could cause dizziness themselves, Mr. Whitman is still at risk. I go out of my way to alert susceptible patients to this side effect because it can be frightening, leading to discontinuation, and dangerous, if it leads to a fall. A few moments of education can do wonders to help patients tolerate and minimize this problem.)* There is a very good chance you won't get lightheadedness, but if you do, you won't be frightened by it. You will know how to deal with that.

You have, if I'm recalling correctly, you have no heart condition, and you had a recent ECG that was normal. I would like to contact your regular MD, if that is okay with you. *(As time permits, it is always a good idea to touch base with the patient's primary care physician. This request also reassures the patient that the new medicine will be used safely with the blessing of his or her long-term physician. At this point, I am doing everything I can to help ensure that Mr. Whitman will not abruptly discontinue the medication before our next appointment, an all too common occurrence, often resulting from inadequate psychoeducation and communication during this critical phase of the initial interview.)*

Patient: Okay.

Dr. Shea: I want to make sure he *(referring to the primary care physician)* is comfortable with this. I would be surprised if he isn't. I will start you on the medication now, and I'll get back to you if there is a problem. I would actually like to see you again in about 1 to 2 weeks. *(pause)* Will you notice anything in 1 to 2 weeks? Well it usually takes 1 to 2 weeks, sometimes even 4 weeks, for the antidepressant to effectively kick in. *(By once again alerting Mr. Whitman to the potential delay in benefits, I am trying to proactively decrease the risk of frustration or disappointment that could lead him to prematurely stop the medication, especially if side effects show up early.)*

I have more than a small number of people who, within several days, feel a little bit better and a little calmer. I don't want to get your expectations up. It could take a while, but you might notice something right away too. Very, very good medicine. It has been used enormously. *(Building confidence in the medication)* It is an older drug, not one of the newer ones, so we know the side effects. One other advantage of it is that, if we are trying to gauge how much needs to be in your system, I can get a blood level of it for you. Then we'll know exactly where it is. Any thoughts about trying the medication?

Patient: Whatever you say.

Dr. Shea: Do you feel that you are sensitive to medicines? Or are you fairly . . . *(This is a great question to ask almost all patients. Even if the patient is not sensitive to medications, but he or she thinks such a sensitivity exists, it is important to listen carefully. If the patient feels that he or she is particularly sensitive to medications, it is often wise to start the medication at a lower than normal dose and let the patient know that you are doing so. Such a respectful response from the physician to patient input greatly enhances the patient's sense of safety. It also lowers his or her anxiety level, thus probably decreasing the risk of "imagined" side effects that can lead to abrupt and unnecessary medication discontinuation.)*

Annotation: A few comments on time management are in order here. This interview ran about 15 minutes overtime, which is one of the reasons why I chose to include it, because it demonstrates that even a seasoned clinician can run overtime. It is important, however, to note that around 10 minutes of that overtime was secondary to the medication psychoeducation and contracting. If this was gone, as it would be for non-psychiatrists during their initial intakes, and I had made some better choices (e.g., to decrease the time spent on past alcohol use and to defer much of the cognitive examination to the second session), the interview would have been performed easily in less than 60 minutes. Indeed, if I had just limited the exploration of past alcohol abuse and shortened the formal cognitive examination, the interview would have lasted almost 60 minutes as is.

But there is one thing I would seldom shorten—the psychoeducation regarding medications. As one can tell, there is a real art to prescribing medications in a way that leads to high patient interest and motivation. A managed care system, or any system, that pushes physicians to shorten this step is "shooting itself in the foot" from a cost perspective. Noncompliance with medications is one of the leading causes of treatment failure, symptom return, increased emergency room and clinic visits, and increased hospital days. The introduction of a medicine to a patient needs to be done well, and physicians need adequate time to do it.

In this regard, at the community mental health center where I was working at the time of this interview, I was expected to complete a full intake, prescribe medicines, and dictate the written document in 60 minutes. Using the principles outlined in this book, I was frequently able to accomplish this task within the desired 60-minute time frame, plus or minus 10 minutes. But this is really "pressing it." I do not feel that it is an appropriate time frame, and it can result in a disservice to the patients, clinicians, and costs of the center.

Considering the critical nature of the initial assessment, both for treatment planning, and patient engagement, combined with the difficult task of creating sound written documents, which are both clinically informative and forensically sound in our litigious society, I believe that the appropriate time allotment for an initial intake, by any mental health professional, should be at least 1½ hours. This provides the clinician with 60 minutes for the actual interview, followed by 30 minutes to write the assessment document. It also provides some flexibility, if the clinician requires, in occasional cases, more than 60 minutes for the interview itself. I believe that it is up to our professional societies, as well as ourselves, to push for such adequate time standards.

Having made my one and only political comment in this book, let us see how the final minutes of our interview unfold.

> **Patient:** If I'm told I need it, I take it.
>
> **Dr. Shea:** Okay. Well let's give it a try and see what happens with it. I would like to see you in about 2 weeks. We'll set that up with the secretary outside. What do you feel after we have talked here? How are you feeling?
>
> **Patient:** I learned something.
>
> **Dr. Shea:** You mean that you have a biological depression? *(Mr. Whitman nods.)* By the way, an enormous number of people get this over the course of a lifetime. Frequently there is only one episode for people, so once we get this thing in remission, you are going to feel a lot better. Sometimes it comes back and, if it does, we will deal with it. There is tremendous hope, Gary.
>
> **Patient:** I hope so. I just can't take it any more.
>
> **Dr. Shea:** I can't tell you how many people we've helped with this. There is a lot of hope and a lot of good medicines out there. And Phil is a fantastic therapist, so he can really help you to put this in perspective and not get down on yourself.
> He'll help you to figure out how to pace yourself with the depression. Now it is a little bit like a person coming back from a track injury, who is a runner. You have to learn how to pace yourself until your brain catches up and starts firing right

again. So take it easy on yourself for a little bit. Don't expect yourself to feel normal because you literally have a biologic disease that, until we get it reversed, you are going to feel a little bit out of sorts.

If this doesn't help in 2 weeks, there are other things we can do. Especially if you are particularly anxious, there are other medicines I could add that could help with the anxiety. But I like to use this principle. Use the smallest number of drugs at the smallest doses to get the most benefit. That will be what you need. So let's try this first. Let me get a prescription pad. *(Begins to write prescription)*

Remember how I said to take it—one in the morning and one at night. This is a relatively low dose of the drug to start off with. If there are any problems with it you can call. I am here Monday, Tuesday, and Wednesday. On Thursday and Friday there is another doctor taking med coverage for me, and on the weekends we even have that number, I already gave you, to get a doctor, even on a Saturday night. So if there are any unexpected side effects or something you are wondering about—whether this is a side effect—you can call. *(Hands Mr. Whitman the prescription, making good eye contact)* Pamelor 10 mg, 1 tablet twice a day. I have a really good feeling about this with you. I think it is going to help you. It is important. If this one doesn't, we'll go on to another one, okay? *(Mr. Whitman nods and smiles.)*

Patient: Any pharmacy?

Dr. Shea: Yes. It is a very common drug. They might give it to you in generic form, which would be cheaper and is fine. *(pause)* What was it like talking with me today?

Patient: I enjoyed it.

Dr. Shea: In what sense?

Patient: It made me feel relaxed. I came in here very defensive. The girl told me that I was going to have him *(another psychiatrist covering the clinic on a different day)* and, if he wasn't available, she would give me someone else. And I said, "No I won't." I said I won't come. I said I want to deal with somebody one-on-one. I don't want to deal with eight or nine people, and I've got to tell them all again. They don't know me from Adam. I don't know them.

Dr. Shea: Well, you are stuck with me now. *(Said with a smile)*

Patient: *(Mr. Whitman chuckles)* That is just fine.

Dr. Shea: What was it, that talking to me, made you feel more comfortable do you think?

Patient: I don't know. Just the way you explained things. Relaxed. Made me relaxed. Guess that's it.

Dr. Shea: Well, you were a pleasure to talk with, and I'm hoping we can help. *(For some reason, I intuitively sensed that Mr. Whitman felt good about the interview, except for the fact that he had cried. I decided to address this possible area of resistance to follow-up.)* Any time a person has pain like you've had, including me, it can help to cry. I find it helps, you know, to get the tears out.

Patient: You're a kid if you cry. *(Apparently my intuition was on the mark.)*

Dr. Shea: That is a normal adult's response to pain. I'm glad you were able to do it with me, and I'll tell you, the vast majority of men who were sitting in that chair cry. So you are one of many, many men. Okay? Don't give it a second thought. I have done it before, and I'll do it again in the future. *(Mr. Whitman smiles.)* Very good talking with you. *(Shaking hands)*

Patient: I appreciate everything you're doing.

Dr. Shea: I'll see you in 2 weeks.

End of Interview

Annotation: That's it. I hope the interview provided a useful illustration of a full intake, presented from front to back, performed in an actual clinic setting. I think a thorough and useful database has been collected and, as previously noted, with just a few changes in strategy, we would have finished within 60 minutes to boot.

Mistakes were made, but I make mistakes every time I interview. Interviews and humans are far too complicated not to make mistakes in such a complex task. With every mistake, I try to learn. I certainly would have done some things in this interview differently, if given a second chance.

Moreover, this example of an interview is not presented as the only way to have achieved our goals. I am sure that there are things the reader saw that he or she would have done differently. That's good. As long as the goals of the interview are achieved by the end of the 60 minutes, then any strategy used was a successful one. Every clinician will approach each patient uniquely. There is no single "right" way to do an interview with Mr. Whitman or anyone else. But this interview does provide, I think, a window into the principles that we have been discussing throughout this book—principles that can help us to creatively and flexibly structure our initial interviews in an effort to more consistently achieve our goals.

Let's return to these goals, for a moment, which were first presented in Chapters 1 and 2, to see if this particular interview successfully achieved them.

As mentioned earlier, "engagement" is the single most important task in the initial interview. If the patient does not return for a second interview, the most accurate DSM-IV diagnosis in the world will be nothing more than a useless piece of data in a useless clinic chart. Without a patient, there can be no treatment. I think that this interview "did the trick" in this regard. Mr. Whitman entered, brimming with wariness and a smoldering hostility. He left, feeling that the clinician had carefully listened to him, feeling comfortable enough that he could laugh and joke.

What may be more remarkable was that this genuine rapport was achieved while gathering an extensive database, one of our other major goals for the initial interview, described in Chapter 2. Besides delineating a sound diagnosis and "history of the present illness," each of the major DSM-IV categories was explored, so as not to miss treatable disorders that are often hidden (e.g., obsessive-compulsive disorder, post-traumatic stress disorder, and substance abuse). Family history, social history, past psychiatric history, medical history, the mental status, and suicide/violence assessment were all carefully delineated, yielding important clues to both engagement and intervention.

The clinical database pointed towards a powerful treatment intervention—the use of an antidepressant—and this treatment intervention was introduced successfully. The database also gave further support to the important role that continued psychotherapy and psychoeducation could play in helping to bring prompt relief for Mr. Whitman.

Perhaps of even more surprise was the rather pronounced change in the affect of Mr. Whitman, which unfolded as the hour proceeded. There is little doubt that, on an interpersonal level and on a very human level, the interview was therapeutic. Yet no therapy was done. Indeed, if one had attempted to do primarily therapy in the hour, perhaps of a solution-oriented type, a clinician would be hard pressed to have created much more of a therapeutic impact.

In this regard, hopefully, the interview illustrates the power of a clinician to decrease a patients's pain and anxiety, while gathering a thorough and useful database. As stated throughout the book, sensitive structuring is powerfully engaging. Through the use of natural and referred gates, with just a smattering of implied gates, the clinician created a sense of free-flowing movement and natural conversation. The thoroughness of the questioning and the clinician's familiarity with the patient's symptoms conveyed a sense of competence and expertise, which helped to open the pathway towards trust. The sincere effort of the clinician to provide useful education and the genuineness of the clinician's affect and humor did not go unnoticed. Mr. Whitman entered the room with fear. He left with hope.

APPENDIX III

THE WRITTEN DOCUMENT: EFFECTIVE STRATEGIES

The "writing up" of the initial assessment is a somewhat daunting task. In recent years, the task has become even more challenging because of the increased time pressures of managed care and the increasingly litigious nature of the society in which we find ourselves practicing. In this appendix, I will try to share some tips and strategies that I have found useful in training clinicians, over the years, from various mental health disciplines. The principles will hopefully help the reader to meet both of the above challenges, by increasing the speed of preparation, while improving the forensic soundness of the document.

To help with our explorations, I have split this appendix into four subappendices: III A: an appendix describing specific tips and strategies for the write-up: III B: an appendix that outlines quality assurance guidelines and dictation prompts for the assessment: III C: a model write-up of an actual assessment to serve as a prototype (this is the write-up from the annotated interview of Mr. Whitman, allowing you a unique opportunity to see the direct translation of interview data into a written document): and III D: a sample assessment form, if you prefer using a predesigned form for your write-ups.

Before proceeding into Appendix III A, let's talk about some basic principles. We shall begin by asking the single most relevant question: "Who is this assessment being written for?"

In the first place, we are writing the assessment for fellow clinicians, in the hope that our assessment may help some future clinician to provide prompt and valuable treatment. Clinicians, who often look carefully at initial assessments, include: inpatient clinicians, crisis clinicians, therapists to whom we may transfer patient care, and psychiatrists, who may be consulted to begin treatment with medications or for a second opinion on diagnosis and treatment planning.

Lawyers have a nasty penchant for looking at our written intakes. When doing so, these documents are scoured for errors of omission, inconsistent data, formulations that are not supported by the database, evidence that important information was not gathered, evidence of "diagnosis-slapping" from the information that was gathered, and frank errors in clinical formulation and judgment. The best clinical interview ever performed, if documented poorly, is a sure-fire ticket to losing a lawsuit. In the last analysis, often it is not so much what you say in court, but rather, what you wrote in your office, that determines the outcome of a lawsuit.

Insurance companies, state mental health divisions, government disability agencies, and accrediting boards often peruse charts with a keen eye. Internal quality assurance personnel and supervisors are also interested in reviewing initial assessment documents. And both the patient and family members of the patient may be interested in reading the intake report. Next in frequency to a "discharge summary," I believe that an initial assessment is the most-read item in a chart.

But I have left off the single most important person for whom the assessment is written—"you," the clinician. We write the assessment for ourselves. The actual writing of the assessment requires us to review the data that we gathered. In this review, we may discover areas of important, sometimes critical information, that we forgot to ask about. If we notice data regions that we consistently miss from one patient to another, we might discover so-called training "blind-spots" or areas where we lack expertise and can subsequently gain it. The writing of the document allows our intuitions to re-formulate our impressions and diagnoses. The act of writing the document opens the door to creative treatment planning, if it is done as an integral part of good care, not as something that one is forced to do. In this light, the writing of the assessment is not so much a nuisance to be resented but a tool to be used. Nobody, including me, likes paperwork. However, this is one piece of paperwork that can actually help our patients, if we do it well.

Part of the trick to easing the "pain" of writing assessments is to do them as close to the time of the interview as possible. An assessment done immediately after seeing a patient may, literally, take half the time to write up as one done days later or even at the end of the day. A promptly written intake report is also one less chronic stress for the clinician, because few things can burn a clinician out faster than an ever-increasing pile of late paperwork. It is indeed unpleasant to approach such a dreaded pile. It is also potentially unnecessary.

In this regard, I urge administrators to always give clinicians at least 30 minutes (preferably 1 hour) to write up the assessment, immediately after doing the 60-minute interview. If an administrator recognizes how important the written document, in question, may be to winning or losing a future lawsuit, this time block is time well spent. It also ensures that there is no back-up in billing, while cutting down the burnout of the staff.

Most clinicians do not have the luxury of dictation services, but if you do, be sure to use them. If you don't know how to dictate, learn. It is not an exaggeration to say that dictation can decrease the time it takes to prepare a document by 70%. A clinician who is experienced with dictation can often dictate a full intake in 15 to 20 minutes or less, a task that would have taken the same clinician 30 to 60 minutes to write by hand.

Concerning the approach to writing the document itself, it is important to remember that the different regions of the document fall into two broad categories: (1) database, recorded as objectively as possible, because there will always remain a subjective quality to some of this information, and (2) clinical judgment and formulation, both of which are truly subjective. It is critical, from a forensic standpoint, that while attempting to record an objective database, you leave out your clinical judgments.

For instance, in the History of the Present Illness (an area from the objective database), the clinician should avoid statements such as, "for several months, Mr. Jones appeared manic," without providing the supporting behavioral data. Without the raw behavioral data, no reader knows whether the subjective word "manic" is being accurately applied.

If the raw data are not supplied, a prosecuting lawyer can attempt to say that the clinician slapped this diagnostic label on the patient. If the patient had gone on to commit suicide on a lithium overdose, then the lawyer can argue that the whole process began by the clinician slapping on this wrong diagnosis.

It is more sound clinically and forensically for the clinician to write something like, "Mr. Jones displayed, for several months, the following symptoms, which became progressively worse: racing thoughts, marked difficulty falling asleep, loud speech, angry outbursts, hypersexuality, and a marked change in spending habits, resulting in Mr. Jones completely exhausting over 15 years of savings." The clinical descriptor, "manic" (a clinical judgment) is not mentioned here. It will be mentioned later in the document under the heading of "Clinical Summary and Formulation."

With the above distinctions in mind, let us look at the components of the written document listed by either objective database or subjective formulation:

I. Database (objective areas)
   Chief complaint
   History of the present illness
   Past psychiatric history (includes substance abuse history)
   Developmental and social history
   Family history

Medical history
Medical review of systems
Mental status
II. Clinical Formulation and Judgment (subjective areas)
DSM-IV diagnostic listing
Clinical summary and formulation
Triage and treatment plan (some clinicians incorporate this
    information into the Clinical Summary and Formulation)

In Appendix III A, we will take a look at some tips and strategies for the written document. Appendix III A covers three areas, which are prototypically objective, subjective, or both: (1) tips for the history of the present illness (one of the objective regions), (2) tips for the summary and formulation (one of the subjective regions), and (3) tips for addressing the assessment of suicide potential (an area that actually has components in both the objective and subjective regions).

In Appendix III B, the clinician is offered a practical outline of the various components of the written document listed above; however, this time specific suggestions are made, from a quality assurance standpoint, as to what information must appear under each heading. Much of this material is based on the Position Paper from the American Psychiatric Association concerning quality assurance expectations of what should be done during an initial assessment.[1] It is meant to offer sound footing from a forensic standpoint. It is also intended to be used as an easy access reference for the student, while he or she is writing up assessments.

In Appendix III C, the actual written document, immediately dictated after seeing Mr. Whitman, is presented in its entirety. This gives the reader a direct view of how the information gleaned from the interview was translated, by the clinician, into each of the sections of the written document. It is also meant to serve as a prototypical model for the student, while the student is writing up his or her first assessments.

In Appendix III D, an example of a clinical assessment form is given. Feel free to use this form as is, or adapt it for your own needs. There is no such thing as a perfect form, nor one that will even totally satisfy two clinicians; however, this form is practical and useful. It provides user-friendly space for each section and also serves as a good reminder of what areas need to be covered; thus, it helps to catch errors of omission.

APPENDIX III A

Practical Tips for Creating a Good Write-Up

History of the Present Illness

The history of the present illness (HPI) is arguably the most important section of the assessment concerning the raw database. From a clinical standpoint, it provides the reader with the most detailed and accurate picture of the patient's specific set of symptoms. From a forensic standpoint, it is easily attacked, providing the "proof" of clinician negligence and inadequate diagnostic data gathering. We shall look at each of these arenas in turn.

Clinically, the HPI is critical in helping clinicians to gather a sound and accurate database, before making a diagnosis. All diagnoses should be made based on DSM-IV criteria gathered from the patient, corroborative sources, and past clinical records. Poor diagnostic work is, at best, problematic for patients, and, at worst, catastrophic. The most valid picture of a patient's symptom phenomenology is often best seen during the first episode of an illness, before all sorts of distorting factors may appear. Such distorting factors include partial remission of symptoms from medications, medication side effects mistaken for symptoms, and lost information simply because people's memories fail over time. A well-written HPI may stand as the single best record of the patient's naturally occurring symptoms, with this database playing a role in treatment decisions that may occur years after the initial intake has been done.

Clinically, the HPI can also provide a reader with a quick snapshot of the immediate stressors affecting the patient and can play a role in crisis support or therapeutic goals. This information includes the patient's perception of his or her own problems, a perception that may contain key hints to potential roadblocks or potential solutions.

From a legal viewpoint, the HPI is a rich domain, both for attack and defense. If a patient is claiming that he or she has suffered from a misdiagnosis (e.g., the patient received the wrong medications over the years; the patient did not receive medications that were needed; the patient was stigmatized secondary to a diagnosis that he or she did not have; the patient was refused care or disability because of a wrong diagnosis), the HPI may tell the tale. In this regard, the HPI will either contain data that confirm the DSM-IV diagnosis in question or it won't. Put succinctly, for every diagnosis and rule-out that appears later in the clinician's DSM-IV differential at the end of the written assessment, the raw data, from which these diagnoses were made, should appear in the HPI.

If, on the other hand, the patient is claiming that a pivotal diagnosis was missed by the clinician, the HPI may once again tell the tale. This time the defense lawyer will be hoping that his or her client has clearly documented, in the HPI, all pertinent negatives. Pertinent negatives are symptoms that the patient was asked about and clearly denied, which would be reflected by statements in the HPI such as, "The patient denied racing thoughts, hypersexuality, sleep disturbances, agitation, anger, or any other symptoms of mania." Well-documented statements, such as these, make it much easier for a lawyer to argue that no negligence was done. To the contrary, the clinician performed a thorough interview, as evidenced by the pertinent negatives listed in the HPI. The diagnosis made was a sound one based on the best available data.

With the above clinical and forensic considerations in mind, the approach to a well-written HPI follows naturally. I suggest the following as one method of documentation, but it is up to the clinician to explore various strategies to see what works best for him or her.

It is nice to begin the HPI with a single paragraph, describing the patient's stressors and perceptions of his or her problems. This provides the reader with a nice snapshot of the current situation, providing a context from which to understand the symptom picture that will follow. Keep this paragraph short. There is no need to describe details; later therapists will sort out the details for themselves. This is one spot where many clinicians waste a lot of time during the write-up, by going into far too much detail. Restrict this section to one paragraph.

The next paragraph should outline, in a simple chronologic framework, the symptoms that support whatever diagnosis the clinician lists as the primary diagnosis in his or her formulation and DSM-IV differential. It will often contain organizing statements that help the reader to see the pertinent symptoms in context and quickly. Such statements may look as follows, "From January onwards, Mr. Franklin's depressive symptoms became more severe and persistent. These symptoms included: difficulty falling asleep (1 to 2 hours), early morning awakening, decreased appetite (with a 15-lb weight loss), decreased energy, decreased concentration, decreased libido, daily tearfulness, and marked anhedonia." As noted earlier, the clinician does not interpret these data by giving a diagnosis. At this point, just the facts are given.

At the end of this paragraph, some clinicians like to add a sentence listing any pertinent negatives, which would be areas of diagnostic investigation, if a patient reported the above symptoms. In this light, clearly a patient with this set of depressive symptoms may have a bipolar disorder. If these symptoms were denied, the clinician might conclude this paragraph with, "Mr. Franklin denied episodes of racing thoughts, reckless spending, loud speech, angry outbursts, or other manic symptoms."

The rest of the HPI follows the above principles. For each diagnosis or rule-out diagnosis, appearing later in the document, a separate paragraph should appear where the supporting symptoms are described. If the patient has two other diagnoses for certain and two other diagnoses to rule out, then four more paragraphs will be needed. Note that if a personality disorder is a secondary diagnosis, sometimes the supporting data will appear in the Social History not in the HPI. On the other hand, if the Axis II diagnosis is the primary diagnosis or is playing a major role in the immediate presentation, the supporting data should probably appear in the HPI.

This approach to the HPI sometimes provides some surprises that are of immediate help to the patient. I have occasionally begun to dictate my HPI, only to discover that I did not have the adequate data to support my diagnosis. In short, I was jumping to a conclusion. When returning to the patient or family members for more data, I sometimes discover that my assumptions were off base, and the patient did not have the diagnosis that I was assuming, leading to the formulation of a new treatment plan.

The last paragraph in the HPI is dedicated to a short listing of the pertinent negatives that may be left. Some clinicians choose to list all pertinent negatives in this paragraph. It doesn't matter how you do it, just so all the pertinent negatives are listed by the end of the HPI (note that some pertinent negatives may also appear in the Mental Status; see Chapter 9, for a detailed description of the write-up of the mental status).

By the way, there is an easy way to tell if an HPI has been written well. To a clinically experienced reader, there should be no surprises once the reader reaches the DSM-IV listing. The HPI will have nicely presented all of the symptoms for each diagnosis, and the astute reader will have already guessed which diagnoses are present.

Indeed, this is an excellent method of quality assurance for supervisors. When reviewing the supervisee's HPI, the supervisor can write in the margin what diagnosis is being supported by each paragraph. If this is not easy to do, then the quality of the HPI is suspect. Moreover, if these diagnoses do not appear or "surprise diagnoses" appear that are not supported in the HPI, there is a clear-cut problem somewhere, either in documentation or clinical formulation.

At this time, if you are interested in seeing some of the above principles at work, you might want to turn to Appendix III C and take a look at the sample HPI presented there.

Summary and Formulation

This section is called different names by different people (e.g., "Narrative Assessment," "Data Interpretation," "Clinical Formulation"), but the bottom line is that the clinician needs an area devoted to a discussion of his or her clinical formulations and judgments. This is the section in which the clinician "puts it all together." By its very nature, this section is subjective. It will vary from one clinician to another, depending on training background, treatment orientation, and personal bias.

From a legal standpoint, it is important to realize that this is the section of the document in which a lawyer will try to prove the presence of poor clinical judgment, negligence, or even malicious intent (e.g., he or she will look for statements suggesting that the clinician did not like the patient). Consequently, it is critical to carefully explain why one has made the decisions that one has made. It is not enough to simply state the decision. For example, it is not enough to write, "the patient does not appear to be suicidal at present." Instead, the clinician needs to explain why he or she feels the patient is not suicidal as with, "Despite his marked depression, Mr. Stevens does not appear to be acutely suicidal at present, as evidenced by his lack of a history of suicide attempts, denial of current suicidal ideation, ready willingness to make a safety contract, and his eagerness to get follow-up care." It is the soundness of your reasoning that will protect you in court. Be sure to take the time to record it.

In this section the clinician will give a quick summary of the case, support his or her diagnostic impressions, support any decisions regarding safety (e.g., suicide or homicide potential), provide pertinent insight into any psychological or social conflicts needing attention, and describe triage and treatment decisions while providing the clinical reasoning behind these decisions. Some clinicians create a separate section devoted to triage or treatment. I prefer including my treatment recommendations in my formulation, because I think that it fits naturally here, allowing one to tie treatment recommendations directly into diagnoses and stress points.

The Summary and Formulation is one of the most, if not the most, read sections of the Initial Assessment by other clinicians. It offers clinicians, who are unfamiliar with the patient, a quick headstart into the history of the patient. A well-written Summary and Formulation is a prized golden nugget for inpatient clinicians, admitting a patient late on a Friday afternoon. Such a summary is also much appreciated by busy clinic clinicians, who might be covering for the treating therapist or may be seeing the patient in an emergency.

Keeping in mind the practical usefulness of this section for future clinicians, the clinician begins this section with a quick statement of pertinent demographics such as age, sex, and marital status, which help to provide a quick idea of who the patient is. If the patient has a lengthy past psychiatric history or is well known to the system, this may be mentioned along with pertinent diagnoses. If the patient has a history of violence or suicide, this can be mentioned here, serving to immediately alert the reader to these potential problems.

With one or two sentences the clinician can summarize what current factors and stresses brought the patient into care. This can be followed by a brief discussion of the DSM-IV differential. There is no need to repeat symptoms here. Such a repetition is a waste of time. One only needs to refer back to the HPI, where the symptoms are well documented. Instead, in the Summary and Formulation, the emphasis is on explaining why specific diagnoses were given. For example, "Despite the numerous neurovegetative symptoms of depression, as noted in the HPI, these symptoms are fluctuating in nature. Consequently I doubt the presence of a true major depression. At present the patient appears to meet the criteria for a dysthymic disorder, and I am suspicious of some characterologic depressive symptoms, as suggested by his rapid depressive responses to relatively mild interpersonal stresses."

Be sure to take the time to explain why any diagnoses, such as borderline personality or antisocial personality that may be accompanied by stigmatization or have important legal/benefits implications, were made. Such statements may protect you from future charges of "label slapping."

It's nice to include some mention of any specific psychological or situational factors (including family dynamics, financial stresses, etc.) that may need to be a focus of treatment intervention. Building on these factors and the DSM-IV diagnoses, the clinician describes treatment modalities and the reason why they are being chosen, ranging from family therapy to the utilization of medications, case management, or even referral to another clinician. This is also a good spot to note any general medical concerns that may require a consult with a primary care physician or specialist, as well as any lab work that needs to be ordered.

Keeping the above principles in mind, the clinician can write a clinically useful Summary and Formulation, which is also good protection in court. With practice, it is surprising how rapidly this can be done.

Assessment of Suicide and Violence Potential

It goes without saying that this section of the initial assessment is a legal hotspot. In order to create a sound forensic document, the clinician will address these concerns in several different areas of the written assessment, spanning both database areas and areas concerned with formulation and clinical judgment.

In the HPI (objective database), the clinician will describe all suicide and violent ideation and actions that occurred in the current episode of the illness, up until the time frame immediately before the assessment. In the Mental Status (objective database), the clinician will describe all such material from the immediate recent past and that ideation experienced during the interview itself (some clinicians include descriptions of safety contracting here, and others include it in the HPI). In the Past Psychiatric History (objective database), all past suicidal and violent information will be tersely described. Finally, in the Summary and Formulation, the clinician will share his or her decision regarding the patient's immediate safety, heavily emphasizing the reasoning behind these decisions.

Here are a few tips that can help the clinician to address these issues rapidly and effectively, both from the goal of communicating clear clinical information and creating a sound legal document.

In the first place, notice how closely the different regions where suicidal/violent ideation will be recorded, parallel the CASE Approach utilized in gathering the information in the interview. If the clinician has utilized the CASE Approach effectively, all of these data will be neatly waiting to "fall into place" in the written document.

It is often wise to include in the HPI or the Mental Status, any direct quotes made by the patient, suggesting that suicide/violence risk is minimal. For instance, the clinician might document statements such as, "I would never kill myself. I just couldn't do that to my kids" or "As much pain as I'm in, I know I won't kill myself, because it is a mortal sin in my religion. It's just not the right thing to do." In your Summary and Formulation, you will refer back to such statements as supportive evidence for your clinical decision. If you are ever taken to court, both you and your attorney will be greatly pleased by the presence of such concrete documentation. Such concrete information also provides important clues to future clinicians, suggesting areas that they can explore to see if such powerful deterrents to suicide are still active for the patient.

Wherever you decide to document any safety contracting, be sure to describe it carefully, emphasizing behavioral clues indicating that the patient was sincere. Don't simply write, "The patient made a safety contract with me." Instead, write something such as, "Mr. Jones made a sound safety contract with me, showing good eye contact, a firm handshake, and a genuine affect. He seemed very interested in our safety plans and wrote down the number of our crisis team."

Carefully document any contacts made with corroborative sources, indicating what they said that was in support of the patient's safety and that the patient is telling the truth. Such a statement need not be long and may sound something like this, "Mr. Jones' wife was contacted. She supported Mr. Jones' assertion that he has not been talking about suicide and also that he has no history of suicide attempts. She is in agreement with our safety plan, commenting, 'I really feel Bill is safe at home, and I'll check in on him as you suggested.'"

Finally, also document any consultation that you made with a colleague. List everybody that you discussed the case with, and state their agreement with your decision. Such a notation may look like this, "I spoke with the patient's therapist at home and also consulted with the on-call psychiatrist, both of whom are in full agreement with the plan." Consulting is probably the single best defense against the charge of negligence; however, it weakens markedly if not recorded. From a clinical standpoint, consulting is often very beneficial, even for the most experienced clinician. I always use the following rule of thumb: If I'm wondering whether or not it would be a good idea to consult someone, it means it is a good time to do so—and I do.

As stated earlier, in your formulation, take the time to describe your clinical reasoning accurately. If you clearly documented that you took a careful history, contacted corroborative sources if indicated, consulted if necessary, and then used good clinical judgment, you will have significantly increased your protection from a lawsuit. Indeed, a good many lawsuits are probably dropped after a lawyer reads a well-written document and realizes that the chances of winning the case are minimal.

Naturally, the meticulousness of your documentation will vary depending on how potentially dangerous the patient may be. But in all circumstances, an understanding of the above principles can help a clinician to write more effective assessments of risk from both a clinical and forensic standpoint. More important, such an organized way of documenting pushes the clinician to do careful assessments. In this fashion the writing of the document can help the clinician to catch critical errors of omission, such as not contacting an important corroborative source, who might tell a very different story than the patient described. The correction of such an "information gap," triggered by the writing up of the document itself, could help us to save a life.

A P P E N D I X   III B

Dictation Prompts and Quality Assurance Guidelines for the Written Document

Dictation Prompts for the Initial Biopsychosocial Assessment

    I. ID, Chief Complaint, and Reasons for the Evaluation
   II. History of the Present Illness
  III. Past Psychiatric History
  IV. History of Substance Abuse
   V. Past Social and Developmental History
  VI. Current Social History
 VII. Family History
VIII. Medical History and Review of System
  IX. Mental Status Examination
   X. Functional Assessment (Optional)
  XI. DSM-IV Differential Diagnosis
 XII. Narrative Summary and Formulation

Note: Especially with patients dealing with severe, long-term mental illnesses, data that can be utilized to support the need for state funding (sometimes called certification) are often most usefully displayed separately from the Social History. In such instances this information is often inserted after the Mental Status Examination section and would read: X. Functional Assessment.

Quality Assurance Guidelines for the Written Document

  I. ID, Chief Complaint, and Reason for Evaluation
     This section should include the following information:
     a. Age
     b. Sex
     c. Marital status
     d. Referring clinician and telephone number if known
     e. Reason for the referral
     f. Chief complaint (direct quotation from the client)
 II. History of the Present Illness
     This section should include the following information:
     a. One paragraph devoted to presenting stressors and the patient's perception of his or her problems
       1. Generally appears first but can appear later in the history of the present illness (HPI)
       2. Keep it brief

  b. One paragraph devoted to a chronological description of the symptoms of the primary diagnosis and any treatment received for it

   1. Sometimes requires more than one paragraph

   2. If suicidal ideation/attempts are present, they are typically described here at the appropriate chronological point (if extensive, they may warrant a separate paragraph)

   3. Often useful to include pertinent negatives associated with the primary diagnosis here

  c. Paragraphs 2 to 5 (if needed) consist of one paragraph for each additional diagnosis (or rule-out diagnosis), describing the DSM-IV symptoms

   1. Include pertinent negatives

   2. Note that if there is an Axis II diagnosis that is the primary diagnosis or is playing a prominent role in the current problems, then the supporting data for the diagnosis should appear in the HPI in separate paragraphs for each Axis II diagnosis, otherwise these symptoms will appear in the Social History.

  d. One paragraph devoted to any miscellaneous pertinent negatives (e.g., symptoms of mood disorders, anxiety disorders, eating disorders, current substance abuse disorders, and psychotic process) if not already covered earlier in the HPI

III. Past Psychiatric History

 This section should include the following information:

  a. Previous episodes of the current disorder

  b. Episodes of other disorders not described in the HPI

  c. Treatment interventions such as hospitalizations, psychotherapy, case management, and medications

IV. History of Substance Abuse

 This section should include the following information:

  a. Episodes of substance abuse

  b. Previous treatment interventions, including detoxification, rehabilitation, outpatient counseling, and Alcoholics Anonymous (AA)

   (Note that current substance abuse would have been described in the HPI.)

V. Past Social and Developmental History

 This section should include the following information:

  a. Educational history

  b. Occupational and military history

  c. Legal history

  d. Family of origin relationships and abuse history

e. Marital relationships or relationships with children or significant others

f. Religious background and framework for meaning

VI. Current Social History

This section should include the following information:

a. Living arrangements

b. Important relationships (family and friends)

c. Current abuse or domestic violence

d. Employment status

e. Involvement with social agencies (e.g., shelters, food stamps)

f. List of strengths (some clinicians prefer this list in the Narrative Summary and Formulation)

VII. Family History

This section should include the following information:

a. All psychiatric and substance abuse disorders found in blood relatives

b. Any pertinent medical disorders in blood relatives (e.g., seizures, thyroid disease)

VIII. Medical History and Review of System

This section should include the following information:

a. Past and current medical disorders

b. Review of systems: list active medical symptoms

c. Current medications and dosages

d. Primary care physician and any other specialists (include telephone numbers if known)

e. Allergies

IX. Mental Status Examination

This section should include the following information:

a. Appearance and behavior

b. Mood and affect

c. Speech and thought process

d. Thought content (including obsessions, compulsions, delusions, and current suicidal/violent ideation) and perceptions (sensory illusions and hallucinations)

e. Sensorium, cognitive and intellectual functioning

X. Functional Assessment (optional, for use with certifiable patients)

a. Activities of daily living

b. Interpersonal functioning

c. Adaptation to change

d. Concentration and task performance

XI. DSM-IV Differential Diagnosis

This section should include the following information:

a. List confirmed diagnoses on all five axes and include

diagnoses that are being considered as possible, requiring further assessment, so-called "rule-out" diagnoses

XII. Narrative Summary and Formulation

This section should include the following information:

a. Brief client identification
b. Supportive reasoning behind all diagnoses
c. Safety assessment
d. Psychotherapeutic, psychosocial, and medical concerns
   1. Possible target areas for psychotherapy, crisis intervention and solution-focused work, psychodynamic issues to be addressed, social situations to be addressed (e.g., housing, finances), and medical concerns
e. Tentative Treatment Plan
   1. Possible therapeutic modalities to be used (e.g., individual, family, couples, group)
   2. Case management interventions (if applicable)
   3. If not a psychiatrist, then describe reasons for psychiatric referral or medication assessment if indicated. If a psychiatrist, then describe the choice of medications and reasons for such choices. If prescribing for the first time, be sure to include that the side effects and benefits of the medication were discussed with the patient. It is also forensically sound to state that the patient understood and was interested in starting the medication. If possible, include the patient's own words such as, "Mr. Whitman was quite interested in starting the medication stating, 'I had a friend who did great on this medicine, I say we give it a shot.'"
   4. Referrals for further primary care assessment and also list any labs that are being requested and why
   5. Predicted course

APPENDIX III C

Sample Written Assessment

INITIAL BIOPSYCHOSOCIAL ASSESSMENT

Clinician: Shawn Shea, M.D.   <u>Date:</u> April 27, 1998

I Identification, Chief Complaint, and Reason for Referral

Gary Whitman (fictitious name) is a 63-year-old, white, married, male veteran referred by his therapist, Phil Randler, for psychiatric assessment and medication evaluation. His chief complaint is, "My kids don't care about me any more. They're out in Arizona and don't ever call."

II History of the Present Illness

Mr. Whitman reports that he was basically doing fairly well until several years ago. At that time he had some difficulties while attempting to get support from the Veterans' Administration for his chronic headaches, which he feels were secondary to three incidents of head trauma while in the Navy. He started to become progressively more depressed. He implied that he had suicidal ideation back then, but he denies past suicide attempts. In the subsequent years he felt that his depression intermittently worsened, which he also believes to be exacerbated by a lack of communication from his son, who was living in Arizona. Another recent stress has been some angry encounters between his landlady and he and his wife, culminating in the landlady kicking his wife.

About 1 year ago his depressive symptoms became more persistent, including: difficulty falling asleep (1 hour), sleep continuity disorder (five or six times per night), early morning awakening, decreased appetite with some weight loss, decreased energy, decreased concentration, memory difficulties, decreased motivation, anhedonia, and depressed mood. His depressed mood is punctuated by irritability, and he reports almost weekly tearfulness. His anhedonia is marked by an inability to enjoy social activities and his computer. He denies any episodes of bizarre happiness, unusual energy, unusual nighttime excitation, or other common manic symptoms. He may have recently been treated with some type of psychotropic agent, but he was not clear what it was and thought that it did not help.

A couple of months ago, while driving home from the lodge, he had an impulsive desire to drive his car off the road and claimed that he almost did so. By the time that he got home, his suicidal ideation had subsided. He hinted that, in the past week, he may have had some suicidal ideation, after having an argument with his wife, but he claims, "I really can't remember." He denies all current suicidal ideation or intent. He was able to make a sound safety contract with good eye contact, a firm handshake, and a genuine affect.

Concerning other psychiatric symptoms, he denies panic attacks, obsessions, compulsions, eating disorder symptoms, hallucinations, or other psychotic symptoms. He also denies any current drinking. He does have a previous history of alcoholism (See History of Substance Abuse).

III   Past Psychiatric History

Mr. Whitman denies any history of other psychiatric disorders or suicide attempts. He also denies psychiatric hospitalizations, psychotherapy, or medications.

IV   History of Substance Abuse

Mr. Whitman reports that he was close to alcoholism in his 20s and 30s. He was drinking two to three cases of beer per weekend and sometimes a case every 2 to 3 days during the week. He had a couple of blackouts during this time. He would occasionally drink alone at night. He claims to have stopped drinking "cold turkey" almost 20 years ago and hasn't touched a drop since. He also reports that he stopped smoking around that time.

V   Past Social and Developmental History

1. **Education:** Mr. Whitman graduated from high school. He tended to get Bs, although he failed U.S. history. He was never suspended.
2. **Family Relationships, Social Network, and Abuse History:** Mr. Whitman reports a good marriage of many years. He has one sister aged 55. Concerning children, he has five boys and one girl. Three sons live in Philadelphia; one daughter lives in Pittsburgh; one son lives in California; and one son lives in Arizona. He has many concerns about his son in Arizona and is also angry with him for his lack of communication. He has

five grandchildren. He denies any history of psychological, physical, or sexual abuse as a child. For more details, please see the Social History by Mr. Whitman's therapist.

3. **Employment Record and/or Military History:** Mr. Whitman was successfully employed at Franklin Drill and Tools for 29 years. He reports a history of being a hard worker throughout his life. He was in the Navy for about 4 years. No active combat. He received three different head blows while in the service, two of which knocked him unconscious and one of which required 24 stitches. From that time onward he has had severe, intermittent headaches and is currently seeking disability compensation.

4. **Legal Record:** Mr. Whitman denies any problems with the law and denies any record of drinking while intoxicated.

5. **Religious Background:** This information is unknown.

VI   Current Social History

1. **Family Relationships and Other Interpersonal Factors:** As noted earlier, Mr. Whitman has a very good relationship with his wife. He is currently retired and quite active in the Masons. There are some serious problems with his landlady (see HPI). There is no current domestic violence of any kind. For more details, see the Social History by his therapist.

2. **Client's Strengths:** Mr. Whitman is intelligent and verbal. He seemed very interested in psychoeducation about his illness. I suspect that he will follow through with medications and therapy. He has a strong desire to get better and has good marital support. *(Reader please note: It can be argued that the list of strengths is really more of an example of the clinician's judgment, as opposed to a database. If one agrees with this view, it is best to address these strengths in the Summary and Formulation.)*

VII   Family History

Both parents are still alive, but his father has carcinoma. He denies any history of depression, bipolar disorder, schizophrenia, substance abuse, eating disorders, or suicide in his family.

VIII   Medical History and Review of Systems

1. **Disorders:** Mr. Whitman has a history of headaches (possibly secondary to trauma), carpal tunnel syndrome in both hands, upper respiratory

breathing problems, degenerative joint disease and a heart murmur. Concerning infectious diseases, he claims to have had polio and three bouts of pneumonia in a row, the last of which proved to be quite dangerous. These bouts of pneumonia occurred about 5 to 10 years ago. He had an electrocardiogram (ECG) last year, and the results were normal.

2. **Review of Systems:** Mr. Whitman has some shortness of breath, which has been a chronic problem. His headaches remain common. He has intermittent problems with a relatively rapid onset of blurring in both eyes, which resolves spontaneously. He denies any episodes of lightheadedness, dizziness, loss of sensation, or decrease in motor strength. He has no tremor or constipation. The remainder of his ROS was negative.

3. **Medications:** Intermittent use of a Ventolin inhaler, Nifedipine (guesses dose at 60 mg), Hydrochlorothiazide 25 mg bid, Piroxicam qd (dose not known), and Motrin prn. He relates that he takes all of his medications as prescribed.

4. **Physician:** Richard Canton, M.D., at the Stanton River V.A.

5. **Allergies:** None known.

IX Mental Status Examination

1. **Appearance and Behavior:** Mr. Whitman presents casually dressed and with good hygiene. He looks his stated age. At first he appeared cool and somewhat disinterested. By the end of the interview, he was engaged and cooperative.

2. **Mood and Affect:** Mr. Whitman's mood was reported as quite depressed. His affect was sad with intermittent tearfulness. As the interview progressed, his affect improved considerably.

3. **Speech and Thought Process:** His speech rate and volume were within normal limits. He had no loose associations, tangential thought, thought blocking, or other signs of a formal thought disorder.

4. **Thought Content and Perception:** He denied hallucinations and delusions as well as ideas of reference. He has had some recent suicidal ideation (see HPI), but he denies current suicidal ideation or intent. He has had some angry feelings towards his landlady but denies any hostile intent or homicidal ideation. He has no obsessions or compulsions.

5. **Sensorium, Cognitive and Intellectual Functioning:** Mr. Whitman was alert and oriented ×3. He could repeat six digits forwards with appropriate ease. He also recalled three objects after 5 minutes, also with appropriate ease. There was no evidence of gross cognitive dysfunction at any point during the interview. He also demonstrated some insight and seemed motivated for care.

X DSM-IV Diagnosis

Main Formulation   *Alternatives To Be Ruled Out*

Axis I

1. Major depression   Early dementia (not likely)
   (Moderate severity)
   (Without psychosis)

Axis II

1. None

Axis III

1. Headaches
2. Intermittently blurred vision
3. High blood pressure
4. Chronic respiratory problems
5. Degenerative arthritis
6. Carpal tunnel syndrome bilaterally
7. Benign heart murmur

Axis IV

1. Housing problem (Fairly severe interpersonal problems with his landlady)
2. Problems with primary support group (Feeling isolated and alienated from his son in Arizona)
3. Health care access issues (Ongoing friction with the VA over disability issues)

Axis V

Current GAF 50

XI Narrative Summary and Formulation

Mr. Whitman is a 63-year-old, white, married, male veteran. He was referred by his therapist for psychiatric evaluation and possible medication therapy. He believes that his long-standing problem with headaches, which he feels are secondary to trauma suffered while in the Navy, is one of the main causes of his depressed state. He is currently involved in a drawn-out dispute with the VA over issues related to the care of his headaches and disability issues.

For more than 3 years he has suffered from depressive symptoms. In the past year, his depressive symptoms have become persistent. Because of the presence of numerous, persistent neurovegetative symptoms of depression, he meets the criteria for a Major Depression. He also complains of significant problems with concentration and memory. Some brief cognitive testing showed no deficits. His mental alacrity, both during these tests and during the interview itself, suggests that an early dementia is not likely. A Folstein Mini-Mental Status will be done at his next session. At present, the most likely cause of his memory and concentration problems is the severity of his depression.

Concerning his suicide risk, I do not feel that he is acutely suicidal, as evidenced by his denial of immediate ideation or intent, no history of suicide attempts, no current drinking, a sincere interest in getting help, and the genuineness of his safety contracting with both myself and his therapist.

There are some significant stressors relating to his landlady, his son, and his chronic headaches. I feel that some directed problem-solving work with the patient and his wife, regarding their landlady, may be of real value. He is also a good candidate, as witnessed by his ego strength, for supportive, time-limited therapy and perhaps some social service intervention regarding his disability issues. On the other hand, I do not feel that the stressors are the sole cause of his depression but are functioning more as exacerbating factors. I believe that he has developed an endogenous depression, suggesting the benefit of antidepressant intervention.

In this regard, I will begin treatment with Pamelor, because of its reported efficacy with older adults and its ease in blood monitoring. If his agitation persists, I may consider the short-term use of an antianxiety agent. If this regimen fails, I will consider using an SSRI. The side effects, risks, and benefits of using Pamelor were discussed in detail with Mr. Whitman. He understood these issues and is eager to start the medicine, commenting something to the effect of "Whatever you say, let's give it a try."

I'll also contact Dr. Canton to see if he agrees with the above treatment plan and also to see if Mr. Whitman's intermittently blurred vision has been evaluated, as well as an update on what has been done to treat his headaches.

In conclusion, I feel that with the combined use of psychotherapy and medications, Mr. Whitman has a very good prognosis.

APPENDIX III D

INITIAL BIOPSYCHOSOCIAL ASSESSMENT

Client's Name: _____   Clinician's Name: _____

Date: _____ Age: _____ DOB: _____   Sex: _____ Marital Status: _____

Employer: _____   Insurance: _____

Chief Complaint (Record in client's own words) **and Referral Source:**

History of Present Illness

A. **Stressors and Symptoms:** (Include current stressors and detailed chronologic history of symptoms for each diagnosis on Axes I and II. Detail current substance abuse, amount and pattern of use here.)

B. **Recent Suicide and Homicide Database:** (Include all recent [past month] ideation, gestures, and attempts. Also record key material such as hopelessness and extent of actions or plans.)

Client's Name: Page 2

Current Symptom Inventory: (All symptoms checked as mild, moderate, or severe must be described in detail in the HPI.)

	Not Present	Mild	Moderate	Severe	Unknown
1. Depressed Mood	_____	_____	_____	_____	_____
2. Sleep Disturbance	_____	_____	_____	_____	_____
3. Other Vegetative Symptoms of Depression (e.g., appetite)	_____	_____	_____	_____	_____
4. Suicidal Ideation	_____	_____	_____	_____	_____
5. Violent Ideation	_____	_____	_____	_____	_____
6. Panic Attacks / Obsessions	_____	_____	_____	_____	_____
7. PTSD Symptoms	_____	_____	_____	_____	_____
8. Abnormal Eating Behavior	_____	_____	_____	_____	_____
9. Psychosis	_____	_____	_____	_____	_____
10. Substance Abuse	_____	_____	_____	_____	_____

Past History Markers:

	Present	Absent	Not Known
1. Sexual / Physical Abuse	_____	_____	_____
2. Substance / Alcohol Abuse	_____	_____	_____
3. Suicide / Self-Mutilation	_____	_____	_____
4. Violence	_____	_____	_____
5. Psychosis	_____	_____	_____

Past Psychiatric and Drug and Alcohol History:

A. **Episodes and Treatment** (Describe previous episodes of current disorder and all other disorders, including treatment modalities such as hospitalization, psychotherapy, medications, and their dosages. Detail past substance abuse, amount and pattern of use here.)

B. **Past Suicidal / Violent Ideation or Behavior:**

Client's Name:

Substance Abuse Profile:

Alcohol	Current Amount	Last Used (date)
THC		
Cocaine / Crack/Pep Pills / Speed		
LSD / Mescaline / Psilocybine		
Barbiturates / Other Sedatives		
Caffeine / Tobacco		

Psychosocial History

1. Education:

2. Family Relationships / Social Relationships / Abuse History:

3. Employment Record / Military:

4. Legal Record:

5. Religious Background:

6. Client's Strengths:

Family History (History of psychiatric or substance abuse disorders in blood relatives):

Client's Name: _____   Page 4
_____

Medical History (Significant past illnesses or traumas, etc.):

Primary Care Physician: _____   Allergies: _____
_____

Current Medications: Taken as Prescribed?

Medication	Dosage	Yes	No
1. _____	_____	_____	_____
2. _____	_____	_____	_____
3. _____	_____	_____	_____
4. _____	_____	_____	_____
5. _____	_____	_____	_____
6. _____	_____	_____	_____

_____

Mental Status:

1. Appearance and Behavior:

_____

2. Mood and Affect:

_____

3. Speech and Thought Process:

_____

4. Thought Content and Perceptions (Include all current [last 24 hours], suicidal / violent ideation):

_____

5. Sensorium, Cognitive and Intellectual Functioning:

Narrative Summary and Formulation (Present and support, diagnostic and psychosocial formulation and treatment recommendations):

Assessment of Suicide/Violence Risk:

Triage and Treatment Recommendations:

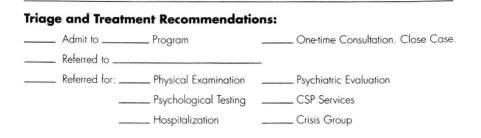

_____ Admit to _____ Program   _____ One-time Consultation. Close Case.

_____ Referred to _____

_____ Referred for: _____ Physical Examination   _____ Psychiatric Evaluation

                       _____ Psychological Testing   _____ CSP Services

                       _____ Hospitalization   _____ Crisis Group

Client's Name: Page 6

Diagnostic Summary:

Axis I: **Clinical Psychiatric Syndromes:**

Main Formulation	Codes	Alternatives to be ruled out
1.		
2.		
3.		
4.		

Axis II: **Personality and Specific Development Disorders:**

Main Formulation	Codes	Alternatives to be ruled out
1.		
2.		
3.		

Axis III: **Physical Disorders:**

Main Formulation	Codes	Alternatives to be ruled out
1.		
2.		
3.		

Axis IV: **Physical Stressors:**

A. Ranked list: 1. _____
2. _____
3. _____

B. Overall Stressor Severity:

1	2	3	4	5	6	0
None	Mild	Moderate	Severe	Extreme	Cat.	Unspecified

Axis V: **Global Assessment of Functioning (GAF):**

Current GAF _____   Highest GAF in past year _____

Clinician's Signature   Date

Psychiatrist and / or Supervisor's Signature   Date

Location of Assessment

Client's Name: _____   Page 7

Genogram (Optional)

APPENDIX IV

TIPS FOR PASSING THE ORAL BOARDS IN PSYCHIATRY

We will begin with understatement. The Oral Boards are not a lot of fun. This is one of the few statements, which I have ever uttered, that has met with universal agreement. The Boards are a "rite of passage" for most psychiatrists: They are always memorable one way or another, and there is a great feeling of relief once one passes them.

In this appendix I will pass on some tips that helped me to pass the Boards and have also helped many of the candidates whom I have assisted with their preparation for the Boards. This appendix is not a replacement for a sound source of overall information about the Boards. The reader should carefully read everything that the Board sends you and also practice a lot. A great source of practical advice and background can be found in the book *Boarding Time, 2nd edition,* by James Morrison and Rodrigo Munoz (APA Press, 1996).

The coaching tips are described under five categories: Successful Attitude, What is Tested, Interview Tips, Presentation Tips, and Preparation Suggestions.

Successful Attitude

One of the biggest hurdles I find, with clinicians having problems with the Boards, arises from an unnecessarily intense fear of the Boards themselves, often generated by a false belief. This anxiety-provoking belief sounds one way or another something like the following statement, "The Boards are extremely difficult and artificial. They don't look like any type of clinical interview that I do."

Don't say this to yourself, because it is very anxiety-producing and suggests that the examinee is being tested on a technique that is unfamiliar. This concept is indeed a frightening thought. Avoid it—it is very counterproductive.

But there is a more important reason to avoid this belief, other than that it is counterproductive. It is patently false. You have successfully performed a similar 30-minute interview many times in your training, under extremely difficult circumstances, and you have done it well. You have carried out this style of interview when you have been "beat tired," harried, and under incredible time pressures.

715

You have done this style of interview successfully many times, when an error does not result in someone failing a test but can result in someone losing his or her life. You have successfully and gracefully done this interview many times, because you have done a very similar interview every single time that you have been "on call." You see, in many respects the "Board interview" is an emergency room interview with a few extras.

When you enter the interview room, don't focus on passing a test. Focus on doing a good clinical interview, much like you have done scores of times in the emergency room. Tell yourself, "I've done this before and I know how to do it." Do a good clinical interview, and you will have done a good "Board interview."

The APBN is trying to ensure that practicing psychiatrists are safe and can soundly perform key clinical skills such as interviewing, case formulation, and treatment planning. They are not trying to see if you can do a comprehensive 60-minute intake in 30 minutes. The Board is attempting to determine whether the interviewer can gather a *reasonable* database in a 30-minute time period that results in a sound formulation and disposition. They do not expect you to do the impossible, but they do expect you to appropriately structure the patient towards giving pertinent information. In a nutshell they want to see if examinees are facile at engagement, practical in choosing areas to explore, and safe in judgment. These skills are exactly the ones that you have used numerous times in the emergency room.

What is Tested

As you are probably already aware, the examination has two parts—a live patient examination and a videotape examination. In the live patient format, the clinician interviews the patient for 30 minutes and then has 30 minutes to present the patient data and formulation and answer the examiner's questions. In the videotape format, you will watch a 30-minute videotape and then have 30 minutes to present the case and your formulation as well as answering the questions of the examiners. With both of these formats, the actual case presentation usually takes about 5 to 10 minutes with the rest of the 30 minutes devoted to questions posed by the examiners.

In the live interview format, the actual grading subcategories are as follows:

1. Physician-patient relationship
2. Conduct of the interview
3. Organization and presentation of data
4. Phenomenology, diagnosis, and prognosis

5. Etiologic, pathogenic, and therapeutic issues (divided into biological, psychological, and social categories)

The subcategories for the videotape are quite similar. Note that although there is no interview for them to grade, they are quite interested in your observations about the patient from the videotape, which you will be presenting in the mental status assessment and in your discussion:

1. Observation of data
2. Organization and presentation of data
3. Phenomenology, diagnosis, and prognosis
4. Etiologic, pathogenic, and therapeutic issues (divided as above)

I believe that one of the most important points to take from the above listing is the fact that, although the actual interview is quite important, much of the grading is done on other fields of evaluation, such as your presentation skills, treatment planning, and core clinical knowledge base.

Pay particular attention to the role of the videotape examination. All of us have been trained for some time in performing interviews and then presenting formulations. Almost none of us have been trained, nor practiced, watching a videotape, culling data from it, and then creating a presentation from the video data. However, you are being tested on this very set of skills. Practice. By the time that you reach the exam room you should feel comfortable with culling data and making presentations from watching a video. It is easy to do once you get used to it, but it feels surprisingly different compared with actively developing the database yourself.

One of the main reasons why I think that clinicians fluster and fail the examination is that they do not allocate enough time to practice culling data from a videotape. I suggest that you should watch at least five 30-minute videos; spend 5 minutes formulating your presentation after each one; and then present your case presentation without interruption. Practice your presentation exactly as it will occur in the Boards. If you don't feel comfortable at the end of five videos, do more. Interviewing videos are available as commercial educational products and at some medical libraries and academic centers. Psychiatric residencies may also have tapes available for training purposes.

Interview Tips

Make no bones about it, time is tight during the Boards, but no tighter than in a busy inner city emergency room (clinicians sometimes have less than 30 minutes in these conditions). However, you already have an understanding of how to successfully create an engaging and sound Board interview if you understand the principles explored in this book.

Just as you do with any other clinical interview, using your understanding of facilics and time utilization, before you even begin the interview, you should enter with an understanding of which topical regions need to be explored and how much material you need to explore in each region. Once within the interview, you start with an open-ended and engaging scouting phase lasting about 5 minutes and then proceed to gather your data region by region. When each region is completed, you gracefully use natural and referred gates to enter the next region and complete it to your satisfaction. If a patient begins to unnecessarily pivot out of a given region, you gently pull the patient back. If the patient shows stylistic resistances, such as being shut-down or wandering, you use the same techniques for transforming these resistances as already described in Chapter 2.

The skills used in the Board interview are identical to your daily interviewing skills. The Board interview is a clinical interview. As with other time-limited interviews, such as an ER interview, the key is that the clinician understands exactly how much material is not sought compared with a standard 60-minute intake. In short, the interviewer needs a very concrete idea of what he or she is not going to ask about in each region.

By way of example, let's take a look at the Family History. In a standard 60-minute intake, this is explored thoroughly. In an ER, and at the Boards, this region is reduced significantly. In the Board-style interview, the clinician will ask only about major psychiatric disorders (e.g., schizophrenia, bipolar disorder, depression, anxiety disorders, substance abuse). The clinician will want to know about any suicides in the family. That's it. That's all there is time for. There is no time to explore for more subtle diagnoses such as cyclothymic disorder or dysthymic disorder and minimal time for details about treatment interventions for family members.

If any of this "unexplored" material may be relevant to treatment planning, this can easily be addressed in your formulation as follows, "I am a bit suspicious that my patient may have some bipolar type II propensities. One thing I would do when I saw this patient in my next session would be to do a more thorough Family History, specifically looking for evidence of cyclothymic disorder or bipolar type II process," or "As I stated, I believe my patient has a panic disorder. One thing I did not have time to explore in detail in this interview was whether or not her mother had a true panic disorder. In my next session I would explore this in more detail and also find out which med seemed to help her mother and at what doses, for this might point me towards the best med to help my current patient." Board examiners will love such awareness of what is important to gather "next time," because it shows sound clinical thinking, which is what the Boards are all about.

REGIONS TO EXPLORE

From our understanding of facilics, we know that the success of a time-limited interview depends directly on how clear the clinician is regarding what specific information he or she wants to obtain in each region of the interview. Bearing this principle in mind, let's take a look at which regions need to be explored in a typical Board examination. These regions are not listed, necessarily, in any special order. As with all clinical interviews, the clinician decides the order that best fits with the defenses and needs of the specific patient, each of whom is unique.

I. The following regions should be explored carefully, essentially exactly as you would explore them in a standard 60-minute assessment:
1. Patient identification, reason for presentation (e.g., what brought the patient into the hospital or clinic), and chief complaint
2. History of the present illness of the suspected primary diagnosis (either Axis I or Axis II)
3. Suicide/violence assessment (the CASE Approach can be very useful here)
II. The following symptom regions should be explored relatively carefully:
1. Mood disturbance symptoms
2. Anxiety disorder symptoms
3. Psychotic symptoms
4. Drug and alcohol symptoms
5. Disorders due to a medical condition, such as dementia
6. Other diagnoses that may appear likely, such as eating disorders, adjustment disorders, or personality disorders
7. Medical history and medical ROS

This does not mean that you are expected necessarily to expand all the diagnoses under each specific symptom cluster. Instead, you want to be certain to enter all of these diagnostic regions at some point during the interview, ask some probe questions, and then decide if a specific diagnosis is likely, at which point you would explore that specific diagnosis more carefully with DSM-IV criteria.

Keep in mind that the examiners want to see if you can intelligently probe in all major areas of psychopathology, wisely choose which areas to expand in more detail, and ultimately defend your decisions. Your goal is to be able to present a good differential diagnosis in your formulation, not necessarily to have identified exactly every diagnosis.

III. You should definitely touch upon the following regions, but they are significantly less thoroughly explored than in a standard 60-minute interview:
1. Past psychiatric history
2. Family history
3. Social and developmental history
4. Cognitive mental status (the noncognitive aspects of the mental status are explored and observed throughout the interview as you would normally do)

By way of example, let us look at the cognitive section of the mental status evaluation. The examinee should always address the cognitive examination at some point in the interview. A nice selection of probe questions could include orientation, digit spans, and three-word recall. That is all that is necessary unless the patient appears to be suffering from a specific cognitive disorder (e.g., delirium or dementia), in which case one would devote more time during the interview to the cognitive examination.

Remember, even if you happen to leave something out of the interview, which you regret omitting, because it ultimately proved to be relevant to your formulation, all is not lost. During your presentation simply say something like, "Because of the time constraints of this setting, I did not do a thorough cognitive exam. But I have become suspicious of the presence of a mild dementia and, in actual practice, I would perform a more thorough cognitive exam, including perhaps a Folstein Mini-Mental Status." Such an explanation would probably satisfy most examiners.

Perhaps the biggest reduction in the amount of data gathered in a Board examination, as opposed to a 60-minute assessment, is in the social history. As with an ER exam, past social history is cut markedly.

I will now list some good probe questions which, time permitting, you can follow up on. If these, or similar, questions are asked, the candidate will probably gather enough social history to present some of the social and psychological factors that help us to understand the patient in a psychosocial context. At a minimum, the questions will probably dig up some material that you can tell the examiners in your formulation are ripe areas for further exploration in future sessions. Keep in mind that during the unstructured scouting phase, at the beginning of the interview, patients will also frequently reveal important social and psychodynamic issues.

1. Tell me a little bit about what it was like growing up in your family.
2. Tell me a little bit about what school was like for you.
3. What are some of the jobs you've had, and what have they been like for you?
4. Have you ever had any troubles with the law?
5. Tell me a little about your wife (substitute words such as significant other, boyfriend, girlfriend for "wife" as appropriate).

You might not even have time for all of these probe questions, therefore just do your best with the time that you have available. If you suspect earlier in the interview that a personality disorder is playing a prominent role in the patient's presentation—especially if you think that it is the primary diagnosis—then you will have needed to have expanded the diagnostic criteria for this disorder fairly carefully, usually during the differential diagnostic component of the interview performed earlier. Such primary personality expansions will inevitably provide even further pertinent social history.

By the way, you don't need to cover all the criteria, you simply should be prepared to discuss your differential diagnosis on Axis II and be able to defend your reasoning. For instance, "With regard to Axis II, I did not have time to gather enough historical information to make a definite diagnosis, but I am suspicious of an antisocial personality disorder. My evidence for this is as follows. In the HPI, he described frequent problems with the law as well as . . . etc."

On the other hand, personality pathology may not show itself until the social history itself is being explored. If such is the case some simple personality screening can be attempted here in the social history, as time permits, enough to give you food for discussion when presenting Axis II. Remember that on Axis II you can discuss personality traits and/or defense mechanisms as well.

TIME SUGGESTIONS

There is no predetermined "right way" to allot time during the Boards, but here is one strategy. Once again these phases are not presented in any fixed order, other than to start with the scouting phase, although most people do like to follow the scouting phase with the HPI and DSM-IV differential diagnosis:

• 5 Minutes   Scouting Phase (Including ID, Chief Complaint, and Reason for Evaluation. Note that the patient may spontaneously provide much of the HPI here.)

- 12 Minutes   HPI, DSM-IV differential diagnoses, and assessment of suicidal/violent ideation
- 4 Minutes   Social History (may include some simple personality exploration)
- 3 Minutes   Medical History, Medical ROS, and Family History
- 3 Minutes   Cognitive Mental Status
- 2 Minutes   Past Psychiatric History
- 1 Minute   Closing (Be sure to tell the patient that he or she did a good job and to thank the patient for participating.)

Good luck with the interview! If you practice the above principles diligently, I think you will be pleasantly surprised at the large amount of data that can be sensitively generated in 30 minutes, if the clinician has a sound understanding of the facilics of the task. Interestingly, you may discover (also to your pleasant surprise) that your practice for the Boards will have made you a better interviewer in the ER as well.

Presentation Tips

In some respects, the candidate's ability to present his or her case data and formulation may represent the single most important skill to practice. A candidate who presents with confidence and organization will project competence. A candidate who presents haltingly or in a disorganized manner will invite failure. Don't deceive yourself; first impressions count. A skilled presenter creates an expectation among the examiners that they are about to see someone who will pass. Everything said from that point onward has the benefit of this positive "lens." On the other hand, a weak presentation creates a negative "filter" through which the examiners unconsciously may be looking for the worse.

For this reason alone, it is wise to practice presenting frequently. However, there is another reason. Clinicians interview daily. Clinicians do not present daily. It is surprising how poorly some psychiatrists are trained in presentation skills, and residencies vary widely regarding how well this skill is taught. In the Boards, you will have only about 5 minutes to prepare your presentation after interviewing the patient or watching the video. Believe me—the 5 minutes pass quickly.

Presenting a case is not particularly difficult, if one has practiced the process a lot. Some people will have been "through the mill" in this regard because of an emphasis upon it in their training. They will not need to practice this skill too much, but even these examinees should practice presenting at least several times in addition to doing their mock Boards.

If your presenting skills are not strong, I urge you to practice interviewing a patient or watching a video at least 10 to 15 times, followed by a 5-minute organization time, and then present the case to a mirror or to a colleague. Another way to practice your presentation skills is to take advantage of the fact that you are probably doing assessments every day in your actual clinic work. Occasionally, instead of dictating your assessment right away, dictate it "after hours." Instead, as soon as you are done with one of your clinic assessments, organize for 5 minutes and then present directly to a colleague or to a mirror non-stop. It's a great way to practice. It doesn't matter that this was a 60-minute assessment: It's the skills of organizing your data rapidly and presenting smoothly that you are practicing.

When practicing your presentations, do not stop. If you make a mistake or pause awkwardly, continue. You must become adept at smoothly covering such errors while maintaining a calm composure. Also, keep in mind that examiners are probably more comfortable with your pauses in presentation than you are. They realize that sometimes we need a moment to organize our thoughts. There is nothing wrong with this process as long as you don't appear flustered.

Concerning time, your presentation should probably last about 5 to 10 minutes at most. Organization is critical both for keeping you calm and for looking like you know what you are talking about. The Board does not officially provide a guide for the outline of the presentation, but the following may be useful. In it, the examinee first provides the database, then proceeds to present a diagnostic formulation, and ends by presenting further labs to be considered and treatment modalities to be utilized. It looks as follows:

I. Database
   A. Identification and Chief Complaint
   B. History of the Present Illness
   C. Pertinent Past Psychiatric History
   D. Pertinent Social History
   E. Pertinent Family History
   F. Medical History and Review of Symptoms
   G. Mental Status
      1. Appearance and Behavior
      2. Speech and Thought Process
      3. Mood and Affect
      4. Perceptual Abnormalities
      5. Thought Content and Lethality
      6. Sensorium and Cognitive Findings

II. Diagnostic Formulation
  A. DSM-IV Differential Diagnosis
      Review all five axes of the DSM-IV in order, listing the most likely diagnoses and rule-outs. (Be sure to mention any organic disorders that may need to be ruled out.)
  B. Psychosocial/Psychodynamic Formulation
      Nothing fancy here—there is no need for "name throwing" of theorists, etc. Just briefly mention any pressing psychosocial and psychological conflicts/defenses that you think are important. Focus on issues that will play a direct role in treatment intervention. If the examiners want more, they will ask for it.
III. Treatment Planning
  A. For each diagnosis list your possible treatment plans and modalities. Be sure to include any future labs or testing that you think are needed. If there are specific psychosocial problems, include your tentative interventions such as case management, help with housing, psychoeducation for family members, and so forth.
      The treatment planning schema, based on systems theory presented in Chapter 4, can be very useful here. Indeed, another way to present the treatment interventions is to simply go from one level to another through this schema. In short, list the treatment interventions that you are considering in the following systems: biological interventions (e.g., meds, labwork, referral to internist), psychological interventions (e.g., individual psychotherapies, readings, hotlines), interpersonal interventions (e.g., social skills training), family interventions (e.g., family therapies, psychoeducation, home outreach, referral to a local NAMI chapter), and social or community interventions (e.g., case management, vocational rehabilitation, support groups, AA).

Practicing your presentations, while using the above guidelines, should help you to present fluidly and concisely, while also increasing your sense of self-confidence. I also suggest that you literally introduce each area as you come to it. For instance, "Concerning the HPI, Mr. Janson reports his symptoms first began . . ." When done with the HPI, one would continue, "Concerning the patient's Past Psychiatric History, the pertinent positives are a hospitalization for schizophrenia at age 18 and a subsequent . . . ." This framing of each section has a nice professional feel to it, and it also helps the presenter to maintain a focused organization.

Be prepared for the fact that some examiners like to interrupt the presentation with questions. If this occurs, simply answer the questions and then return to your presentation. Never look disconcerted by examiner interruptions. Answer openly and with interest. Never bullshit. This will only get you into trouble.

In fact, sometimes it is advantageous to openly admit what you don't know and what you would do about that deficit in real practice. Sound clinicians are recognizable by the degree with which they know what they don't know. By way of example, the following admission would probably impress board examiners, "I'm not entirely certain whether or not the Paxil would impact on the blood level of Serax. Before I would prescribe Serax, I would definitely look that up in the PDR. If I wasn't satisfied there, I would call the pharmacist. But no matter what, I always check into drug-drug interactions before I prescribe."

Examinees often want to know what type of questions are fair game. The examiners are asked to focus their questioning on practical clinical issues that are raised by your case or could be extended into general practice. They are to avoid trivia. They are not trying to stump you. They simply want to see what you know and whether or not you apply your knowledge in a competent fashion. The examiners are urged to help decrease undue stress. In this regard, the examiner instructions state, "It is the examiner's job to help the candidate to display competence in what might be best described as an environment of compassionate collegial neutrality." These examiners remember what it was like to take this test, and they are there to help you do your best.

Preparation Suggestions

For your part, "doing your best" requires three things: (1) Practice, (2) Practice, and (3) Practice. Unfamiliarity with the protocol, and a subsequent freezing up during the examination, is probably the prime reason why competent psychiatrists sometimes fail the boards. This factor can essentially be eliminated by practice. It also helps to remember, as stated before, that you have often done a similar type of interview in the ER.

It is critical that you undergo enough mock Boards to feel comfortable with the protocol and atmosphere of the examinations themselves. Many residencies are now doing a good job of providing mock Boards. If some time has elapsed since you did your mock Boards, or if you want more practice, get a colleague to function as an examiner. Make sure that the colleague acts exactly like an examiner, showing no familiarity with you or your work and following the time schedule of the Boards to a tee. It is best to have two colleagues acting as examiners, just as will occur in the Boards.

In addition to doing mock Boards, as noted earlier, I would

repeatedly practice developing and presenting a case from a 30-minute video, as well as other methods of practicing your presentations mentioned earlier. Board review courses can be very valuable, but make sure that the course you choose includes opportunities for both your interview and presentation to be directly watched and feedback given. For more background and practical tips for passing the Boards, as mentioned earlier, *Boarding Time,* by Morrison and Munoz is an outstanding book. Naturally, you should also do some refresher reading, especially with regard to DSM-IV differential diagnosis and clinical pharmacology.

In closing this Appendix, I hope that the above tips prove to be of some value. Trust in yourself and your skills. With good preparation, sound clinicians tend to do well on the Boards. Good Luck and Good Boarding!

Glossary of Interview
Supervision Terms

Blending

Blending is the subjective and objective evidence, collected from the interview, which suggests that the engagement process is going well. For group discussion and supervision purposes, it is useful to rate blending on a scale from zero (patient is hostile toward clinician) to ten (patient and clinician appear extremely natural together). The degree of blending can be determined from three complementary perspectives: (1) the clinician's subjective feelings, (2) objective evidence from the patient's behavior (e.g., increased eye contact or smiling), and (3) self-report from the patient. The degree of blending depends on two major elements—the clinician's skill and the patient's defenses and psychopathology. Consequently, low blending is not necessarily a sign of poor clinician performance. For instance, a skilled clinician may only achieve a blending of three with a patient who displays active paranoid process.

Closed-Ended Questions

Closed-ended questions are those questions that are extremely easy for a moderately guarded or moderately resistant patient to answer with one word, a short phrase, or a simple "yes" or "no." All inquiries that provide or imply a specific list of answers or ask for specific items, places, dates, numbers, or names are viewed as closed-ended. In patients who are easily engaged, these questions may also tend to decrease interviewee response length, for in many instances the socially appropriate answer is only one word, a short phrase, or a simple "yes" or "no."

Content Region

An area of dialogue in which a specific topic becomes the center of focus. Typical content regions include diagnostic regions, history of the present illness, social history, family history, and the lethality assessment.

Engagement

The actual degree to which the patient feels comfortable and safe with interviewer. It is reflected in the "blending" of the interview.

Facilics

Facilics is the study of the flow and structuring of the interviewing process, including the study of the clinician's time management. In its applied format it includes the study of the methods utilized by clinicians to explore specific topics and processes (delineated as "regions") as well as the study of transitions (delineated as "gates") between these regions. A method of diagramming the various regions and transitions has been developed and is currently utilized as both a supervision and research tool. In a pure research form, facilic analysis can be applied to any dialogue, whether an everyday conversation or a television interview.

Gentle Assumption

A technique for increasing the likelihood that sensitive material will be discussed more openly. The clinician assumes that the suspected behavior is occurring and frames a question based on this assumption. Thus, the clinician does not ask, "Do you masturbate?" but "How frequently do you masturbate during a typical week, if at all?"

Gentle Commands

Gentle commands represent one of the two most powerful open-ended techniques (open-ended questions being the other). They begin with phrases such as "Tell me about your . . ." or "Say something about . . .", which gently direct the patient to discuss a topic. The tone of voice is gentle and nonthreatening. An example of such a statement is "Tell me something about your stress on the job."

Implied Gate

A relatively smooth transition initiated by the clinician, who leaves one topic by discussing a closely related topic that seems to follow the conversation. It does not (as in the case of the natural gate) take its cue from the immediately preceding patient response.

Introduced Gate

These gates do not naturally follow the flow of conversation, but they are relatively smooth, for the clinician verbally notes that a transition is under way. An example is as follows: "For a moment let's change topics to how your mood has been recently."

Manufactured Gate

A technique for setting up a natural transition by bringing up a bridging topic. For instance, let us say that the clinician had finished an expansion of major depression and wanted to enter the region of alcoholism. The clinician might say, "Earlier you had mentioned your father had drinking problems, how about yourself, do you drink much?" Manufactured gates are actually combination gates. This example began as a referred gate into family history, but the clinician immediately used a natural gate to enter the region of alcohol dependence. There is usually a smoother and simpler way to make a transition than a manufactured gate.

Natural Expansion

An exploration of a given topic in which the clinician's questions seem to follow naturally and convey an almost conversational feeling to the interview.

Natural Gate

A smooth transition from one topic to a new topic initiated by the clinician. In a natural gate the clinician cues directly off the patient's immediately preceding statement.

Open-Ended Questions

Open-ended questions are difficult to answer with one word or a short phrase, even if the interviewee is moderately guarded or moderately resistant. It is virtually impossible to respond to these questions with a simple "yes" or "no." Questions that provide or imply possible answers, or ask for specific items, places, dates, numbers, or names, are never viewed as open-ended, because they limit the freedom of answer choice. In patients who are easily engaged, open-ended questions should tend to produce relatively large quantities of speech.

PACE

An acronym representing the four major assessments made by a clinician during the scouting period:

P = Patient's perspective and conscious agenda
A = Assessment of the patient's mental status on an informal basis
C = Clinician's perception of the patient's problems and unconscious agenda
E = Evaluation of the interview process itself (e.g., is the interview shut down, wandering, or rehearsed?)

Phantom Gate

This relatively weak transition occurs when a new topic is introduced with an abrupt entrance that seems to come from nowhere. Such gates may convey a sense of awkwardness or disinterest on the part of the clinician, especially if his or her style is frequently characterized by such blunt transitions.

Pivot Points

A pivot point occurs when a patient spontaneously changes topics. If the clinician is consciously aware of a pivot point, then a decision can be made regarding the wisdom of following or gently refocusing the patient. Uncontrolled wandering interviews frequently result when clinicians miss pivot points and consequently never appropriately focus the patient.

Process Regions

An area of dialogue in which the focus is on the manner in which the patient answers, not the content of what is said. Classic process regions include facilatory regions, psychodynamic regions, and regions in which specific types of resistance are addressed. Other process regions include phenomenological inquiries and educational regions. Sometimes process regions may also function as content regions, as is the case with phenomenological and educational regions.

Referred Gate

A graceful transition in which a new topic is entered by referring to a previous topic raised earlier in the interview. These transitions convey a sense of careful listening and concern. They frequently begin with phrases such as, "Earlier you had mentioned . . ." or "At one point you had talked about . . . ."

Region

A region is a facilic analysis term referring to an area of interview in which a specific topic is being explored or in which the clinician is utilizing a specific interviewing tool focused on the process as opposed to the content of the interview (see Content Region and Process Regions).

Rehearsed Interview

This interview is characterized by a moderate to large production of spontaneous speech that focuses only on topics of interest to the patient. It is a method by which the interview is controlled by the patient.

Responsive Zone

The range of distances between the clinician and the patient in which both participants feel comfortable and seem to be aware, at least at an unconscious level, of each other's movements. Once within the responsive zone (RZ), nonverbal behaviors of the clinician have the potential to effectively impact upon the patient. Inside the RZ, nonverbal behaviors may be intimidating or overwhelming. Outside the RZ, nonverbal behaviors may seem insignificant and noneffective.

Scouting Period

Generally the first 5 to 7 minutes of a 50- to 60-minute interview. This period is composed of both the introduction and the opening phase of the interview. Open-ended verbalizations tend to predominate, for the main goal of the clinician is the development of a sound engagement with the patient. One or two empathic statements are frequently useful.

Shame Attenuation

A technique for increasing the validity of the patient's response by maintaining a nonthreatening stance. The question tends to be phrased in such a fashion that a positive reply does not feel incriminating to the patient but suggests a specific problem to the clinician. A classic example would be the question, "Do you find that other men pick fights with you when you're trying to enjoy a drink at the bar?" If the patient answers yes, it is easy to discover the number of fights and whether the patient actually plays a role in their initiation, as seen in sociopathy.

Shut-Down Interview

In this type of interview, the patient answers tersely and shows little spontaneity or interest in engagement. Eye contact is frequently poor, and gesturing is at a minimum. A variant of this style is the hostile interview, in which the patient's tone of voice may be angry and the content of the patient's responses may be sharp or antagonistic. In the hostile interview, eye contact may be prolonged and glaring.

Side-Tracking

Side-tracking is a method of handling resistance in which the clinician switches topics away from the issue raised by the patient. It can be very effective with tangential patients, especially if the clinician chooses a topic about which the patient is invested in talking. If the patient returns to the original resistance, it suggests that side-tracking will not work.

Spontaneous Gate

A smooth transition from one topic to another that is initiated by the patient. The clinician completes the transition by asking questions of relevance to the new topic.

Statement of Inquiry

These statements follow the declarative pattern of subject/verb. They represent statements, but the tone of voice suggests that they are intended to be inquiries and are followed by a question mark. Two examples are as follows: (1) "You were always late for work?" and (2) "So you were hesitant to go to college?" In shut-down interviews these statements of inquiry can be answered tersely. On a positive side, they may function to effectively clarify questions or to summarize the patient's story. On a negative side, they are leading questions.

Stilted Expansion

An exploration of a given topic in which the clinician's questioning seems highly structured and awkward. It is sometimes seen when clinicians utilize a checklist approach to symptoms or when the transitions between questions are repeatedly abrupt or odd. Stilted expansions can create a "Meet the Press" style of interaction.

Swing Questions

Questions that essentially ask the interviewee whether he or she would like to answer or not. They begin with phrases such as, "Could you tell me . . .", "Would you say something about . . .", or "Can you describe . . ." If engagement is high, such swing questions function essentially as open-ended questions. But if engagement is low, they can easily be answered tersely and hence tend to further shut down the interviewee, functioning as closed-ended inquires.

Symptom Amplification

A technique for increasing the validity of a patient's response by setting the upper limits of a question at such a high level that when the patient downplays the amount, the remaining sum still suggests a problem. For example, "How much liquor can you hold at one time, say a pint or a fifth?" If the patient responds "Oh no, not that much, maybe a pint, perhaps a pint and a half at most" then the clinician is still aware that a significantly high tolerance is present.

Tracking

The ability of the clinician to sensitively follow the patient's train of thoughts with appropriate clarifying questions. The clinician can track both the affect of the patient or the content of the patient's speech.

Unipolar Blending

A specific type of blending that occurs when the patient appears immediately and unusually at ease with the clinician. This "high engagement" is in reality relatively superficial and arises essentially independently of the clinician's engagement techniques. The patient is often talkative and may be dramatic. The presence of unipolar blending frequently suggests underlying psychopathology such as histrionic traits, a hypomanic or manic state, or acute intoxication.

Type A Validity Errors

These errors are related to the content of the interviewer's questions and include leading questions, negative questions, multiple questions, and other phrasing errors.

Type B Validity Errors

These errors are related to paralanguage and nonverbal activity. They include processes such as a curt tone of voice, a horizontal head nod while asking a question, or inappropriately cutting patients off.

Wandering Interview

An interview characterized by a patient with verbose speech production and tangential or circumstantial thought. A variant of this interview type is the loquacious interview, in which the patient produces large amounts of speech but the speech stays on the chosen topic. The wandering interview is furthered by poor structuring techniques on the part of the clinician.

Note: Page numbers in *italics* refer to illustrations; page numbers followed by (t) refer to tables.

Psychosis *(Continued)*
family system in, 356–360
hallucinations in, 301, 344–346, 446–447
and suicide risk, 447
hard signs of, 313, *315,* 321
elicitation of, in patient with soft signs
of psychosis, 317
head trauma and, 297, 330
hypochondriacal, monosymptomatic, 310
illogical thought in, 347
interview approach in presence of, 73–
74, 317, 349, 353–356
behavioral incident–based, 203–204
countertransference complicating, 354
gate-based, 348, 350, 469
patient's requests for clinician's opinion and, 610–613
invasion experiences in, 339–340
"micro"-episodes of, 332–333
nonverbal behavior in, 155–156
PCP (phencyclidine) use and, 298
personality disorders and, 333, 384–387
probe questions for, 422
physiologic system in, 337–343
porous ego in, 339, 340
predicative thinking in, 347
psychological system in, 344–353
racing thoughts in, 346–347
religious preoccupation in, 360
and homicide risk, 499
and suicide risk, 448
broaching of subject of, in interview,
350–351
Schneiderian symptoms of, 339–340
sleep disturbances in, 337
soft signs of, *315,* 317, 321
elicitation of hard signs of psychosis
in presence of, 317
somatic passivity experiences in, 340
subculture of patients with, 359–360
thought blocking in, 347, 527
thought broadcasting in, 340
Psychosis-prone personality disorders,
384–387
probe questions for, 422
Psychotherapy, patients suitable for,
552–561
Psychotic structure, in Kernberg's model
of development, 563
Public distance, 150. See also *Space,
interpersonal.*

Qualitative questions, 82(t), 84
Quality assurance guidelines, for
documenting biopsychosocial
assessment, 698–701
Question(s), clinician's, 35–36, 81, 82, 82(t),
83
"cannon" delivery of, 45–46

Question(s) *(Continued)*
closed-ended, 82(t), 83, 727
ratio of open-ended queries to, varying with type of interview, 80(t)
concerning adolescence, 47
concerning behavioral incidents. See
Behavioral incident.
counter-productive, 85, 87, 89–90
covering patient's coping skills, 203
demographic, in bridge between 1st
and 2nd phases of interview, 66
devoted to depressed patient's family
relationships, 279
fact-oriented, 36–39
interpretative, 558
leading, 84–85
"miracle" posited in, 560
negative bias in, 45
open-ended, 81, 82, 82(t), 729
in opening phase of interview, 65,
66
over-reliance on, consequences of,
39
ratio of, to closed-ended queries,
varying with type of interview,
80(t)
pertaining to past diagnoses, 196
probe, for personality disorders, 420–
423
qualitative, 82(t), 84
replying to resistant patient's queries,
590
seeking specific denials, 400–401
suicide assessment aided by, 481,
482
soliciting thoughts of lethality,
expressed as homicidal/violent
ideation, 502–511
expressed as suicidal ideation. See
*Suicide, risk factor(s) for, inter-
view of patient with.*
swing, 82(t), 84, 733
topics for, 88
transitional, 117, 118
formulation of, by interviewee, 131–132
resistance-handling based on, 590
Quiet delirium, 324

Racing thoughts, in agitated depression,
267
in psychosis, 346–347
Reaction time latency (RTL), in interview,
11, 12, 80(t)
effect of deceptive responses on, 164
Reality, sense of estrangement from, in
psychosis, 339
Reciprocal kinesic behaviors, 167–168, 181,
185, 186
Recurrent depression, DSM-IV criteria for,
231. See also *Depression.*